D0892042

Alternative Medicine for the Elderly

Springer

Berlin
Heidelberg
New York
Hong Kong
London
Milan
Paris
Tokyo

P. Cherniack · N. Cherniack (eds.)

Alternative Medicine
for the Elderly

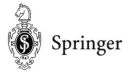
Springer

Library of Congress Cataloging-in-Publication Data
Alternative medicine for the elderly / Paul Cherniack, Neil Cherniack (eds.).
    p.; cm.
  ISBN 3-540-44169-7 (hard cover : alk. paper)
    1. Alternative medicine. 2. Aged – Diseases – Alternative treatment.
    I. Cherniack, Paul, 1959- II. Cherniack, Neil S.
    [DNLM: 1. Complementary Therapies – methods – Aged. WB 890 A46558 2003]
    R733.A469 2003
    615.5'47–dc21
    2003041540

ISBN 3-540-44169-7   Springer Verlag Berlin Heidelberg New York

Springer-Verlag Berlin Heidelberg New York
a member of BertelsmannSpringer Science+Business Media GmbH

http://www.springer.de/medizin

© Springer-Verlag Berlin Heidelberg 2003
Printed in Germany

Cover Design: design & production, Heidelberg
Typesetting: Hilger VerlagsService

SPIN 10878049   3109 – 5 4 3 2 1 0   Printed on acid free paper

Foreword

The explosion of information about complementary and alternative medicine (CAM) has demanded the attention of health professionals and responsible consumers, including the elderly. Increasingly, medical schools are providing education about CAM.

This book brings together for academicians and interested mainstream practitioners much of the current information on CAM and its role in the health of the elderly. The individual chapters are thoroughly researched and quite readable, even for patients and the lay public concerned with the state of the evidence and art supporting CAM's role in prevention and management of illness and well-being. This book provides educators with much necessary information needed to prepare coursework and learning activities.

Although definitive data are lacking regarding efficacy and even safety of CAM methodologies, many chapters in this book summarize the existing evidence in a usable way. The topics analyzed range from well-accepted therapies, such as vitamin E for dementia and zinc tablets for the common cold, to far less conventional therapies such as transcendental meditation. The conclusions are often surprising, but well-presented and defended. Even the most highly controversial areas, such as the use of acupuncture to treat low back pain and osteoarthritis of the knee, are thoroughly and fairly reviewed.

Finally, the chapters address some of the political issues that challenge CAM. These issues include who should be allowed to practice a CAM discipline whose efficacy is not based on the scientific method, and some of the state-to-state variations in practice standards and licensure.

Clearly, more research on CAM is needed. This book provides the information needed to guide both future investigational efforts and the attitudes that health care practitioners, grounded in conventional science but aware of its limitations, and older individuals, attracted by the promise of preservation of function and greater control over their own care, ought to have toward CAM as new evidence becomes available in the decades ahead.

Spring 2003

Bernard A. Roos, MD, Director
Division of Gerontology and Geriatric Medicine
University of Miami School of Medicine
Miami, Florida

Table of Contents

19 Looking After Our Elders: Healthcare and Well-being of the Elderly from the Perspective of Gwich'in and Other First Nations of Canada 287
R. WELSH, N.J. TURNER

20 Complementary and Alternative Medicine Use Among Latinos 301
D. SALAS-LOPEZ, A. NATALE-PEREIRA

C Common Medical Problems of the Elderly and CAM

List of Contributors

J. Astin, PhD
University of Maryland, Complementray Medicine Program, 2200 Kernan Drive,
3rd Floor, Kernan Mansion, Baltimore, MD 21207, USA

Brent Bauer, MD
Dept. of Medicine, Mayo School of Medicine, Division of General Internal Medicine,
200 First St. SW, Rochester, MN 55905, USA

E. Paul Cherniack, MD
Division of Geriatrics, University of Miami School of Medicine, Miami VA,
Medical Center (11A), 1201 NW 16th St., Miami, FL 33125, USA

Neil Cherniack, PhD
University of New Jersey-Newark, School of Medicine and Dentistry of New Jersey
at Newark University Hospital, 150 Bergen Street, Newark, NJ 07103, USA

Prof. Edzard Ernst
Department of Complementary Medicine, University of Exeter, 25 Victoria Park Road,
Exeter EX2 4NT, UK

Steven Farrell, MD
Dept. of Rehabilitation, Medical College of Ohio, 3065 Arlington Ave., Toledo,
OH 43614, USA

Adrian Furnham, PhD
Dept. of Psychology University College London, 26 Bedrord Way, London WC1 0AP,
UK

Glenn Gerber, PhD
Division of Urology, University of Chicago SBRI J653, 5812 Ellis Ave., Chicago,
ILL 60637, USA

Seth Kaufman, PhD
Department of Neurology, Weill Medical College of Cornell University and New York,
Presbyterian, Hospital- Cornell Medical Center, 1300 York Ave., New York, NY, USA

Peter Komesaroff, MD
Baker Medical Research Inst., Monash Universtiy Medical School, P.O. Box 6492,
St. Wilda Centre, Melbourne 8008, Australia

YUAN LIN, PhD.
Marco Polo Technologies, 5900 Conway Road, Bethesda, MD 20817, USA

ROBERT MCCARNEY, PhD
Academic Unit at Royal London Homeopathic Hospital, 60 Great Ormond Street,
London WC1N 3HR, UK

PROF. J. MCELNAY
Chairman, School of Pharmacy, The Queen's University of Belfast, 97 Lisburn Road,
Belfast, BT9 7BL, UK

LEWIS MEHL-MADRONA, PhD
Coordinator, Integrative Psychiatry and Systems Medicine, Program in Integrative
Medicine, University of Arizona College of Medicine, 1650 E. Fort Lowell Rd.,
Suite 201, Tucson, AZ 85719, USA

FELISE MILAN, MD
Montefiore Medical Center RBM, Albert Einstein School of Medicine,
3544 Jerome Ave., Bronx, NY 10467, USA

KOJI MIYAMOTO, BS, MD, PhD
Prof. and Director, Dept. of Bioregulatory Function, Molecular Science and Applied
Medicine, Yamaguchi University School of Medicine, 1-1-1 Minami-kogishi, Ube City,
755–8505 Yamaguchi, Japan

ARSHAG MOORADIAN, MD
St. Louis University School of Medicine, Dept. of Endocrinology,
1402 South Grand Blvd, Saint Louis, Missouri 63104, USA

HASAN MUKHTAR, PH.D.
Evan P Helfaer Professor and Director of Research Department of Dermatology,
University of Wisconsin,Medical Science Center, 1300 University Avenue, Madison,
WI 53706, USA

I. RAMAKRISHNA, PhD
Nagamalli, 23–23–60/A, Majetivari St., S.N. Puram, Vijayawada-11, Andra Pradesh,
India

MICHAEL RUBIN, MD
Department of Neurology, Weill Medical College of Cornell University and New York
Presbyterian, Hospital- Cornell Medical Center, 1300 York Ave. New York, NY 10021,
USA

DEBBIE SALAS-LOPEZ, PhD
MSB 1 550, Department of Medicine UMDNJ-Newark, 185 S. Orange St., Newark,
NJ 07103, USA

ROBERT SCHNEIDER, PHD
College of Maharishi Vedic Medicine, Maharishi University of Management,
504 N. Fourth St, Suite 207, Fairfield, IA 52556, USA

ANNA L. SILBERMAN
CEO, Lifestyle Advantage, Highmark Blue Cross/Blue Shield, Fifth Ave. 120,
Fifth Ave. Pl., Suite 2110, Pittsburgh, PA 15222, USA

JEROME THURMAN, MD
St. Louis University School of Medicine, Dept. of Endrocrinology,
1402 South Grand Blvd, Saint Louis, Missouri 63104, USA

NANCY TURNER, PHD
University of Victoria, School of Environmental Studies, Sedgewick Bldg. C135,
P.O. Box 1700, Victoria, BC V8W 2Y2, Canada

WEN-HSIEN WU, MD, MS
Pain Management Center, Doctors Office Center, 90 Bergen Street, Suite 3400,
Newark, NJ 07103, USA

A Epidemiology

1 Patterns and Predictors of CAM Use Among Older Adults

J.A. Astin

Introduction

Studies in the United States, Europe, and elsewhere continue to document the growing interest in and use of complementary/alternative (CAM) therapies by the general public. Some of this research has suggested that CAM use is higher among middle-aged, "Baby Boomers" [6, 7] and therefore less frequently used by both younger and older populations [3]. While in general, across surveys, this pattern tends to hold true, Astin [1] failed to find a significant association between age and extent of CAM use in his multivariate analysis of predictors of utilization. While relatively few studies have specifically examined use of CAM by elderly persons, several recent reports have appeared in the literature. In this chapter, I will summarize this literature examining frequency of CAM use by older adults; highlight which specific CAM therapies are most commonly employed by these populations; and examine specific demographic and attitudinal characteristics that might account for elderly persons decision to utilize CAM.

Patterns of CAM Use

One of the first published studies that specifically examined CAM use among elderly persons involved a survey of 728 Californians enrolled in a Medicare risk product that offered coverage for acupuncture and chiropractic [2] The authors reported 41% overall CAM use (use being defined somewhat more narrowly than in the most oft cited studies [1, 7] in the U.S.) The most commonly employed modalities were herbs (24%), chiropractic (20%), massage (15%), and acupuncture (14%). It should be noted that estimates of utilization in this study may have been inflated since the sample was from a geographic region of the country known to have significantly higher rates of CAM use.

Drawing from a more representative, national sample (a secondary analysis of the Eisenberg et al. 1997 data [7]), Foster et al. [8] examined CAM use among adults aged 65 and older (*n*=311). Overall, 30% of these individuals reported use of at least one CAM therapy in the previous year, significantly less than the figure of 46% reported for those persons less than 65 years of age in that same study. The most commonly used therapies by this subgroup of older adults were chiropractic (11%), herbal medicine (8%), relaxation techniques (5%), mega-vitamins (5%), and religious/spiritual healing by others (4%). The authors found that 6% of older adults reported taking herbs in addition to their prescription medications and that 57% did not discuss their use of CAM with their conventional physicians. The most common clinical conditions for which older adults sought CAM treatment were arthritis, back pain, heart disease, allergy, and diabetes.

In a similar secondary analysis of CAM use by older adults drawn from Astin's national data set [1] 35% of those respondents aged 65 and older (n=185) reported use of at least one CAM therapy in the previous year. Chiropractic (19%), prayer/spiritual practice (9%), and lifestyle diet (7%) were the most frequently employed therapies. It should be noted that in this sample, use of herbal therapies was considerably lower (2%) than the 8% reported by Foster et al. This likely reflects the explosion of public interest in and use of herbal medicines and dietary supplements in the U.S. following the passage of DSHEA, which effectively de-regulated and opened up commercial markets for these products. In both the Foster et al and Astin analyses, older adults were less likely to report use of relaxation techniques and massage. For example, only 2.7% of elderly respondents reported use of relaxation therapies compared with 8% of non-elderly subjects in the Astin study.

Dello Buono and colleagues [5] recently published a paper examining use of alternative therapies among community dwelling elderly persons in Padua, Italy. In this sample (n=655), 29% reported use of at least one CAM therapy in the past year (the precise definition of "CAM" was not clear in this study). Most frequently used therapies were herbs/phytotherapeutics (14%) and acupuncture (10%) while relaxation therapies were used by 4% of respondents. As with other general population studies [4], the vast majority of subjects in this study (96%) did not rely exclusively on CAM therapies but instead used these approaches alongside more conventional medical approaches. In a convenience sample of 421 elderly patients being seen in a geriatric primary care practice and a veteran's medical clinic (both in New York City), Cherniack et al. [4] found that 58% of subjects reported some use of CAM. Data were not available, however, on survey response rate or the specific CAM modalities utilized.

Several studies have also examined CAM use for specific clinical conditions. In a population based study of 480 elderly arthritis patients, Kaboli et al. [9] reported that 66% of respondents used one or more CAM therapies; 28% stated that they had seen a CAM provider. Ramsey et al. [11] found that 47% of older osteoarthritis patients participating in a clinical trial stated that they had tried at least one type of CAM therapy over the course of the 20-week trial. The most commonly employed modalities were massage, chiropractic, and "non-prescribed alternative medications."

In a relatively small study (but one that had a high response rate of 81%), Lippert et al. [10] examined rates of CAM use by patients with localized prostate carcinoma. Forty-three percent of those surveyed reported use of alternative therapies with vitamins, prayer/religious practice and herbal treatments being the most common. Wyatt et al. [13] in a study of 699 heterogeneous cancer patients aged 64 and older found that 33% reported using CAM therapies with exercise, herbal medicine, and spiritual healing the most frequently employed.

Predictors of CAM Use

Studies have also begun to examine a variety of demographic, attitudinal and health related factors that might account for (or are at least associated with) use of CAM by elderly persons. While one study failed to find an association between education level and CAM utilization [9], studies have more typically found that older adults who have higher levels of education are more likely to use CAM therapies [1, 2, 4]. As with general population studies in which CAM use tends to be associated with poorer overall health status, research also suggests that those elderly persons with poorer health and who make more frequent visits to conventional providers [2, 8] are more likely to use CAM therapies as well. Specific medical conditions that are most frequently associated with CAM use in older populations include arthritis [2, 4, 9], depression or anxiety [2, 5], thyroid, and chronic obstructive pulmonary disease [4]. While some studies have found elderly CAM use to be higher among females, others have failed to find such an association [2].

While studies do tend to show an association with poorer health status and the presence of various chronic medical conditions (e.g., arthritis) and CAM use, research also suggests that elderly CAM users are more likely to be health conscious. For example, Astin et al. [2] found that those respondents who reported using CAM therapies were also more likely to engage in physical exercise and practice meditation, and there was also a non-significant trend toward their being less likely to smoke cigarettes and drink alcohol. These findings suggest that the relationship between use of CAM and health status may be somewhat of a curvilinear one in that CAM use is highest among those with the poorest health *and* those who are the most health conscious.

One of the largest, most comprehensive examinations of predictors of CAM use was carried out by Astin [1]. In this study, three broad factors that might account for utilization were examined: dissatisfaction with conventional medicine, desire for control over health-related matters, and philosophical congruence. In this general population sample of U.S. adults, only the third factor – philosophical congruence – emerged as a significant predictor in the multivariate analysis suggesting that people were motivated to use CAM, in part, because they perceived these therapies to be more closely aligned with their own philosophies of health and life, particularly in terms of acknowledging the importance of non-physical (i.e., psychospiritual) factors.

The relatively small number of elderly persons in the Astin study (n=185) precluded doing any comprehensive multivariate analyses to examine predictors of CAM use in this subpopulation. However, what follows is an analysis comparing respondents aged 65 and older with those aged 18–64 on a number of factors that emerged as significant predictors in the original study. As I will argue, these preliminary findings suggest a somewhat different attitudinal/psychological profile for the elderly CAM user than that typically found among middle and younger aged users of CAM.

In the Astin study [1] three variables emerged as significant predictors of CAM use. And taken both separately and together, these offer support for the "philosophical congruence" hypothesis. These were:

▶ a holistic orientation ("the health of my body, mind and spirit are related and however cares for my health should take that into account"),

▶ reporting having had a "transformational experience that changed the way I view the world"), and

▶ being classified in a value subculture – the "Cultural Creatives" characterized by one's interest in personal growth psychology, esoteric forms of spirituality, feminism, environmentalism, a love for things foreign and exotic and for mastering new ideas [1, 12].

Table 1.1 compares older adults with the rest of the sample on each of these variables, highlighting the percentage within each attitudinal/value category that used CAM.

In general, it was the case that older adults were less likely to be categorized as "cultural creatives," (12% compared with 26% of non-elderly respondents), and somewhat less holistic in their orientation toward health (45% endorsing this orientation compared with 53% of the non-elderly). However, what is of particular interest is that these factors seem to be significantly *less* predictive of CAM use among the elderly. For example, differences in CAM use between those classified as "Cultural Creatives" and those who were not was quite marked among the non-elderly population (57% and 36% respectively), However, these differences were significantly less pronounced among those aged 65 and older (41% of elderly cultural creatives used CAM compared with 34% of those not in this value subculture). In other words, among the elderly, being a cultural creative was not as strongly associated with use of CAM.

This pattern was even more pronounced when one looks at the variable of "holding a holistic orientation." Among non-elderly subjects, 49% of those who subscribed to a holistic philosophy of health were CAM users compared with 33% among the non-holistically inclined. However, among the elderly, there were no differences in CAM use (35% and 36% respectively) between those who subscribed to a holistic orientation and those who did not.

Again, a similar pattern emerged in the question "I've had a transformational experience that's changed the way I view the world." The percentage of elderly and non-elderly respondents who answered this question in the affirmative was quite similar (17% and 19% respectively). However, there was no association between such a positive response and use of CAM among the elderly subjects whereas among non-elderly, this question was strongly associated with use of CAM. Among non-elderly respondents, 58% of those who answered "yes" to this item used CAM while only 38%

Table 1.1 Percentage of attitudinal/value category that used CAM

	Elderly (n=185) [%]	Rest of Sample (n=847) [%]
Holistic	35[a]	49
Non-holistic	36	33
Cultural creative	41	57
Non-cultural creative	34	36
Transformational experience	29	58
Non-transformational experience	36	38

[a] % of subgroup using CAM.

of those who responded negatively to this item reported CAM use. However, among the elderly, *fewer* people (29% to 36%) actually used CAM who answered this question in the affirmative.

In terms of demographic variables, slightly different patterns also emerged when elderly respondents were compared to the rest of the sample. Among those less than 65 years of age, women were somewhat more likely to be CAM users (43%) than men (40%). However, among elderly subjects, men actually reported slightly higher rates of use (38%) than women (33%). In terms of health status, those reporting poorer health were more likely to report use of CAM irrespective of age.

No clear pattern emerged between the desire to maintain control over health decisions and use of CAM although among non-elderly subjects, there was a trend toward those desiring greater control being more likely to use CAM. It is interesting to note, however, that elderly respondents were more inclined (18%) to say that in health care decisions, they would prefer to "leave it in the doctor's hands" compared with non-elderly (4%). Similarly, 9% of older adults stated that they would prefer to "keep control in their own hands", compared with 20% of non-elderly respondents. There was also a non-significant trend in both elderly and non-elderly participants suggesting that those with more of a passive and unquestioning faith in Western medicine ("I take my body to the doctor's office, and I expect the doctor to 'fix it'") were less inclined to use CAM. Again, what is interesting to note about this item is that elderly respondents were significantly more likely to indicate such unquestioning faith (47% to 21%) compared with non-elderly subjects.

Summary and Conclusions

While general population studies suggest the highest rates of CAM use are by middle-aged adults, use of complementary/alternative therapies *is* considerable among those aged 65 and older with rates ranging between 30–66% across surveys. However, CAM is a very heterogeneous category and not surprisingly there do appear to be significant differences in the types of therapies used. While chiropractic and herbal medicine tend to be the most frequently employed modalities irrespective of age, therapies such as relaxation and massage tend to be used less frequently by the elderly [8].

One possible explanation for these apparent differences in the types of CAM therapies used by older adults might be found in their unique attitudinal and value profiles. For example, the secondary analyses of the Astin 1998 study [1] suggests that greater alignment with a holistic-spiritual orientation to health and life may be less of a motivating factor among elderly CAM users since these variables while strongly associated with CAM use among younger respondents, were not correlated with CAM use among the elderly and fewer older adults subscribed to such beliefs. It may be the case that for older adults, a stronger motivating factor underlying the decision to use CAM may be a more pragmatic one – i.e., in part as a result of their age, they are more likely to suffer from various chronic conditions that often fail to respond well to conventional approaches which therefore draws them to experiment with alternatives. However, it should be noted that as is the case in general population studies, the vast majority of older adults who use CAM do so along with (i.e., as a complement to rather than alternative or substitute for) conventional therapeutic approaches. That being said, the data also suggest that many older adults (like their younger counterparts) are disinclined to discuss their use of CAM with their conventional medical providers [2, 8] Because some CAM therapies (e.g., herbals and nutritional supplements) may interact negatively with conventional (particularly pharmacologic) approaches, it is vital that physicians and other medical providers create a climate where patients feel safe and are encouraged to discuss their use of these less conventional approaches.

It is quite possible that as the baby boomers age, we will see a marked explosion of interest in and use CAM therapies since many of the values associated with greater use of CAM (e.g., holism, viewing of health within the larger context of personal/spiritual growth) are more prominent among this generational cohort. Also, as others have noted, as the baby boomers age, we will undoubtedly see significant increases in the numbers of people living longer and therefore facing more chronic medical conditions. And this will likely as not lead to increasing rates of CAM use among those older adults who are facing such difficult to treat medical conditions.

References

1. Astin JA (1998) Why patients use alternative medicine: results of a national study. JAMA 279(19): 1548–1553
2. Astin JA, Pelletier KR, Marie A, Haskell WL (2000) Complementary and alternative medicine use among elderly persons: one- year analysis of a Blue Shield Medicare supplement. J Gerontol A Biol Sci Med Sci 55(1): M4–9
3. Bausell RB, Lee W, Berman BM (2001) Demographic and health-related correlates of visit s to complementary and alternative medical providers. Medical Care 39: 190–196
4. Cherniack EP, Senzel RS, Pan CX (2001) Correlates of use of alternative medicine by the elderly in an Urban population. J Altern Complement Med 7(3): 277–280
5. Dello Buono M, Urciuoli O, Marietta P, Padoani W, De Leo D (2001) Alternative medicine in a sample of 655 community-dwelling elderly. J Psychosom Res 50(3): 147–154
6. Eisenberg DM, Kessler RC, Foster C, Norlock FE, Calkins DR, Delbanco TL (1993) Unconventional medicine in the United States. Prevalence, costs, and patterns of use. N Engl J Med 328(4): 246–252
7. Eisenberg DM, Davis RB, Ettner SL et al. (1998) Trends in alternative medicine use in the United States, 1990–1997: results of a follow-up national survey. JAMA 280(18): 1569–1575
8. Foster DF, Phillips RS, Hamel MB, Eisenberg DM (2000) Alternative medicine use in older Americans. J Am Geriatr Soc 48(12): 1560–1565
9. Kaboli PJ, Doebbeling BN, Saag KG, Rosenthal GE (2001) Use of complementary and alternative medicine by older patients with arthritis: a population-based study. Arthritis Rheum 45(4): 398–403
10. Lippert MC, McClain R, Boyd JC, Theodorescu D (1999) Alternative medicine use in patients with localized prostate carcinoma treated with curative intent. Cancer 86(12): 2642–2648
11. Ramsey SD, Spencer AC, Topolski TD, Belza B, Patrick DL (2001) Use of alternative therapies by older adults with osteoarthritis. Arthritis Rheum 45(3): 222–227
12. Ray P, Ray SA (2000) The cultural creatives: how 50 million Americans are changing the way we live. Harmony Books, Nevada City
13. Wyatt GK, Friedman LL, Given CW, Given BA, Beckrow KC (1999) Complementary therapy use among older cancer patients. Cancer Pract 7(3): 136–144

2 Why Do the Elderly Use Complementary and Alternative Medicine?

A. Furnham

Introduction

Many forms of the complementary and alternative medicine (CAM) can trace their history back literally hundreds of years. Acupuncture, herbalism and homoeopathy all claim a long lineage in terms of practice. But it has been particularly in the last fifty years (and more particularly in the past 20 years) that have seen a dramatic and sustained growth in interest in the area throughout the western world and people from many different age groups. Growth in the use of an increasingly wide variety of CAM therapies has quite naturally led to increasing research endeavour to answer questions about the efficacy and choice of CAM [60, 62, 72] compared to orthodox, western, medicine.

In the United States Eisenberg et al. [19] found that 34% of Americans had used at least one conventional therapy or remedy in the past year, and a third visited "unconventional therapists". More visits were made to providers of unconventional therapy than to all U.S. primary care physicians (general practitioners) of orthodox medicine (O.M.). The expenditure on unconventional therapists ($ 13.7 billion) is enormous and growing. In Europe, surveys suggest that a third of people have seen a complementary therapist or used complementary remedies in any one year. The popularity of CAM throughout Europe is growing rapidly. In 1981, 6.4% of the Dutch population attended a therapist or doctor providing CAM, and this increased to 9.1% by 1985 and 15.7% in 1990. The use of homoeopathy, the most popular form of complementary therapy in France, rose from 16% of the population in 1982 to 29% in 1987 and 36% in 1992 [28]. In Britain there are more CAM practitioners than OM practitioners. Ernst and Kaptchuk [24] found that around 25% of the British population have used some form of CAM. Further around 80% of the public are satisfied with CAM therapies compared to 60% of OM therapy, and around 65% of the British hospital doctors believe that CAM has a place in mainstream medicine. More recently White and Ernst [76] noted that annual expenditure on CAM for the whole UK was in the region of £1.6 billion per annum which is spent "out-of-pocket" and is in addition to the $ 40 million expenditure of the National Health Service.

We know that from more recent figures that 1 in 5 of the British adult population consults a CAM therapist or takes CAM treatments regularly. Further around £500,000,000 is spent on CAM products annually. There seems little doubt that there is considerable rise in public and research interest in complementary medicine [73]. One index of this is the "theme issue" of the *Journal of the American Medical Association* (JAMA) 1998, Vol. 280, No. 18 which included results of a follow-up study looking at trends in America [20]. Extrapolating to the population as a whole, they found a 47.3% increase in total visits to CAM practitioners from 427 million in 1990 to 629 in 1997 exceeding visits to primary care physicians.

It is dangerous and foolhardy to talk about the "typical" patients as CAM rejoices in differences and individuality and the uniqueness of people's lives. However there have been patterns and higher probability that particular types of people are likely to seek out, use, and benefit from CAM, and their recommended treatment.

Demography. Although it clearly depends on various issues it seems that CAM patients are more likely to be: women rather than men; aged 30–40 rather than older or younger; middle rather than working class; well-educated, above average levels; urban rather than rural.

Medical History. There are things that seem to characterize patients. First they have chronic problems rather than acute. Secondly they are often non-specific or have a heavy psychological (i.e. non physical) component. Thirdly, many patients have a "thick file" in the sense that their interest in health issues has led them to seek out various remedies from many different sources.

Beliefs, Attitudes and Values. Many patients seem to be sympathetic with green issues, ideas and understanding. These include environmentalism, one worldism and amaterialism and issues around inequality, alienation, and social exclusion. Patients also seem interested and sensitive to business ethic issues that are frequently discussed. CAM patients also seem to be interested in general consumer affair issues and may even belong to bodies that attempt to lobby in favor of a certain position. They appear to be sensitive to consumer rights, bad practice and poor treatment. CAM patients appear to be particularly interested in the "life of the mind". They certainly believe the maxim of "a healthy mind and a healthy body". CAM patients are likely to be inquisitive and open to new ideas. This may mean they are interested in aesthetics (music, art) as well as new ideas in web sites. CAM patients are, because of their own medical condition, likely to be very empathic to the plight of others, and hostile to the "uncaring" attitude of certain specialists (e.g. surgeons).

What is CAM?

The incredible range of varieties of CAM inevitably means there is a considerable diversity of theories, philosophies and therapies. The arcane diagnostic system of the iridologist stands in dramatic contrast to the osteopath's up-to-date knowledge of human anatomy. Equally, the bizarre explanations of gem therapy bear little or no relationship to that of homoeopathy. Yet there are common themes in the philosophies of CAM. Aakster [1] argued that they differ from orthodox medicine in terms of five things. Inevitably, these sorts of contrasts exaggerate both the differences and the within-group homogeneity, but they are nonetheless worth considering:

▶ *Health:* Whereas conventional medicine sees health as an *absence* of disease, alternative medicine frequently mentions a *balance* of opposing forces (both external and internal).

▶ *Disease:* The conventional medicinal interpretation sees disease as a specific, locally defined deviation in organ or tissue structure. CAM practitioners stress many wider signs, such as body language indicating disruptive forces and/or restorative processes.

▶ *Diagnosis:* Regular medicine stresses morphological classification based on location and etiology, while alternative interpretations often consider problems of everyday functionality to be diagnostically useful.

▶ *Therapy:* Conventional medicine often aims to destroy, demolish or suppress the sickening forces, while alternative therapies often aim to strengthen the vitalizing, health-promoting forces. CAM therapies seem particularly hostile to chemical therapies and surgery.

▶ *Patient:* In much conventional medicine the patient is the passive recipient of external solutions, while in CAM the patient is an active participant in regaining health.

Aakster [1] described three main frames of medical thinking: the *pharmaceutical* model, which sees disease as a demonstrable deviation of function or structure that can be diagnosed by careful observation. From this perspective the causes of disease are mainly germ-like and the application of therapeutic technology is all-important. The second was the *integrational* model which resulted from technicians attempting to reintegrate the body. This approach is not afraid of allowing for psychological and social causes to be specified in the etiology of illness. The third model was labeled *holistic* and does not distinguish between soma, psyche and social. It stresses total therapy and holds up the idea of a natural way of living.

Indeed the above five characteristically may hold the key for understanding why elderly people maybe attracted to CAM and to particular certain branches of it. Older people may have different views on causes of health and illness as well as treatment and the role of the patient. They may in turn make them more or less attracted to CAM.

Gray [45] argued there are currently four quite different perspectives on complementary medicine:

The Biomedicine Perspective

This is concerned with curing of disease and control of symptoms where the physician-scientist is a technician applying high level skills to psychological problems. Assumptions which thus permeate biomedicine include

▶ that the natural order is autonomous from human consciousness, culture, morality, psychology and the supernatural;

▶ that truth or reality resides in the accurate explanation of material (as opposed to spiritual, psychological or political) reality;

▶ that the individual is the social unit of primary importance (as opposed to society); and

▶ that a dualistic framework (e.g. mind/body) is most appropriate for describing reality, and is antagonistic toward and sceptical of CAM, believing many claims to be fraudulent and many practitioners unscrupulous.

The Complementary Perspective

Though extremely varied, those with this perspective do share certain fundamental assumptions

▶ believing in the importance of domains other than "the physical" for understanding health,
▶ viewing diseases as symptomatic of underlying systematic problems,
▶ a reliance on clinical experience to guide practice and
▶ a cogent critique of the limits of the biomedical approach. Interventions at the psychological, social and spiritual level are all thought to be relevant and important supporting the idea of a biopsychosocial model.
▶ Many advocates are critical of biomedicine's harsh and often unsuccessful treatments, and paradoxically not being based on "solid scientific evidence".

The Progressive Perspective

Proponents of this perspective are prepared to support either of the above, depending entirely on the scientific evidence in favor. They are hardened empiricists who believe it is possible to integrate the best of biomedicine and unconventional approaches. Like all other researchers, their approach is not value free – the advocates of this approach welcome the scientific testing of all sorts of unconventional therapies.

The Post-Modern Perspective

This approach enjoys challenging those with absolute faith in science, reason and technology and deconstructing traditional ideas of progress. Followers are distrustful of, and cynical toward, science, medicine, the legal system and institutionalized religion and even parliamentary democracy. Postmodernists see truth as a socially and politically constructed issue and believe orthodox practitioners to be totalitarian persecutors of unconventional medicine. Proponents of this position argue

▶ to have a complementary perspective in any debate is healthy,
▶ that CAM practitioners are also connected to particular economic and theoretical interest,
▶ that the variety of values and criteria of assessing success is beneficial and
▶ that the ill people themselves should be the final *arbitrators* of the success of the therapy.

Gray [45] concludes: "It has been argued above that the biomedical and complementary perspectives tend to be characterized by strongly held beliefs about the nature of health, illness and reality, while the proponents of the progressive perspective subjugate such beliefs to the test of scientific method, which in itself is characterized by values. Postmodernists argue that all perspectives are value-based and socially constructed, and that no one perspective will have all the truth about health practices, or anything else. They encourage the articulation of multiple perspectives as a basis for fully informed decision-making, with the individual ill person as final arbitrator" (p.70). There remains much more diversity than unity within CAM. Whilst there have been calls to find regulatory bodies to oversee all CAM practices this has proved very difficult because of the theoretical, historical and political differences between the various CAM specialties.

This chapter will examine the extent social science literature that has attempted to ascertain why people chose to use CAM. It will first examine the limited, but growing, literature on CAM use among the elderly. It will then consider research on choice of CAM followed by an examination of the OM and CAM consultation. Finally it will speculate in why CAM may be a particularly attractive alternative or supplementary form of therapy for older people.

CAM in the Elderly Patient

There has been a dearth of studies looking specifically at CAM use among the elderly. Ernst [25] noted that CAM was used by the elderly in Britain at least, for psychological and musculoskeletal problems particularly back pain which seems ubiquitous. He notes: "The attraction for senior citizens of CAM is undoubtedly the image of being gentle and (largely) free of adverse reactions. The constraints lie in the fact that CAM is usually paid for privately and that contraindications might apply (e.g. osteoporosis for spinal manipulation). Survey data suggest that a significantly larger proportion of patients older than 60 years prefer CAM to mainstream medicine compared with younger patients, and a recent Mirtel report shows that 54% of the British population aged 65 and over agree with the notion that CAM is effective" (p. 358).

Very few studies have actually looked at the use of CAM usage among the elderly. However, there is an exception in the study of Astin et al. [3]. The population surveyed in this study were enrolled in a Medicare risk product which offers coverage for acupuncture and chiropractic care. Surveys were mailed to 1597 members in 1997 but 728 received in reply which is above average being 45%. Health risk assessment data were also obtained 21–15 months following enrolment in the plan. Forty-one percent of elderly people reported use of CAM: Herbs, chiropractic, massage, and acupuncture were the most frequently cited therapies. CAM users tended to be younger, more educated, report either arthritis and/or depression/anxiety, not be hypertensive, engage in exercise, practice meditation, and make more frequent physician visits. This data looks similar to those found in middle aged samples. Use of CAM was however not associated with any observed changes in health status which was not expected. Respondents also expressed considerable interest in receiving third-party coverage for CAM. Although 80% reported that they had received substantial benefit from their use of CAM, the majority did not discuss the use of these therapies with their medical doctor which is not unusual.

They note: "Although previous research has suggested that complementary/alternative medicine is primarily used by those aged 35–50, the present study suggests that a substantial number of seniors are:

▶ using CAM therapies to address a variety of health-related problems as well as prevent illness and optimise health and well-being;

▶ perceive these therapies to be efficacious;
▶ are not discussing such use with their physicians; and
▶ are interested in having their health plans offer coverage for such therapies.

Significant use of, and interest in, approaches such as chiropractic, acupuncture, and herbal medicine by seniors – a segment of the population that is both growing exponentially as well the largest consumers of health care – suggest the need for more well-controlled studies examining the potential efficacy of these therapies. As the 35–50 year old postwar Baby Boomers continue to use CAM with greater frequency into their advanced years, both the promise and perils of these therapies need to be further researched. Clinical and cost outcomes based on longitudinal studies need to focus on Medicare-eligible populations to determine if CAM versus conventional versus an integrated model of CAM and conventional care results in decreased disability and improved health status. Addressing such clinical, financial, and public policy questions becomes ever more pressing as over 15,000 people per day become Medicare-eligible" (p. 118).

Another Italian study looked specifically at the use and satisfaction with herbal/homeopathic, acupuncture and relation techniques. Buono et al. [10] found herbs (phytotherapeutics [(47%)]) and acupuncture (34%) were the most cited therapies. The most heavy users were females with depressive symptoms, pain and discomfort but not suffering from chronic somatic disease. They note "The majority of our users also reported turning to practices such as acupuncture or relaxation techniques on their own initiative or on the advice of relatives and friends, although referral to such alternatives was in some cases by a G.P. or specialist. albeit to a lesser extent.

Further, a noteworthy finding is that elderly consumers of exclusively alternative medicines seem to be younger, less likely to be physically ill and to report functional disorders and chronic somatic diseases. The percentage of elderly persons in this group who positively perceived subjective physical health was over 95%, while the percentage of respondents with scores exceeding the cut-off for depressive symptoms was similar to those who also used a combination of orthodox and non-orthodox practices and higher than the same percentage in other groups. This finding is worth special attention. Depression also proved to be a significant predictor of alternative medicine use in the recent survey on the elderly by Astin et al. [3] (p. 152).

Only further research on the above issue will help explain why older people are more or less attracted to CAM in general or particular branches of it compared to younger people. However there are things to note from studies in the area. First elderly people maybe more secretive than others with their GP about their use of CAM. That is, they are less willing to admit using OM and CAM simultaneously. Second they are a quickly growing sector of the population and an increasingly politically active one and hence they maybe expected to put pressure on governments to have subsidized CAM treatment. Third they seem to be interested in a broader range of CAM therapies than hitherto to expected. Certainly this is an important and currently neglected area of research.

Why Do People Choose CAM?

Sociological Speculations

Researchers and reviewers have come up with various lists of the possible motives of CAM patients seeking out treatment. Anthropologists and sociologists have stressed the importance of cultural variables and shifts such as the growth of post modernism [77]. Economists have in part accounted for the rise of interest in CAM as a function of the costs to patients, doctors and health insurance companies. Psychologists and psychiatrists have focused more on interpersonal and intrapsychic explanations for why certain individuals seek out CAM [72]. Medical practitioners stress the medical history of particular patients (and chronicity of their illness) or indeed differences in the average consultation between the CAM practitioner and the GP [21, 22].

Willliams and Calnan [77] believe that as people generally live longer and in a more pain-free environment, there is increasing ambivalence about modern, technological medicine such as transplantation surgery, new reproductive technologies and the use of modern drugs. It is seen as cold, invasive and unnatural. Modern medicine is both a fountain of hope *and* despair. Growing concern about *risk* (and litigation) encourages a subtle balance between active trust and radical doubt in medical experts of all kinds. The *media* often attempt a demystification role in putting modern medical practices on trial by encouraging the audience to be the jury. Lay people particularly middle aged and older educated people are acquiring more sophisticated technical knowledge which makes them more medical educated and demanding consumers. "... one thing remains clear: namely that lay people are not simply passive or active, dependent or independent, believers or sceptics, rather they are a complex mixture of all these things (and much more besides)" [77].

Lupton [55] found that in the doctor's surgery, patients pursue the "consumerist" and "passive patient" position simultaneously depending on context. People shop for health while accepting the benefits of modern high-tech medicine. She believes that the consumerist movement is counter productive as it undermines the faith and trust in conventional medical practitioners that is central to the healing and comfort very ill people desperately seek in the medical encounter.

Cassileth [15] believes that the popularity of any specialist CAM treatment is, in part, a function of how well it fits into the sociocultural context of the (our) time. He believes that there are five underlying social trends of our time that render certain treatments popular. They are: Various rights movements (including patients' rights); Consumer movements that shift patients from the dependent role to a partnership/active consumer role; The holistic medicine movement; Self-care and fitness emphases; Disaffection with, and mistrust of, organized orthodox medicine.

The belief in the power and supremacy of the individual and his/her overriding need to understand and control, leads people to the "mind has the power to heal" philosophy. Frustration with a lack of ability to cure and control various diseases leads to attempts to achieving control, healing and understanding via less intrusive or toxic therapies. Patients are attracted to alternative therapies whose ideologies fit the current spirit of the times. Indeed with older people it maybe that therapies that reflect the "zeitgeist" of their times rather than the modern "zeitgeist" have particular attractions. Further it maybe that some CAM therapies and philosophies echo an earlier time making them particularly attractive to elderly people.

McKee [57] argued that the CAM holistic health movement can be accused of promoting both an *individualistic* rather than a social analysis of health, and a *victim-blaming* ideology which serves to transfer the burden of health costs from the state and corporations to the individual. She argues that holistic health serves the interest of capital accumulation, while Western medicine promotes capitalism. Short-term treatment of disease is profitable and medical practice is oriented to crisis intervention and pathology correction, not prevention or health maintenance. This is a particularly interesting issue with older people as it maybe argued that their personal life-style was a major factor in their current health. That is, they have been largely personally instrumental in their current health status.

Lynse [56] noted two reasons why patients in general choose alternative medicine: push and pull: *disappointment* with currently available health care (push) and *curiosity* (pull). First, alternative practitioners use new, unaccepted controversial concepts. Second, empirical data in support of CAM therapies may be impossible to understand against the background of the prevailing paradigm; that is, effects have not been well recorded or documented, *but are real*. Third, the development of a new paradigm provides the opportunity for reinterpreting pre-scientific terms and data in a new light.

There remains many interested philosophical and sociological explanations as to why people may be attracted to CAM. These explanations have not been focused on elderly people specifically though it is not difficult to see how this maybe done. These speculations to account for the general rise of interest in CAM in the general public rather than focusing on one specific group, though it is unlikely that the motives differ radically between different groups.

Empirical Studies

As well as socio-historical and theoretical speculations about the cause of the rise of interest in CAM there have also been a number of empirical studies that set out to test various very specific hypotheses.

Thomas and her medical colleagues in the UK [65] specifically set out to discover whether CAM patients had turned their backs on conventional medicine. The majority of adult patients in their sample (64%) reported having received conventional treatment for their main problem from their general practitioner or a hospital specialist before receiving their present CAM treatment; just under a quarter of those who had received conventional treatment continued it while receiving CAM treatment. The remaining 36% had not received any conventional medical treatment, but they may have received advice on their condition from their general practitioner who may also have suggested CAM therapy. It is also noteworthy that 3% of the patients were recommended to visit their general practitioner by the CAM therapist whom they had been consulting at the time. They found that the use of prior conventional medical treatment was dependent on the type of problem for which patients were seeking help. Patients reporting atopic conditions, headaches and arthritis were more likely to report a combination of previous and concurrent conventional treatment, usually drugs. Thomas rejected the view that patients attending CAM therapists do not understand or appreciate the benefits of conventional medicine or that the popularity of complementary medicine represents a "flight from science".

Ernst et al. [21] asked three groups of everyday medical patients (68 Austrians, 89 Britons and 54 Germans) why they thought "people seek treatment by alternative methods like acupuncture, homoeopathy and chiropractic" They were offered 9 explanations and asked to tick all that applied. Because

▶ they are disappointed by orthodox medicine: 31.8%
▶ it is their last hope: 37.9%
▶ they are not really ill: 4.3%
▶ they are inclined to unscientific ideas: 8.1%
▶ they feel they will be better understood: 28.9%
▶ they want to use all possible options in healthcare: 57.8%
▶ they previously had a good experience: 37.9%
▶ they hope to be cured without side-effects: 47.9%
▶ it usually costs extra: 3.8%

They concluded that disenchantment with mainstream medicine is *not* the most prominent reason for choosing CAM. A more positive motivation (e.g. wanting to try all options of health care) may play a prominent role. Second, they noted that few patients are opponents of CAM.

Vincent and Furnham [72] asked over 250 patients from three CAM therapies – acupuncture, osteopathy and homoeopathy – to complete a questionnaire rating 20 potential reasons for seeking complementary treatment. The reasons that were most strongly endorsed were "because I value the emphasis on treating the whole person"; "because I believe complementary therapy will be more effective for my problem than orthodox medicine"; "because I believe that complementary medicine will enable me to take a more active part in maintaining my health"; and 'because orthodox treatment was not effective for my particular problem'. Five factors were identified, in order of importance:

▶ A positive valuation of complementary treatment;
▶ the ineffectiveness of orthodox treatment for their complaint;
▶ concern about the adverse effects of orthodox medicine;
▶ concerns about communication with doctors;
▶ the availability of complementary medicine.

Osteopathy patients' reasons indicated they were least concerned about the side-effects of conventional medicine and most influenced by the availability of osteopathy for their complaints. Homoeopathy patients were most strongly influenced by the ineffectiveness of medicine for their complaints, a fact which was largely accounted for by the chronicity of their complaints. Three of the factors showed significant differences between the three patient groups. Acupuncture and homoeopathy patients seemed "put off" by the potential side-effects of medicine more than the osteopathy group.

This was probably due to the nature of the problems they presented with, and possible use of drugs by their physicians. A second difference between the groups indicated that the osteopathy patients rated the availability of their therapy as more important than the other two groups. The final factor, which referred to the ineffective nature of conventional medicine, was rated most highly by the homeopathic group, who may have complaints that are particularly resistant to conventional treatment.

Hertschel et al. [48] interviewed 419 German patients, half currently using and half not using CAM, through a 168 item questionnaire. They were interested in how the two groups differed on socio-demographic lifestyle, and illness-related data as well as their illness-preventing behaviors, their psychological makeup, doctor-patient relationship and particular doctor preference. Their study was exploratory rather than hypothesis testing, though it yielded some very interesting findings. CAM patients were more likely to be women, and were also less likely to smoke and drink and more likely to follow particular (and medical) diets. Many in the CAM group claimed to have been seriously ill, with chronic complaints. They were more likely to change their medical doctor if dissatisfied and to visit their doctor more frequently. CAM patients also spent more on everyday medication and were more willing to do so, if they believe it worked. Many reported being much more dissatisfied with conventional medicine than OM patients.

The CAM patients in the study had had more experience of various types of CAM (homoeopathy, natural therapy) as well as psychotherapy than the medical patients. There was no difference in the preventative health measures of either group, however. CAM patients were also more likely to worry about contracting a serious illness and were found to be more prone to boredom, depression, loneliness and alienation. They also tended to be more pessimistic about life. CAM patients who went to GP as well as to CAM practitioners appeared to expect and receive more empathy from their GP and to have more faith in them than conventional medical patients. Overall patients seemed to seek CAM for migraine, depression, allergies, and skin diseases and medical care for life-threatening conditions like heart attacks, diabetes and cancer.

Kelner and Wellman [50] interviewed 300 Canadian patients in total, 60 each of family physicians, chiropractors, acupuncturists, naturopaths and Reiki patients. They were from very different demographic groups. Overall, the CAM patients, compared to the medical patients, were more likely to be female, educated, working, relatively well off and agnostic. Patients clearly went to the different specialists for different things: the chiropractor for musculoskeletal problems, the GP for cardiovascular problems and the Reiki specialist for emotional issues. Four patients of the CAM practitioners were also very frequent patients of the GPs. Indeed all patients were users of multiple therapies. The patients of chiropractors were most different, consulting for very specific problems. They conclude: "Alternative therapies are flourishing alongside conventional medicine. What we are seeing here is a pluralistic and complementary system of health care in which patients choose the kind of practitioner they believe will best be able to help their particular problem. What we do not see is an either/or decision about which kind of practitioner is the one to consult for everything pertaining to health care" (p. 139).

Finally Furnham and Vincent [43] have set out nine testable, and in some instances tested, hypotheses for why people seek out CAM.

▶ *Mental health*: The psychologically less stable are attracted to the quasi-psycho-therapeutic methods and philosophy of CAM [61]. Furnham and Smith [32] and Furnham and Bhagrath [34], using different instruments, both found evidence for the fact that matched homeopathic patients were less well adjusted than GP patients. However the direction of causality is unclear: Chronic illness maybe just as likely to increase mental illness as the possibility that the mentally unstable are attracted to CAM therapies.

▶ *Beliefs about health* (prevention of illness, resistance to disease, staying healthy): CAM is as much about prevention as cure and appeals to healthy lifestyle groups. Furnham and Smith [32], Furnham and Bhagrath [34] and Furnham et al. [39] found CAM (homoeopath) patients believed more than conventional medical patients that changes in lifestyle (diet, sleep, relaxation) were related to prevention of illness. In this sense CAM patients have different health beliefs than OM patients. CAM patients are often better informed and more interested in health issues.

▶ *Health consciousness* (interest in health related issues): Those interested in all aspects of health (mental, physical, spiritual) are attracted to CAM [45]. Furnham and Bhagrath [34] found much evidence that CAM patients took a more active interest in health matters to all ages.

▶ *Perceived susceptibility (vulnerability) to illness*: Those who feel they may be particularly vulnerable to specific illnesses (possibly psychosomatic) are attracted to CAM. Furnham and Bhagrath [34] and Furnham and Smith [32] found no evidence that CAM patients thought they were more susceptible to a large number of everyday illnesses. That is, there is little evidence of neurotic hypochondriacs.

▶ *Beliefs in the efficacy of treatment*: Are CAM patients naive, uninformed, optimistic or simply gullible because they do not know the lack of acceptable evidence for the efficacy of the treatment [16]? Furnham and Smith [32] and Furnham and Bhagrath [34] found CAM (homoeopathy) patients rather more sceptical than medical patients about their treatment. Indeed, CAM patients believe less in the efficacy of their practitioner and the rapid termination of treatment – no doubt because of the chronic nature of their illness and many disappointments in the past.

▶ *Personal control over health*: Conventional medical patients are health fatalists and CAM patients health instrumentalists. That is, CAM patients believe they have more personal control over their health than other patients. Although results do not replicate perfectly, there does seem sufficient evidence that CAM patients believe more strongly in self, rather than provider control, over personal health [34, 39, 71]. The CAM patient feels that he/she is "captain of their ship and master of their fate"; namely that in a major way they (not God, doctors, or luck) determine their state of health.

▶ *Medical history and career*: The particular medical history of patients characterized by chronic, painful and unsuccessfully treated problems (e.g. back pain) leads them, in desperation, to seek out CAM cures. This is a seriously under-researched area and may well give the greatest clues as to why people seek out CAM practitioners. Indeed this maybe the most important single cause for elderly people and suggests that all research in this area would do well to explore each person's medical history for clues.

▶ *Beliefs about scientific (evidence-based) Medicine*: Patients are postmodernists [11]: they are highly sceptical of the approaches, motives and success rate of conventional biomedicine. Furnham et al. [39] and Vincent et al. [71] found that CAM patients had not lost their faith in science but compared to medical patients, did indeed believe less in the scientific basis of medical science. Further, CAM patients stressed more than medical patients the role of psychological factors in illness and the many potential harmful side effects of modern medicine.

▶ *Attitude to physicians*: Deep disenchantment about the style and efficacy of GPs, particularly their bedside manner and poor communication skills. Furnham et al. [39] found that compared to medical patients, CAM patients were less likely to believe that GPs are sympathetic, have time to listen, are sensitive to emotional issues and are good at explaining the nature of the treatment or why an individual is ill.

Thus both speculation and research have provided a list of possible factors that lead patients to seeking out CAM, and presumably, staying with a CAM practitioner. However this research has, to date, not really considered why certain specific and definable groups like the elderly maybe particularly attracted to CAM therapies.

The Consultation

One fundamentally important but neglected area of research is the doctor-patient encounter and more particularly how it differs between OM and CAM practitioners. This maybe part reason for the attractiveness of CAM. Taylor [64] focused on the doctor-patient encounter and the nature of the relationship between practitioner and client which the alternative system offers. Earlier, Hewer [49] stressed the importance of the nature of the consultation and the relationship between doctor and patient. Taylor [64] argued that scientific medicine sees the human body as a machine, like any other, which needs servicing. Patients, who are described as cases, should not distract the doctor by their unique personal feelings and experiences. Taylor [64] believed that the orthodox doctor is teacher and facilitator, while the alternative practitioner is therapist. Too many people have become accustomed to the sort of medicine which "relies on magic bullets administered by harassed physicians who cannot distinguish us one from another as we flow from waiting room to examination room to billing office" (p. 197). Conventional medicine concentrates on sickness and alternative medicine concentrates on wellness. CAM practitioners seem to characterize orthodox medical practices as technological and aggressive and their own as natural and non-invasive. Taylor offers four explanations for the growing popularity of CAM. First a change in the cultural mood. Second, medicine has not changed and still sees itself as "restoring people to productivity within a certain form of society". Third, alternatives expand and contract in popularity in proportion to the successes and failures of conventional medicine. Finally, fear of iatrogenic diseases which are problems which stem from medical intervention and drugs which are supposed to cure, but in fact often exacerbate, the problem.

The rise and fall of different healing systems is contingent in large part on the changing nature of the medical encounter the traditional 6–8 minute clinical consultation. When medicine can promise neither relief nor cure, the quality of the individual doctor-patient relationship is paramount. The consumer movement, the women's movement and the more general demand for participation all focused on the medical encounter, but some traditional medical schools and practizing doctors have resisted populist demands and the pressure for democratization and customer service. Not only did medicine resist change, but for many there was a perceptible deterioration of the medical encounter in terms of "quality time" for the patient. Malpractice lawsuits (particularly in America) have made doctors more cautious; there are fewer generalists and more specialists so a long-term relationship is less likely; and the increase in technological "breakthroughs" has alienated many "modern" patients. Patients have neither a "voice option" in the medical encounter, nor an "exit option" to leave. Changing doctors, getting second opinions, paying for insurance are very difficult particularly for older and less education people, hence patients have to confront the many problematic aspects of the relationship with a conventional medical doctor.

What the modern Western patient (of all ages) wants, and appears not to be getting, is to be treated with individual respect; not to have to endure crowded waiting rooms, or being patronized. Being processed as a "case" not a person is a common complaint among many patients. Patients want to be treated as educated consumers, yet find they still being met by a wall of clinical autonomy and a refusal to share information. Patients resent being faced by doctors who claim to have nothing to offer and do nothing, either because in their view treatments don't work or because the best policy is judged to be to do nothing. Many patients now want a consumer contract with equal responsibilities. Many patients complain that doctors do not trust them to make appropriate decisions about their health care.

Thus for Taylor, medicine is basically a professional relationship. The fate of CAM is determined not so much by the proven efficacy of its methods, but rather by orthodox practitioners being either unwilling or unable to deliver what the modern patient wants.

It is possible to compare and contract the stereotypic CAM and OM consultation (Table 2.1).

Sixteen differences are noted many of which suggest the CAM consultation would be more attractive to patients particularly the elderly: they get more time, with a more sympathetic doctor, who appears to have tremendous faith in his or her speciality. It is readily acknowledged that the table encourages stereotypes and is not empirically based.

It may be argued that the idea of comparison is essentially flawed for what is essentially an analysis of variance problem. That is that the variation is consultations *within* either OM or CM is of necessity greater than the variation *between* them. It concerns whether one could legitimately talk about any typical or average consultation. Thus it is inevitable and expected that an aromatherapist's consultation differs widely from that a homoeopath. Similarly an osteopath will do quite different history taking and treatment from a iridologist. The same is true for conventional medicine: Consider how a psychiatrist and an orthopedic surgeon operates. Consider for instance the nature of the patients problem means that they may well be significantly similarities between branches of CAM and OM in the treatment by osteopath and orthopdedic surgeon.

Table 2.1. The stereotype CAM and OM consultation. A compare and contrast exercise

	CAM	OM
Time	More	Less
Touch	More	Less
Money	More	Less
History taking	Holistic	Specific
	Affective	Behavioural
Language	Healing	Cure
	Holistic	Dualistic
	Subjective	Objective
	Personal story	Case history
	Wellness	Illness
Patient role	Consumer	Sick role
Decision making	Shared/consumer	Doctor/paternalistic
Bedside manner	Charismatic	Cool
	Empathic	Professional
Sex ratio/role	F=M; feminine	M>F; masculine
Time spent talking	Patient >or = to practitioner	Practitioner >patient
Style	Authoritative	Authoritarian
	Supportive	Information/advice giving
	Counselling	
Confidence in methodology/outcome	Very high	High
Client relationship	Long term	Short term
Consulting rooms	Counselling	Clinical
Practitioner history	Second profession	First profession
Ideology	Strong	Moderate
	Left wing	Middle way

There are two further problems which make comparisons problematic. The first is that there may be within each CAM or OM specialty different "schools of thought" which results in different types (styles) of consultations. Secondly and inevitably there is the issue of individual differences of practitioner (their personality, biography, education, experience). In this sense it is difficult to suggest that there is ever such a thing as a typical consultation. However, despite these acknowledged problems it maybe that it is the medical encounter which "sells" the treatment best. There is considerable research to suggest that patient compliance is best predicted by the patient evaluation of the consultation. Certainly the consultation may account for why patients stay with, and/or leave, a particular practitioner of a specific problem.

Elderly people in particular maybe attracted to the CAM therapist precisely because of their consultation style. They have more time with a more sympathetic practitioner and one with a more empathetic bedside manner. The authoritative, supportive and counseling style of many CAM practitioners may be particularly attractive to older people though this has yet to be empirically tested.

The fact that patients in most countries have to pay money for CAM therapy (whilst OM is often free) may be both a source of advantage and disadvantage. It may naturally constitute a problem for old people on a reduced or restricted income. On the other hand we have long known that people value things they pay for more than things they do not.

Suffice it to say, that the consultation per se may be an important but as got seriously under-researched reasons while all, but particularly old people seek out, and appear to benefit from, CAM.

References

1. Aakster C (1986) Concepts in alternative Medicine. Soc Sci Med 22: 265–273
2. Astin J (1988) Why patients use alternative medicine: Results of a national study. J Amer Med Assoc 279: 1548–1953
3. Astin J, Pelletier K, Marie A, Haskell W (2000) Complementary and alternative medicine use among elderly person: One-year analysis of a Blue Shield Medicare Supplement. J Gerontol 55: 4–9
4. Bakx K (1991) The "eclipse" of folk medicine in western society. Sociol Health Illness 13
5. Baum M (1989) Rationalism versus irrationalism in the care of the sick: science versus the absurd (editorial). Med J Aust 151(11–12): 607–608
6. BMA (1993) Complementary medicine. Report of the Board of Science and Education
7. Boon H (1998) Canadian naturopathic practitioners: Holistic and scientific world views. Soc Sci Med 46: 1213–1225
8. Budd C, Fisher B, Parruder D, Price L (1990) A model of co-operation between complementary and allopathic medicine in a primary care setting. Brit J Gen Pract 40(338):376–378.
9. Bullock M, Pheley A, Kiresuk T, Lenz S, Culliton P (1997) Characteristics and complaints of patients seeking therapy at a hospital-based alternative medicine clinic. J Altern Complement Med 3: 31–37
10. Buono M, Urauli O, Marietta P, Padoanik W, Leo D (2001) Alternative medicine in a sample of 655 community-dwelling elderly. J Psychosom Res 50: 147–154
11. Cant S, Calnan M (1991) On the margins of the medical market place? An exploratory study of alternative practitioners' perceptions. Sociol Health Illness 13: 46–66
12. Canter D, Nanke L (1989) Emerging priorities in complementary medical research. Complement Med Res 3: 14–21
13. Canter D, Nanke L (1991) Psychological aspects of complementary medicine. Paper presented at University of Keele, January
14. Cassileth BR (1986) Unorthodox Cancer Medicine. Cancer Invest 4(6): 591–598
15. Cassileth B (1998) The social implications of questionable cancer therapies. Cancer 63(7): 1247–1250
16. Cassileth BR, Zuphis RV, Sutton-Smith K, March V (1980) Information and participation preferences among cancer patients. Ann Intern Med 92 (6): 83206
17. Donnelly W, Spykerboer S, Thong Y (1985) Are patients who use alternative medicine dissatisfied with orthodox medicine? Med J Aust 142(10): 539–541
18. Downer S, Cody M, Mcluskey P, Wilson P, Arnott S, Lister T, Slevin M. (1994) Pursuit and practice of complementary therapies by cancer patients receiving conventional treatment. Br Med J 309: 86–89
19. Eisenberg D, Kessler RC, Foster C, Norlock F, Calkins D, Del Banco T (1993) Unconventional medicine in the United States. N Engl J Med 328: 246–252
20. Eisenberg D, Davish R, Ettner S, Appel S, Wilkey S, Van Rompay H, Kessler R (1998). Trends in alternative medicine use in the United States, 1990–1997. J Amer Med Assoc 289: 1569–1575
21. Ernst E, Resch K-L, White A (1995) Complementary medicine: what physicians think of it. Arch Intern Med 155: 2405–2408
22. Ernst E, Willoughby M, Weihmayr T (1995) Nine possible reasons for choosing complementary medicine. Perfusion 8: 356–359
23. Ernst E (1996) Complementary medicine: An objective appraisal. Butterworth Heinemann, London
24. Ernst E, Kaptchuk T (1996). Complementary Medicine – the case foe dialogue. J Royal College Physicians London 30: 410–412
25. Ernst E (1997) Complementary medicine: does it have a role in the medical care of elderly people. Rev Clini Gerontol 7: 353–358
26. Ernst E, Furnham A (1998) BMW sales and complementary medicine: Cause or correlation. Unpublished paper
27. Finnigan M (1991) The Centre for the Study of Complementary Medicine: An attempt to understand its popularity through psychological, demographic and operational criteria. Complement Med Res 5: 83–88
28. Fischer P, Ward A (1994) Complementary Medicine in Europe. Br Med J 309: 107–111
29. Foucault M (1979) Discipline and Punishment. Penguin: Harmondsworth, Middlesex

30. Fulder SJ, Munro RE (1985) Complementary medicine in the United Kingdom: patients, practitioners, and consultations. Lancet 2 (8454): 542–545
31. Furnham A (1986) Medical students' beliefs about five different specialties. Br Med J 293: 1067–1680
32. Furnham A, Smith C (1988) Choosing alternative medicine: a comparison of the beliefs of patients visiting a GP and a homoeopath. Soc Sci Med 26: 685–687
33. Furnham A (1993) Attitudes to alternative medicine: a study of the perception of those studying orthodox medicine. Complement Ther Med 1: 120–126
34. Furnham A, Bhagrath R (1993) A comparison of health beliefs and behaviours of clients of orthodox and complementary medicine. Br J Clin Psychol 32: 237–246
35. Furnham A (1994) Explaining health and illness. Soc Sci Med 39: 715–725
36. Furnham A, Forey J (1994) The attitudes, behaviours and beliefs of patients of conventional vs. complementary (alternative) medicine. J Clin Psychol 50: 458–469
37. Furnham A, Kirkcaldy B (1995) The health beliefs and behaviours of orthodox and complementary medicine clients. Br J Clin Psychol 25:49–61
38. Furnham A, Hanna D, Vincent C (1995) Medical students' attitudes to complementary medical therapies. Complement Ther Med 3: 212–219
39. Furnham A, Vincent C, Wood R (1995) The health beliefs and behaviours of three groups of complementary medicine and a general practice group of patients. Journal of Alternative and Complementary Medicine 1:347–359.
40. Furnham A (1997a) Why do people choose and use complementary therapies? In: Ernst E (ed) Complementary Medicine: An Objective Approach. Butterworth-Heinemann, London, pp 71–88
41. Furnham A (1997b) Flight from science: alternative medicine, post modernism and relativism. In: Fuller R, Walsh P, Mcginley P (eds) A century of psychology. Routledge, London
42. Furnham A, Baguma F (1999) Cross-cultural differences in explanations for health and illness. Mental Health, Religion and Culture 2: 121–134
43. Furnham A, Vincent C (2000) Reasons for using CAM. In: Kelner M, Wellman B, Pescosolido B, Saks M (eds) Complementary and alternative medicine: challenge and change. Harwood Academic Publisherr, Amsterdam
44. Gaus W, Hogel J (1995) Studies on the efficacy of unconventional therapies: Problems and design. Drug Research 45: 88–92
45. Gray R (1998) Four perspectives on unconventional therapies. Health 2: 55–74
46. Greenblatt R, Hollander H, McMaster J, Henke C (1991) Polypharmacy among patients attending an AIDS clinic. J Acquir Immune Defic Syndr 4: 136–143
47. Gursoy A (1996) Beyond the orthodox: Heresy in medicine and the social sciences from a cross-cultural perspective. Soc Sci Med 43: 577–592
48. Hertschel C, Kohnen R, Hauser G, Lindner M, Haln E, Ernst E (1996) Complementary medicine today: Patient decision for physician or magician. Eur J Phys Med Rehabil 6: 144–150
49. Hewer W (1983) The relationship between the alternative practitioner and his patient. A review. Psychother Psychosom 40(1–4): 172–180
50. Kelner M, Wellman B (1997) Who seeks alternative care? A profile of the users of five modes of treatment. J Altern Complement Med 3: 127–140
51. Knipschild P (1988) Looking for gall bladder disease in the patient's iris. Br Med J 297(6663): 1578–1581
52. Knipschild P, Kleijnen J, Ter-Riet G (1990) Belief in the efficacy of alternative medicine among general practitioners in The Netherlands. Soc Sci Med 31(5): 625–626
53. Levin J, Coreil J (1986) "New age" healing in the U.S. Soc Sci Med 23(9): 889–897
54. Lewith GT, Aldridge DA (1991) Complementary medicine and the European Community. C.W. Daniel, Saffron Walden, Essex
55. Lupton D (1997) Consumerism, reflexivity and the medical encounter. Soc Sci Med 45: 373–381
56. Lynse N (1989) Theoretical and empirical problems in the assessment of alternative medical technologies. Scand J Soc Med 17: 257–263
57. McKee J (1988) Holistic health and the critique of Western medicine. Soc Sci Med 26: 775–785
58. Moore J, Phipps K, Marcer D, Lewith GT (1985) Why do people seek treatment by alternative medicine? Br Med J 290(6461): 28–29
59. Murray J, Shepherd S (1988) Alternative or additional medicine? An exploratory study in general practice. Soc Sci Med 37: 983–988
60. Sharma U (1992) Complementary medicine today: Practitioners and patients. Routledge, London
61. Skrabanek P (1988) Paranormal health claims. Experientia 44(4): 303–309
62. Stalker D, Glymore L (1989) (eds) Examining Holistic Medicine. Promotheus, Buffalo, NY
63. Strong P (1979) Sociological imperialism and the medical profession. Soc Sci Med 13: 199–211
64. Taylor R (1985) Alternative medicine and the medical encounter in Britain and the United States. In: Salmon J, Warren P (eds) Alternative medicine: prejudice and policy perspectives. Tavistock, London, pp. 191–221
65. Thomas KJ, Carr J, Westlake L, Williams BT (1991) Use of non–orthodox and conventional health care in Great Britain. Br Med J 302(6770): 207–210
66. Turner B (1987) Medical Power and Social Knowledge, Sage, London
67. Vecchio P (1994) Attitudes to alternative medicine by rheumatology outpatient attenders. J Rheumatol 21: 145–147

68. Verhoef M, Sutherland L, Birkich L (1990) Use of alternative medicine by patients attending a gastroenterology clinic. Can Med Assoc J 142: 121–125

69. Vincent C, Furnham A (1994) The perceived efficacy of complementary and orthodox medicine. Complement Ther Med 2: 128–134

70. Vincent C, Furnham A (1995) Why do patients turn to complementary medicine? An empirical study. Br J Clin Psychol 35: 37–48

71. Vincent C, Furnham A, Willsmore M (1995) The perceived efficacy of complementary and orthodox medicine in complementary and general practice patients. Health Educ Res 10: 395–405

72. Vincent C, Furnham A (1997) Complementary Medicine: A Research Perspective. Wiley, Chichester

73. Vincent C, Furnham A (1999) Complementary Medicine: state of the evidence. J R Soc Med 92: 170–177

74. Visser E, Peters L, Rasker J (1992) Rheumatologists and their patients who seek alternative care: An agreement to disagree. Br J Rheumatol 31: 488–490

75. Wharton R. and Lewith G. (1986) Complementary medicine and the general practitioner. Br Med J 292(6534): 1498–1500

76. White A, Ernst E (2000) Economic analysis of complementary medicine: a systematic review. Complement Ther Med 8: 111–118

77. Williams S, Calnan M (1996) The "limits" of medicalization? Modern medicine and the lay populace on "late" modernity. Soc Sci Med 42: 1609–1620

3 The Use of Alternative Medicine by the Elderly and the Doctor-Patient Relationship

E.P. Cherniack

Introduction

The use of complementary and alternative medicine (CAM) may have important implications for the relationship between the elderly patient and physician. As CAM treatments are often obtained by the patient in the absence of knowledge or at times disapproval of the patient's physician, they have the potential for causing harm to the relationship, whose integrity is necessary to ensure that the older patient, who is more likely to be in need of medical care and require detailed instruction, receives adequate treatment. This chapter will review what is known about the use of influence of alternative medicine on the doctor-patient relationship.

Characteristics of the Elderly Outpatient

The elderly often bring to the doctor-patient relationship attitudes which greatly influence their relationship with physicians. The formation of relationships by patients with their practitioners is a multifaceted process [50] that includes overcoming initial fears, identifying a physician who meets a patients needs, searching for evidence of caring, and comparison of the patient's physician with other doctors, all of which might be influenced by a patients use of CAM.

On one hand, the physician is a person who possess certain knowledge not generally available to most people, requiring the patient to defer to the greater medical understanding of the physician in order to be cured of illness [29, 64, 97, 98]. However, as the level of the general education of the layperson has increased, the gap in understanding of medicine between physician and patient has narrowed [61, 64, 100]. This has resulted in with enhanced power for the patient and new emphasis on the legitimacy for his concerns [8, 64, 75, 93]. The patient brings to the relationship certain attitudes and experiences that might help influence his desire to use CAM for treatment of his health concerns, or their willingness to follow a doctor's advice about treatment, and both a of the lesser degree of knowledge, but a greater demand for information about their own health by patients, an increased willingness to challenge a physician's authority, often referred to as "consumerism" [10, 11, 62, 64–66, 78, 105]. This emphasis on the health perrogatives of the patient has been codified in law with the Patient Self-Determination Act of 1990 [85]. The decline in the paternalistic model of a relationship between physician and patient may be associated with increased interest in CAM among users of health care [46, 82].

Nevertheless, this trend among the general public may not have influenced the elderly as much as the young. Beisecker noted that both young and old individuals avidly seek health information, but the old are more likely to defer to the opinions of their physicians [11]. Older persons tend to be less educated, literate, and, as will be described in greater detail later, more passive [7, 66, 112, 119, 137].

Unfortunately, the number of formal studies of this relationship is surprisingly few, and the largest recent study is approximately twenty years old. Marie Haug conducted face-to-face interview of a population of young and old patients from communities of varying size in Ohio [64]. The sample was stratified to account for sex, race, and socioeconomic status. The interview asked questions to determine how willing subjects were to challenge the authority of their physicians. When rated on a 20 point scale, the young (below 60) were quite significantly more likely to be willing question the authority of the physician or actually have challenged that authority in the past as measured on several indices specifically designed to measure these variables [64]. The young were also more likely to question any authority in general, be more knowledgeable about health, believe they had a right to know information about their health, and were more likely to have actually experienced an error by their practitioners [64]. The older the patient was, the less likely he was to question his physician [63, 65]. In a Spanish survey, the elderly were more satisfied with care and more compliant with carrying out medical advice [124].

Older age was noted to be most likely correlated between a patients preferring a passive and dependant relationship, more so than other correlates, such as lower income, lower occupational achievement, and large gap in education and socioeconomic status between patient and physician [7, 13, 17, 25, 31, 34, 66, 112, 122, 123, 128, 137]. Roter suggests that older patients may find a paternalistic relationship with a doctor comforting [112]. Old patients often opt to concur with their physicians out of belief in a physician's knowledge or authority [63, 119]. The support that an elderly patient may acquire from such a relationship may be significant for an ill dependent patient, granting him increased freedom from worry [31]. In addition, elderly people in general are characterized by asserting themselves less in conversation, complaining less, interrupting less, and asking questions [21, 59, 76, 109, 121]. However, in one study in which the interactions of 140 family physicians and patients were audiotaped noted that older patients more often displayed antagonistic sentiments [119].

Other demographic factors did make some difference; the elderly over 65 (but also the young below 35) who were big-city dwellers, and fee-for-service patients, were least likely to follow their doctor's recommendations [124]. Higher income and occupational level were also associated with greater propensity to challenge authority [39, 65, 112], in some studies, but others have found older patients with high out of pocket expenses were less likely to remain passive [64, 68]. Sex, race, and health status was not correlated with belief in physician authority in one study [97], but less healthy individuals, particularly those with chronic health problems felt less satisfied with their medical care in others [59, 60, 109, 112]. While older persons may be more overtly compliant with physicians, there is also evidence that they do not communicate as well with doctors or younger patients. The research of Greene et al. noted that the elderly not only participated less in decision-making, in agreement with the work of Haug and the

Medical Outcomes Study, but, when surveyed, disagreed with physicians more frequently than younger patients on the purpose of outpatient visits and focus of discussion during these visits [3, 4, 45, 51–53, 104, 107, 121]. Older patients perceived themselves as participating less in decision-making during physician visits than the young [77, 121]. An investigation of more than 8000 patients, the Medical Outcomes Study, observed that the elderly, as well as males, individuals with less education, and minorities, participated less in discussions with doctors than other patients [77]. Individuals who were over than 75 had fewer visits to a physician in which they took part in the decision making than all but the youngest patients. The interactions between 126 physicians and approximately 550 patients were audiotaped and analyzed for content. The conversations of older patients were characterized as being more directed and dominated by the physician and patient than those of younger patients. Both physician and older patients believed that their conversations were less likely to achieve their goals and less satisfying than the interactions between doctors and younger individuals [111, 121]. In another survey, older patients and physicians agreed less than half the time about what problems should be discussed in patient visits [104].

In addition for the tendency of older individuals to be more passive patients, the elderly may have other barriers to interaction with their physicians. Aged persons may have more extensive medical histories, and have sensory deficits, such as loss of hearing and vision, and cognitive deficits, that may make it more difficult for them to make their needs known to their doctors [4, 74, 115, 121]. Physical problems may lead to loss of function [60], such as mobility, that enable the elderly less able to visit the physician [4].

Elderly patients may need to be accompanied by caregivers, which influences the dynamic of the doctor-patient relationship. While doctor-patient interactions during third party visits have been not been studied in great detail, at least one study in which visits were audiotaped noted that patients make their needs known even less frequently and are less assertive when a third party is present during a physician visit [4, 54]. However, other investigations have observed that caregivers' roles can be helpful, providing history, and encouraging compliance with medication regimens [23, 30].

Older persons' physical, communicative, and educational deficits may influence how physicians view elderly patients. The physician may have a negative bias toward the elderly ("ageism") that affects their interaction with older persons [4]. Firstly, some studies suggest that the speech of an older-sounding person alone may induce stereotypical, "ageist" responses in younger individuals [48]. Physicians may be dissatisfied by the extra time and effort needed to comprehend the more complex medical histories elderly people have and obtain necessary medical information from older people with severe communicative, mental, or educational deficits. This is manifest by doctors minimizing the concerns of the elderly, attributing them to the inevitable process of aging [4, 52], utilizing less preventive medicine [4, 56], spending less time with the elderly [4] generalizing that elderly patients are more difficult to treat [3, 4], or even being disrespectful and using derogatory language when speaking to them [4].

Furthermore, many physicians have been shown to resent sicker patients, and the elderly more frequently have illness [59]. Audiotape investigations of conversations have noted physicians disagree more with individuals who are more ill, feel less satisfied with their interactions, and speak to them in a more negative tone of voice [4]. Physicians may possess biases against the older persons with common illnesses of the elderly, such as cognitive impairment, which has been referred to as "dementiaism" [3, 4].

However, there have been few formal studies as to the degree of "ageism" present in physicians. In a Swiss study, doctors' ages and the percentage of elderly in a practice influenced attitudes toward older persons [79]. Older doctors spent more time with elderly patients. Physicians who were more interested in caring for elderly patients, who were more concerned with preventive medicine, and who had less conservative personalities, spent more time on home or nursing home visits with the elderly.

There may be differences in attitudes of physicians toward aged persons depending on the demographic characteristics of the physicians. Approximately 800 physicians including residents and medical students at two Midwestern university medical centers were questioned as to their attitudes toward elderly patients. Physician dominance in decision-making was preferred by ninety percent of physicians. More physicians, however, believed in greater input for the elderly than the young patient. Younger physicians and medical students were more favorably disposed to granting decision-making authority, to the aged individual [12].

Impediments to the doctor-patient relationship in the elderly might have an important influence on the health of the elderly. One review of the effect of the doctor-patient relationship on health outcomes noted that a relationship in which a patient can ask questions and express opinion was associated with positive outcomes [120]. Patients who were invited to participate more after physicians received training on how to elicit patient involvement felt less anxious, had a greater degree of symptomatic relief, and better health and functional outcomes [41, 55, 76, 110, 120]. Physician recognition of patient concerns was also associated with improved symptom control and health [58, 67, 96, 103, 120]. In another survey of more than 8000 recipients Medicare recipients, elderly people were shown to have longer ties with physicians than younger persons [133]. This longer relationship was correlated with lower rates of hospitalization and decreased costs. Other studies have also indicated that patients who have longer ties with their doctors have less lengthy hospital stays [133], fewer emergency room visits [73], and use fewer laboratory tests [71], greater satisfaction [9, 43, 72, 73, 81, 132] and are more likely to follow practitioner directions [71]. Whether the use of CAM alters these benefits has yet to be determined.

One aspect of patient care upon which practitioner-patient communication may be especially significant is in the maintenance of compliance with medication regimens. Rost and Roter observed that more than half of all elderly patients forgot lifestyle recommendations immediately after doctor visits, and more than half of all medications were also not recalled [108]. The more medications older patients use, and the more frequently they must take a given medication per day, the less likely they are to be compliant with medication regimens [47, 87]. Patient satisfaction, which can be influenced by the physician's attitude, can alter compliance.

Several studies have stressed the role of good communication with increased compliance [30, 87, 121]. Roter noted that the style of communication by the physician was noted to be related to patient recall [112]. Physician who asked fewer open-ended questions and gave more information during visits were more likely to have patients remember what transpired [108]. The time a physician spends explaining a medication regimen has a significant influence on whether patients will comply with it [92].

Theoretically, the use of CAM therapies, which patients may not tell physicians about because persons seeking medical care might feel doctors have limited knowledge of, or might disapprove of, may add to confusion about the use of conventional therapies. Time limits on physician visits may discourage patients and physicians from discussing CAM. However the exact effect of CAM therapies on compliance with medication regimens remains uncertain.

Physicians' Attitudes Towards CAM

Many studies have outlined physicians' attitudes toward CAM. Most surveys, however, have described in little detail the opinions of small numbers of doctors. Physicians in certain European countries, such as the United Kingdom and Germany, have generally positive attitudes toward CAM, often referring patients to CAM practitioners or utilizing it themselves. In other parts of the world, such as the United States, physicians remain more skeptical, although many also refer patients to CAM practitioners.

Berman et al. tried to identify beliefs among approximately 300 family practitioners in several mid-Atlantic states about CAM [14]. A written survey was given to physicians inquiring as to their knowledge, use of, interest in, and referrals for CAM. They noted that almost three-quarters of the physicians believed many forms of CAM, such as forms of counseling, biofeedback, diet, exercise, and hypnotherapy were "legitimate medical practices". More than fifty percent also included acupuncture and massage therapy, and almost fifty percent deemed chiropractic and vegetarianism as "legitimate". Most had referred patients to CAM practitioners for chiropractic, biofeedback, diet, exercise or counseling. However, non-Western and Native American forms of CAM and homeopathy were not recommended by the physicians. Two-thirds or more had knowledge of biofeedback, behavioral medicine, and exercise, and at least have were interested in training about all CAM therapies surveyed, including homeopathy, prayer, Oriental and Native American CAM, and electromagnetism. Physicians considered both their own and their colleagues' person experiences and patients' reports as well as published evidence important to their acceptance of treatments, whether CAM or conventional.

The largest survey of US physician attitudes, a randomized mail survey of close to six hundred family practitioners found that many had positive attitudes toward CAM [18]. When physicians were asked how they would advise patients who were interested in individual CAM therapies, approximately eighty percent of patients would encourage relaxation techniques, seventy percent biofeedback, and more than half would encourage meditation and therapeutic massage. Over eighty percent would also refer a patient to a practitioner of relaxation techniques or biofeedback, roughly two-thirds for massage or hypnosis and slightly more than half for meditation or acupuncture. A majority would discourage patients from pursuing energy healing, megavitamin or herbal remedies, however. Physicians remained divided or neutral if patients were interested in other therapies surveyed such as chiropractic, imagery, spiritual healing, lifestyle and diet therapies, hypnosis, acupuncture, homeopathy, yoga, or rolfing. More than half sent their patients for CAM treatments. The older the physician was, the less likely he would encourage a patient to use a CAM treatment.

In this study, very few physicians practiced CAM therapies themselves. Approximately one-quarter offered relaxation techniques, and seventeen percent used lifestyle and diet modification, but less than then ten percent used any of the other therapies surveyed [18].

Roughly 500 family practitioners were questioned as to their beliefs and referral practices with regards to chiropractors in Washington state. Nearly sixty percent did refer patients to chiropractors for low back pain [27].

Approximately one hundred practitioners in Ohio were also questioned as to attitude about CAM by Crock et al. in 1999 [33]. Approximately three-quarters believed the CAM therapies assessed were beneficial. When asked to rate on a scale of 1–5 (1 – harmful, 5 – beneficial) the average ratings for CAM therapies were close to four. Of those physicians who had actually applied CAM in patient care, at least half found all the therapies considered to be of benefit to patients. Physicians rated therapies as more helpful when therapies were used as complementary to conventional medicine rather than as replacements. In most cases, there was no difference in the evaluations of CAM between generalists and specialists. Younger physicians judged CAM therapies more favorably than older physicians and were more familiar with the different modalities of CAM.

Attitudes toward CAM have been surveyed in several other countries. In a study of 200 general practitioners(GPs) in Western Canada by mail survey, most believed it was a important to know something about the most important CAM therapies, but a small majority did not agree that it was necessary for a physician to be able to answer questions or give advice about CAM [126]. The vast majority of practitioners surveyed did not claim to know a great deal about any of the forms of CAM surveyed [127]. Most felt that acupuncture and chiropractic care were very useful for musculoskeletal problems such as soft tissue injuries, acute back pain, joint disorders, and tension headaches, but acupuncture was not considered useful to treat asthma. Hypnosis was deemed quite worthwhile for insomnia, eating disorders, stress control, smoking cessation, relaxation, and other psychological disorders. Only a minority believed that other forms of CAM such as osteopathy, herbal medicine, reflexology, faith healing, homeopathy, and naturopathy were valuable [127]. Domestically-trained general practitioners referred patients to CAM practitioners significantly more than foreign-trained practitioners. Some ambivalence about CAM was also discerned by the survey; on one hand, a majority concurred that CAM contained concepts from which conventional medicine could benefit, and disagreed with the belief that CAM was dangerous to public health, but, on the other hand, most believed treatments that were not scientifically recognized should be discouraged, and most did not feel that CAM was useful as a supplement to conventional medicine. Although many conventional medical practitioners who are opposed to the use of CAM claim that CAM proponents rely on anecdotal evidence to support their claims, most physicians in this survey reported that anecdotal evidence was most critical to their formation of opinions about CAM. Surprisingly, older physicians claimed to have greater knowledge and use of CAM than younger physicians. Older physicians also were more likely to perceive that the use of CAM was increasing among their patients [127].

In a small study of physicians in Israel, there was also ambiguity [114]. Most doctors wanted to know more about CAM and a small majority felt it was useful, but most also thought it was unscientific. Most did not practice CAM and slightly less than half referred patients for CAM, although most claimed they would refer patients to CAM practitioners under certain circumstances.

In Norway, more negative attitudes towards CAM by physicians have been examined in several studies. However, in one survey by written questionnaire, these beliefs of physicians about CAM were not shared by other health professionals, such as nurses and clerks [106]. In a small sample nurses and clerks were twice or more likely to use CAM and had a far more positive attitude to CAM than physicians. The use of and attitude toward alternative medicine was correlated with age. Elderly and female professionals were less likely to use or maintain a positive attitude toward CAM, want more information about CAM, or believe that CAM had something valuable to contribute to conventional medicine. A majority of nurses studied believed that CAM might be useful to treat musculoskeletal disorders, migraine headaches, allergies, and rheumatic diseases. Another investigation noted negative attitudes by physicians toward CAM, observed that few knew much or felt CAM therapies to be valuable [1]. Only ten percent of Norwegian physicians wanted to have CAM therapies introduced into hospitals [106]. An additional Norwegian mail survey of physicians noted, however, that one-third of doctors would give favorable advice to patients about homeopathy, and half thought homeopathy might be useful to treat at least one medical problem [99]. Physicians who had tried CAM were more likely to opt to refer patients to use CAM [1, 99].

An investigation of several hundred randomly selected physicians in Sweden explored attitudes toward selected types of alternative medicine [89]. Most did have positive feelings about the forms of CAM surveyed, but more felt favorably than unfavorably toward traditional Chinese acupuncture, and a vegetarian diet.

In England, CAM was also frequently used by GPs, according to one study [101]. When GPs were compared to medical students, the GPs were also far more likely to have heard of or understand CAM therapies. Half or more at one time made referrals to chiropractors, osteopaths and acupuncturists, and half or more referred patients to CAM practitioners for these therapies and homeopaths when a patient requested it. However, CAM practitioners were consulted five percent of the time or less by the physicians in the survey.

In a random mail survey of approximately 150 general practitioners, about a third had training in CAM techniques, and sixty percent found such techniques useful [135]. While approximately sixty to eighty percent of the respondents rated their own knowledge of CAM as poor, approximately ninety percent rated spinal manipulation, sixty-five percent acupuncture, and eighty percent hypnosis as useful. Twice as many found homeopathy and spiritual healing to be as useful as not useful. Approximately fifty percent referred patients to CAM practitioners for spinal manipulation, roughly forty percent referred them for homeopathy or hypnosis. Personal experience or and observed benefit to patients were the most important influences on use.

Several hundred English general practitioners surveyed by mailed questionnaire almost fifteen years ago were found to exhibit a low degree of CAM use for some modalities and of self-reported knowledge by physicians [6]. Almost all had discussed CAM with at least one patient; and approximately sixty percent had referred patients at some point to a CAM practitioner. Eighty percent of practitioners had discussed spinal manipulation, sixty percent acupuncture and forty percent homeopathy with their patients, resulting in half of all physicians referring patients for spinal manipulation, twenty percent referring for acupuncture, and almost twenty percent referring for homeopathy. However, the absolute number of patients for whom CAM had been discussed or referred was small: an estimated 1.8% of patients had discussed CAM and 0.5% had been referred for CAM therapies. Sixteen percent of the physician surveyed actually practiced a form of CAM.

That most physicians, had at one time referred any patients was surprising considering the degree of skepticism about CAM expressed in the survey. Less than half believed alternative medical systems had a valid basis in theory. Only thirty percent felt spinal manipulation had a valid theoretical basis, fifteen percent acupuncture, and less than ten percent felt hypnotherapy homeopathy or any of the other therapies surveyed had any validity.

In some parts of the world, many GPs actually practice CAM. In a study of several hundred, physicians in Auckland, New Zealand, thirty percent of general practitioners utilized CAM, the majority of which used acupuncture [90]. Two thirds of the physicians referred patients for CAM therapies, the vast majority of which were again for acupuncture. More than one quarter also referred patients for osteopathy, homeopathy, and massage. The group of physicians not practicing CAM therapies considered acupuncture, and massage as more useful than average treatments. A second survey from New Zealand, a mail survey send to more than two hundred GPs, uncovered that twenty-seven percent practice at last one form of CAM. Three-quarters of GPs also referred patients to others for CAM therapies [57].

High acceptance of certain forms of CAM, was found in a survey of Australian GPs by Pirotta et al. [102]. Most believed acupuncture, chiropractic medicine, hypnosis, and osteopathy either moderately or highly effective. The majority felt that it was reasonable for trained GPs to offer these forms or CAM and that Medicare should cover the costs of these as well as herbal, vitamin or mineral therapy. A majority was interested in learning meditation and hypnosis, approximately one-quarter trained in the use of hypnosis and acupuncture, and a third trained in the use of meditation. Most would also encourage a patient's suggestion to use any of these three therapies. Those who used the therapies practiced them on less than one-quarter of their patients.

The beliefs of medical specialists have also been assessed. Newell and Sanson Fisher surveyed oncologists in Australia and notes that meditation, hypnotherapy and acupuncture were most likely to be deemed helpful [95]. Treatments deemed harmful were diets, "psychic surgery" Iscador therapy (a treatment using a derivative of the mistletoe plant which will be discussed more completely in another chapter), and coffee enemas.

Visser and Peters found a very high rate of acceptance among general practitioners in the Netherlands [129]. A survey that was mailed out to 360 determined that almost half had actually treated patients with CAM themselves, and that ninety percent referred patients for CAM therapies, although the actual number of patients that had actually been referred was low. However, only fifty-seven percent had received formal teaching in using the CAM techniques. Virtually all had discussed the possibility of utilizing CAM therapies with patients at some point during their care. Approximately three quarters believed that a GP be knowledgeable about the most important therapies. Most felt that there were techniques and concepts that were part of CAM that conventional medicine could benefit from applying, but nearly half believed that the efficacy of CAM was primarily due to placebo effect.

General practitioners in the Netherlands favored some therapies but not others in an earlier survey by Knipschild. Techniques of physical therapy, acupuncture, homeotherapy, yoga, and hot baths were favorably regarded, but other treatments were not [84].

Ernst et al. did a meta-analysis on investigations of physicians' attitudes towards CAM in parts of the world outside the United States [40]. In this meta-analysis, six experts on topics of CAM were asked to evaluate the efficacy of CAM based on physicians' perceptions of efficacy in twelve studies between 1986 and 1993. There appeared to be no major difference in perception of efficacy between physicians of different nationalities. In most studies, CAM was deemed modestly to moderately effective. They noted however, that many studies were conducted by known proponents of CAM, and these investigations reported a higher degree of CAM efficacy, suggesting a possible selection bias. They also noted that in many investigations physicians did not specify why they may perceive CAM therapies as valuable, theorizing that some may find them merely useful placebo treatments. Over the time period studied, 1982 to 1994, the perception of the utility of CAM declined slightly.

Patients' Attitudes Towards CAM

The impact of CAM on use on patients' perceptions of their relationship with practitioners have been outlined in a small number of surveys. One major concern is whether patients are willing to disclose CAM use to their physicians, which patients theoretically may believe physicians will dislike and earn the patient disapproval. In a study of slightly more than one hundred individuals in a family practice, fifty percent used CAM, of which half used CAM for reasons other than that for which they saw the physician [37]. The rationale for CAM use was important in determining whether or not they disclosed CAM use; three quarters of those who utilized CAM for the same reason they visited the doctor told them about it, approximately forty percent of CAM users who had a different reason did not.

In a survey in Germany, attitudes of patients and doctors were compared and their influence on the doctor-patient relationship analyzed [70]. Only a small number of physicians (forty) answered the mail survey sent to them, and, of these, eighty-five percent used CAM to treat patients. Almost eight-five percent of these utilized CAM because they felt the treatments were successful, about half also employed them because of low incidence of side-effects, and one third because individuals requested it.

About half of the physicians believed the benefits of CAM and conventional medicine for the conditions treated were equal, and minorities of doctors deemed the CAM either better or worse than conventional remedies. A large majority of German practitioners in the study used CAM to treat people with chronic illnesses. Most felt CAM therapies should become a part of conventional medicine after an appropriate evaluation. Half felt they were responsible for recommending CAM to their patients, more commonly in rural than in urban areas. Three-quarters of the physicians in rural areas claimed they refer patients for CAM several times a week, while only about a third of urban physicians did. Slightly more than two thirds of the physicians noted people who had refused CAM treatments, more commonly urban patients.

Approximately 300 patients were also interviewed, one third of whom were older than sixty. One third of the older persons were treated with CAM, and almost half of these patients preferred CAM whether they were treated with it or not. Women and younger persons were more commonly given CAM treatments than then. Almost seventy percent preferred to be treated more often by CAM, and slightly more than half preferred CAM to conventional medicine. Seventy percent of patients treated with CAM methods perceived greater benefit for CAM than for conventional medicine. One-third noted that practitioners had recommended a CAM therapy at least once, more commonly rural patients. A small minority claimed they had asked their doctor for CAM treatment. There was not a statistically significant difference in patient satisfaction with physicians who did or did not utilize CAM therapies.

It is very difficult to generalize from a small number of patients and physicians from a region of Germany. As the authors pointed out, there may have been a selection bias in that practitioners and patients using CAM may have been more likely to respond. In this population, there were some interesting findings. There was great interest in and acceptance of CAM by both doctors and those they treat, although greater by the latter. The authors noted there had been a long tradition in the use of certain forms of CAM among the subjects, such as herbal medicines and mineral water. The employment of CAM did not create dissatisfaction in care by patients, although doctors perceived patients requested CAM therapies more frequently than patients believed they were asking for them.

There have been numerous other surveys of use of CAM among patients which have implications for the doctor patient relationship. In these, use of CAM ranges from approximately one-quarter to one-half of patients surveyed [138]. The topic most frequently considered by such investigations has been whether or not patients discuss use with their physician. Other very important topics, such as whether or not users of CAM are less compliant with conventional medications, or less willing to follow the advice of physicians who disagree with the use of CAM therapies, have not been addressed.

In the landmark study of CAM use by Eisenberg in 1993, 1500 individuals across the US were interviewed by telephone as to their use of CAM [35]. A third of the total population was using CAM, but only one quarter of users disclosed to their physicians that they were utilizing CAM. Five years later, in a second study of 2000 persons, of whom more than forty percent were using CAM, the CAM disclosure rate was no greater in the first survey [6].

In an analysis of the subgroup of the 1998 study who were elderly, slightly less than half did not tell their physician [42]. Only one third of elderly patients seeing chiropractors told their conventional practitioners about their alternative therapy.

Several studies of selected populations of CAM users have considered the question of disclosure of use to physicians. In an investigation of approximately 90 women with breast cancer, half of whom were elderly, roughly three quarters used CAM therapies [5]. Of these, only about one-third told their physicians that they were utilizing CAM. The most common explanation given for failure to inform physicians of CAM use was that patients felt that their physicians would not be interested. Other reasons included concern of physician disapproval, skepticism that the physician could contribute anything helpful, use of CAM treatments for purposes unrelated to the reason for the patient visit, and the belief that utilization of CAM was part of an effort to self-treat that did not involve the physician. Unfortunately, the number of women who held each belief was not quantified.

In a previously cited study of approximately 300 general practitioners in England, ninety-five percent stated that they had discussed CAM with at least one patient. However, as mentioned, the total percentage of patients with whom CAM was discussed was quite small, less than two percent of the total patient population of each practitioner [6].

Bernstein analyzed the CAM use by 122 Israelis (six percent of those surveyed) who consulted with CAM practitioners, aged 45 to 75 from face-to-face interviews in an urban communities [15]. Only 30 percent were also visiting conventional practitioners. Forty-five percent went to CAM practitioners because they were dissatisfied with the conventional treatments, twelve percent specifically wanted to try CAM treatments, eleven percent were concerned with polypharmacy, and six percent did not want to receive invasive procedures. Almost two-thirds felt that the CAM treatments had helped. When answers to questions were rated on a seven-point scale, users of CAM practitioners believed slightly, but statistically significantly more often than non-users that conventional practitioners were unwilling to spend enough time with them, had inconvenient schedules and waiting times, provided inadequate amounts of information, and provided poorer quality of care.

Wellman et al. explored the differences between elderly patients who visited either conventional or alternative practitioners in a small sample of seventy-seven urban patients in Canada. Using lengthy face-to-face interviews, they noted several differences between patients of CAM and conventional practices [134]. CAM practitioner patients were more likely to have been to many other practitioners before their current doctor, and were more likely to be skeptical about the ability of physicians and medications to help their conditions.

Twemlow et al. analyzed the relationship between patient attitudes and use and satisfaction with medical care in a patient population in Kansas [125]. They noted that while more than ninety percent of patients felt satisfied with their medical care, there was a correlation between CAM use and lack of sense of control over one's life. These patients were also noted to have a greater fear of dying and lesser sense of responsibility about one's health and therapies.

Some surveys have delineated the use of CAM among individuals who suffer from age-related disorders common among the elderly. These have included persons with neoplasms, coronary artery disease, arthritis, dementia, and other mental illness.

The attitudes of oncology patients towards CAM has been the subject of much investigation [2, 22, 24, 26, 32, 38, 49, 86, 140]. While the use of CAM to treat neoplasms will be addressed more extensively in another chapter, a the contribution of few studies towards understanding the influence of CAM on the doctor-patient relationship will be mad mention of here. Boon et al. investigated the attitudes of approximately 400 women with breast cancer using CAM about their treatment by postal survey [19]. The CAM users were slightly younger (average age 56.4 versus 61.3) than women who did not use CAM. Approximately half of the women informed physicians that they were using CAM. Slightly but statistically significantly fewer CAM users felt conventional therapies would work or prevent the spread of cancer. Only one-quarter felt that conventional therapies were perfectly safe, whereas about half of the non-CAM users did. More individuals utilizing CAM believed conventional therapies had side effects. Significantly more people employing CAM felt conventional therapies do not allow the body's "natural forces" to heal, improve immune function and weaken the body's "natural reserves". Only one-quarter to one-third of CAM users believed CAM treatments would actually cure, prevent the spread of or reduce the incidence of recurrence of cancer, but two-thirds felt that they would relieve the symptoms of cancer. More than seventy percent felt that CAM therapies were perfectly safe, increased quality of life and gave a person a feeling of control over one's cancer. Approximately eight-five percent of people using CAM believed that CAM methods assist the bodies "natural forces" to heal and improve immune function.

Warrick et al. interviewed 200 patients with head and neck cancer [131]. Each subject was personally interviewed by the same investigator. Approximately forty percent had used CAM therapies. Among those who did not, more than half stated that the absence of physician support was the reason they did not use CAM, the most common reason for not using such treatment. Slightly fewer than half believed there was insufficient medical research to try CAM. Only one percent of patients sought CAM therapy initially for their symptoms, which resulted in a delay in their cancer being diagnosed for several months. Most felt that physicians were useful in providing knowledge about CAM, twenty percent or less felt that CAM practitioners such as herbalists, homeopaths, naturopaths, and chiropractors were reliable. Other potential sources of information such as books, other patients, the media were considered informative by less than half of all subjects. However, only eleven percent, were introduced to CAM by physicians; two-thirds had been introduced to CAM by family or friends. Most used CAM for reasons other than their cancer. Less than half believed that CAM helped them; even fewer derived benefit when CAM was used to treat their cancers.

Cassileth et al. surveyed over than six hundred oncology patients who used CAM more than fifteen years ago. Most CAM users given these treatments by physicians, and forty percent terminated their use of conventional medicine entirely after obtaining CAM treatment. Slightly more than half of the patients using conventional therapies also used CAM [26].

Liu et al. interviewed almost 400 patients awaiting cardiac surgery, more than fifty percent of whom were over sixty-five, as to their attitudes toward CAM [88]. Subjects were asked to rate responses to four questions asked on a scale from one to ten. Three-quarters of the respondents had in fact used CAM, and of those, a significantly greater number believed that CAM therapies assisted conventional treatments in curing illness, and that CAM therapies promoted general health and well being. Only seventeen percent had discussed CAM with their physicians, and, of the remaining eighty-three percent who had not, only thirty-six percent were willing to discuss the subject with their practitioners.

Visser et al. explored the use of alternative medicine by rheumatology patients in the Netherlands and the attitudes of their physicians [130]. Surveying the patients of all Dutch rheumatologists, it was found that slightly less than half utilized CAM. The majority of these approximately 1500 patients did tell the rheumatologists about these treatments, despite the fact that most rheumatologists disapproved of them. Patients did sense a greater sense of satisfaction from visits of rheumatologists who accepted CAM than from those who did not approve of CAM. While the primary reason for patients to seek CAM treatments was failure of conventional care, the patients found conventional therapy to be more effective than CAM.

The influence of CAM on the physician-caregiver relationship in patients with cognitive disorders has not been extensively explored. Coleman et al. examined the use of CAM among patients with Alzheimer's disease as administered by the patients' caregivers [31]. More than half of all caregivers had given CAM to the patients, most at the onset of the illness. The perception of physician approval of CAM was not correlated with the use of CAM by caregivers.

An interesting issue is how the use of alternative medicine might influence the relationship between therapists and patients with mental illnesses.

The second telephone survey of Eisenberg et al. previously cited was analyzed to ascertain details of the use of CAM by these patients [36, 80]. A high rate of use was revealed; slightly more than half of all individuals with anxiety and depression used CAM during the previous twelve months before they participated in the survey. Substantial numbers of individuals with mental disorders using CAM was also noted in several other studies, however none of these studies delineates the impact of this use on the doctor-patients relationship [83, 136, 139]. In Spain, a high rate of use was observed among patients with somatization disorders, and the use of CAM was thought to be related to the desire of such patients to have a more intense doctor-patient relationship with more time spent with physicians [44].

Three hundred elderly veterans who attended a large urban hospital outpatient clinic who used CAM were surveyed about their discussions about CAM with their physicians. Demographic characteristics of the individuals and details of the questionnaire have been described elsewhere [28].

Those subjects who had discussed CAM use with their physicians were asked to use 1–5 scales to rate perceptions of physician attitudes towards CAM, (1 – most positive), whether the discussions changed the patients' use of CAM (1 – much change), how important such discussions were to the patient (1 – very important) how willing the physician was to discuss CAM (1 – very willing) and how satisfied patients were with the discussions (1 – very satisfied). The results can be found in Table 3.1.

In this population, the elderly ascribed a great deal of importance to discussions about CAM with physicians. They perceived physicians as being willing to discuss CAM and maintaining a positive attitude about CAM therapies. These older individuals were satisfied with their discussions, which often resulted in a change in how patients used CAM. However, less than half actually did discuss CAM use with their practitioners.

In Table 3.2, we examined the reasons for elderly CAM users' failure to discuss CAM with physicians. In fact, in this sample, more often it was the patient who opted not to bring up CAM with the physician than the physician who failed to elicit the information.

Table 3.1. Patients' attitudes toward discussions of CAM with MDs[a]

Discussed CAM[b]	MD Attitudes[c]	Change in use[a]	Importance[e]	Willingness to discuss[f]	Satisfaction[g]
44	1.9	2.4	1.9	1.5	1.5

[a] $n = 99$, [b] % patients who discussed CAM with physicians, [c] average rating by patients of physician attitudes toward CAM (1–5 scale, 1=most positive), [d] average rating by patients of whether discussions resulted in a change in use of CAM (1–5 scale, 1=much change), [e] average rating by patients of importance of discussion of CAM with MDs (1–5 scale, 1=very important), [f] average rating by patients of physician willingness to discuss CAM (1–5 scale, 1=very willing), [g] average rating by patients of satisfaction with discussion (1–5 scale,1= very satisfied).

Table 3.2. Reasons why elderly did not discuss CAM with physicians (%)[a]

Physician did not bring up	25
Patient did not think important or necessary	27
Patient did not think of it	19
Patient thought physician would think negatively about patient	8
No time	7
Other	13

[a] $n=99$.

Sleath et al. analyzed demographic characteristics of patients and physicians that made middle aged and older patients more likely to discuss alternative medicine, among medical residents interviewing a predominately minority patient population (approximately two-thirds Hispanic) in a New Mexico medical school clinic [117]. Patient visits were audiotaped by research assistants, who interviewed the subjects after their visits. In the roughly 200 taped conversations, a relatively low number of patients 17.5% of total population, had CAM, and only 10% had discussed CAM with physicians. Younger, female physicians, white patients, and individuals who perceived themselves to be sicker were more likely to speak about CAM use. It is uncertain how physicians' advance understanding that investigators would be monitoring the clinic visits and the audiotaping of conversations might have influenced the content of these conversations.

In a small study done among women aged sixty-five or older, Yoon and Horne ascertained that approximately forty percent of all subjects reported use of herbal products to their physicians [141]. The investigators reported that the subjects commonly believed that the products they used were safe, and therefore, did not discuss their use with physicians.

While it has commonly been suggested that the use of CAM is deleterious to the relationship between the patient and physician practicing conventional medicine, such as the concern that the disclosure by the patient that he uses CAM might evoke the disapproval of the physician, there has also been the suggestion that CAM disclosure might, in fact, improve the doctor-patient relationship. Bignami proposed that, because the rationale for CAM therapies approximate common-sense notions more than conventional, science-based remedies do, they are especially appealing to patients [16]. He asserts that the discussion of CAM between patients and physician fosters a more patient-focused interaction between patient and practitioner.

Older individuals belonging to cultures and societies in which a tradition of folk medicine exists may have particular affinities for certain types of CAM. Older women, in particular, who have in many societies been the practitioners and reservoirs of the traditions of folk medicine, may have predilections to use CAM [20, 46, 118].

The influence of folk medicine use on the relationship between doctor and patient has seldom been studied. One investigation was performed on immigrants to Israel from Yemen [94] in which over three hundred subjects, all over seventy, were interviewed in percent by investigators. Most of the users of folk remedies were self-treated. Two-thirds of the individuals used conventional physicians, and the younger the person, and the longer the person had resided in Israel, the less likely he was to use traditional medicine.

Other studies of the use of traditional folk healers were performed among Mexican immigrants to the United States [69, 116]. These showed at least constant, if not increasing use, over recent decades.

While the association between CAM use and income is controversial, with some studies showing higher use by the more affluent, and others showing no difference in CAM use by income, Wooten and Sparber have suggested that there may be a bimodal distribution of CAM use with both higher and lower-income persons utilizing CAM more frequently [70]. It is unknown whether less affluent elderly, who may have worse access to conventional medical care, use more CAM nor if that influences their relationship with physicians.

It is very difficult to generalize from small samples of elderly patients.

Nevertheless, from the relatively small numbers of studies based on very limited information, there is no evidence yet that the use of alternative medicine does, in fact, significantly alter the doctor-patient relationship. Larger studies will be needed to verify this conclusion. While acceptance of CAM by physicians appears to vary according to type of CAM and geographic location, physicians do appear to accept many forms of CAM.

However, there are many questions studies have yet to consider to truly ascertain that CAM does not influence the physician-patient relationship. Firstly, it remains uncertain whether visits to alternative practitioners change the way in which patients perceive conventional physicians. Nor is it clear whether use of CAM alters how individuals regard or utilize medications given simultaneously for the same conditions. Do patients respect the opinions of conventional practitioners to the same degree if they perceive CAM therapies as more effective than conventional therapies or as effective supplements to conventional therapies that conventional physicians disapprove of? Is there a difference between young and old patients who use CAM therapies in the perception of conventional medicine and its practitioners? Do patients who use both confuse conventional and CAM therapies? Such questions might prove the basis for a more detailed examination of the influence of CAM on the physician-patient relationship.

References

1. Aasland OG, Borchgrevink C, Fugelli (1997) Norwegian physicians and alternative medicine. Knowledge, attitudes and experience. Tidsskrift for Den Norske Laegeforen Jun 30: 117(17): 2464–2468.
2. Abu-Realh M, Magwood G, Narayan M, et al. (1996) The use of complementary therapies by cancer patients. Nursing Connections 9: 3–12.
3. Adelman R, Greene M, Charon R (1991) Issues in physician-elderly patient interaction. Ageing and Society. 127–48.
4. Adelman R, Greene M, Ory M (2000) Communication between older patients and their physicians. Clinics in Geriatric Medicine 16(1): 1–24.
5. Adler S, Fosket J (1999) Disclosing complementary and alternative medicine use in the medical encounter: a qualitative study in women with breast cancer. Journal of Family Practice 48(6): 453–463.
6. Anderson E, and Anderson P (1987) General practitioners and alternative medicine. Journal of the Royal College of Physicans 37: 52–55.
7. Arntson P, Makoul G, Pendelton D, et al. (1989) Patients' perceptions of medical encounters in Great Britain: variations with health loci of control and sociodemographic factors. Health Communication 2: 75.
8. Becker H (1962) Nature of a profession. In: Henry N (ed) Education for the Professions, part 2. Univ of Chicago, Chicago
9. Becker M, Drachman R, Kirscht J (1974) A field experiment to evaluate various outcomes of continuity of physician care. American Journal of Public Health. 64: 1062–1070.
10. Beisecker A (1988) Aging and the desire for information and input in medical decisions: patient consumerism in medical encounters. Gerontologist 28:330–335.
11. Beisecker A, Beisecker T (1990) Patient information-seeking behaviors when communicating with doctors. Medical Care 28: 19–28.
12. Beisecker A, Murden, R, Moore W, et al. (1996) Attitudes of medical students and primary care physicians regarding input of older and younger patients in medical decisions. Medical Care 34(2): 126–136.
13. Benbassat J, Pilpel D, Tidhar M. (1998) Patients' preferences for participation in clinical decision making: a review of published surveys Behavioral Medicine 24: 81–88.
14. Berman B, Singh, B, Lao L, et al. (1995) Physicians' attitudes toward complementary or alternative medicine regional survey. Journal of the American Board of Family Practice 8(5): 361–6.
15. Bernstein J, Shuval J (1997) Nonconventional medicine in Israel:consultation patterns of the Israeli population and attitudes of primary care physicians. May;44(9): 1341–8.
16. Bignami G (1999) The physician-patient relationship in the contexts of different medicines. Annuale 1st Super Sanita 35(4): 499–504.
17. Blanchard C, Labrecque M, Ruckdeschel J, et al. (1988) Information and decision-making preferences of adult hospitalized cancer patients. Social Science and Medicine 27: 1139–1145.
18. Blumberg D, Grant W, Hendricks S, et al. (1995) The physician and unconventional medicine. Alternative Therapies, Health, and Medicine 1(3): 31–5.
19. Boon H, Stewart, M, Kennard, M, et al.(2000) Use of complementary and alternative medicine by breast cancer survivors in Ontario: prevalence and perceptions. Journal of Clinical Oncology 18(13): 2515–2521.
20. Boulding E (1975) The underside of history. A view of women through time. Boulder, CO: Westview Press.
21. Breemhaar B, Visser A, Kleijnen J (1990) Perceptions and behaviour among elderly hospital patients: description and explanation of age differences in satisfaction, knowledge, emotions and behavior. Social Science and Medicine 32: 853.
22. Brigden M (1995) Unproven (questionable) cancer therapies. Western Journal of Medicine 153: 463–469.
23. Brown J, Brett P, Stewart M, et al. (1998) Roles and influence of people who accompany patients on visits to the doctor. Canadian Family Physician 44: 1644–1650.
24. Burstein H Gelber S, Guadagnoli E (1999) Use of alternative medicine by women with early-stage breast cancer. New England Journal of Medicine 340(22): 1733–1739.
25. Cassileth B, Zupkis R, Sutton-Smith K, et al. (1980) Information and participation preferences among cancer patients. Annals of Internal Medicine 92: 832–836.
26. Cassileth B, Lusk E, Strouse T. et al. (1984) Contemporary unorthodox treatments in cancer medicine. A study of patients, treatments, and practitioners. Annals of Internal Medicine 101(1): 105–112.
27. Cherkin D, MacCormack F, Berg A (1989) Family physicians' views of chiropractors: hostile or hospitable. American Journal of Public Health 79: 636–637.
28. Cherniack E, Senzel R, and Pan C (2001) Correlates of use of alternative medicine by the elderly in an urban population. Journal of Complementary and Alternative Therapies 7(3): 277–80.
29. Coe R (1970) Sociology of medicine. McGraw-Hill: New York.
30. Coe R, Prendergast C, Psathas G (1984) Strategies for obtaining compliance with medications regimens Journal of the American Geriatrics Society 32: 589.
31. Coleman L, Fowler L, Williams M. (1995) Use of unproven therapies by people with Alzheimer's disease. Journal of the American Geriatrics Society 43(7): 747–750.
32. Coss R, McGrath P, Caggiano V. (1998) Alternative care: patient choices for adjunct therapies within a cancer center. Cancer Practice 6: 176–181.
33. Crock, R, Jarjoura D, Polen A, et al. (1999) Confronting the communications gap between conventional and alternative medicine: a survey of physicians' attitudes. Alternative Therapies 5(2): 61–6.

34. Degner L, Sloan J (1992) Decision making during serious illness: what role do patients really want to play? Journal of Clinical Epidemiology 45: 941–950.

35. Eisenberg D Kessler R, Foster C et al. (1993) Unconventional medicine in the United States: prevalence, costs, and patterns of use. New England Journal of Medicine 328: 246–252.

36. Eisenberg D, Davis R, Ettner S. et al. Trends in alternative medicine use in the United States. Journal of the American Medical Association 1998; 280: 1569–1575.

37. Elder N, Gilcrist A, Minz. Use of alternative health care by family practice patients. Archives of Family Medicine 1997; 6: 181–4.

38. Eliason B, Kruger J, Mark D, et al. (1997) Dietary supplement users: demographics, product use and medical system interaction. Journal of the American Board of Family Practice 10: 265–271.

39. Ende J, Kazis, L Ash A, et al. (1989) Measuring patients' desire for autonomy: decision making and information-seeking preferences among medical patients. Journal of General Internal Medicine 4: 23–30.

40. Ernst E, Resch K-L, White A (1995) Complementary medicine: what physicians think of it. Archives of Internal Medicine 155: 2405–8.

41. Evans B, Kielleru F, Stanley R, et al. (1987) A communication skills programme for increasing patients' satisfaction with general practice consultations. British Journal of Medical Psychology 60: 373–378.

42. Foster D, Phillips R, Hamel M et al. (2000) Alternative medicine use in older Americans. Journal of the American Geriatrics Society 48: 1560–1565.

43. Freeman G, Richards S (1994) Is personal continuity of care compatible with free choice of doctor? Patients' views on seeing the same doctor. British Journal of General Practice 43: 493–497.

44. Garcia-Campayo J, Sanz-Carrillo C (2000) The use of alternative medicines by somatoform disorder patients in Spain. British Journal of General Practice 50(455): 487–488.

45. Garms-Homolova V (1985) Not at all or too much: patterns of inadequate use of health and social services by the elderly. Paper presented at the XIII International Congress of Gerontology July 12–17, New York.

46. Gaylord S (1999) Alternative therapies and empowerment of older women. Journal of Women and Aging 11(2/3): 29–47.

47. German P, Klein L, McPhee S, et al. (1982) Knowledge of and compliance with drug regimens in the elderly. Journal of the American Geriatrics Society 30(9) 568–571.

48. Giles H, Coupland N, Williams A, et al. (1992) Intergenerational talk and communication with older people. International Journal of Aging and Human Development 34(4):271–297

49. Goldstein J, Chao C, Valentine E et al. (1991) Use of unproved cancer treatment by patients in a radiation oncology department: a survey. Journal of Pschosocial Oncology 9: 59–66.

50. Gore J, Ogden J (1998) Developing, validating and consolidating the doctor-patient relationship: patients' views of a dynamic process. British Journal of General Practice 48(432): 1391–4.

51. Greene M (1987) The physician-elderly patient relationship: An examination of the language and behavior of doctors with their elderly patients. Final report to the AARP Andrus Foundation.

52. Greene M, Hoffman S, Charon R et al.(1987) Psychosocial concerns in the medical encounter. A comparison of the interactions of doctors with their old and young patients. Gerontologist 27: 164–8

53. Greene M, Adelman R, Friedmann E, et al.(1989) Concordance between physicians and their older and younger patients in the primary care medical encounter. Gerontologist 19: 808–13.

54. Greene M, Majerovitz S, Adelman R, et al. (1994) The effects of the presence of a third person on the physician-older patient medical interview. Journal of the American Geriatrics Society 52: 413–419.

55. Greenfield S, Kaplan S, Ware J (1984) Expanding patient involvement in care-effects on patient outcomes. Annals of Internal Medicine 102: 520–528.

56. Greenfield S, Blanco D, Elashoff R, et al. (1987) Patterns of care related to age of breast cancer patients Journal of the American Medical Association 257: 2766–2770.

57. Hadley CM (1988) Complementary medicine and the general practitioner: a survey of general practitioners in the Wellington area. New Zealand Medical Journal 101(857): 766–768.

58. Haezen-Clemens I, Lapinska E (1984)Doctor-patient interaction, patient's health behavior and effects of treatment. Social Science and Medicine 19: 9–18.

59. Hall J, Epstein A, DeCiantis M, et al. (1993) Physicians' liking for their patients: more evidence for the role of affect in medical care. Health Psychology; 12: 140–6.

60. Hall J, Milburn M, Roter D, et al.(1998) Why are sicker patients less satisfied with their care? Test of two explanatory models. Health Psychology 17: 70–5.

61. Haug M (1973) De-professionalization: an alternate hypothesis for the future. In: Halmos P (ed) Professionalization and and social change, The Sociological Review Monograph No 20, Univ of Keele, UK.

62. Haug M (1976) The erosion of professional authority: a cross-cultural inquiry in the case of the physician. Milbank Q 54: 83–106.

63. Haug M, Lavin B (1978) Method of payment for medical care and patient attitudes to physician authority. Journal of health and social behavior 19, 279–291.

64. Haug M. Doctor patient relationships and the older patient (1979) Journal of Gerontology 34(8): 852–9.

65. Haug M, Lavin B (1979) Public challenge of physician authority. Medical Care 17(8): 844–858.

66. Haug M, Lavin B (1983) Consumerism in medicine: challenging physician authority, Beverly Hills CA, USA, Sage.

67. Headache Study Control Group of the University of Western Ontario (1986) predictors of outcome in headache patients presenting to family physicians -a one year prospective study. Headache 26: 285–294.

68. Hibbard J (1987) Consumerism in health care. Prevalence and predictors. Medical Care 24(1): 52–66.

69. Higginbotham J, Trevino F, Ray L (1990) Utilization of curanderos by Mexican Americans: prevalence and predictors. Findings from HHANES. American Journal of Public Health 80(suppl): 32–35.
70. Himmel W, Schulte M, Kochen M. Complementary medicine: are patients expectations being met by their general practitioners? British Journal of Gen eral Practice 1993; 43: 232–5.
71. Hjortdahl P, Borchgrevink C (1991) Continuity of care: influence of general practitioners' knowledge about their patients on use of resources in the community. British Medical Journal 303: 1181–1184.
72. Hjortdahl P, Laerum E. (1992) Continuity of care in general practice: effect on patient satisfaction. British Medical Journal 304: 1287–1290.
73. Hurley R, Gage B, Freund D (1991) Rollover effects in gatekeeper programs: cushioning the impact of restricted choice. Inquiry 21: 375–384.
74. Irish J (1997) Deciphering the physician-older patient relationship. International Journal of Psychiatry and Medicine 27(3): 251–267.
75. Jackson J (1970) Professions and professionalization-editorial introduction. In: Jackson J (ed) Professions and professionalization, Cambridge Univ Press, Cambridge, UK.
76. Kaplan S, Greenfield S, Ware J Jr (1989) Assessing the effects of physician-patient interactions on the outcomes of chronic disease. Medical Care 27 (suppl 3): S110–127.
77. Kaplan S, Gandek B, Greefield S, et al. (1995) Patient and visit characteristics related to physicians' participatory decision-making style: results from the Medical Outcomes' Study. Medical Care 33: 1176–87.
78. Kasteler J, Kane R, Olsen D, et al. (1976) Issues underlying prevalence of "doctor-shopping" behavior. Journal Health and Social Behavior. 17: 329–339.
79. Kern K (1990) Some aspects of doctor-patient relationships and the older patient. Zeitschrift fur Gerontologie 23(6): 354–360.
80. Kessler R, Soukup J, Davis R, et al. (2001) The use of complementary and alternative therapies to treat anxiety and depression in the United States. American Journal of Psychiatry 158(2): 289–294.
81. Kibbe D, Bentz E, McLaughlin C (1993) Continuity quality improvement for continuity of care Journal of Family Practice 36: 304–308.
82. Kleinman A (1978) Concepts and a model for the comparison of medical systems as cultural systems. Social Science and Medicine 12; 85–93.
83. Knaudt P, Connor K, Weisler R, et al. (1998) Alternative therapy use in psychiatric outpatients. Journal of Nervous and Mental Disease 187(11): 692–695.
84. Knipschild P, Klejnen J, Riet G (1990) Belief in the efficacy of alternative medicine among general practitioners in the Netherlands. Social Science and Medicine 31: 625–626.
85. LaPuma J, Orientlicher D, Moss R (1991) Advance directives on admission, clinical implications and analysis of the Patient Self-Determination Act of 1990. Journal of the American Medical Association 266: 402–405.
86. Lerner I, Kennedy B: The prevalence of questionable methods of cancer treatments in the United States. CA Cancer Journal for Clinicians 42: 181–191.
87. Linn MW, Lynn BS, Stein SR. Satisfaction with ambulatory care and compliance in older patients. Medical Care 1995; 33: 1176–87.
88. Liu E, Turner L, Lin S, et al.(2000) Use of alternative medicine by patients undergoing cardiac surgery. Journal of Thoracic and Cardiovascular Surgery 120: 335–41.
89. Lynoe N, Svensson T. Physicians and alternative medicine-and investigation of attitudes and practices. Scan J Soc Med 1992; 20: 55–60.
90. Marshall R, Gee R, Israel M, et al. (1990) The use of alternative therapies by Auckland general practitioners. New Zealand Medical Journal 103: 213–5.
91. McCormick W, Insui T, Roter D (1996) Interventions in physician-elderly patient interactions. Research in Aging 18(1): 103–136.
92. McLane C, Zyzanski S, Flocke S. (1995) Factors associated with medication noncompliance in rural elderly hypertensive patients. American Journal of Hypertension 8: 206–209.
93. Moore W (1970) The professions and the rules. Russell Sage Foundation: New York.
94. Nakar S, Vinker S, Kitai E, et al. (2001) Folk, traditional, and conventional medicine among elderly Yemenite immigrants in Israel. Israeli Medical Association Journal 3(12): 928–931.
95. Newell S, Sanson-Fisher R (2000) Australian oncologists' self-reported knowledge and attitudes about non-traditional therapies used by cancer patients. Medical Journal of Australia 172(3): 110–3.
96. Orth J, Stiles W, Scherwitz L, et al. (1987) Interviews and hypertensive patients' participation in medical care-effects on blood sugar control and quality of life in diabetes. Health Psychology 6: 29–42.
97. Parsons T (1951) The social system. The Free Press: New York.
98. Parsons T (1975) The sick role and role of the physician reconsidered. Milbank Memorial Fund Quarterly, Health and Society 53: 257–278.
99. Pederson E. Norheim A, Fennebe V (1996) Attitudes of Norwegian physicians to homeopathy: A questionnaire among 2,019 physicians on their cooperation with homeopathy specialist. Tidsskrift for Den Norske Laegeforen Aug 10; 116(18) 2186–2189.
100. Pellegrino E (1977) Medicine and human values. Yale Alumni Magazine and Journal, 41: 10.
101. Perkin M, Pearcy R, Fraser J (1994) A comparison of the attitudes shown by general practitioners, hospital doctors, and medical students towards alternative medicine. J Royal of the Society of Medicine 87: 523–5.

102. Pirotta M, Cohen M, Kotsirilos, V, et al. (2000) Complementary therapies: have they become accepted in general practice? Medical Journal of Australia 172: 105–9.
103. Putnam S, Stiles W, Jacob M. et al. (1985) Patient exposition and physician explanation in initial medical interviews and outcomes of clinic visits. Medical Care 23(1): 74–83.
104. Rakowski W, Hickey T, Dengiz A (1987) Congruence of health and treatment perceptions among older patients and providers of primary care. International Journal of Aging and Human Development 25: 67–81.
105. Reeder L (1972) The patient-client as a consumer: some observations on the changing professional-client relationship. Journal of Health and Social Behavior, 13: 406–412.
106. Risberg T, Kolstad A, Johansen, et al. (1999) Opinions on and use of alternative medicine among physicians, nurses and clerks in Northern Norway. In Vivo 13: 493–8.
107. Rost K, Frankel R. (1993) The introduction of the older patient's problem in the medical visit. Journal of Aging and Health 5: 387–401.
108. Rost K, Roter D. (1987) Predictors of recall of medication regimens and recommendation for lifestyle changes in elderly patients. Gerontologist 27(4): 510–515.
109. Roter D (1994) Patient question asking in physician-patient interaction. Health Psychology 3(5): 395–409.
110. Roter D, Hall J (1991) Improving psychosocial problem address in primary care: is it possible and what difference does it make? [lecture] International Consensus Conference on Doctor-Patient Communication, Toronto, Nov 14–16.
111. Roter D, Stewart M, Putnam S, et al. (1997) Communication patterns of primary care physicians. Journal of the American Medical Association 270: 350–355.
112. Roter DL (2000) The outpatient medical encounter and elderly patients. Clinics in Geriatric Medicine 16(1): 95–107.
113. Salzman C. (1995) Medication compliance in the elderly. Journal of Clinical Psychiatry 56 (suppl 1): 18–22.
114. Shachter L, Weingarten M, Kahan E (1993) Attitudes of family physicians to nonconventional therapies. Archives of Family Medicine 2: 1268–70.
115. Sillman R (1989) Caring for the frail older patient: the doctor-patient-family caregiver relationship. Journal of General Internal Medicine 4: 237–241.
116. Skaer T, Robison L, Sclar D. et al. (1996) Utilization of curanderos among among foreign-born Mexican American women attending migrant health clinics. Journal of Cultural Diversity 3; 29–34.
117. Sleath B. Rubin R, Campbell W. et al. (2001)Ethnicity and physician-older patient communication about alternative therapies. Journal of Complementary and Alternative Therapies 7(4): 329–35.
118. Stein D (1990) All women are healers. Freedom, CA: The Crossing Press.
119. Stewart M (1984) Patient characteristics which are related to doctor –patient interactions. Family Practice 1(1): 30–36.
120. Stewart M (1995) Effective physician-patient communication and health outcomes: a review. Canadian Medical Association Journal 152(9): 1423–1433.
121. Stewart M, Meredith L, Brown J, Galajada J (2000)The influence of older patient-physician communication on health and health related outcomes. Clinics in Geriatric Medicine 16(1):25–36.
122. Strull W, Lo B, Charles G (1984) Do patients want to participate in medical decision making? Journal of the American Medical Association 252: 2990–2994.
123. Thompson S, Pitts J, Schwankowsky L (1993) Preferences for involvement in medical decision-making: situational and demographic influences. Patient and Education Counseling 22: 133–140.
124. Torio Durantez J, Gardia Tirado M (1997) The physician-patient relationship and the clinical interview (I): the opinion and preferences of users. Aten Primaria 19(1): 18–26.
125. Twemlow S, Bradshaw S, Coyne L, et al. (1995) Some interpersonal and attitudinal factors characterizing patients satisfied with medical care. Psychology Reports 77(1): 51–59.
126. Verhoef M, Sutherland L (1995) General practitioners' assessment of and interest in alternative medicine in Canada. Social Science and Medicine 41(4): 511–3.
127. Verhoef M, Sutherland L Alternative medicine and general practitioners (1995) Canadian Family Physician 41: 1005–11.
128. Vertinsky I, Thompson I, Uyeno D (1974) Measuring consumers' desire for participation in clinical decision making Health Services Research 9: 121–134.
129. Visser G. Peters L (1990) Alternative medicine and general practitioners in the Netherlands: toward acceptance and integration. Family Practice 7(3): 227–232.
130. Visser G, Peters L, Rasker J (1992) Rheumatologists and their patients who seek alternative care: and agreement to disagree. British Journal of Rheumatology 3(7): 485–490.
131. Warrick P, Irish J, Morningstar M, et al. (1999) Use of alternative medicine among patients with head and neck cancer. Archives of Otolaryngology and Head and Neck Surgery 125: 573–9.
132. Wasson J, Sauvigne A, Mogielnicke R, et al. (1984) Continuity of outpatient medical care in elderly men: a randomized trial. Journal of the American Medical Association 252: 2413–2417.
133. Weiss L, Blustein J (1996) Faithful patients: the effect of long-term physician-patient relationships on the costs and use of health care by older Americans. American Journal of Public Health: 86(12); 1742–7.
134. Wellman B, Kelner M, Wigdor B (2001) Older adults' use of medical and alternative care. Journal of Applied Gerontology 20(1): 3–23.

135. Wharton R, Lewith G (1986) Complementary medicine and the general practitioner. British Medical Journal 292: 1498–500.
136. Wong A, Smith M, Boon H (1998) Herbal remedies in psychiatric practice. Archives of General Psychiatry 279: 1548–1553.
137. Woodward N, Wallston S (1987) Age an health care beliefs: self-efficacy as a mediator of low desire for control. Psychology and Aging 2: 3–8.
138. Wooten J, Sparber A (1999) Surveys of complementary and alternative medicine. In Micozzi M, (ed.) Current review of complementary medicine (Philadelphia: Current Medicine).
139. Yager J. Landsverk J, Edelstein C (1989) Help seeking and satisfaction with care in 641 women with eating disorders, I: patterns of utilization, attributed change, and perceived efficacy of treatment. J Nervous and Mental Disease 177: 632–637.
140. Yates P, Beadle G, Clavarino A, et al. (1993) Patients with terminal cancer who use alternative therapies: their beliefs and practices. Sociology of Health and Illness. 15: 199–217.
141. Yoon S-J, Horne C. (2001) Herbal products and conventional medicines used by community residents. Journal of Advanced Nursing 33(1): 51.

4 Alternative Medicines and the Elderly

J.C. McElnay and C.M. Hughes

Definitions and Remit of the Chapter

The term alternative medicine is one that can cover a range of topics and can mean many things to different audiences. For this particular chapter, focus has been placed on the use of "medicinal products" within alternative medicine such as herbal products, homoeopathic remedies and aromatherapy agents [21]. This chapter will examine utilization patterns of such products in the elderly population, the types of products which are or could be used, and usage issues which can arise in this patient group, notably adverse effects and drug interactions. Recommendations are made by way of attempting to promote the more rational use of alternative medicines in the elderly.

Utilization Trends of Alternative Medicines by the Elderly

The use of herbal and other forms of traditional medicine has been the dominant form of medical treatment in developing nations for centuries [29]. However, over recent years, the usage of alternative medicines within the general population has been increasing dramatically in Western countries. For example, the current market for herbal supplements in the United States is approximately $4 billion [33] and a recent survey of medication use in the ambulatory population of the USA indicated that alternative medicines (as defined above) were taken by 14% of the population [47]. Such widespread use of herbal products is not restricted to the USA and indeed, one research study indicated that herbal medicine accounted for over 25% of all alternative medicine usage in a South Australian population [60] while a further study has indicated that herbal medicine is widely used to treat many conditions in Japan [46].

The extent of alternative medicine usage by the elderly population (by convention, over the age of 65) is less clear. In one recent study, Astin et al. [2] surveyed Californian residents (*n*=675) who were enrolled in a health care plan for those over 65 years (Medicare Shield 65). Herbal medicines were used by 24% of the sample. In a further large US survey published in 2002, the prevalence of use of alternative products was higher in those aged between 45–64, but men and women over the age of 65 were more likely to consume certain products e.g. glucosamine and Gingko bilioba [47]. Dello Buono et al. [25] found that the use of alternative medicines was widespread in an Italian sample of community dwelling elderly (over 65 years old), with herbal products being used by almost half of those who used any form of alternative medicine. However, what has given rise to concern is that elderly patients also consume more conventional drugs than other age groups [22] and the concomitant use of alternative medicines may give rise to interactions and other adverse effects. In many developed countries, alternative medicines are widely available in community pharmacies, health food shops, via complementary/alternative practitioners and via mail order, therefore access is relatively easy [69]. Furthermore, since many of these products are unlicensed, untested and may be of dubious quality, healthcare professionals must be prepared to advise patients accordingly.

Why Does the Elderly Population Consume Alternative Medicines?

The rationale for use of these products by elderly patients is no different to that in the rest of the adult population. In Western society, there has been a drive towards self-care [43] and coupled with this, there has been a trend towards the increased use of "natural" alternative approaches to healing and disease management [11]. The efficacy of conventional medicines is increasingly being questioned and the side-effects associated with many conventional drugs may also have led patients to seek alternative modes of treatment [11]. It is also important to bear in mind that there is a strong cultural influence in the use of alternative medicines and this may be accentuated in an elderly population. Cappuccio et al. [15], in a cross-sectional population based study in South London, found that people of African origin were more likely to use alternative medicines than Caucasians or those from South Asia. Patients of Asian descent with Type II diabetes were more likely to use herbal and other alternative medicines to treat their illness compared to other patients attending the same our-patient clinic in London [41]. Ma [59] found high rates of alternative medicine usage in Chinese immigrant communities in two cities in the USA, although this was not differentiated by age. Liu et al. [57] noted that in Chinese cancer patients, alternative medicines were consumed in the hope that they may be of some benefit to their well-being or disease control or even in the production of a miracle cure.

There are large regional differences in the use of homoeopathy. This mode of treatment is extremely popular in France, where products are routinely dispensed on prescription rather than being bought over the counter, while the United Kingdom has one of the lowest per capita spending in Europe on this type of health care [35]. More widespread availability of homoeopathic products in community pharmacies and health food stores in the UK may lead to changes to in these statistics. Little data are available about the usage of homoeopathic remedies in the USA and epidemiology studies to date have not specifically focused on this form of alternative therapy in the elderly.

Marshall et al. [61] surveyed New Zealand general practitioners (GPs) and found that the most common reason for referring a patient for an alternative therapy was failure of conventional therapy. The use of alternative medicines in self-care is often driven by the fact that patients perceive alternative medicines to be safer than conventional therapies. Wagner et al. [88] interviewed patients who were using St. John's Wort in the management of depression; they found that patients reported that it was a safe treatment option. Weiss et al. [89] surveyed emergency department patients' knowledge of alternative medicines and found that 16% ($n=350$) considered all alternative medicines to be safe. The public has therefore often been led to believe that alternative medicines are less toxic than conventional medicines or completely free from side-effects [57].

Elderly patients may also appreciate the time spent with alternative medicine practitioners, which, in contrast to mainstream medical practice, may be unhurried and as such, may engender a good patient-practitioner relationship [34]. As many elderly people are retired with more free time, the experience of this type of health care, coupled with the view that side-effects will be absent, may motivate them to invest in alternative therapies and perhaps reduce their contact with their doctors and other conventional health care professionals.

Products Used and Their Indications

The range of alternative medicines which are available and the conditions for which they have been used is extensive. Table 4.1 is by no means exhaustive, but provides an overview. Such products are not exclusively used in the elderly, but as will be seen in

Table 4.1. Common medical conditions and alternative medicines which have been used in their treatment

Condition	Alternative medicine
Depression	St. John's Wort [37]
Insomnia	Melatonin [37]
	Valerian [37]
	German chamomile [37]
Dementia	Ginkgo [53]
	Thiamine [8]
Migraine	Feverfew [53]
Hyperlipidaemia	Garlic [53]
Asthma	Ginkgo [90]
	Magnesium sulphate [13]
Chronic obstructive pulmonary disease	Sobrerol [16]
	Magnesium sulphate [80]
Diabetes mellitus	Garlic [74]
	Echinacea [74]
Osteoarthritis	Extract of avocado and soya bean [10]
	Capsaicin [16]
	Ginger [9]
	Stinging nettle [71]
	Glucosamine sulphate [19]
	Rhus toxicodendron [86]
Leg cramps	Cuprum [86]
Cystitis	Cantharis [86]

later sections in this chapter, the use of such products in this vulnerable population needs to be considered carefully. Furthermore, in many cases, there is little evidence from well-designed trials to support the efficacy of these substances in the management of the conditions for which they are recommended.

Many of the conditions listed above are common in the elderly. Perceived poor control by conventional prescription medications may lead patients to purchase alternative medicine products to supplement conventional treatments. This raises the possibility of drug interactions. Although drug interactions are a valid concern, there are also a number of adverse effects which need to be considered before alternative medicines are initiated in the elderly.

Changed Pharmacokinetics and Pharmacodynamics in the Elderly

Ageing results in a number of physiological changes, such as reduced gastrointestinal motility, reduced liver size and blood flow, a reduction in renal tubular secretion and reabsorption, a reduction in glomerular filtration and an increase in body fat [78]. It is well-known that these changes impact on the pharmacokinetic handling of conventional drugs, i.e. absorption, distribution, metabolism and elimination. Age-related changes in pharmacodynamic parameters in elderly patients in terms of the effects exerted by the drug on the body have also been clearly demonstrated. In conventional medicine, these changes in kinetics and dynamics often necessitate a reduction in the daily dose of a drug that is required by elderly patients. It may also be necessary to reduce the dose of some alternative medicines to counter these changes, otherwise adverse effects may be manifested. Although this is a logical extension of existing knowledge about conventional therapy, there is a lack of published data on the handling of the individual active components of alternative medicines in the ageing body.

One of the main reservations held by health care professionals regarding alternative medicines' usage is the public perception of their safety, despite numerous reports in the literature which would suggest otherwise. There are also concerns about the lack of safety information and regulation of such products, including quality control/assurance associated with their production. Many of the adverse reactions which have been reported to date arise from case studies, rather than from large trials and therein lies a problem of a lack of evidence base for rational use of many alternative medicines. The following sections focus on issues relating to adverse effects of alternative medicines in the elderly.

Adverse Effects Associated with Alternative Medicines

A classification system for adverse effects associated with alternative medicines offers a useful framework to monitor and chart such events. Drew and Myers [29] provided such a classification system (Table 4.2) which has been adapted for the present discussion.

Table 4.2. Classification of adverse effects associated with alternative medicines (adapted from [29])

Intrinsic effects	Extrinsic effects
Type A effects:	Effects associated with production or regulation issues
Predictable toxicity, overdosage, interactions with conventional medications, excess morbidity and mortality	Misidentification
Type B effects:	Contamination
Idiosyncratic, arising from allergy or anaphylaxis	Unsupported claims
	Lack of standardization of products
	Other extrinsic effects:
	Discontinuation of conventional treatments

Intrinsic Effects

Predictable Toxicity and Overdosage. Although more likely to be used in a younger age population, a Chinese herb product containing aristolochic acid which is used as part of a slimming regimen has been associated with fibrosing interstitial nephritis. Such a condition was identified in 1992 and has been described as Chinese herb nephropathy (CHNP; [82]). Yang et al. [94] reported that from January 1995 to July 1998, 12 Chinese patients in Taiwan developed this condition following herbal medicine use in the form of plant extracts, tablets or powders. A 69 year old woman who had taken the product for arthralgia was included in this series of case studies. Since 1999, the Committee on the Safety of Medicines (CSM) has banned the import, sale and supply of products in the United Kingdom (UK) which contain aristolochia followed the report of end stage renal failure in patients who had taken the herb for eczema [58, 65]. In a further study, patients with CHNP were also found to have developed urothelial carcinoma; all patients had been exposed to aristolochia [66]. The latter is a well-known nephrotoxin, but the precise mechanisms of action giving rise to CHNP and carcinoma are unknown [94].

Herbal remedies may also be hepatotoxic. Sho-saiko-to is used extensively in Japan to treat chronic viral hepatitis, but also causes hepatic necrosis, steatosis and fibrosis [20]. A similarly named product, dai-saiko-to, which has been used to treat dyspepsia and gallstones in Japanese patients has been implicated in an idiosyncratic (Type B) reaction. A 55 year old women developed auto-immune hepatitis following treatment with the herb [45].

Many naturally occurring products are used to make herbal teas and again, the natural and perceived innocuous nature of these has led to serious toxicity and death. Foxglove is the original source of cardiac glycosides, notably digoxin, and some leaf preparations are still available [77]. There has been a report of an elderly man who consumed tea prepared from the leaves of a foxglove plant found in his garden; cardiotoxicity resulted [28].

St. John's Wort (also known as *Hypericum perforatum*) has been used extensively as an antidepressant and is the most extensively studied herbal remedy used in this condition [70]. A meta-analysis has indicated that it is superior to placebo and as effective as conventional antidepressants [56] and Woelk et al. [91] reported that it was therapeutically equivalent to imipramine in treating mild to moderate depression following testing in a randomized controlled trial in 40 German outpatient clinics. Although it is generally well-tolerated, there have been a number of reports which im-plicate the product in mania or hypomania. One pertinent case relates to an elderly woman with a history of recurrent depression, but with no bipolar disorder, who developed manic symptoms soon after starting St. John's Wort [95]. However, the authors did caution that the patient discontinued her prescribed medications and the presence of antidepressant-withdrawal mania could not be discounted.

Another well-known psychoactive agent is valerian, derived from the valerian root [76]. With its sedative and anxiolytic action, it may be a popular choice for older people who are reluctant to use conventional medications like benzodiazepines. However, it is not without side-effects, with adverse effects from chronic use including headache, cardiac disturbances and mild agitation. In overdosage, patients may experience fatigue, abdominal pain, dizziness, mydriasis, tremor, and of course, marked sedation [76].

Melatonin has also been used in insomnia, by purportedly regulating sleep and improving circadian rhythms [76]. Adverse effects associated with chronic ingestion include severe headaches, abdominal cramps, loss of libido and excessive sedation.

Ginseng is one of the most popular alternative remedies with approximately 120 million capsules sold in the USA every year [42]. It has been prescribed by alternative practitioners for conditions as wide-ranging as hypertension, diabetes, congestive heart failure, dementia and anemia, conditions which are prevalent in the elderly [50]. Chronic excessive consumption of ginseng in its many forms can give rise to diarrhea, agitation, insomnia, hypertension and tachycardia, a syndrome known as ginseng abuse syndrome [79]. Clearly such effects would be of concern in elderly patients with cardiac conditions. Much larger doses (in excess of 15 grams) can result in a psychotic manifestation [76].

Zinc is a mineral which has become popular in the management of the common cold [63]. In order to avoid non-prescription remedies which may contain drugs e.g. sympathomimetic amines, that would be contra-indicated in certain medical conditions or which could not be taken in combination with prescribed drugs, elderly people may opt for a zinc preparation. Adverse effects associated with chronic excess ingestion of zinc include gastro-intestinal upset, a metallic taste in the mouth and rarely hematuria or lethargy [76].

Glucosamine sulphate is taken by many people for osteoarthritis and some studies have indicated that it can prevent joint structure changes in patients with osteoarthritis of the knee with a significant improvement in symptoms [72]. However, it may be best avoided in patients with diabetes as it can result in insulin resistance [1].

Essential oils used in aromatherapy are pharmacologically active and in high concentrations are potentially carcinogenic, but adverse effects are extremely rare when used externally and in concentrations ranging from 1–3% [87].

The National Poisons Unit in London carried out a pilot survey to investigate the frequency and severity of adverse effects/toxicity from exposure to alternative medicines, including food supplements [69]. Over the time period surveyed (8 years), 5536 enquiries were recorded and symptoms were reported in 12% of these. A notable point raised by the authors was that patients taking products such as kelp and digestive aids appeared to consider that amounts greater than the recommended dose would have an increased therapeutic effect and were absolutely unaware that excessive intake might be toxic.

Interactions with Conventional Medications. Elderly patients consume more conventional medications than their younger counterparts and the addition of an alternative medication will further complicate the situation. Again, due to the perceived safety of alternative medicines, the assumption that is often made is that they can be freely taken with prescribed or other purchased conventional medications. Furthermore, because many patients do not perceive alternative products to be medications, they do not inform doctors or pharmacists that they are taking these products. One study showed that 72% of respondents who used alternative medicines did not inform any health care professionals of their use [31].

Reports of interactions between alternative medicines and conventional products are now being documented in the literature. Some interactions are well-defined and understood, whereas others still require clarification. Vickers and Zollman [85] recommended that if patients are taking conventional drugs, alternative medicines should be used with caution; this advice will certainly apply to elderly patients who may be less resilient to the adverse events resulting from such an interaction.

Table 4.3 lists some clinically significant interactions involving herbal preparations and conventional prescribed drugs. This is not exhaustive by any means, but serves to illustrate the possible resultant effects of herbal products being taken with conventional drugs commonly used by elderly patients.

Excess Morbidity and Mortality. Such events can result from the consumption of alternative medications. Lin and Lin [55] carried out a retrospective cohort study of over 2500 patients admitted to a Taiwanese hospital over a 10 month period to determine the incidence of drug-related admissions. The incidence of admissions was much higher in the elderly and the third most common group of products responsible for these admissions was herbal medicines. This was attributed to the population's enthusiasm for such products, social custom, cultural tradition and poor regulation.

Bensoussan et al. [5] investigated the frequency of adverse events that occurred as a result of the practice of traditional Chinese medicine (acupuncture and herbal medicine) in Australia. Although this does not fall strictly within the realms of our definition, this study was notable in that practitioners were experiencing an average of 1 adverse event every 8–9 months of full-time practice. The authors emphasized that Chinese herbal medicine was not without risks and fatalities had occurred.

Table 4.3. Clinically significant drugs interactions involving alternative medicines and conventional drugs (adapted from [12, 37, 85, 81])

Herbal Drug	Conventional Drug	Resultant Effect
St. John's Wort	SSRI antidepressants	Serotonin syndrome-delirium, cardiovascular instability, myoclonic seizures and death
	Digoxin	Decreased digoxin serum levels
Garlic	Warfarin	Enhanced anticoagulant effect
Ginkgo	Warfarin	Enhanced anticoagulant effect
Valerian	Benzodiazepines	Enhanced sedation
Kava kava	L-dopa and other Parkinson's disease treatment	Possible antagonism of dopamine effects
	Codeine and other opiates	Enhanced sedation
Kelp	Thyroxine	Reduction in thyroxine efficacy
Ginseng	Insulin, biguanides, sulphonylureas	May potentiate hypoglycemia
	Tamoxifen	May stimulate estrogenic activity and opposed effects of tamoxifen
	Phenelzine	Enhanced psychoactive effects resulting in sleeplessness, nervousness and euphoria
Liquorice	Thiazide diuretics	Risk of hypocalemia

Extrinsic Effects

As with conventional medicinal substances, factors unrelated to the pharmacological action of an alternative medicine may also lead to adverse effects (see Table 4.2). Due to poor regulation, such outcomes are much more likely with alternative medicines.

Misidentification. Misidentification can result from nomenclature problems as there can be much similarity in names. Ginseng is also known as renshen, radux ginseng and Panax ginseng [77]; Panax ginseng is also known as Chinese ginseng which differs from Siberian ginseng, the latter being a completely different species [81]. Hence, patients may be unaware that they are consuming the same substance by using different products. Cohosh is used in one area of the USA to describe the baneberry which is toxic, while in the Appalachian mountains, cohosh can be used to describe another range of plants which exhibit different patterns of toxicity [75]. Misidentification can also arise by simply mistaking one product for another, with serious consequences. A good example of this involved a marketer of herbs who misidentified deadly nightshade as comfrey, with resultant atropine poisoning in consumers [44]. The complex nature of crude herbs can also make identification of individual components very difficult. One case series involved an unidentified herbal tea which was consumed by four women, one of whom developed a skin rash and 3 of whom had venoocclusive disease of the liver. The tea contained pyrrolizidine alkaloids at a high concentration [51, 52].

Contamination. During growth and storage, crude plant materials can become contaminated by a range of substances [29]. Lead, cadmium, mercury, arsenic and other heavy metals have been found in a range of herbal medicines [49, 92], with the obvious potential for severe toxicity. Lead has been found in concentrations ranging from 6–60% weight/weight in Asian traditional remedies with resultant lead poisoning in recipients [4]. The CSM recently reported that random testing of Chinese medicines available for purchase in the UK were contaminated with mercury and arsenic [38].

Contamination may also be intentional in which case the content of a product is adulterated deliberately. Keane et al. [48] analyzed 11 herbal creams supplied to patients by Chinese herbalists for the treatment of eczema. Eight products contained dexamethasone, a potent steroid, in varying concentrations. All patients were unaware of the content of the creams, although they had assumed that they were steroid-free. Further investigations by a UK parliamentary group revealed that a mail order product called Skincap, marketed for the treatment of psoriasis, was also adulterated with steroid, despite claims from the company that the active ingredient was zinc pyrithione [9]. Gupta et al. [39] screened 120 samples of alternative medicines available in India used in the treatment of asthma and arthritis; almost 40% of them contained steroids. In a series of case reports, herbal products which were recommended for arthritic conditions were found to be adulterated with mefanamic acid and diazepam; acute interstitial nephritis, renal failure and peptic ulceration resulted in elderly patients who took these products [27, 36].

Unsupported Claims. Because of the lack of rigorous research evidence and the inadequate regulation of alternative medicines, many of these products are marketed on the basis of unsupported claims. Such claims can give vulnerable patients false hope which is often not realized. Hainer et al. [40] documented the case of a 55 year old man with cancer who had obtained hydrazine sulphate which had been described as a chemotherapeutic agent on an alternative medicine website. The patient took hydrazine during the first 4 months after diagnosis, before being admitted to hospital where he died of hepatic and renal necrosis. A previous randomized trial had failed to show any benefit of this substance in patients with cancer [50]. Drew and Myers [29] described how seaweed patches were being advertised as an aid to weight loss on the basis that the patches would reverse hypothyroidism by releasing iodine into the body, thereby increasing metabolism. The claim was entirely without foundation.

Lack of Standardization of Products. One important issue with alternative medicines and especially those derived from plant origin, is that their therapeutic efficacy cannot be attributed to just one compound [14]. Complete characterization of a product requires multiple chemical analyses. Furthermore, the quantities of active ingredients and thus effects may vary substantially from one sample to another. The therapeutic or toxic components of plants will vary depending on the part of the plant used, stage of ripeness, where the plant was grown and storage conditions after harvesting [29]. Several herbs may often be included together, which practitioners claim improves efficacy and reduces adverse effects, although there is little evidence to support this [85]. Again, this complicates analysis and may lead to variation in the content of active ingredients. The content of ginsenoside, to which most of the activity of ginseng has been attributed, was analyzed in 50 commercial brands available in 11 countries [23]. In 44 of these products, the concentration of ginsenoside ranged from 1.9% to 9% weight per weight. Six products contained no ginsenoside. It has also been reported that herbal medicines containing aconite root may vary greatly in their alkaloid content dependent on the origin of the plant, the time of harvest and method of processing [17]. Furthermore, products are often poorly labeled, with little indication of content and concentration of active ingredients as reported by Cui et al. [23].

Discontinuation of Conventional Treatments. Homoeopathy has gained much popularity and has often been promoted on the basis that there are no serious direct risks of highly dilute remedies, which of course is the central tenet of this form of alternative therapy [34]. However, in terms of the elderly, the concern is that some practitioners believe that conventional drugs reduce the efficacy of homoeopathy and adverse events have resulted when patients have discontinued conventional treatment when receiving homoeopathic therapy [86]. This type of practice is not peculiar to homoeopathic treatment and indeed, patients may abandon conventional drugs during treatment with other alternative medicines. Doctors and pharmacists need to take this into account, particularly if patients present with symptoms which suggest poor control of their medical conditions or if they fail to collect refills of prescribed medicines.

How Can the Elderly Patient Achieve Benefit from Alternative Medicine?

Alternative forms of health care are here to stay as evidenced by their increasing popularity, in tandem with a growing lack of trust of mainstream medicine [34] and a desire for less invasive forms of health care [18]. Elderly patients may be particularly vulnerable to the philosophy of alternative medicine, especially in terms of its perceived safety and natural origins. However, as outlined above, elderly patients may also be at increased risk of adverse effects which they may not attribute to the use of such products and which conventional health care professionals may not be aware they are using. A concerted effort must be made to ensure that the elderly and other users can achieve the most from these products and the following points represent some guidelines for the future.

Regulation of Alternative Medicines

Because of the safety concerns which have been outlined in section 1.3, there have been many calls for the stricter regulation of the alternative medicines industry and associated practitioners. The House of Lords in the UK have issued a report on complementary and alternative medicines. They concluded that the public was not protected due to the lack of regulation and called for tighter controls of both products and practitioners [62]. Benzi and Ceci [6] noted that there were marked differences in the approaches adopted by different countries in the scrutiny of herbal medicines, and no European criteria had been established regarding the scientific assessment of the safety and efficacy of these products. There is also much confusion on the process by which a product is classified as a food or as a drug and this has implications for where it can be sold. The Irish Medicines Board (the body responsible for licensing drugs in the Republic of Ireland) have proposed new regulations governing the sale of herbal medicines which will require manufacturers to prove that their products are of sufficient quality, safe for use and appropriate for the medical benefit claimed [24]. The same body ruled that St. John's Wort could only be obtained on a prescription. As detailed earlier, there is often a lack of standardization in content between samples of purportedly the same product [14] and there have been calls to force manufacturers to adhere to pharmaceutical industry standards of quality and safety [26].

Monitoring of adverse reactions on a systematic basis would form part of any quality assurance mechanism. Chan [18] described a system in operation in Hong Kong by which reports on adverse effects to alternative medicines have been gathered through on-going surveillance of patients treated in hospitals, and via reports and enquiries received by the Drug and Poisons Information service. The UK National Poisons Unit in London has also implemented a similar surveillance system [69] and the CSM (UK) accepts reports of adverse events resulting from alternative medicines through its Yellow Card scheme [65]. For such surveillance systems to work, health care professionals must be vigilant and ask patients about their use of alternative medicine products.

Of course, regulation of products will only go so far in promoting safety and it has been recognized that practitioners of alternative medicine also require regulation along the same lines as conventional health care professionals. Many alternative medicine practitioners work alone, few have other healthcare qualifications and they are not obliged to join any official register before setting up practice [85, 86]. The House of Lords Report [62] recommended that each profession should lay down its own standards and that there should be greater collaboration between professional bodies. Within the UK, there is marked variation in the content and teaching of herbalist courses. However, the National Institute of Medical Herbalists, which maintains a register of qualified herbalists, will only accept practitioners who have undertaken an approved course and a strict code of ethics is maintained [85]. Similarly, the Society of Homoeopaths maintains a register for practitioners who do not have conventional health care qualifications [86]. Patients who wish to try alternative medicines should be encouraged to use practitioners who are included on such registers.

Building the Evidence Base for Alternative Medicines

One of the main reservations that many conventional health care professionals have regarding the use of alternative medicines is the lack of research evidence to support claims of efficacy and effectiveness. In this era of evidence-based medicine, provision of an evidence base is as essential to the assessment of alternative medicine as any other intervention. Importantly, both the quantity and quality of research studies on alternative medicine is increasing [84], with a greater focus on randomized controlled trials, which are considered to be the gold standard in terms of assessing clinical efficacy and effectiveness [83]. Many of these trials are also finding their way into highly regarded journals which is a testimony to their quality [30, 54, 67, 91]. An increasing number of systematic reviews are also available which provide guidance on the value of products and interventions [32]. While it has been argued by some that this alternative form of health care cannot be assessed by conventional research techniques, this is seldom the case. However, there are obstacles in the form of a lack of research culture in alternative therapy practice and research funding has been difficult to obtain [34]. In the USA, the federal government has shown a degree of commitment to research in this area by the establishment of the National Center for Complementary and Alternative Medicine with an annual budget of approximately $70 millions [64]. The inclusion of elderly patients in research trials should also be recommended. It has been highlighted that this patient population has generally been excluded from trials on drugs which are extensively used in the elderly [3]. These trials may demonstrate the impact of physiological changes due to ageing on the pharmacokinetics and pharmacodynamics of alternative products.

The demand for evidence will grow from health care provider organizations as they attempt to distribute resources cost-effectively and if research findings support the use of certain products, as in the case of St. John's Wort for mild depression [91], this will increase the likelihood of alternative therapies being available and paid for through national and/or local drug benefit systems.

The Role of Conventional Health Care Professionals in Promoting the Safe and Effective Use of Alternative Medicines

Many mainstream health professionals feel ill-prepared to offer advice to patients on alternative medicines due to their lack of training and knowledge of the field and this has been a major barrier to their appropriate use [7]. This is changing to some extent with undergraduate courses in both medicine and pharmacy starting to include material on alternative medicine [68, 73]. Although such courses do not provide a definitive training in the provision of this type of health care, they do represent a base from which conventional health care professionals can develop and build upon. Postgraduate courses are also available and are likely to be increasingly popular as conventional practitioners are faced with demand for information from patients. This type of training may also alter attitudes of mainstream clinicians, who have often viewed the field of alternative medicine with scepticism and suspicion. Bouldin et al. [11] reported that a survey of pharmacists revealed that the profession had little confidence in herbal medicines. The authors speculated that such attitudes may change if pharmacists had greater familiarity with the topic and if they were able to access balanced and objective information [11]. Zollman and Vickers [97] commented that doctors generally regard alternative therapies as being of unproven benefit.

Indeed, conventional health care professionals must demonstrate increasing awareness that their patients may be taking alternative medicines, perhaps in place of prescribed or recommended medicines. Professions who are responsible for prescribing medication, either through a formal prescription or through the supply of a non-prescription product, must ask appropriate questions. Pharmacies often stock a wide variety of alternative medicines, hence, pharmacists, in their role of health advisors, must become more familiar with the products they recommend and supply and in addition ask patients about their use of alternative products, to avoid potential drug interactions or to ascertain underlying causes of new signs or symptoms.

Conclusions

This chapter has provided an overview of some of the main challenges which must be considered in the use of alternative medicines in the elderly. Many of the issues, such as adverse effects and drug interactions, are not unique to this section of the population, but such problems may be magnified due to changes in physiology brought on by ageing, and the perennial problem of polypharmacy and decreased resilience to adverse effects in elderly patients. Regulation, research and training represent a number of strategies which can promote safe, effective and appropriate use of alternative medicines in this unique patient group.

References

1. Adams ME (1999) Hype about glucosamine. Lancet 354: 353–354
2. Astin JA, Pelletier KR, Marie A, Haskell WL (2000) Complementary and alternative medicine use among elderly persons: one-year analysis of a Blue Shield Medicare Supplement. J Gerontol 55A: M4–M9
3. Avorn J (1997) Including elderly people in clinical trials. BMJ 315: 1033–1034
4. Bayly GR, Braithwaite RA, Sheehan TMT, Dyer NH, Grimley C, Ferner RE (1995) Lead poisoning from Asian traditional remedies in the West Midlands-report of a series of five cases. Hum Exp Toxicol 14: 24–28
5. Bensoussan A, Myers S, Carlton AL (2000) Risks associated with the practice of traditional Chinese medicine. Arch Fam Med 9: 1071–1078
6. Benzi G, Ceci A (1997) Herbal medicines in European regulation. Pharmacol Res 35: 355–362
7. Berman BM (2001) Complementary medicine and medical education. BMJ 322: 121–122
8. Blass JP, Sheu KF, Cooper AJ, Jung EH, Gibson GE (1992) Thiamine and Alzheimer's disease. J Nutr Sci Vitaminol 20: 401–404.
9. Bliddal H, Rosetzky A, Schlichting P et al. (2000) A randomized placebo-controlled cross-over study of ginger extracts and ibuprofen in osteoarthritis. Osteoarthritis and Cartilage 8: 9–12
10. Blotman F, Maheu E, Wulwik A, Caspard H, Lopez A (1997) Efficacy and safety of avocado/soybean unsaponifiables in the treatment of symptomatic osteoarthritis of the knee and hip. A prospective, multicenter, three-month, randomized, double-blind, placebo-controlled trial. Revue du Rhumatisne, English Edition 64: 825–834
11. Bouldin AS, Smith MC, Garner DD, Szeinbach SL, Frate DA, Croom EM (1999) Pharmacy and herbal medicine in the US. Soc Sci Med 49: 279–289
12. Braun L (2001) Herb-drug interactions. Aust Fam Physician 30: 473–476
13. Britton J, Pavord I, Richards K, Wisniewski A, Knox A, Lewis S, Tattersfield A, Weiss S (1994) Dietary magnesium, lung function, wheezing and airway hyper-activity in a random adult population sample. Lancet 344: 357–362
14. Capasso R, Izzo AA, Pinto L, Bifulco T, Vitobello C, Mascolo N (2000) Phytotherapy and quality of herbal medicines. Fitoterapia 71: S58–S65
15. Cappuccio FP, Duneclift SM, Atkinson RW, Cook DG (2001) Use of alternative medicines in a multi-ethnic population. Ethnicity and Disease 11: 11–18
16. Castiglioni CL, Gramolini C (1986) Effects of long-term treatment with sobrerol on the exacerbations of chronic bronchitis. Respiration 50: 202–217
17. Chan TYK, Critchley JAJH (1996) Usage and adverse effects of some Chinese herbal medicines. Hum Exp Toxiocol 15: 5–12
18. Chan TYK (1997) Monitoring the safety of herbal medicines. Drug Safety 17: 209–215
19. Chard J, Dieppe P (2001) Glucosamine for osteoarthritis: magic, hype or confusion. BMJ 322: 1439–1440
20. Chitturi S, Farrell GC (2000) Herbal toxicity: an expanding but poorly defined problem. J Gastroenterol Hepatol 15: 1093–1099

21. Cohen M (2000) What is complementary medicine? Aust Fam Physician 29: 1125–1133
22. Compendium of Health Statistics. 11ᵗʰ edition, Office of Health Economics, London 1999
23. Cui J, Garle M, Eneroth P, Bjorkhem I (1994) What do commercial ginseng preparations contain? Lancet 344: 134
24. Cullen P (2001) IMB wants strict checks on all herbal medicines. Irish Times, Wednesday, November 21
25. Dello Buono M, Urciuoli O, Marietta P, Padoani W, De Leo D (2001) Alternative medicine in a sample of 655 community-dwelling elderly. J Psychosom Res 50: 147–154
26. DeSmet PAGM (1995) Should herbal medicine-like products be licensed as medicines? BMJ 310: 1023–1024
27. Diamond JR, Pallone TL (1994) Acute interstitial nephritis following use of tong shueh pills. Am J Kidney Dis 24: 219–221
28. Dickstein ES, Kunkel FW (1980) Foxglove tea poisoning. Am J Med 69: 167–169
29. Drew AK, Myers SP (1997) Safety issues in herbal medicine: implications for the health professions. Med J Aust 166: 538–541
30. Drew S, Davies E (2001) Effectiveness of Ginkgo biloba in treating tinnitus: double-blind, placebo controlled trial. BMJ 322: 1–6
31. Eisenberg DM, Kessler RC, Foster C, Norlock FE, Calkins DR, Delbanco TL (1993) Unconventional medicine in the United States: prevalence, costs and patterns of use. N Engl J Med 328: 246–252
32. Ernst E (2000) Data supplement. Full list of systematic reviews of herbal medicinal products. BMJ 395: 1–3
33. Ernst E (2000) Herbal medicines: where is the evidence? BMJ 321: 395–396
34. Ernst E (2000) The role of complementary and alternative medicine. BMJ 321: 1133–1135
35. Fisher P, Ward A (1994) Medicine in Europe: complementary medicine in Europe. BMJ 309: 107–111
36. Gertner E, Marshall PS, Filandrinos D, Potek AS, Smith TM (1995) Complications resulting from the use of Chinese herbal medications containing undeclared prescription drugs. Arthritis Rheum 38: 614–617
37. Goethe JW, Price AL (2000) Herbal medicines with psychiatric indications: a review for practitioners. Connecticut Med 64: 347–351
38. Gould M (2001) Patients warned of dangers of Chinese medicines. BMJ 323: 770
39. Gupta SK, Kaleekal T, Joshi S (2000) Misuse of corticosteroids in some of the drugs dispensed as preparations from alternative systems of medicine in India. Pharmacoepidemiol Drug Safety 9: 599–602
40. Hainer MI, Tsai N, Komura ST, Chiu CL (2000) Fatal hepatorenal failure associated with hydrazine sulfate. Ann Intern Med 133: 911–913
41. Hawthorne K (1990) Asian diabetics attending a British hospital clinic: a pilot study to evaluate their care. Br J Gen Pract 40: 243–247
42. Herbal roulette. Consumer reports (1995): 698–705
43. Hughes CM, McElnay JC, Fleming GF (2002) Benefits and risks of self-medication. Drug Safety 24: 1027–1037
44. Huxtable RJ, Awang DVC (1990) Pyrrolizidine poisoning. Am J Med 89: 547–548
45. Kamiyama T, Nouchin T, Kojima S, Murata N, Ikeda T, Sato O (1997) Autoimmune hepatitis triggered by administration of a herbal medicine. Am J Gastroenterol 92: 703–704
46. Kanba S, Yamada K, Mizushima H, Asai M (1998) Use of herbal medicine for treating psychiatric disorders in Japan. Psychiatry Clin Neurosci 52: S31–S333
47. Kaufman DW, Kelly JP, Rosenberg L, Anderson TE, Mitchell AA (2002) Recent patterns of medication use in the ambulatory adult population of the United States. The Slone Survey. J Am Med Assoc 287: 337–344
48. Keane FM, Munn SE, du Vivier AWP, Taylor NF, Higgin EM (1999) Analysis of Chinese herbal creams prescribed for dermatological conditions. BMJ 318: 563–564
49. Kew C, Morris C, Aihie A, Fysh R, Jones S, Brooks D (1993) Arsenic and mercury intoxication due to Indian ethnic remedies. BMJ 306: 506–507
50. Kosty MP, Fleishman SB, Herndon JE et al. (1994) Cisplatin, vinblastine and hydrazine sulfate in advanced non-small-cell lung cancer: a randomized placebo-controlled, double-blind phase III study of the Cancer and Leukemia Group B. J Clin Oncol 12: 1113–1120
51. Kumana CR, Ng M, Lin HJ, Ko W, Wu PC, Todd D (1983) Hepatic veno-occlusive disease due to toxic alkaloid herbal tea. Lancet 2: 1360–1361
52. Kumana CR, Ng M, Lin HJ, Ko W, Wu PC, Todd D (1985) Herbal tea induced hepatic veno-occlusive disease: quantification of toxic alkaloid exposure in adults. Gut 26: 101–104
53. LaFrance WC, Lauterbach EC, Coffey CE et al. (2000) The use of herbal medicines in neuropsychiatry. J Neuropsych Clin Neurosci 12: 177–192
54. Lewith GT, Watkins AD, Hyland ME, Shaw S, Broomfield JA, Dolan G (2002) Use of ultramolecular potencies of allergen to treat asthmatic people allergic to house dust mite: double blind randomised controlled clinical trial. BMJ 324: 520–523
55. Lin SH, Lin MS (1994) A survey on drug-related hospitalization in a community teaching hospital. Intern J Clin Pharmacol Ther Toxicol 31: 66–69
56. Linde R, Ramirez G, Mulrow CD, Pauls A, Weidenhammer W, Melchart D. (1996) St. John's Wort for depression: an overview and meta-analysis of randomised clinical trials. BMJ 313: 253–258
57. Liu JM, Cgu HC, Chin YH, Chen YM, Hsieh RK, Chiou TJ, Whang-Peng J (1997) Cross-sectional study of use of alternative medicines in Chinese cancer patients. Japan J Clin Oncol 27: 37–41
58. Lord GM, Tagore R, Cook T Gower P, Pusey CD (1999) Nephropathy caused by Chinese herbs in the UK. Lancet 354:481–482
59. Ma GX (1999) Between two worlds: the use of traditional and Western health services by Chinese immigrants. J Com Health 24: 421–437

60. MacLennan AH, Wilson DH Taylor AW (1996) Prevalence and cost of alternative medicine in Australia. Lancet 347: 569–572

61. Marshall RJ, Gee R, Israel M et al. (1990) The use of alternative therapies by Auckland general practitioners. N Z Med J 103: 213–215

62. Mills SY (2001) The House of Lords report on complementary medicine: a summary. Complement Ther Med 9: 34–39

63. Mossad SB, Macknin ML, Medendorp SV, Mason P (1996) Zinc gluconate lozenges for treating the common cold-a randomized double-blind, placebo-controlled study. Ann Intern Med 125: 81–89

64. Nahin RL, Straus SE (2001) Research into complementary and alternative medicine: problems and potential. BMJ 322: 161–164

65. Northern Ireland Regional Medicines and Poisons Information Services, The Royal Hospitals, Belfast Northern Ireland (2001) Safety concerns with alternative medicines. Drug Data 53, June

66. Nortier JL, Matinez M-CM, Schmeiser H et al. (2000) Urothelial carcinoma associated with the use of a Chinese herb (*Aristolochia fanchi*). N Engl J Med 342: 1686–1692

67. Oken BS, Storzbach DM, Kaye JA (2001) The efficacy of Gingko biloba on cognitive function in Alzheimer's disease. Arch Neurol 55: 1409–1415

68. Owen DK, Lewith G, Stephens CR (2001) Can doctors respond to patients' increasing interest in complementary and alternative medicine? BMJ 322: 154–158

69. Perharic L, Shaw D, Colbridge M, House I, Leon C, Murray V (1994) Toxicological problems resulting from exposure to traditional remedies and food supplements. Drug Safety 11: 284–294

70. Pies R (2000) Adverse neuropsychiatric reactions to herbal and over-the-counter "antidepressants". J Clin Psych 61: 815–820

71. Randall C, Randall H, Dobbs F, Hutton C, Sanders H (2000) Randomized controlled trial of nettle sting for treatment of base-of-thumb pain. J R Soc Med 93: 305–309

72. Reginster JY, Deroisy R, Rovati LC et al. (2001) Long-term effects of glucosamine sulphate on osteoarthritis progression: a randomised, placebo-controlled clinical trial. Lancet 357: 251–256

73. Royal Pharmaceutical Society of Great Britain (2001) Consultation on revised requirements for accreditation of pharmacy degrees. Pharm J 267: 172–173

74. Ryan EA, Pick ME, Marceau C (2001) Use of alternative medicines in diabetes mellitus. Diabet Med 18: 242–245

75. Saxe TG (1987) Toxicity of medicinal herbal preparations. Am Fam Physician 35: 135–142

76. Shannon M (1999) Alternative medicines toxicology: a review of selected agents. Clin Toxicol 37: 709–713

77. Sheehan DM (1998) Herbal medicines, phytoestrogens and toxicity: risk:benefit considerations. Exp Biol Med 217: 379–385

78. Shetty HGM, Woodhouse K (1999) Geriatrics. In: Walker R, Edwards C (eds) Clinical pharmacy and therapeutics, 2nd edn. Churchill Livingstone, Edinburgh, pp 119–131

79. Siegal R (1979) Ginseng abuse syndrome. Problems with the panacea. J Am Med Assoc 241: 1614–1615

80. Skorodin MS (1995) Magenesium sulfate in exacerbation of chronic obstructive pulmonary disease. Arch Int Med 155: 496–500

81. Stockley I (2001). Drug interactions, 5th edn. Pharmaceutical Press, London

82. Vanherweghem JL, Depierreux M, Tielemans C et al. (1993) Rapidly progressive interstitial renal fibrosis in young women: association with slimming regimen including Chinese herbs. Lancet 341: 387–391

83. Vickers A (1998) Bibliometric analysis of randomised controlled trials in complementary medicine. Complement Ther Med 6: 185–189

84. Vickers A (2000) Recent advances. Complementary medicine. BMJ 321: 683–686

85. Vickers A, Zollman C (1999) ABC of complementary medicine. Herbal medicine. BMJ 319: 1050–1053

86. Vickers A, Zollman C (1999) ABC of complementary medicine. Homoeopathy. BMJ 319:1115–1118

87. Vickers A, Zollman C (1999) ABC of complementary medicine. Massage therapies. BMJ 319:1254 –1257

88. Wagner PJ, Lester D, LeClair B, Taylor T, Woodward L, Lambert J (1999) Taking the edge off. Why patients choose St. John's wort. J Fam Pract 48: 615–619

89. Weiss SJ, Takakuwa KM, Ernst AA (2001) Use, understanding and beliefs about complementary and alternative medicines among Emergency Department patients. Acad Emerg Med 8: 41–47

90. Wilkens JH (1990) Effects of PAF-antagonist (BN 52063) on bronchoconstriction and platelet activation during exercise induced asthma. Br J Clin Pharmacol 29: 85–91

91. Woelk H for the Remotiv/Imipramine Study Group (2000) Comparison of St. John's wort and imipramine for treating depression: randomised controlled trial. BMJ 321: 536–539

92. Wu MS, Hong JJ, Lin JL, Yang CW, Chien HC (1996) Multiple tubular dysfunction induced by mixed Chinese herbal medicines containing cadmium. Nephrol Dialysis Transplant 11: 867–870

93. Yamey G (2000) Inquiry discovers fraudulent skin treatments. BMJ 320: 76

94. Yang CS, Lin CH, Chang SH, Hsu HC (2000) Rapidly progressive fibrosing interstitial associated with Chinese herbal drugs. Am J Kidney Dis 35: 313–318

95. Zajecka J, Tracy KA, Mitchell S (1997) Discontinuation symptoms after treatment with serotonin reuptake inhibitors: a literature review. J Clin Psychiat 58: 291–297

96. Zhang WY, Li Wan Po A (1994) The effectiveness of topically applied capsaicin. A meta analysis. Eur J Clin Pharmacol 46: 517–522

97. Zollman C, Vickers A (1999)-ABC of complementary medicine. Complementary medicine and the doctor. BMJ 319: 1558–1561

5 Ethical Issues Associated with CAM Use Among the Elderly

P. Komesaroff

The therapeutic use of complementary and alternative medicines (CAM) and the conduct of research into them raise a wide range of social and ethical issues. These issues, which have a special intensity in the case of elderly populations, concern the balance of benefits and harms associated with the practices, the extent to which consent can validly be given when evidence for efficacy and safety is lacking, the responsibility of the community as a whole to protect vulnerable people, and the lessons to be learnt by conventional medicine from the popularity of complementary therapies.

This article will review some of these issues, with a special focus on their implications for elderly people. It will consider in turn, implications of CAM for the individuals who use them, for their relationships with their health care team, and for the society more broadly. The question of the need for, and the problems confronting, research into complementary medicines will also be briefly addressed.

In the discussion that follows "ethics" is used in a broad sense to refer to the complex fields of values associated with complementary medicines and the problems of plotting trajectories through them, rather than in the more limited, frequently employed sense of a set of fixed "principles" or universal rules for action [29, 50]. We believe that it is only with such an approach that the richness of the problems to be addressed can be fully appreciated.

Ethical Issues in Relation to Individuals

The variety and importance of the ethical and social issues associated with the use of complementary medicines in part derive from the diversity of complementary medicines themselves and their widespread use. As is well recognized, the expression "complementary medicines" covers a wide range of practices, from historically well-established therapies, such as traditional Chinese medicine, to more exotic practices, such as color therapy and psychic healing [15]. Taken together, the precise extent of their use is unknown, but it is clear that the industry is a very large one, with evidence suggesting that in the U.S. and Australia about one fifth of the population visit alternative practitioners each year and up to half use complementary medicines on a regular basis [3, 18, 19, 36]. Evidence concerning use among elderly people is even more limited, although one study of older Americans estimated that about 30% are regular users [23], with a survey in Italy suggesting a similar figure [11]. As with younger people using complementary medicines, elderly people often use them in conjunction with, and not merely as a substitute for, conventional therapies [11, 23, 46]. Whatever the true figures and details of use, there is no doubt about the fact that very substantial numbers of elderly people are using complementary medicines, so that the issues raised are likely to carry large scale implications for both individuals and society.

It is well recognized that for many complementary therapies the evidence regarding clinical effectiveness and the risks associated with their use is limited [17, 39], a fact which itself raises important ethical issues, as discussed below. Randomized clinical trials have been few, and it is sometimes even argued that complementary therapies in general are in principle not susceptible to assessment using randomized trial designs. While significant insights have been achieved into physiological mechanisms of action, the clinical studies that have been performed have often been flawed by poor design, inadequate measures and statistical analysis, and lack of follow up data [3, 19].

There are a few settings in which credible evidence for the effectiveness of complementary medicines exists. Vitamin therapy in the case of dietary insufficiency is an obvious example. There is some evidence from randomized controlled trials suggestive of positive effects of various complementary therapies in the elderly: for example, therapeutic touch reduces chronic pain in osteoarthritis [17]; massage reduces anxiety [24]; music-based therapy is effective in the management of depression [26]; acupressure may assist with the treatment of sleep disturbances [8]; and Alexander technique may enhance functional reach [12]. Of course, these examples reflect only a trivial component of the actual use of these therapies and emphasize the need for further rigorous and wide ranging study. Nonetheless, they do emphasize the fact that many complementary treatments are likely to be effective and that, at least in cases where the risks are minimal and with the provisos mentioned below, there is often little harm done by patients choosing to use them.

People take complementary medicines for many reasons, including to treat disease, to control symptoms, and to manage side-effects of conventional medicines. Users of CAM generally consider that they obtain benefit from them, although there appears sometimes to be a degree of doubt [33]. Lack of evidence from randomized controlled trials is not always a disincentive to use, as is shown by the example of the many conventional medicines that have never been subjected to such testing; this is probably based at least partly on the recognition that knowledge gained from personal experience and passed on from practitioner to practitioner is a valuable and indispensable form of evidence within all medical traditions. In the case of the elderly, resort to CAM use may also reflect the lack of efficacy of conventional medicines in relation to their specific medical conditions. For example, limited treatments only are available for dementia, general malaise and frailty; for individuals suffering from these conditions complementary medicines may provide actual relief, or – perhaps more importantly in some cases – may offer hope or other psychological or social benefits.

Avoidance of conventional medicines may in many cases save the community money and allow elderly people to avoid unpleasant side effects and interactions commonly associated with conventional pharmaceutical agents in this age group; this can still be the case even if control of symptoms is incomplete. In this context, the costs of adverse effects of conventional drugs should not be underestimated: for example, it has been estimated that on average one in 1200 persons taking NSAIDs for at least 2 months will die from gastroduodenal complications who would not have died had they not taken NSAIDs [47]; it is unlikely that the morbidity of complementary therapies could rival this result. This issue is likely to be of particular importance for the elderly as it is well recognized that in older age groups drug interactions and side effects are more common [9].

These considerations are relevant to the assessment of the overall balance of harm and benefit of CAM. However, they are by no means sufficient to allow the possibility of serious harm associated with either lack of efficacy or significant toxicity of complementary medications to be dismissed. Individuals who are sick are always vulnerable as a result of their illnesses. Those who seek out complementary medicines may be particularly vulnerable if they are doing so in response to a perception that conventional medicine is unable to meet their needs; elderly people may be additionally vulnerable if they are suffering from diminished cognitive capacity and have little access to sources of information on which they can rely.

The risks associated with the use of complementary medicines, as with orthodox ones, may be considerable. Use of complementary treatments might lead to withdrawal from appropriate medical therapy or delays in diagnosis or treatment of underlying conditions [1, 10 42]. CAM diagnostic methods may result in falsely positive diagnoses that generate anxiety and which may incur their own treatment costs [21]. In most countries, complementary practitioners are not required to complete formal medical training and instead undergo training programs that are essentially unregulated. This raises the possibility of wide variations in levels of competence and the ability to identify serious underlying illnesses or contraindications for CAM therapies.

Physical treatments can cause adverse effects and herbal therapies can be either toxic themselves or contaminated with toxic substances: serious reactions and even death can occur [14, 19, 30, 37]. Complications of acupuncture have included pneumothorax and puncture of other vital organs, spinal cord lesions, and infections, including HIV and hepatitis B [25, 41], once again associated with possible death [38]. Such misadventures are well documented in the medical literature. Diagnostic techniques themselves are often associated with risk, and those employed in complementary medicines are unlikely to represent an exception. Excessive use of X-ray diagnosis by some chiropractors may carry some degree of hazard [20]. In many cases, interactions of complementary medicines with each other, or with conventional medicines, are poorly understood but, as the recent example of St John's Wort has shown, are potentially serious [44]. Accordingly, it is likely that the elderly are at particular risk of adverse effects of complementary medicines. The substances and techniques promoted as "complementary" can vary widely in quality and effectiveness. While efficacy may be limited [39, 48], direct adverse or toxic effects of medicinal substances or contaminants may be so severe as to cause serious, including lethal, reactions [14, 30, 37]. Contaminants recorded in herbal medical preparations include heavy metals, infectious agents and pesticides, but of particular concern is the prevalence of contamination with non-declared herbs or conventional pharmaceutical agents [28]. It is sometimes argued that where therapies have been in use for many years it can be taken for granted that they are safe and effective; however, while this is no doubt true in many cases, it cannot be generally assumed, as the examples above and those of many orthodox drugs have shown. It is not known to what extent elderly people suffer adverse events from herbal medications, either as direct toxic effects or as the results of interactions with other herbals or with conventional drugs, although it might be expected that, as with drug treatments in general, the elderly would be particularly susceptible. This is made more likely by the fact that elderly people are in many cases already taking multiple medications and may suffer from chronic conditions that alter drug metabolism or excretion.

If they were to offer effective and safe alternatives to expensive conventional treatments complementary medicines could potentially result in reduced costs of medical care. However in many cases, the costs of complementary medicines are very considerable and cost benefits are uncertain [6, 49]. With respect to overall expenditures in Western countries incomplete data only are available, but it is estimated that in the U.S., expenditure on complementary therapies in 1990 was about $14 billion [15] and a later estimate suggests that the figure is now closer to $27 billion [19]. In the U.K., the annual expenditure on CAM for the whole U.K. population was estimated to be in the region of £ 1.6 billion per annum [22], about 4% of the public expenditure on health. For Australia, the figure is also likely to be in the billions of dollars [24, 50, Alastair MacLennan, pers. communication]. In many cases – especially in countries like the U.K. and Australia, where the costs of pharmaceuticals is heavily subsidized by the community – the costs of CAM significantly exceed those of conventional medications. Clearly, these costs may carry ethical implications. Individuals with serious or chronic diseases are more likely to be indigent than other members of the population, and the additional cost of complementary medicines may cause real hardship. This applies particularly to elderly people, who are on average less well off than younger people. Furthermore, resources devoted to complementary medicines are resources diverted from other uses, and adverse effects may lead to additional expenses by increasing demand for health care facilities; it is appropriate that these potential costs are also taken into account.

In additional to their actions – positive or negative – in the treatment of disease and their financial costs, there are also possible more subtle effects of complementary medicines. They may, for example, have an impact on the relationships between patients and their careers which are either beneficial or harmful, which is the case depending on the specific circumstances of the relationship. On the one hand, it is possible that negotiation around the use of conventional or complementary medicines may offer an opportunity for constructive dialogues about alternative health care strategies and lead to an increased emphasis on lifestyle and dietary factors in the prevention and treatment of disease; thus patients may feel empowered by their ability to direct their own health care decisions independently of representatives of established authority; and doctors may recognize in the growing interest in complementary medicines an expression of dissatisfaction by their patients and respond to it by greater openness and more effective communication. On the other hand, it is possible that the use of these therapies may undermine the relationship by eroding the openness and trust that is essential for effective medical care [32]: indeed, there is evidence that in many cases patients – perhaps about half [18, 36] and maybe up to 60% of older persons [43] – do not tell their doctors that they are using complementary therapies, largely because they fear disapproval, which, in some cases at least, appears justified [4, 16]. Lack of disclosure may lead to confusion, guilt, embarrassment and hesitation to seek medical care when required, and may disrupt finely balanced caring networks; where serious illness is present this may result in significant risk [34].

In view of all these risks and uncertainties, the ethical arguments in favor of rigorous clinical testing of complementary therapies are compelling. Indeed, few would contest the proposition that consumers should have access to reliable information about the safety and efficacy of treatments they are considering using, or that the systematic collection of data is an effective way of obtaining useful information. However, even here ethical complexities arise. Testing of pharmaceutical agents using clinical trials, which to many appears a transparent, objective exercise, is in fact itself subject to philosophical problems and biases [31]. The use of placebo controls, for example, has been questioned, especially where an accepted therapy exists. Randomized clinical trials have been criticized because they test only a narrow range of specifically designated end-points, as a result of which qualitative variables that assess issues relating to values, such as patient experience, are systematically omitted. It is argued that through this technique only information about average effects among large groups of people can be produced, overlooking individual differences and excluding therapies – like many complementary ones – that tend to be highly individualized. These arguments emphasize the need for the development of testing strategies that are appropriate to the specific practices under investigation and to the fact that formal study using randomized controlled trials does not replace traditional forms of communication, including the sharing of clinical experience amongst practitioners, the reporting of individual cases documenting successes, failures and adverse events, or basic research into physiological processes. This point is especially important in relation to elderly patients, who may experience particular difficulty understanding technical data. This will obviously be the case where the patient is suffering from dementia or cognitive impairment for outer reasons [27]. In these cases, special care needs to be taken to ensure that adequate communication is established either with the patient or with the person legally responsible for him or her.

In summary, as with orthodox medical practices, the possibility of significant harm associated with the use of complementary therapies, either because of adverse effects of the medications themselves or indirectly, due to disruption of established caring practices and networks, raises complex ethical considerations. As a general rule, it should be accepted that individual consumers ought to be able to know what the effects of the substances or treatments they are considering using are likely to be. However, testing processes themselves are not free of value-related assumptions, and this also must be taken into consideration when assessing the nature and the quality of the available evidence and the range of possibilities for obtaining new information. The complexity of these issues emphasizes both the importance of careful communication with patients about all aspects of complementary medicine use, including the current status of the evidence and limits of knowledge and the underlying reasons for seeking these therapies in the first place, and the extent to which in elderly patients the process of "consent" can be very finely balanced.

Ethical Issues in Relation to Society

The widespread use of complementary medicines raises ethical questions of a broader, social kind. Why have risk and lack of evidence not deterred potential patients and practitioners? Even if is widely accepted that individuals should be free to make their own choices with respect to health care, are not claims of cures matters of public interest affecting public health? Further, does the community have an obligation to protect vulnerable citizens from exploitation by practitioners with uncertain qualifications who apply practices with dubious benefits and unknown risks? Should special measures be introduced to protect such citizens from practices that may lead to their being denied conventional therapies of proven efficacy [40]? Should the training and rights to practise of complementary therapists – at present largely unrestricted – be subject to a formal system of regulation? And should the application of public funds be directed by consumer demand, or should it be limited to practices – orthodox or complementary – for which reasonable evidence of effectiveness and safety can be provided?

The question of why people use complementary therapies is an important one which may have ethical implications of its own. Some of the reasons are mentioned above: there is also evidence that people turn to alternatives because they are disillusioned with orthodox medicine, as a result of dissatisfaction either with doctor patient interaction patterns or with medicine in general [45]. In the latter case, declining public support for hospitals and the introduction of economic practices such as managed care that promote cost saving in the face of potentially deleterious implications for the clinical encounter may well exacerbate this process. In general, elderly people are especially vulnerable to changes in health policy and escalating costs of health care and may be particularly susceptible to such disillusionment.

Broader philosophical and sociological considerations may also be of importance. It is widely held that complementary therapies may appeal to philosophical perspectives not accessible to orthodox practices: for example, they may incorporate systems of embodiment at variance with – and maybe even contradictory to – those of a medicine based on the principles of the biological sciences. Further, interest in complementary medicines at least in part reflects a reaction in the community against the social role of orthodox medical institutions and the value systems they are thought to represent. It is likely, therefore, that at least some of the interest in complementary therapies can be understood in terms of the development of a more heterogeneous and diverse cultural environment, in which a multiplicity of philosophical and ethical perspectives, of concepts of the body, of truth and of values coexist. Like other patients, elderly people conceptualize their use of drugs in moral terms, even if they commonly adopt the language of medicine to formulate and legitimate their perspectives. They therefore make decisions about their treatments in relation to philosophical variables [5, 7, 35] and will use complementary therapies if they are seen as compatible with their values, worldviews and beliefs about health and illness [2].

These considerations lead naturally to the question of the regulation of complementary medicines. If complementary health practices are associated with significant potential risks to individuals and may carry widespread social implications it is appropriate for the community as a whole to develop policies for their regulation and control. Classically, the question here has been formulated in terms of an ethical dilemma: should individuals be allowed to make their own decisions about the medical practices they utilize, unconstrained by paternalistic intrusions by government or government controlled agencies, or should medical therapies be subject to rigorous processes of surveillance, regulation and control in order to protect the community from unsafe practices and prevent the exploitation of vulnerable citizens? This dilemma is presented as a decision between unrestrained choices of individuals on the one hand and mutual responsibilities of the members of a community to each other on the other; or, in legal terms, between rights of individuals and their social obligations.

In the case of orthodox medicine a similar argument was conducted long ago, with the question being decided forcefully in favor of regulation. An elaborate system of legally based processes restricts the ability of untrained and unscrupulous individuals to present themselves as practitioners of conventional medicine and so exploit the weak and the vulnerable for the sake of profit. Medical education, medical practice and medical pharmaceutics are all tightly controlled to prevent this. Not surprisingly, it is often argued – especially by orthodox practitioners – that similar processes should apply to complementary medicines, since the ethical arguments about regulation are general ones. Such a regulatory regime would require the development of an apparatus to control the selection and education of complementary practitioners, to oversee the specific details of the practice of complementary medicines, and to scrutinize the administration and availability of drugs. Although the case for such a system has been strongly put, however, it is by no means universally accepted, and many argue that the value of individual freedom should be regarded as stronger than the putative obligations of citizenship. As a result, although governments have generally recognized the need for some level of regulation of complementary medical practices this has been instituted at a rather restrained level, at least in comparison with the restrictions imposed on orthodox medicine. While in the latter case, the emphasis has been placed on controlling the actions of individual practitioners, in the former it has been on informing the patient or consumer and allowing him or her to make the choice.

The basis for this discrepancy between the approaches to regulation of conventional and complementary medicines is itself a matter of ongoing debate. On one side, it is argued that similar standards should be applied to all forms of medical practice. On the other, it is claimed that the two are in fact sufficiently different to justify divergent regulatory strategies: complementary medicines are – so it is said – inherently less dangerous, and in any case the level of public demand and the variety of complementary therapies means that tight control would simply not be possible. But – the proponents of regulation rejoin – conclusions about safety are difficult to draw in the absence of carefully conducted clinical trials, and anyway the fact that any claim for effective medical treatment, no matter how outlandish or improbable, will attract people willing to subject themselves to it, often in desperation and without careful analysis, is an argument in favor of regulation rather than against it.

Both arguments have considerable cogency, and indeed, it is impossible to make a clear choice between them. This however, merely demonstrates that the regulation question is more complex than the classical formulation suggests. Freedom and justice, here presented as mutually exclusive possibilities, are not independent of each other but are intimately related in the social and cultural context in which they are identified as problems and subsequently interpreted and theorized. Similarly, the reasons people choose to utilize complementary medicines – or, for that matter, orthodox ones – are themselves complicated and invariably incorporate varying cultural, philosophical, ethical, and maybe psychological, factors. The question of the regulation of medical practices raises fundamental issues about the nature of both orthodox and complementary medicines, the cultural contexts in which they are embedded, and their relationships with each other. The task of devising an appropriate framework within which different medical cultures can coexist – however it is ultimately resolved – must take into account all these levels of complexity.

Conclusion: The Need for a New Paradigm

The ethical problems associated with the use of complementary medicines in the elderly are diverse and complex, reflecting the interplay of social and cultural issues and sometimes the clash of philosophical perspectives. They may include fundamental questions about the nature of the different medical cultures available, their conceptual structures, the broader contexts in which they are embedded, and their relationships with each other. Furthermore, the problems raised in connection with CAM use in the elderly are not qualitatively different from those raised with respect to different age groups, although some particular issues may be of special importance, so that the emphases may be different. The problems are epitomized in the very terms that are used to describe the practices of CAM, which refer to their fluctuating relationships with conventional medicines as either "complementary" or as "alternative". For reasons that have in part been discussed above, neither paradigm is fully adequate: the notion of alternativeness suggests that the two medical cultures are independent and that individuals simply need to make a choice of one or the other, but this is misleading because they stand in a dynamic relationship and may serve different purposes, even for a single individual; and the concept of complementarity suggests that they stand in a relationship not of rupture but of continuity, which is problematic too, because it elides the – sometimes radical – differences between them and obscures the possibility of qualitative choice.

This article has argued implicitly that there are no straightforward solutions to the ethical and social perplexities raised by the popularity of CAM, but that what is required is a proper appreciation of the range of issues and perspectives involved. Such an appreciation itself requires a more adequate account of the relationships between different medical practices, which allows simultaneously for the coexistence of both continuity and difference, cohesion and opposition, interchangeability and incommensurable difference. While there is no established concept for such a category of dynamic relations, the philosophical idea of the "supplement" may provide some assistance. As in the case of contending medical approaches, a supplement provides something additional, something that is lacking, but in the process also retains a critical difference that may stimulate the mutual recognition of underlying assumptions and deficiencies. It adds itself, it is a surplus, a "plenitude, enriching another plenitude", while at the same time it intervenes or insinuates itself in the place of something else, it fills a gap that without it remains invisible [13].

The clear articulation and elaboration of a concept that retains the key ideas underlying both complementarity and alternativeness while preserving their mutual tension and fecundity is more than a mere matter of language. It emphasizes the practical task of respecting and actively promoting divergent sets of possibilities, and thus of opening up a "third way" between the established polarities. It sets the scene for a dynamic interplay of ideas that may stimulate critical reflections on strengths and weaknesses, achievements and deficiencies, and – hopefully – new insights and therapeutic possibilities. It also well represents the challenge presented by the problem of regulation of medical practices in general: the challenge to develop a cultural and legal framework that can simultaneously promote the achievement of mutually held goals and preserve radical and critical oppositions between them, that encourages the exchange of ideas based on both deep complexity and radical difference.

In conclusion, complementary medicines raise a range of ethical issues which bear on both their clinical applications and their social implications. These issues in turn are intertwined with scientific and philosophical questions and questions of social policy. The use of complementary medicines among elderly people focus many of these issues intensely, and it raises some additional ones of its own. In many cases, as with ethical debates in general, there are no clear answers. However, the debate itself is of value, as is the process it engenders of rich, ongoing dialogue within the community across different value perspectives.

References

1. Angell M and Kassirer JP (1998) Alternative medicine – The risks of untested and unregulated remedies. New Eng J Med 339: 839–840
2. Astin J (1998) Why patients use alternative medicine. Results of a national survey. JAMA 279: 1548–1553
3. Ban E (1998) Australian alternatives. Nat Med 1998; 4: 8
4. Berman B, Singh BK, Lao L, Singh BB, Ferenz KS, Hartnoll SM (1995) Physicians' attitudes towards complementary or alternative medicines: a regional survey. J Am Board of Family Practitioners 8: 361–366
5. Britten N (1994) Patients' ideas about medicines: a qualitative study in a general practice population. Brit J Gen Practice 44: 465–468
6. Carey TS, Garrett J, Jackman A, McLaughlin C, Fryer J, Smucker DR (1995) The outcomes and costs of care for acute low back pain among patients seen by primary care practitioners, chiropractors, and orthopaedic surgeons. The North Carolina Back Pain Project. New Engl J Med 333: 913–917
7. Cartwright A, Smith C (1995) Elderly people, their medicines and doctors. Routledge, London
8. Chen ML, Lin LC, Wu SC, Lin JG (1999) Effectiveness of acupressure in improving the quality of sleep of institutionalised residents. J Gerontol Med Sci 54A: M389–M394
9. Conrad KA, Bressler R (1982) Drug therapy for the elderly. CV Mosby, St Louis
10. Coppes MJ, Anderson RA, Egeler RM, Wolff JEA (1998) Alternative therapies for the treatment of childhood cancer. New Engl J Med 339: 846
11. Della Buono M, Urciuoli O, Marietta P, Padoani W, De Leo D (2000) Alternative medicine in a sample of 655 community dwelling elderly. J Psychosomatic Res 50: 147–154
12. Dennis RJ (1999) Functional reach improvement in normal older women after Alexander technique instruction. J Gerontol Biol Sci Med Sci 54: 8–11
13. Derrida J (1967) Of Grammatology. Johns Hopkins UP, Maryland pp 144–145
14. Drew AK, Myers SP (1997) Safety issues in herbal medicine: implications for the health professions. Med J Aust 166: 538–541
15. Eagle R (1978) Alternative Medicine. Futura, London
16. Easthope G, Tranter B, Gill G (2000) General practitioners' attitudes toward complementary therapies. Soc Sci Med 51(10): 1555–1561

17. Eckes Peck SD (1997) The effectiveness of therapeutic touch for decreasing pain in elders with degenerative arthritis. J Holistic Nurs 15: 176–198
18. Eisenberg DM, Kessler RC, Foster C et al. (1993) Unconventional medicine in the United States: prevalence, costs and patterns of use. New Eng J Med 328: 246–252
19. Eisenberg D M, Davis R, Ettner S L, Appel S, Wilkey S, Rompay M V (1998) Trends in alternative medicine use in the United States, 1990–1997. JAMA 280: 1569–1575
20. Ernst E (1998) Chiropractors' use of X-rays. Br J Radiol 71: 249–251
21. Ernst E (2000) Iridology – not useful and potentially harmful. Arch Ophthalmol 118: 120–121
22. Ernst E, White AR (2000) The BBC survey of complementary use in the United Kingdom. Compl Ther Med 8: 32–36
23. Foster DF, Phillips RF, Hamel MB, Eisenberg DM (2000) Alternative medicine use in older Americans. J Am Geriatr Soc 48: 1560–1565
24. Fraser J, Kerr JR (1993) Psychophysiological effects of back massage on elderly institutionalised patients. Nursing 18: 238–245
25. Halvorsen TB, Anda SS, Naess AB, Levang OW (1996) Fatal cardiac tamponade after acupuncture through congenital sternal foramen. Lancet 345: 1175
26. Hanser SB, Thompson LW (1994) Effects of music therapy strategy on depressed older adults. J Gerontol 49: 265–269
27. Hogan DB, Ebly EM. Complementary medicine use in a dementia clinic population. Alzheimer Dis Assoc Disord 1996;10(2):63–67.
28. Huang WF, Wen KC, Hsiao ML (1997) Adulteration by synthetic therapeutic substances of traditional Chinese medicines in Taiwan. J Clin Pharmacol 37: 334–350
29. Humber JM, Almeder RF (1998) Alternative medicine and ethics. Humana Press, New Jersey
30. Kelly S (1990) Aconite poisoning. Med J Aust 153: 499
31. Komesaroff PA, Wiltshire J (1994) Drugs in the health marketplace. Arena Publications, Melbourne
32. Komesaroff PA (1995) From bioethics to microethics. In: Komesaroff PA (ed) Troubled bodies. Duke UP, Durham
33. Lam K (2001) Use of CAM among patients with HIV/AIDS. Monash University BSc (Hons) thesis
34. Liu EH, Turner LM, Lin SX, Klaus L, Choi LY, Whitworth J, Ting W, Oz MC (2000) Use of alternative medicine by patients undergoing cardiac surgery. J Thorac Cardiovasc Surg 120(2): 335–341
35. Lumme-Sandt K, Hervonen A, Jylha M (2000) Interpretative repertoires of medication among the oldest-old. Soc Sci Med 50(12): 1843–1850
36. MacLennan A, Wilson D, Taylor A (1996) Prevalence and cost of alternative medicine in Australia. Lancet 347: 569–573
37. Mullins RJ (1998) Echinacea-associated anaphylaxis. Med J Aust 168: 170–171
38. National Health and Medical Research Council (1989) Acupuncture Working Party. NHMRC, Canberra
39. National Institutes of Health (1998) Acupuncture. NIH Consensus Statement
40. Neeley GS (1998) Legal and ethical dilemmas surrounding prayer as a method of alternative healing for children. In: Humber JM, Almeder RF (eds) Alternative medicine and ethics. Humana Press, New Jersey, pp 163–194
41. Norheim AJ, Vinjar Fønnebø (1995) Adverse effects of acupuncture. Lancet 345: 1576
42. Oneschuk D, Bruera E (1999) The potential dangers of complementary therapy use in a patient with cancer. J Palliat Care 15: 49–52
43. Pan CX, Pinderhughes S, Ek K, Senzel R, Cherniak P, Ness J (1999) Conversations between older patients and their physicians about use of alternative medicines. J Am Geriatr Soc 47(9): S104
44. Rey JM, Walter G (1998) Hypericum perforatum (St John's Wort) in depression: pest or blessing? Med J Aust 169: 583–586
45. Siahpush M (1998) Postmodern values, dissatisfaction with conventional medicine and popularity of alternative therapies. J Sociology 34: 58–70
46. Thomas K, Westlake L, Williams BT (1991) Use of non-orthodox and conventional health care in Great Britain. BMJ 302: 207–210
47. Tramèr MR, Moore RA, Reynolds DJ, McQuay HJ (2000) Quantitative estimation of rare adverse events which follow a biological progression: a new model applied to chronic NSAID use. Pain 85: 169–182
48. Vincent C, Furnham A (1997) Complementary medicine: A research perspective. Wiley, ###, pp 181–182
49. White AR, Ernst E (2000) Economic analysis of complementary medicine: a systematic review. Compl Ther Med 8: 111–118
50. Yezzi R (1988) Prescribing drugs for the aged and dying. In: Humber JM, Almeder RF (eds) Biomedical ethics reviews. Humana Press, Clifton, NJ, pp 31–57

6 Future Trends in Use – Focus on Transcendental Meditation as a Traditional System of Natural Medicine

R.H. Schneider, J.W. Salerno and S.I. Nidich

with a Preface by E.P. Cherniack

Preface

Prediction of the future can be a daunting task. It is unlikely that 20 years ago many physicians would have predicted the explosive growth in the use of complementary and alternative medicine (CAM) that has occurred in the past two decades. Nevertheless, there are certain trends in the use of CAM that may be important to note.

Firstly, the use and interest in CAM among the elderly by physicians and patients is expected to grow. As has been discussed in other chapters, several large demographic studies of CAM use [2–4, 6], but not all [1] have found the greatest utilization among middle-aged users. However, in the next few decades, those users will become elderly, and there is no reason to predict that their enthusiasm for CAM will lessen. In fact, as they start to develop, if they have not already done so, chronic illnesses more prevalent with age, such as depression or arthritis, that are correlated with CAM use, they may become more likely to use CAM. Furthermore, many may already be or become caregivers of elderly relatives, and they may recommend CAM to these older individuals.

The use of CAM by the elderly, although it should increase, should also become more selective. While sales of CAM herbal products, for example skyrocketed in the mid 1990 s, there has been more recent reduction in increased purchasing. Demand for herbal substances increased by seventeen percent in 1997, by twelve percent in 1998, but only by one percent in 2000 [11]. Speculation about reasons for the drop in demand for CAM more recently include a negative study that appeared about the efficacy of St. John's Wort, and disappointment over exaggerated claims of supplement efficacy [1]. When adverse publicity or negative studies become available about CAM therapy, there may be a major impact on how patients use various treatments, including the elderly. Consumers and their physicians, however, may be becoming more educated as more information about CAM is being disseminated, and the older individual may be become more sophisticated about his use of CAM products. Seventy-six medical schools offered courses in 2001 about CAM up from 46 in 1996 [9]. Certain products, that have an appeal in that they might address problems that concern the elderly, yet have not yet been shown to have a high incidence of side effects, or at least not had a popularized account of major adverse reactions, may become more popular among the elderly. Such products as gingko or glucosamine, may become more common, while others, such as kava, may be less frequently used. Medicare may chose to reimburse popular therapies under pressure from older consumers, which may also influence use.

As patients and physicians learn more about CAM, the more certain therapies may become accepted as part of conventional treatment. For years, a popular form of CAM therapy has been the use of large doses of vitamins recognized. With the publication of trials that imply the benefit of certain vitamins for certain disorders prevalent among the elderly, such as vitamin E for dementia, the utilization of such vitamins, in these circumstances becomes part of conventional medicine. Many trials of CAM therapies for indications important to the elderly are currently ongoing, such as the use of acupuncture to treat low back pain and osteoarthritis of the knee. As the results of such trials become available. It would not be surprising if certain forms of CAM became accepted as conventional medicine.

There is a trend toward the increased regulation of CAM. CAM has already been more strictly regulated in Europe than in the North America for many years. In Germany, for example, the German Medicines Act of 1976, in addition to European Union and World Health Organization regulations, subject certain CAM therapies, such as homeopathic medications, to certain standards regarding quality and efficacy [5]. In 1999, Canada established an federal office, The Office of Natural Health Products to regulate CAM treatments [8]. The limitations of the United States law that regulates many CAM substances, the Dietary Supplement Health and Education Act of 1994 (DSHEA), has been One year ago a report by the United States Department of Health and Human Services inspector general said US does a poor job of regulating dietary supplements and called for increased regulation [10]. Federal and local governments will also have to address the difficult task of determining how to regulate CAM practitioners.

Governments have also had to and will continue to address the issue of who should be allowed to practice a CAM discipline whose efficacy is not based on the scientific method. In Germany, there has been federal legal and medical opinion that the CAM practitioners not be held to a different standard as conventional medical practitioners [7].

In the United States, the issue is left up the states, and a number of states license some but not all types of practitioners, such as acupuncturists.

In order to determine how much regulation is necessary, which will depend on the safety and efficacy of CAM, more research will have to be done, including research on the efficacy of therapies whose theoretical foundation is not based on conventional science. In the following chapter, transcendental meditation (TM) is discussed. TM is one of a number of such disciplines not originally based on conventional science which is being investigated, the reports of which are beginning to appear in peer-reviewed journals.

References

1. Astin J (1998) Why patients use alternative medicine: results of a national study. J Am Med Assoc 279: 1548–1553
2. Bausell R, Lee W, Berman B (2001) Demographic and health-related correlates of visits to complementary and alternative medical providers. Med Care 39: 190–196
3. Eisenberg D, Kessler R, Foster C et al. (1993) Unconventional medicine in the United States. Prevalence, costs, and patterns of use. N Engl J Med 328: 246–252
4. Eisenberg D, Davis R, Ettner S et al. (1998) Trends in alternative medicine use in the United States, 1990–1997: results of a follow-up national survey. J Am Med Assoc 280: 1569–1575

5. Keller K (1997) Special therapeutic guidelines from the viewpoint of BfArM (Federal Institute for Drug and Medical Products). Z Ärztl Fortb Qualitätssicherung 91: 669–674
6. MacLennan A, Wilson W, Taylor A (1996) Prevalence and cost of alternative medicine in Australia. Lancet 347: 569–573
7. Ostendorf GM (1994) Expert assessment of naturopathy, alternative treatment methods and homeopathic practitioners. Versicherungsmedizin 46: 174–177
8. Sibbald B (1999) New federal office will spend millions to regulate herbal remedies, vitamins. CMAJ 160: 1355–1357
9. USA Today April 18, 2001
10. USA today, Apr 17, 2001
11. USA Today, May 9, 2001

Focus on Transcendental Meditation as a Traditional System of Natural Medicine

The perspectives and practices of healthcare in the U.S. and globally are fundamentally changing rapidly due to ever evolving technological, social, economic and spiritual influences as we stand at the dawn of a new millennium. As an unprecedented large and rapidly aging US population, the baby-boomers, are a mounting pressure on health care policy makers, healthcare insurers, and medical providers to give greater attention to their unique healthcare needs. Technological innovations of the new information age such as the Internet have made patients more knowledgeable, savvy and assertive in their quest for greater insight, self-control, empowerment and personal attention regarding their healthcare needs [1, 38]. These changing times are requiring a new approach to healthcare delivery and the growing trend in complementary and alternative medicine (CAM) is promising to play a enormous role in the integration and transformation of our existing healthcare system [1, 17].

It is the elderly population over age 65 that stands to benefit most from this sweeping CAM trend. Between 1990 and 1997, CAM usage by the general U.S. population increased from 34% to 42% with the older age groups (over 50) reporting higher rates of CAM usage (39–50%) [20]. In a more recent survey targeted at the elderly (over age 65), 41% reported use of CAM [6] with a follow-up study finding an 80% satisfaction rate with their particular CAM therapy and a considerable expressed interest in third party coverage for CAM therapies in general [7]. This growing prevalence of CAM usage was found to be similar across all sociodemographic sectors of a large study sample [34]. Moreover, this CAM usage trend among elderly is anticipated to explode upwards in the coming 10–20 years as the next generation – the baby boomers – move into their retirement years [34, 57].

The growing disillusionment with the conventional allopathic healthcare system has been an important contributing factor in the escalating use of CAM therapies – both prescribed and unprescribed. It has been reported that over 45% of the general US population suffer from at least one chronic disease with an alarmingly high prevalence of 88% among the elderly [26]. Attempts to treat these chronic conditions through allopathy alone have given rise to an epidemic of iatrogenic diseases – hazards caused by the adverse side effects of modern medicine (i.e. pharmaceuticals, surgery and other medical diagnostic errors) [36]. It has been estimated that iatrogenic diseases caused by pharmaceuticals alone account for over 10 percent of all hospital admissions [27].

National policy makers and gerontological experts have established national health objectives that call for studies of innovative health promotion strategies for the elderly [30, 58, 63, 82]. These experts have suggested the following eight points:

▶ Utilize treatment strategies that address the causes of disease, not just the symptoms;
▶ provide the elderly with a health care choice that is holistic;
▶ ensure cost-effective medical care;
▶ provide preventative as well as curative approaches;
▶ incorporate positive lifestyle changes in treatment planning;
▶ incorporate treatments that have high acceptability and compliance rates;
▶ close the health gap for the underserved including ethnic minorities and the elderly;
▶ consider natural alternatives or complements to pharmacological/surgical procedures when appropriate and feasible.

Although healthcare professionals have acknowledged that CAM therapies can help broaden the spectrum of healthcare and enhance overall quality of life in the elderly as both prevention-oriented care and as an adjunct to conventional medical care [17, 38], many CAM approaches are often applied in an unsystematic framework that has yet to be adequately subjected to rigorous empirical verification. It would be reasonable to suggest that an ideal CAM healthcare system responding to the eight national policy points above for the elderly might be one that has been time-tested and is a comprehensive and fully integrated traditional approach that has already been subjected to substantial empirical investigation. Such a system might hold the most promise in attracting healthcare insurers and influence policy makers. The notable successes with meditation and traditional approaches such as the use of Chinese and Ayurvedic herbs indicate that an integrated holistic healthcare system may contribute to the increasing public and professional interest in CAM treatments for chronic diseases common to the aged [19, 20] and provide impetus for investigating whole "unfragmented" traditional systems of medicine with a holistic conceptual framework. Consensus guidelines from the NIH-OAM Workshop on Alternative Medicine [88] and the British Initiative on Integrated Medicin [79] now clearly recommend that traditional systems of medicine be studied in their original intact, and integrated form as clinically used, rather than as isolated components for clinical efficacy and overall safety [83]. In this next section we will introduce Maharishi Vedic Medicine and discuss why this particular traditional system of healthcare shows enormous potential for fulfilling future healthcare needs of the aging population. We will also focus on the more well-known modalities or therapies within this medical system such as the Transcendental Meditation (TM) program and why the elderly might be particularly motivated in its long-term goal-oriented approach for compliance and benefits.

Maharishi Vedic Medicine – Introduction and Theory

A traditional system of healthcare known as "Maharishi Vedic Medicine" (MVM) which has been reported to slow aging, extend longevity and markedly improve well being and quality of life has recently been re-evaluated for its application and integration in the context of modern healthcare [42, 45, 66]. To date, a considerable body of research has shown that several key therapies within this healthcare system reduce chronic stress-related diseases, promote health, vitality, mental well-being and cognitive functioning in older people which are consistent with the concept of prevention of "usual" aging and promotion of "successful" aging [61, 62].

Maharishi Vedic Medicine (MVM) has been described as the most time-tested, comprehensive system of prevention-oriented natural medicine in the world today [42, 45, 66] since it is reported to be the oldest continuously practiced medical system, having its heritage in the ancient Vedic civilization of India [8, 35, 77, 8, 89]. "Veda" in Sanskrit translates as "knowledge" [45, 41]. Vedic medicine, which includes but extends considerably beyond Ayur-Veda – "knowledge of life" –, has been recognized by the World Health Organization as a sophisticated system of natural medicine with a detailed scientific literature consisting of classical medical texts, an uninterrupted oral tradition of classical knowledge predating the written texts, a comprehensive *materia medica*, and a wide breadth of clinical procedures relevant to the prevention and treatment of acute and chronic diseases [8, 81]. The recent availability of Vedic Medicine especially in the West is due to a recent worldwide revival and restoration to its Vedic authenticity by Maharishi Mahesh Yogi in collaboration with leading traditional physicians, scholars and modern scientists (hence, the name Maharishi Vedic Medicine) [42, 45, 66]. Over the last thirty years, more than 600 scientific research studies have been published on various MVM treatment and prevention modalities at over 200 research institutions and universities in 33 countries [11, 53, 74, 86].

In Maharishi Vedic Medicine, therapeutic, diagnostic and preventive modalities are drawn from a broad range of Vedic modalities and are said to holistically enhance the body's innate self-repair and homeostatic mechanisms, thereby preventing disease and promoting health. MVM goes beyond of scope of Ayurveda to encompass other important branches of the Vedic literature to facilitate the development of the full potential of the individual-body, mind, and environment [77].

Approaches of MVM include techniques to reduce psychosocial stress; non-invasive methods of diagnosis (e.g. through pulse), diet and herbal food supplements for the systematic detection and treatment of physiological imbalances. Other strategies involve physiological purification and behavioral recommendations. Still others take advantage of knowledge of the effects of the near environment (Vedic architecture) and distant environment (Vedic approach to chronobiology and chronomedicine) on health. Finally, there are technologies for reducing social stress and enhancing collective health (group practice of the TM and advanced TM-Sushi programs). These approaches are largely missing from modern medicine [66].

From the theoretical perspective of MVM, diseases are reportedly addressed by treating their ultimate causes – disruptions of the body's "inner intelligence" [45]. It is this "inner intelligence" which structures and governs the human body and is seen as a lively and orderly expression of the same intelligence of Natural Law which structures and governs the entire universe [42, 66].

This ancient Vedic perspective of an underlying field of "intelligence" is consistent with modern theories of quantum physics [25]. For example, Einstein originally postulated a single unified field of natural law at the basis of all the force fields and matter fields in the universe [25]. In the quantum mechanical view, the physical particles which structure the universe are ultimately frequencies of wave functions of the self-interacting dynamics of the unified field. Similarly, from the Vedic perspective, the universe, including the human body, is the expression of self-interacting impulses of intelligence [25, 45]. MVM further identifies this unified field as being identical to the field of human consciousness [24].

The experimental data relevant to aging and the elderly on these different MVM approaches are briefly reviewed below. In the last 30 years, the majority of studies on MVM have been on

▶ the TM program;
▶ herbal nutritional supplements and
▶ traditional physiological purification procedures.

Newer data on Vedic sound/vibration are also highlighted. This next section of this chapter briefly reviews the scientific research focusing on older subjects using these traditional MVM modalities that demonstrates its feasibility and effectiveness in this growing population.

The Transcendental Meditation Program

Introduction. Over 6 million individuals worldwide have learned the TM program over the last 40 years–many of them older adults. The TM technique is described as a simple, natural and effortless procedure practiced twice a day for 20 minutes while sitting comfortably with eyes closed [60]. It requires no changes in beliefs, philosophy, religion or life-style, which may be a particularly attractive feature for our growing elderly population. Clinical reports indicate that this technique can easily be learned by individuals of any age, level of education, occupation, or cultural background [3, 60].

During the practice of the TM technique, one's awareness gradually settles down to states of lesser excitation until a least excited state is experienced [39, 60]. TM practitioners report the attainment of this state, which is one of restful alertness, as an experience in which the ordinary thinking process is "transcended". This state also serves to distinguish the TM technique from other meditation and relaxation techniques that use contemplation and concentration and thus may increase mental activation [56].

Effects of the TM Program on Physiological Correlates of Aging. A study by Wallace et al. [86] compared the differences between biological and chronological age on 84 subjects (mean age = 53 years) using a previously validated and standardized index of biological aging known as the Morgan Adult Growth Examination (auditory discrimination, near-point vision accommodation, and systolic blood pressure) [44]. Findings showed that the long-term TM practitioners (>5 years meditating) had a mean biological age 12 years younger than their mean chronological age. Short-term TM meditators were 5 years younger while the non-meditator controls were 2 years younger. These differences were significant for the TM groups compared to the age-matched controls. This study statistically controlled for potentially confounding effects of diet and exercise.

It is known that levels of serum dehydroepiandrosterone sulfate (DHEAS) have been shown to decline with age [51]. A study by Glaser et al. compared DHEAS levels in 328 TM practitioners to 1462 controls. Findings shown that both male and female TM subjects had significantly higher levels of DHEAS with the difference being especially pronounced for older subjects (age >45) whose DHEAS levels were comparable to levels in controls 5–10 years younger [23]

Effects of the TM Program on Neurophysiological Correlates of Aging. Practice of the TM program in adults was associated with improved neurocognitive function including reaction times [12, 29], efficiency of reflex responses [86, 87] and auditory thresholds [86]. TM practice has been shown to increase alpha power and coherence in the EEG which are correlated with enhanced cognitive performance [13]. Using measures of electrodermal activity, adult TM practitioners had larger skin conductance responses along with faster habituation to loud stressful tones [52]. These studies suggest a more adaptive style of functioning characterized by initially faster and greater orienting responses to novel or significant stimuli, followed by faster habituation. In contrast, progressive aging is associated with less adaptable, less flexible neurophysiologic patterns of response [9].

Effects of the TM Program on Cognitive Correlates of Aging. Long term practice of the TM program also appears to produce long-term changes in cognitive functioning that appear to be opposite in direction to those associated with aging. These TM-induced changes include enhanced short-term and long-term memory, organization of memory as evidenced in learning tasks [14, 43]; incremental gains on fluid intelligence [12], improved perceptual flexibility [14]; and increased perceptual motor speed [31]. Elderly TM practitioners (average age 67 years) have been shown to exhibit significantly higher levels of fluid reasoning, verbal intelligence, long-term memory, and speed of processing than age and demographically matched controls [49].

Effects of the TM Program on Healthcare Utilization. Healthcare utilization of individuals with several clinical conditions and diseases which commonly afflict older persons has been shown to improve with TM practice. An epidemiological study investigated the health insurance records of more than 2000 people practicing the TM program over five years. Findings demonstrated significantly less health care utilization by the TM practitioners for all major disease categories when compared to other groups (n~400,000) of similar age, gender, profession, and insurance terms [54]. This included 87% less hospitalization for heart disease, 55% less for cancer, and 87% less for nervous system disorders. When the data was analyzed by age group, it was found that older TM subjects(>40 years) had the greatest reductions in need for both inpatient services (68% less) and outpatient medical services (74% less).

A later study [55] of archival medical utilization and expenditures data from a major health insurance carrier confirmed and extended this research to persons using, in addition to the TM program, a variety of other MVM modalities including herbal supplements and physiological purification. The 4-year total medical expenditures per person in the MVM group, for all ages and all disease categories, were 59% and 57% lower, respectively, than the norm (n = 600,000) and a demographically matched control group (n = 4,148). The greatest savings were seen among older MVM users (age >45 years) who had 88% fewer inpatient days compared to controls. For example, hospital admissions were 11.4 times higher for the controls than the MVM group for cardiovascular disease, 3.3 times higher for cancer, and 6.7 times higher for mental health and substance abuse [55].

Effects Of The Transcendental Meditation Program on Cardiovascular Disease in the Aging. A review and quantitative meta-analysis of 26 studies indicated that the TM technique produced a significantly larger reduction of high blood pressure than did other forms of meditation or meditation-like techniques [56]. For example, in a prospective randomized controlled study by Alexander et al. on the effects of TM in the elderly (mean age = 81), the TM group showed a mean reduction of 12 mmHg over a 3-month period compared to modest change or no change for the two other relaxation treatment conditions [2].

In the most rigorous study to date on TM and hypertension in the elderly, Schneider et al. [5, 65] conducted a randomized controlled, single-blind clinical trial on 127 African Americans (average age 66 years) with mild hypertension. This included a three month follow-up period in a primary care, inner city health center. Compared to a lifestyle modification education control (EC), TM intervention significantly reduced systolic blood pressure by 10.7 mmHg and diastolic blood pressure by 6.4 mmHg. A parallel progressive muscle relaxation (PMR) intervention lowered systolic blood pressure by 4.7 mmHg and diastolic blood pressure by 3.3 mmHg, but, TM lowered BP significantly greater than PMR. Regularity of practice for the TM group was high: 97% (81% for PMR).

In a study of oxidized lipids and stress reduction, Schneider et al. [67] found significantly lower levels of serum lipid peroxides in elderly long-term TM practitioners (average age = 67 yrs.) compared to age/education/gender matched controls while controlling for meat intake and nutritional supplements. These results suggest that oxidative stress, which has been implicated in aging processes including coronary artery and cerebrovascular disease, may be reduced by this stress reduction approach.

Effects of the Transcendental Meditation Program on Mortality in the Elderly. A randomized controlled study exclusively targeted the effects of TM to the advanced elderly (mean age = 81 years at onset of study) [2]. Over a three-year period, the TM group improved most, followed by mindfulness meditation, and then the no-treatment and generic relaxation groups, for the following measures: paired associate learning, two measures of cognitive flexibility, systolic blood pressure, self-ratings of behavioral flexibility and aging, multiple indicators of treatment efficacy, and mental health after 18 months. After three years, survival rate for TM was 100% and mindfulness 87.5% in contrast to a generic clinically devised form of mental relaxation (65%) and no treatment (77%).

A follow-up study reported that the mean survival time was 65% higher in the TM group than all other comparison groups combined after eight years and 22% higher after 15 years [4]. These findings may suggest not only lower mortality rates but also more favorable long-term compliance rates among the elderly with the TM program than other stress management techniques.

According to the MVM model, the consideration of "consciousness" is the fundamental element missing from modern medicine. In the MVM system, development of higher states of human consciousness is achieved through practice of the Transcendental Meditation (TM) and the advanced TM-Sidhi programs [45, 60, 39, 67]. The prevention and health promotion effects of these programs for aging are thought to occur through the enhancement of the body's inner intelligence, thereby allowing physiology to eliminate accumulated stress. This, in turn, is proposed to promote mental, emotional and physiological balance, as well as mind/body integration (homeostasis).

It has been suggested by some CAM researchers that traditional forms of meditation which are long term goal-oriented towards "enlightenment" – i.e. liberation of the egocentric self, developing a sense of harmony with the universe and the ability to increase ones compassion, sensitivity and service to others might be more attractive to the elderly population than clinically devised forms of meditation which are often more short-term process oriented towards improved health [68]. In traditional forms of meditation that have been practiced for thousands of years in a religious/spiritual setting or context, improved health has been considered a by-product or side benefit of the evolutionary process of the meditating practitioner's nervous system toward higher states of consciousness.

Maharishi Vedic Medicine Herbal Supplements

The classical Vedic medicine texts describe certain herbal preparations for specific physiological disorders, and other herbal preparations, which are proposed to promote general health by increasing resistance to disease, activating tissue repair mechanisms, and arresting or reversing deteriorative effects associated with aging [69]. Each herbal preparation contains various herbs or plant parts, each herb having hundreds or thousands of phytochemicals [76]. According to traditional Vedic and modern theories, by using the combined herbal preparation rather than using the isolated chemical active ingredients, the various chemical constituents may function synergistically and mitigate adverse side effects associated with individual components [75].

To date, the majority of research on these herbal preparations called "rasayanas" has involved two compounds collectively called "Maharishi Amrit Kalash" (MAK), its commercially available name. MAK-4 and MAK-5 contain distinctly different combinations of herbs. MAK-5, available in tablet form, consists of Gymnema aurantiacum, Hypoxis orchiodes, Tinospora cordifolia, Sphaeranthus indicus, butterfly pea, licorice, Vanda spatulatum, Lettsomia nervosa, and Indian wild pepper. MAK-4, available as a "fruit paste", consists of raw sugar, ghee (clarified butter), Indian gallnut, Indian gooseberry, dried catkins, Indian pennywort, honey, nutgrass, white sandalwood, butterfly pea, shoeflower, aloewood, licorice, cardamom, cinnamon, Indian cyperus, and turmeric. Although quantitative chemical analyses has not been performed, both MAK-4 and MAK-5 have been shown on a qualitative chemical analysis to include a mixture of low-molecular weight substances and antioxidants, such as alpha-tocopherol, beta-carotene, ascorbate, bioflavonoids, catechin, polyphenols, riboflavin, and tannic acid [18, 32, 33, 59]. In the classical literature, MAK has been reported to promote longevity, vitality, physiological balance, youthfulness, and resistance to disease [69, 75]. Below are reviewed several studies relevant to the prevention and treatment of age-related disorders.

Antioxidant Properties of MAK. Analysis of MAK components has identified a large number of natural antioxidants [10]. Investigators have reported that both MAK-4 and MAK-5 scavenge oxygen free radicals in a dose-dependent manner, thereby minimizing their deleterious effects. Reactive Oxygen Species (ROS) scavenged by MAK-4 and MAK-5 include superoxide, hydroxyl, and peroxyl radicals, and hydrogen peroxide generated both in cellular (neutrophil) and noncellular (xanthine-xanthine oxidase) systems [10, 50]. MAK-4 and MAK-5 have also been shown to reduce levels of lipid peroxide, a marker of free radical damage, and inhibit oxidation of low-density lipoproteins (LDL) [72], reduce platelet activation [70] and reduce angina pectoris [16] and the development of atherosclerotic lesions [80].

Cardiovascular disease (CVD) and MAK. A study by Sundaram et al. [80] found that hyperlipidemic patients supplemented with MAK-4 for 6 months had a profound time-dependent reduction in their LDL oxidation by Cu^{+2} and endothelial cells. Lee et al. found significant reductions in lipid peroxides, increased glutathione peroxidase, resistance of LDL to endothelial cell-induced and cupric ion-catalyzed oxidation and a significantly lower percentage area of atheroma in Wantanabe Heritable Hyperlipidemic (WHHL) rabbits receiving MAK-4 for 6 months (6% diet) [37].

Effects of MAK on Immune system. Weakened immune function has been implicated in the detrimental effects of aging [84]. Dilleepan et al. [15] used animal and cell models to study the effects of MAK under a number of different conditions of immune challenge. There were increases of 100% to 160% in T-lymphocyte proliferation depending on the MAK dosage. This study suggests that MAK may have an anti-aging effect on the immune system.

Effects of MAK on Nervous System. It is known that neurological functions decline with age. Central nervous system mechanisms underlying the effects of MAK may involve interactions with a wide range of important neurotransmitter receptors or uptake sites including opioid receptors [71]. A double-blind placebo controlled study was conducted to test the effect of MAK on an age-related alertness task [22]. Forty-eight men over 35 years of age were randomly assigned to receive MAK-5 tablets or a closely matched placebo twice daily for six weeks. The MAK group improved significantly more in their performance of this task after three and six weeks of treatment relative to the placebo group. Performance, which required an unrestricted flow of homogeneous attention as well as focalized concentration, was highly correlated with age. This study suggests that MAK may enhance attentional capacity or alertness, and therefore reverse some of the detrimental effects of aging on cognitive abilities.

Physiological purification techniques

MVM recommends multimodality physiological purification therapies on a seasonal basis for enhancement of physiological homeostasis, removal of impurities (toxins) that accumulate over time, promotion of mental and emotional well-being and overall physical health [75]. These procedures have been recently and collectively termed Maharishi Rejuvenation Therapy (MRT). These procedures are all prescribed and supervised by trained physicians. Proposed physiological mechanisms of action for several of these procedures have been described [78].

In a controlled study, Schneider and coworkers found that 142 patients undergoing MRT had reported, after a one week treatment period, significantly greater improvements in well-being, energy-vitality, strength-stamina, appetite and significantly less anxiety, depression and fatigue than 60 control subjects who participated in a didactic class on MVM [64]. A more recent study found that following a typical 5 day purification program of MRT, total cholesterol, lipid peroxides, diastolic blood pressure and anxiety levels fell acutely and HDL cholesterol rose significantly three months following treatment. Vasoactive intestinal peptide (VIP), a coronary vasodilator, rose significantly by 80% [73].

Research shows that speed of processing mediates memory processes, is associated with physical frailty and mortality in adult populations. This study assessed the effects of MRT on speed of processing ability in middle-aged adults. Findings indicated significant improvement in speed of processing, using a visual matching test, for the MRT group compared to controls over a one-week period [48].

Maharishi Vedic Vibration Technology (MVVT)

MVVT is a technique of consciousness recently revived from the Vedic tradition by Maharishi Mahesh Yogi. It makes use of impulses of Natural Law in the form of sound which are silently projected at the finest and simplest level of human awareness. Physically sitting in close proximity to the patient, an expert practicing this technique silently directs his/her attention toward the patients problem area during a session of approximately 30 minutes. To date, experts have been trained to attend to many but not all diseases. In a randomized double blind placebo controlled study, 174 patients with chronic arthritis participated [46]. Findings showed significant reductions of pain and stiffness, and improvement in range of motion with the most commonly reported category of improvement being 100%. Given that arthritis is the leading cause of disability in the elderly and medical authorities acknowledge that no cure exists for both osteo- and rheumatoid arthritis, such a treatment program is worthwhile investigating further in preparation for wider implementation in a modern clinical setting.

In a second published study, MVVT has also been reported to improve the quality of life in individuals with chronic disorders in categories including neck pain, respiratory, digestive, mental health, arthritis, insomnia, back pain, headaches, cardiovascular, and eye problems. Results showed that self-reported improvement averaged 41% with significant reductions in frequency of pain or discomfort, intensity of discomfort and disabling effects in activity, in addition to overall improvement in mental health and vitality [47].

Multimodality MVM in the elderly

This recent controlled clinical trial in elderly subjects (mean age = 74) tested the effect of a multimodality MVM, on carotid intima-media thickness (IMT) using a non-invasive measure of atherosclerosis [21]. Fifty-seven healthy seniors were randomized among 3 treatment groups: MVM, modern, and usual care. The MVM group learned the TM technique were given MAK herbal supplements, received Ayurvedic diet recommendations – one that varies with the seasons but is generally low in fat and high in fruits and vegetables and learned the daily exercise routine incorporating two types of Vedic exercises (yoga asanas and surya namaskara) each for 10 minutes a day, and walking for 30 minutes a day. The modern group learned a physical exercise program consisting of aerobic walking 3 times a week and comprehensive stretching and isotonic exercises 2 times a week with a design and intensity appropriate for seniors. Subjects in the modern group participated in the same number of meetings as the MVM group, but these meetings focused on the dietary information and recommendations of conventional medicine as well as on the dangers of negative lifestyle habits such as excessive alcohol consumption and cigarette smoking. This group also was given a standard multivitamin supplement (without vitamins A and D) to take twice daily. Carotid IMT was determined by B-mode ultrasound before and after treatment. After 1 year of treatment, carotid IMT had decreased in a higher proportion of MVM subjects than in the modern and usual care subjects combined (odds ratio = 3.7, p = 0.05). For subjects with multiple CHD risk factors, IMT decreased more in the MVM than in the usual care (p = 0.009) or modern (p = 0.10) groups. Within-group reductions in IMT were significant for the MVM subjects both in the larger group (n = 20, p = 0.004) and in the high-risk subjects (n = 6, p = 0.01). For the first 3 months and the last 9 months in all MVM subjects, compliance rates averaged 86% and 90%, respectively, for the TM technique and 43% and 72%, respectively, for mean compliance rates to all components of the program. The evidence provided here for regression of atherosclerosis in elderly patients suggests that MVM would be useful for elderly persons especially those with marked CVD risk.

Conclusion

It has been reported that older patients reasons for seeking CAM therapies include health promotion and disease prevention, disillusionment with conventional therapies with their adverse side effects and high costs, ineffectiveness of conventional medicine to relieve their chronic condition, no emotional or spiritual benefit (i.e. lack of holism, treating the whole person – mind, body and spirit – and treating the root causes not just alleviating symptoms [20]). This present overview suggests the potential for a recently revived, traditional and most comprehensive approach to natural medicine to respond to and fulfill the perceived healthcare needs of our ever-growing elderly population in the US. Given the considerable social, political and economic burden that our older population have now begun to exert on our fragile healthcare system as we enter the new millennium, the implications of establishing and integrating such a promising healthcare system in the US with our current conventional system appears timely, highly pertinent and worthy of widespread implementation.

References

1. Adams LL, Gatchel RJ, Gentry C (2001) Complementary and Alternative Medicine: Applications and implications for cognitive functioning in elderly populations. Altern Ther Health Med 7: 52–61
2. Alexander CN, Langer EJ, Newman RI, Chandler HM, Davies JL (1989) Transcendental Meditation, mindfulness, and longevity: an experimental study with the elderly. J Pers Soc Psychol 57: 950–964
3. Alexander CN, Sands D (1993) Meditation and relaxation. In: Mcgill RH (ed) Mcgill's survey of the Social Sciences: Psychology. Salem Press, Pasadena, CA, pp 1499–1504
4. Alexander CN, Barnes VA, Schneider RH, Langer EJ, Newman RI, Chandler HM, Davies JL, Rainforth M (1996) A randomized controlled trial of stress reduction on cardiovascular and all-cause mortality in the elderly: Results of 8 and 15 year follow-ups. Circulation 93: P19
5. Alexander CN, Schneider R, Staggers F et al. (1996) A trial of stress reduction for hypertension in older African Americans (Part II): Sex and risk factor subgroup analysis. Hypertension 28: 228–237
6. Astin JA, Pelletier KR, Marie A, Haskell WL Complementary and alternative medicine use among elderly persons: one-year analysis of a blue shield medicare supplement. J Gerontol Med Sci 54A: M1–M6
7. Astin JA, Pelletier KR, Marie A, Haskell WL (2000) Complementary and alternative medicine use among elderly persons: one- year analysis of a Blue Shield Medicare supplement. J Gerontol A Biol Sci Med Sci 55: M4–9
8. Bannerman RH, Burton J, Wen-Chien C (1983) Traditional medicine and health care coverage: reader for health administrators and practitioners. World Health Organization, Geneva
9. Birren JE, Fisher LM (1995) Aging and speed of behavior: possible consequences for psychological functioning. Annu Rev Psychol 46: 329–353
10. Bondy S, Hernandex T, Mattia C (1994) Antioxidant properties of two Ayurvedic herbal preparations. Biochem Arch 10: 25–31
11. Chalmers R, Clements G, Schenkluhn H, Weinless M (1990) Scientific research on the transcendental meditation program: collected papers (vol 2–4). MVU Press, Vlodrop
12. Cranson RW, Orme-Johnson DW, Gackenbach J, Dillbeck MC, Jones CH, Alexander CN (1991) Transcendental Meditation and improved performance on intelligence-related measures: a longitudinal study. Pers Ind Differ 12: 1105–1116
13. Dillbeck MC, Bronson EC (1981) Short-term longitudinal effects of the Transcendental Meditation technique on EEG power and coherence. Int J Neurosci 14: 147–151
14. Dillbeck MC (1982) Meditation and flexibility of visual perception and verbal problem solving. Memory and cognition 10: 207–215
15. Dilleepan KN, Patel V, Sharma HM, Stechschulte DJ (1990) Priming on splenic lymphocytes after ingestion of an Ayur-Vedic herbal food supplement: Evidence for an immunomodulatory effect. Biochemistry Archives 6: 267–274
16. Dogra J, Grover N, Kumar P, Aneja N (1994) Indigenous free radical scavenger MAK-4 and 5 in angina pectoris. It is only a placebo? JAPI 42: 466–467
17. Dossey BM (1997) Complementary and alternative therapies for our aging society. J Gerontol Nursing 23: 45–51
18. Duke JA (19885) CRC handbook of medicinal herbs. CRC Press, Boca Raton
19. Eisenberg D, Kessler R, Foster C, Norlock F, Calkins D, Delblanco T (1993) Unconventional medicine in the United States: Prevalence, costs, and patterns of use. N Engl J Med 328: 246–252
20. Eisenberg DM, Davis RB, Ettner SL, Appel S, Wilkey S, Van Rompay M, Kessler RC (1998) Trends in alternative medicine use in the United States, 1990–1997: results of a follow-up national survey. J Am Med Assoc 280: 1569–1575
21. Fields JZ, Walton KG, Schneider RH et al. (2002) Effect of a multimodality natural medicine program on carotid atherosclerosis in older subjects: a pilot trial of Maharishi Vedic Medicine. Am J Cardiol, in press
22. Gelderloos P, Ahlstrom HHB, Orme-Johnson DW, Robinson DK, Wallace RK, Glasser JL (1990) Influence of a Maharishi Ayur-Vedic herbal preparation on age-related visual discrimination. Int J Psychosom 37: 25–29
23. Glaser JL, Brind JL, Vogelman JH, Eisner MJ, Dillbeck MC, Wallace RK, Chopra D, Orentreich N (1992) Elevated serum dehydroepiandrosterone sulfate levels in practitioners of Transcendental Meditation (TM) and TM-Sidhi programs. J Behav Med 15: 327–341
24. Hagelin J (1987) Is consciousness the unified field? A field theorist's perspective. Modern Science and Vedic Science 1: 29–88
25. Hagelin J (1989) Restructuring physics from its foundation in light of Maharishi's Vedic Science. Modern Science and Vedic Science. 3: 3–72

26. Hoffman C, Rice D, Sung H (1996) Persons with chronic conditions: Their prevalence and costs. J Am Med Assoc 276: 1473–1479
27. Holland EG, Degruy F (1997) Drug-induced disorders. Am Family Phys 56: 1781–1788
29. Holt WR, Caruso JL, Riley JB (1978) Transcendental Meditation vs. pseudo-meditation on visual choice reaction time. Perceptual and Motor Skills 46: 726
30. Institute of Medicine Division of Health Promotion and Disease Prevention (1990) The second fifty years: Promoting health and preventing disability. In: Berg R, Cassels J (eds) National Academy Press, Washington, D.C.
31. Jedrczak A, Clements G (1984) The TM-Sidhi programme and field independence. Percept Mot Skills 59: 999–1000
32. Kapoor LD (1990) CRC handbook of Ayurvedic plants. CRC Press, Boca Raton
33. Kar DK, Sen S (1986) Content of sapogenins in diploid, tetraploid, and hexaploid asparagus. Int J Crude Drug Res 23: 131–133
34. Kessler RC, Davis RB, Foster DF, Van Rompay MI, Walters EE, Wilkey SA, Kaptchuk TJ, Eisenberg DM (2001) Long-term trends in the use of complementary and alternative medical therapies in the United States. Ann Int Med 135: 262–268
35. Kurup PNV, Bannerman RH, Burton J, Ch'en WC (1993) Traditional medicine and health care coverage. World Health Organization, Geneva, Switzerland
36. Leape L (19949 Error in medicine. J Am Med Assoc 272: 1851–1857
37. Lee J, Hanna A, Lott J, Sharma H (1996) The antioxidant and antiatherogenic effects of MAK-4 in WHHL rabbits. J Altern Complement Med 2: 463–478
38. Longino CF (1997) Beyond the body: an emerging medical paradigm. American Demographics 19: 14–19
39. Maharishi Mahesh Yogi (1963) Science of being the art of living. New American Library, New York
40. Maharishi Mahesh Yogi (1967) On the Bhagavad-Gita a new translation and commentary: Chapters 1–6. Penguin Books, Baltimore
41. Maharishi Mahesh Yogi (1994) Vedic knowledge for everyone. Maharishi Vedic University Press, Vlodrop, Netherlands
42. Maharishi Mahesh Yogi, Maharishi Forum of Natural Law and National Law for Doctors (1995) Perfect health for everyone disease-free society. Age of Enlightenment Publications, India
43. Miskman DE (1977) Performance on a learning task by subjects who practice the Transcendental Meditation technique. In: Orme-Johnson DW, Farrow JT (eds) Scientific research on the transcendental meditation program: Collected papers. MERU Press, Rheinweiler, pp 382–384
44. Morgan RF, Fevens SK (1972) Reliability of the adult growth examination: a standardized test of individual aging. Percept Mot Skills 34: 415–419
45. Nader T (1995) human physiology-expression of veda and the Vedic literature. Maharishi University Press: Vlodrop, pp 6–11
46. Nader T, Smith D, Dillbeck M et al. (2001) A double blind randomized controlled trial of Maharishi Vedic Vibration Technology in subjects with arthritis. Frontiers Biosci 6: h7–17
47. Nidich S, Schneider R, Nidich R et al. (2001) Effects of Maharishi Vedic vibration technology on chronic disorders and associated quality of life. Frontiers Biosci 6: h1–6
48. Nidich SI, Nidich RJ, Sands D, Schneider RH, Sharma HM, Barnes VA, Jossang S, Smith DE (2002) Maharishi Rejuvenation program and speed of processing ability. J Soc Behav Pers, in press
49. Nidich SI, Schneider RH, Nidich RJ, Foster G, Sharma H, Salerno JW, Goodman R, Alexander CN (2002) Effect of the transcendental meditation program on intellectual development in community-dwelling older adults. J Soc Behav Pers, in press
50. Niwa Y (1991) Effects of Maharishi 4 and Maharishi 5 on inflammatory mediators-with special reference to their free radical scavenging effects. Indian J Clin Prac 1: 23–27
51. Orentreich N, Brind JL, Rizer RL, Vogelman JH (1984) Age changes and sex differences in serum dehydroepiandrosterone sulfate concentrations throughout adulthood. J Clin Endocrinol Metabol 59: 551–555
52. Orme-Johnson D (1973) Autonomic stability and transcendental meditation. Psychosom Med 35: 341–349
53. Orme-Johnson DW, Farrow J (1977) Scientific research on the transcendental meditation program: Collected Papers, vol. 1. MERU Press, Rheinweiler
54. Orme-Johnson DW (1987) Medical care utilization and the transcendental meditation program. Psychosom Med 49: 493–507
55. Orme-Johnson DW, Herron RE (1997) An innovative approach to reducing medical care utilization and expenditures. Am J Managed Care 3: 135–144
56. Orme-Johnson D, Walton K (1998) All approaches to preventing or reversing effects of stress are not the same. Am J Health Prom 12: 297–299
57. Perry D (1999) Healthy aging in the national interest: the politics of research. In: Dychtwald K (ed) Healthy aging: challenges and solutions. Aspen Publishers, Gaithersburg
58. Rakowski W (1992) Disease prevention and health promotion with older adults. In: Ory MG, Abeles RP, Lipman PD (eds) Aging, health, and behavior. Sage Publications, Newbury Park
59. Rao PS, Rao KVP, Raju KR (1987) Synthesis and antibacterial activity of some new embelin derivatives. Fitoterapia 58: 417–418
60. Roth R (1994) Maharishi Mahesh Yogi's Transcendental Meditation. Primus, Washington, DC, pp 90–102
61. Rowe J, Kahn R (1997) Successful aging. The Gerontologist 37: 433–440
62. Rowe JW, Kahn RL (2000) Successful aging and disease prevention. Adv Renal Replace Ther 7: 70–77

63. Schmidt RM (1994) Preventive health care for older adults: Societal and individual services. Generations 18: 33–38
64. Schneider RH, Cavanaugh K, Rothenberg S, Averbach R, Robinson D, Wallace RK (1990) Health promotion with a traditional system of natural medicine: Maharishi Ayur Veda. J Soc Behav Pers 90: 1–27
65. Schneider RH, Staggers F, Alexander C, Sheppard W, Rainforth M, Kondwani K, Smith S, King CG (1995) A randomized controlled trial of stress reduction for hypertension in older African Americans. Hypertension 26: 820–827
66. Schneider RS, Charles B, Sands D, Gerace DD, Averbach R, Rothenberg S (1997) The Maharishi Vedic Approach to Health and Colleges of Maharishi Vedic Medicine-Creating perfect health for the individual and a disease-free society. Mod Sci Vedic Sci 7: 299–315
67. Schneider R, Nidich S, Salerno J, Sharma H, Robinson C, Nidich R, Alexander C (1998) Lower lipid peroxide levels in practitioners of the Transcendental Meditation program. Psychosom Med 60: 38–41
68. Shapiro D (1995) Meditation. In: Strohecker JTL, Lewis D, Florence M (ed) Alternative medicine: the definitive guide. Future Medicine Publishing, Fife, Washington, pp 339–345
69. Sharma P (1984) Charaka Samhita. Chaukhambha Orientalia, Varanasi
70. Sharma H, Feng Y, Panganamala RV (1989) Maharishi Amrit Kalash (MAK) prevents human platelet aggregation. Clinica and Terapia Cardiovascolare 8: 227–230
71. Sharma HM, Hanissian S, Rattan AK, Stern SL, Tejwani GA (1991) Effect of Maharishi Amrit Kalash on brain opioid receptors and neuropeptides. J Res Edu Indian Med: 1–8
72. Sharma HM, Hana AN, Kaufman EM, Newman HA (1992) Inhibition of human LDL oxidation in vitro by Maharishi Ayurveda herbal mixtures. Pharmacol Biochem Behav 43: 1175–1182
73. Sharma HM, Nidich SI, Sands D, Smith DE (1993) Improvement in cardiovascular risk factors through Panchakarma purification procedures. J Res Edu Indian Med 12: 2–13
74. Sharma H, Alexander CN (1996) Maharishi Ayurveda: Research Review. Altern Med J 3 :21–28
75. Sharma HM, Alexander CN (1996) Maharishi Ayurveda: Research Review-Part 2. Altern Med J 3: 21–28
76. Sharma H (1997) Phytochemical synergism: Beyond the active ingredient model. Altern Ther Clin Pract 4: 91–96
77. Sharma H, Clark C (1998) Contemporary Ayurveda: Medicine and Research in Maharishi Ayur-Veda. Churchill Livingston, New York
78. Smith DE, Salerno JW (1992) A model for extraction of both lipid and water soluble toxins using a procedure from Maharishi Ayurveda. Medical Hypotheses 39: 1–5
79. Steering Committee for the Prince of Wales' Initiative on Integrated Medicine (1997) Integrated healthcare: A wave forward for the next five years? Foundation for Integrated Medicine
80. Sundaram V, Hanna AN, Lubow GP, Koneru L, Falko JM, Sharma HM (1997) Inhibition of low-density lipoprotein oxidation by oral herbal mixtures Maharishi Amrit Kalash-4 and Maharishi Amrit Kalash-5 in hyperlipidemic patients. Am J Med Sci 314: 303–310
81. Thatt UM, Dahanukar SA (1986) Ayur-Veda in contemporary scientific thought: Trends in Pharmacology. Science 7: 247–251
82. US Department of Health and Human Services (1990) Healthy People 2000. National Health Promotion and Disease Prevention Objectives, Washington, DC
83. Vickers EA, Cassileth B, Bernst E et al. (1997) How should we research unconventional therapies? Panel report from the conference on Complementary Therapies and Alternative Medicine, National Institute of Health, USA. Int J Tech Assess Healthcare 13: 111–121
84. Walford R (1969) The immunological theory of aging. Munksgaard, Copenhagen
85. Wallace RK, Dillbeck M, Jacobe E, Harrington B (1982) The effects of the Transcendental Meditation and TM-Sidhi program on the aging process. Int J Neurosci 16: 53–58
86. Wallace RK, Orme-Johnson DW, Dillbeck MC (1990) Scientific research on the transcendental meditation program: collected papers, vol. 5. MIU Press, Fairfield, Iowa
87. Warshal D (1980) Effects of the transcendental meditation technique on normal and jendrassik reflex time. Percept Mot Skills 50: 1103–1106
88. Workshop on Alternative Medicine (1994) A report to the National Institutes of Health on alternative medical systems and practices in the United States, 1994. Alternative Medicine – Expanding Medical Horizons. Chantilly, VA
89. World Health Organization (1978) The promotion and development of traditional medicine. World Health Organization Technical Report Series 622, Geneva, Switzerland

B Types of CAM Used

7 Alternative Therapy: Vitamin Use in the Elderly

J.E. Thurman, A.D. Mooradian

In the next 30 to 40 years, the population of adults over the age of 65 years of age is estimated to double [1]. As the population of the United States ages, there is a concurrent need to address the morbidity associated with ageing. Rudman et al. [2], examined a population of nursing home residents and found that nearly 70% of the residents had a reduced body mass index (BMI), a 50% incidence of anemia, and a majority had a serum albumin <3.5 g/dl. They also found that all of the study group had a dietary intake <50% of the recommended dietary allowance (RDA) of several essential nutrients including: zinc, magnesium, manganese, copper, vitamin E retinol, nicotinic acid, pyridoxine, and folic acid. With this in mind, it is important to consider that institutionalized elderly may be deficient in their dietary intake of several essential vitamins. This dietary deficiency may lead to further health complications.

While the data of nursing home residents may seem concerning, it is also important to note that a significant percentage of the population of independently living elderly do not consume the RDA for many essential nutrients. In fact, 22 to 56% of aged men and 17 to 60% of elderly women consume <75% of the RDA of many essential vitamins and minerals [3]. Of note, the Baltimore Longitudinal Study of Aging [5] showed that healthy, college-educated men, regardless of age met the current RDAs of nutrient intake.

Fortunately, those partaking in the Western diet rarely see overt deficiencies in vitamin and mineral status. As we age, our health status changes as does our nutritional and physiologic requirements. It is plausible that some age-related disease processes such as cancer formation and cardiovascular disease may be reduced with dietary intervention. The goal of nutritional therapy is to recognize and retard these age-related processes and intervene with dietary and/or supplemental modalities however possible. The current RDAs, however do not account for this. It is best to consider changing the RDA for elders, especially those over 65 years of age [1] keeping in mind the potential benefits and consequences of dietary intervention.

Vitamin use amongst the elderly is often self-prescribed and without medical basis. Often, vitamin and dietary supplement use is an attempt to prevent disease. This may be fueled by vitamin manufactures or those that support the use of supplements for personal gain. People may take over-the-counter preparations in an effort to prevent or modify disease processes and take control of their own health [5]. Vitamin use is very common. It is second only to analgesics amongst over-the-counter medications [6].

Since vitamins and dietary supplements are over-the-counter in the United States, they may be conceived as "safe" [6]. The most commonly self-prescribed vitamins are ascorbic acid (vitamin C) and vitamin E [7]. Despite the general public's preconceived notions that all over-the-counter preparations are "safe" many vitamins and other supplements may have potential toxicities. The medical community has yet to educate the public of the possible adverse effects of excessive vitamin and dietary supplement use [6]. The theme of this chapter is to discuss the potential uses and toxicities of vitamin supplementation.

Antioxidant Vitamins

Ascorbic Acid (Vitamin C)

Ascorbic acid is the most commonly self-administered vitamin in the United States. Often, despite evidence to the contrary [8], ascorbic acid is taken in large doses to prevent or relieve the symptoms of the common cold [9]. The current RDA of vitamin C is 60 mg/day for non-smokers. Tobacco smokers have a reduced renal threshold for ascorbic acid excretion and thus the RDA has been increased in this population to 100 mg/day. Despite this increase in the RDA, smokers need to consume >200 mg/day to attain plasma ascorbic acid levels that of non-smokers [10–12].

The ideal source of ascorbic acid is from fruits and vegetables. The daily ingestion should be equivalent to five servings of fruits and vegetables ($\approx$200 mg/day). While this is in excess of current RDA guidelines, it is considered "safe" under current nutritional guidelines. Supplemental ascorbate should be less than 500 mg/day to avoid potential side effects [13]. Nursing home residents may not be able to ingest 200 mg/day from dietary sources. Their portions are commonly small and their vegetables are often cooked thereby reducing the available ascorbic acid from their food source. Twenty percent of nursing home residents have a dietary intake <75 percent of the current RDA (60 mg/day) of ascorbic acid [2]. Supplementation of 50 percent of the RDA of ascorbic acid (30 mg/day) as fruit juice can significantly increase plasma ascorbic acid levels [14]. It is interesting to note that persons with decreased ascorbic acid intake have higher incidence rates of cervical cancers and squamous epithelial carcinomas of the upper airways [15].

Ascorbic acid is a potent antioxidant. Production of oxygen free radicals and oxidative stress are reduced with ascorbate supplementation. The reduction in oxidative stress may improve cell membrane qualities allowing for an improvement in glucose transport [16]. Persons with type 2 diabetes mellitus have reduced plasma ascorbic acid levels as compared with non-diabetic controls [17]. Supplementation with vitamin C in type 2 diabetics may reduce fasting insulin levels, glycated hemoglobin, and low-density (LDL) cholesterol [18]. Vitamin C may also improve carbohydrate metabolism, increase non-oxidative glucose disposal [16] and have a modest blood pressure lowering effect [19–22]. The modest blood pressure lowering effect of vitamin C is of questionable clinical significance. However, supra-physiologic doses of vitamin C have been demonstrated to reduce super-oxide anions thereby restoring endothelium-derived nitric oxide (EDNO) activity in hypertensive patients [23]. Long-term prospective studies are necessary before ascorbic acid therapy can be shown to be well tolerated and efficacious in improving glycemic control and blood pressure control.

Ascorbic acid is essential in the formation of connective tissues. Supplementation is effective in improving vascular integrity in nursing home patients. As a result, these patients may have reduced purpura and petechial hemorrhages [24]. Ascorbic acid may be useful in the prevention and treatment of decubitous ulcers [19].

While the current RDA for ascorbic acid is 60 mg/day, the most common over-the-counter dosage is 500 mg. This large dose is very well tolerated [25, 26]. Dosages in excess of one gram are largely unabsorbed. The intestinal absorption of ascorbic acid is energy dependent and the transporters are easily saturated. Once the GI ascorbic acid transporters are saturated, ascorbic acid pools in the intestines leading to the most common side effects namely abdominal bloating and an osmotic diarrhea. Excess ascorbic acid in the GI tract may interfere with stool occult blood testing [27]. Absorbed ascorbic acid in excess of physiologic requirements is filtered, unchanged via the kidneys into the urine providing for a systemic means of regulation of ascorbic acid status [27]. This filtration of excess ascorbic acid has been used in some to acidify the urine of nursing home patients to manage and prevent urinary tract infections. However, vitamin C is not clinically effective in these situations [20].

Despite being generally well tolerated, ascorbic acid supplementation may have some insidious adverse events. Rarely, ascorbic acid may precipitate an acute hemolysis in persons with glucose-6-phosphatase deficiency [28]. Previously it was held that ascorbic acid might precipitate urinary oxalate stones. Healthy persons supplemented with large (1 to 10 grams/day) of ascorbic acid did not experience an increase in oxalate stone formation. However, those with a history of oxalate stones should refrain from its use [29].

Ascorbic acid may interfere with some glucose test meters resulting in a falsely lower reading thereby leading to a perceived improvement in diabetic control [30]. In addition, vitamin C may deplete plasma cyanocobalamin (vitamin B_{12}) levels [31, 32].

Abrupt discontinuation of large doses of vitamin C may lead to rebound scurvy. Relative deficiencies following its discontinuation may result in the classic scurvy symptoms gum bleeding and sub-periosteal bleeding [33].

Despite significant circumstantial evidence supporting its use as a supplement, ascorbic acid use has yet to have been proven in large clinical trials. Considering its potential toxicity in some persons, supplementation should be limited to no more than 200 mg/day. A larger dose (500 mg/day) may be justified in individuals with vascular fragility and open skin ulcers.

Tocopherols (Vitamin E)

The most active form of vitamin E is alpha-tocopherol. Vitamin E acts as an antioxidant. It is found in cell membranes where it neutralizes free radicals. Vitamin E is a lipid soluble vitamin found in dietary vegetable and seed oils. Vitamin E status is not affected by aging [34]. However >60 percent of institutionalized elderly persons consume <50 percent of the ideal dietary intake (12–15 IU/day) [2]. As an antioxidant vitamin E may, theoretically be useful in situations where oxidation and free radical formation may be the inciting event in a disease process. Therefore, vitamin E may be helpful in the prevention of atherosclerosis, cataract formation [35], retinal degeneration [36], and carcinogenesis [37].

Diets high in fruits, vegetables and fiber are associated with a reduced incidence of colo-rectal cancer. The typical Western diet, higher in fats and carbohydrates, is linked to increases in colo-rectal, ovarian, breast and prostate cancer [38]. The addition of dietary fiber, fruits and vegetables may have a protective effect for colo-rectal carcinoma [39]. Theoretically, the addition of antioxidants, found predominately in fresh fruits and vegetables would reduce the incidence of new cancer formation.

While laboratory models suggest a negative effect of antioxidants upon new cancer formation, persons with high intakes of carotenes, ascorbic acid and vitamin E appear to have lower rates of new cancers [40]. This, however, has not been borne out in large direct trials in humans. A large placebo-controlled trial, the Polyp Prevention Study [41] failed to demonstrate a reduction in the incidence of colonic adenomas in patients with previous history of colon polyps after supplementation with ascorbic acid or vitamin E. Likewise in a study group of smokers, vitamin E supplementation had no effect in reducing lung cancer incidence [42], or in the reduction of the incidence of breast cancers in post-menopausal women [43]. Therefore, supplementation with vitamin E and other antioxidants may not be as efficacious in reducing the incidence of cancers as does dietary and lifestyle modification.

A small study [44] in persons with type 1 diabetes mellitus of short duration (less than 10 years) demonstrated normalization of retinal and renal blood flow when supplemented with large doses (1,800 IU/day) of vitamin E. The clinical significance of this is not known until larger studies involving persons with both type 1 and type 2 diabetes mellitus have been undertaken.

Vitamin E supplementation may improve the immune response by reducing free radical and eicosanoid expression from macrophages. These factors are associated with reduced lymphocyte proliferation [45]. Large dose supplementation of vitamin E (2000 IU/day) may delay the progression of Alzheimer's disease [46] but long-term studies will be necessary before it will be acceptable as a therapy.

While the role of Vitamin E in the prevention of cancers is questionable, its use in the prevention and treatment of coronary artery disease (CAD) and angina pectoris [47] is showing promise. The Health Profession Follow-Up Study [48] indicated that vitamin E supplementation may reduce the risk of CAD by 35% in men. Similarly, in women, the Nurses' Health Study indicated that supplementation with ≥100 IU of vitamin E on a daily basis allows for a 40% risk reduction in CAD. A dietary intake of vitamin E in excess of 250 IU/day can reduce the risk of CAD by 50% in elderly-post-menopausal women [49]. In order to achieve this level of vitamin E intake, one would need to eat 5 servings of fruits and vegetables on a daily basis. This is not possible for many elderly persons as 74% of nursing home residents consume <50% of the current RDA of vitamin E (15 IU/day) [50].

Vitamin E appears to have its effect on the cardiovascular system by inhibiting the oxidation of low-density lipoprotein (LDL). LDL particles contain polyunsaturated fats. These polyunsaturated fats are degraded by lipid peroxidation. These oxidized LDL particles are taken up by macrophages to form foam cells which make up, in part, atherosclerotic plaques [51, 52].

The Cholesterol Lowering Atherosclerosis Study (CLAS) [53] demonstrated angiographic evidence that supplementation with vitamin E (≥100 IU/day) reduced progression of coronary artery plaques as compared to men who did not receive vitamin E. However, large dose supplementation with vitamin E had no effect on the restenosis rate of coronary arteries following angioplasty [54]. The Cambridge Heart Antioxidant Study (CHAOS) [55] showed a 77% reduction in the risk of nonfatal myocardial infarction in patients with known CAD that were supplemented with 400 to 800 IU of vitamin E per day. Of note, there was no reduction in total mortality or risk of cardiovascular death in this group.

While previous studies suggest a benefit of vitamin E supplementation in those with known CAD recent, large placebo-controlled trials have failed to support the notion that vitamin E can reduce the incidence of CAD in high-risk individuals. The Alpha-Tocopherol, Beta-Carotene Cancer Prevention Study (ATBC Study) [56] showed low dose vitamin E to have only a marginal reduction in the incidence of fatal CAD in male smokers with no prior history of myocardial infarction. Moreover, there was no reduction in on non-fatal MI in this group. A small study [57, 58] examining the combination of simvastatin, niacin, and antioxidants (800 IU vitamin E, 1000 mg vitamin C, 25 mg β-carotene, and 100 µg of selenium) demonstrated limited benefit of antioxidants in persons with heart disease and normal LDL but low HDL. In addition, the Heart Outcomes Prevention Evaluation (HOPE) Study [59] failed to produce an effect on cardiovascular outcomes in persons that have had prior myocardial infarctions supplemented with vitamin E for four to six years. However, the researchers suggested that vitamin E supplementation may require more than five years to have an effect upon cardiovascular disease.

Vitamin E supplementation may have an effect of primary prevention of CAD in persons that are not of high risk. However, short-term vitamin E supplementation may not necessarily have a role in the secondary prevention of CAD.

Vitamin E supplementation is largely without side effects. However, vitamin E can worsen the deficiency in vitamin K deficient states such as those treated with warfarin [60]. It is very well tolerated, long term, at a variety of dosages in excess of the RDA [61]. While vitamin E as an anti-oxidant may have no anti-cancer effects, it may have a favorable effect upon LDL cholesterol oxidation and subsequent atherosclerotic plaque formation. However, further long-term (>5 year) studies are necessary before vitamin E can be considered a therapeutic agent in the prevention or treatment of cardiovascular disease.

Retinoids and Carotenoids

Retinol is a naturally formed, lipid-soluble vitamin found in dairy products and liver. The current RDA for retinol for individuals [3] is 800 to 1000 µg/day (approximately 5000 IU/day) [62]. Many elderly (nearly 40%) [3] have dietary deficiencies of retinol this can become more evident in the winter when fresh fruits and vegetables are less in supply or more expensive [63]. The metabolites of retinol are part of the visual cycle. Retinol deficiency has been associated with night blindness. In addition to its role in the retina, retinol plays a significant role in cellular differentiation and in the structural integrity of epithelial cells [64]. Retinol deficiency can lead to xerophthalmia and night blindness which are usually reversible with supplementation [65]. Women with cervical dysplasia have been demonstrated to have lower serum retinal levels when compared to control groups [66]. Similarly, low serum β-carotene levels have been associated with an increase in all-cause mortality [67].

β-carotene, found in fresh fruits and vegetables, is partially converted to retinal during gastrointestinal absorption. β-carotene and other carotenoids have anti-oxidant properties that may make them useful in the prevention of cancers, particularly those of the gastrointestinal tract [68]. Considering retinol's role in cellular differentiation as well as the anti-oxidant properties of β-carotene it is reasonable to consider that supplementation of either of these compounds will reduce the formation of new cancers. Increased β-carotene intake has been associated with a reduction in stomach cancer risk [70]. Similarly, ingestion of large doses of retinal (>10,000 IU/day) has been shown to reduce the age-adjusted risk for breast cancer in women [71]. However, large placebo-controlled studies have yet to have demonstrated any promising evidence supporting their use in cancer prevention. β-carotene supplementation did not reduce any risk of malignancy, death from cardiovascular disease or all cause mortality in the Physicians Health Study [72]. Nor did β-carotene supplementation have any effect on lowering the incidence of major coronary events in smokers [56, 73] . The β-Carotene and Retinol Efficacy Trial (CARET) [74] as well as the α-Tocopherol, β-Carotene Cancer Prevention Study [75] failed to show any benefit from supplementation of retinol or β-carotene in the prevention of lung cancers in persons at high risk (i.e. smokers and those with asbestos exposure). In fact, the CARET study showed a surprising increase (28%) in lung cancers and a 17% increase in deaths the group of smokers that were supplemented with β-carotene as compared to those who did not [74, 76].

Despite any evidence supporting the efficacy of either retinol or β-carotene in cancer prevention or reduction in overall mortality, their use continues. Retinol is available without a prescription at doses of 25,000 IU (5-fold the current RDA) [26]. Acute retinol toxicity is manifested by increased intra-cranial pressure, headache and possible pseudo-tumor cerebri. Chronic toxicity with doses of only 5,000 to 10,000 IU/day can lead to liver toxicity, skin dryness or desquamation [77]. β-carotene supplementation is largely without severe adverse effect although supplementation can lead to hyper-carotenosis leading to yellowing of the skin saving the sclera [78, 79]. Most elders are able to consume adequate retinol to avoid deficiency. It is important to remember that there is an increased risk of deficiency during the winter months when fresh fruits and vegetables may be in short supply or simply more expensive [63].

Vitamin B Complex

The vitamin B complex is composed of thiamin (vitamin B_1), riboflavin (vitamin B_2), nicotinic acid, pyridoxine, panthenic acid, biotin, folate, cyanocobalamin, choline, inositol and p-aminobenzoic acid. While these are chemically and functionally discrete compounds, they were originally stratified as a single group as they are found naturally in similar dietary sources (liver and yeast) [80].

Vitamin B_1 (Thiamin)

As one ages, there is a tendency to have decreased thiamin levels [81]. Thiamin is necessary for carbohydrate metabolism and neurologic function [82]. The current RDA for thiamin is 1.2 mg/day for elderly men and 1.0 mg/day for women. It is surprising that nearly 30% of non-institutionalized elderly in the New England area [2] and 40% of nursing home residents consume <70% of the current RDA of thiamin. Deficient thiamin intake can be seen in patients with chronic alcoholism and in states were there is decreased absorption [83].

Chronic thiamin deficiency may lead to cardiac (wet) beriberi, which is rare in the United States. Mild thiamine deficiency states may exacerbate underlying cardiac failure. Certainly, supplementation with thiamin may be beneficial in those who are prone to deficiency with co-existing cardiac failure [84]. Oral thiamin has not been shown to be toxic. Excess thiamin is quickly cleared via the kidneys [62].

Vitamin B₂ (Riboflavin)

The RDA for riboflavin is 1.2 to 1.4 mg/day [62]. Approximately 40% of dietary riboflavin is derived from milk and dietary products. The incidence of riboflavin deficiency is between 10 and 27% while >40% of elders do not consume adequate riboflavin. This is even more evident in Blacks and those in lower socio-economic groups [85].

Riboflavin is essential for the metabolism of pyridoxine (vitamin B₆) and folic acid [86]. Deficiency is typically manifested by angular stomatitis, chelosis, angular lingual papillae, glossitis and seorrheic skin lesions. These oral and dermatological findings are thought to be due to impaired pyroxidine formation [86, 87].

Diets high in fat, like the Western diet, increase riboflavin requirements [88] as does exercise in elderly women [89]. Avoidance of dairy products as seen in individuals with lactose intolerance can result in riboflavin deficiency. Supplementation is advisable in situations where adequate dietary intake is not possible. Riboflavin supplementation is well tolerated and should provide the minimum RDA of 1.2 mg/day [90].

Pyridoxine (Vitamin B₆)

Pyridoxine in its active coenzyme form [pyridoxal 5'-phosphate (PLP)] has several metabolic activities. Pyridoxine supplementation and the subsequent increase in PLP may, in the elderly, result in an improvement in storage and processing of new information. Pyridoxine is a necessary co-factor in neurotransmitter formation. PLP is involved in the production of: nor epinephrine, dopamine, serotonin, γ-amino butyric acid and turbine [91]. As a result of increased PLP activity, supplementation may inhibit the age-related reduction of processing and storage of verbal information and long-term memory [92].

Pyridoxine deficiency can lead to increases in lactic acid concentrations leading to early fatigue during exercise. Pyridoxine has a very important role in the citric acid cycle. Deficiency of pyridoxine leads to inhibition of pyruvate dehydrogenase activity leading to lactic acid accumulation [93].

Deficiency of pyridoxine can also play a role in the progression of coronary artery disease (CAD). Pyridoxine, folate and cyanocobalamin have roles in the metabolism of homocysteine. Pyridoxine deficiency may lead to elevated homocysteine levels [94] which has been implicated in CAD [95–97]. Therefore, supplementation with pyridoxine and folic acid supplementation may have a role in inhibiting the furtherance of CAD [95].

Since pyridoxine (PLP) is involved in the synthesis of serotonin, deficiency of pyridoxine may play a role in the pathogenesis of hypertension. Low serotonin levels can lead to general stimulation of the sympathetic nervous system [98]. Subtle changes in pyridoxine status can affect blood pressure.

Pyridoxine also appears to play a role in the function of calcium channels. Low pyridoxine levels can lead to calcium channel dysfunction again resulting in elevated blood pressure [99].

Elderly individuals with a low pyridoxine status may have impaired humoral and cell mediated immunity. Deficiency my reduce circulating lymphocyte numbers and antibody production [100]. Cell-mediated and humoral immunity may be improved with pyridoxine supplementation [101]. Some rheumatolgic disorders such as: periarticular synovitis of the fingers, stenosing tenosynovitis (trigger finger), and de Quervain's disease may, occasionally respond to pyridoxine therapy [102]. Deficiency of pyridoxine and PLP has also been associated with an increased risk of hip fracture in the elderly [103]. In addition, some movement disorders, such as tardive dyskinesia may be response to pyridoxine therapy [104].

The clinical symptoms of pyridoxine deficiency include stomatitis, cheilosis and glossitis [105]. Nearly 10% of independent elderly and over 50% of institutionalized elderly have low pyridoxine levels [106]. Elderly persons with diabetes mellitus may have an associated pyridoxine deficiency. Low PLP levels may contribute to the non-enzy-matic glycation of proteins leading therefore to tissue damage. This subsequent protein glycosylation may play a role in several complication of diabetes mellitus such as neuropathy, retinopathy, cataract formation, neuropathy, and peripheral artery disease [107].

While many disease processes may be affected by pyridoxine supplementation, mega-dose (>200 mg/day) supplementation is not without side effects. Pyridoxine therapy is generally well tolerated in the elderly at doses of ≤100 mg/day [108]. This dose limit is 50 fold the current RDA [62]. Pyridoxine toxicity is associated with a progressive sensory ataxia and impairment of positional and distal vibratory sensation. Toxicity is also associated with diminished, if not loss of tendon reflexes [109] and photosensitivity [110]. High dose pyridoxine therapy may also cause large and small nerve fiber dysfunction. The neurotoxic effects of high dose pyridoxine therapy may be reversible several weeks after cessation of therapy [111]. Therefore, high dose pyridoxine therapy (>100 mg/day) should be avoided [109].

Nicotinic Acid and Nicotinamide (Niacin)

Nicotinic acid deficiency is rare even in institutionalized elderly [2]. Although not a vitamin by the strictest definition, nicotinic acid can be absorbed from the diet or synthesized from dietary tryptophan. Deficiency can lead to pellagra, which is typically manifested by wasting, dementia, dermatitis and diarrhea [112].

Nicotinic acid a common supplement in high dosages (2 to 3 grams daily) as a therapy for hyper-lipidemia. It is important to note that nicotinamide supplementation has no effect on serum cholesterol. Nicotinic acid can reduce triglycerides and very-low-density lipoprotein (VLDL) production from the liver [113], reduce lipoprotein (a) levels [114], and increase high-density lipoprotein (HDL) levels [115]. To achieve adequate therapeutic response, the dose requirement of nicotinic acid is approximately 3 grams daily [116]. The Coronary Drug Project [117] demonstrated a 10% reduction in total cholesterol. The researchers also found a 20% reduction in the recurrence of myocardial infarction after five years. Similarly, the Stockholm Ischemic Heart Disease Study [118] showed that combination therapy with niacin and clofibrate reduced total mortality by 26% in patients with previous coronary artery disease. The combination of simvastatin and niacin demonstrated a 90% reduction in the rate of major clinical events in patients with CAD, who have normal LDL and low HDL levels. This combination also showed slight regression in proximal coronary artery stenosis. The risk reduction was thought to me mediated by an increase in HDL levels [57].

Nicotinic acid would be an ideal and cost-effective agent in treating hyper-lipidemia would it not be for its quite bothersome side effects. The most noticeable side effect is a prostaglandin-mediated flushing. Often, this effect can be alleviated with the co-administration of aspirin (salicylic acid) [113]. Newer, sustained-release formulations (Niaspan) can reduce the flushing symptoms. Prior sustained-release preparations had associated hepatic-toxicity and a potential for liver failure [119]. Other common side effects of nicotinic acid include: gastric irritation, headaches, postural hypotension, gout, and glucose intolerance [120] and elevated liver function tests. Therefore, patients with underlying diabetes mellitus, glucose intolerance or liver disease should avoid nicotinic acid therapy or watch closely for worsening of their underlying condition.

Cyanocobalamin (Vitamin B$_{12}$)

Cyanocobalamin is synthesized by intestinal bacteria and can be absorbed from dietary sources. The vitamin is absorbed in the small intestine bound by intrinsic factor, which is formed in the stomach. Pernicious anemia is the classic deficiency state that is caused by a lack of intrinsic factor [121]. It is estimated that between 20 and 40% of independently living elders may have undiagnosed cyanocobalamin deficiency [122, 123]. Overt deficiency results in anemia and macrocytosis. However, elderly with dementia and cyanocobalamin deficiency may not display these symptoms [124]. Low serum cyanocobalamin levels may not necessarily be a marker or cause of dementia in the elderly [125].

Although common, cyanocobalamin deficiency can lead to several disorders. Long-term deficiency can lead to several neurological disorders resulting in peripheral neuropathy and gait disturbances [123, 126]. These neurological manifestations are believed to be caused by alterations in myelin structure as cyanocobalamin plays an essential role in fatty acid metabolism. As a result, chronic deficiency may lead to demyelinization [127].

As with many vitamin deficiencies, cyanocobalamin deficiency may occur from poor intake, an increase in metabolic requirements or poor utilization at the tissue level. Since cyanocobalamin is dependent upon a healthy gastrointestinal system, other causes of deficiency may include: decreased parietal cell mass as a result of atrophic gastritis [123], auto-immune disease, total or partial gastrectomy leading to reduced intrinsic factor synthesis and achlorhydria, pancreatic insufficiency, gastrointestinal stasis or bacterial overgrowth [128].

The Schillings' test is the standard procedure for detecting the etiology of cyano-cobalamin deficiency [129]. The Schillings' test, however, is not reliable [130]. Nearly 50% of patients with unexplained low serum cyanocobalamin levels have malabsorp-tion of food-bound or protein-bound cyanocobalamin. This malabsorption of cyano-cobalamin is not necessarily a result of gastric disorders or those with achlorhydria such as those receiving H_2 receptor antagonists. These patients will have a normal Schillings' test as free crystalline cyanocobalamin will be absorbed in the gastrointes-tinal tract [123, 131].

It is not uncommon that a physician or caregiver may prescribe a vitamin B_{12} injec-tion for patients complaining of fatigue. Often, this is merely for a placebo effect. The current RDA for cyanocobalamin is 2.0 µgrams daily [62]. Despite large body stores of cyanocobalamin, deficiency is common as absorption decreases with age. This chronic malabsorption and resultant deficient state may have an effect upon many organs, particularly the nervous system [132]. As atrophic gastritis is more common in the eld-erly, periodic serum measurement of vitamin B_{12} is warranted to evaluate the need of cyanocobalamin supplementation in those >55 years of age. Oral crystalline cyanoco-balamin may suffice for some, however intra-muscular administration may be neces-sary as atrophic gastritis and decreased intrinsic factor may occur in some elderly patients [133]. Monitoring of serum cyanocobalamin levels should become more rou-tine as the consequences of mild deficiency may lead to significant neurologic deficits [131].

Folic acid

Folic acid is necessary for the metabolism of homocysteine to methionine as are py-ridoxine and cyanocobalamin. Deficiencies of these vitamins can lead to an accumu-lation of homocysteine [132]. Higher levels of homocysteine has been associated with increases in CAD [97], peripheral vascular disease [134], and carotid artery disease [135].

Homocysteinuria is a group of rare metabolic diseases that results in high levels of circulating homocysteine and urinary homocysteine. Patients with this disorder have a high incidence of thrombotic events and premature coronary artery disease [136]. This has lead investigators to believe that the elevated homocysteine may contribute to the pathogenesis of vascular disease [137]. Lowering serum cholesterol, smoking ces-sation and blood pressure control are a few of several modifiable risk factors that can reduce CAD. However, modification of these risk factors cannot explain why some in-dividuals may develop CAD while others do not when also considering non-modifi-able risk factors such as age, sex and family history. Other risk factors have been discovered including elevated serum homocysteine levels [96].

The Framingham Heart Study [135] identified that over 50% of elders have folic acid deficiency. This high prevalence of folate deficiency may contribute to the increase in cardiovascular disease. Those elderly with the lowest folic acid levels had higher homocysteine levels and were thus at a presumed greatest risk for developing cardiovascular disease. Schnyder et al. [138] showed the combination of folic acid (1 mg), vitamin B$_{12}$ (400 µg) and pyridoxine (10 mg) daily significantly reduced homocysteine levels and decreased the rate of restenosis of coronary vessels following coronary angioplasty. This combination may potentially be an inexpensive and effective treatment to reduce the incidence of major cardiac events. However, larger prospective studies are necessary before the combination can be accepted as medical practice.

The ideal source for folic acid is via a diet high in fresh fruits and vegetables [139]. The current RDA for folate is approximately 200 µg/day. However, an intake of folic acid in excess of 400 µg per day is necessary to suppress high levels of serum homocysteine [140, 141]. Supplementation with high dose folic acid without the addition of cyanocobalamin should be avoided. Folic acid supplementation may correct the megaloblastic anemia as seen with cyanocobalamin deficiency. While correcting the anemia of cyanocobalamin deficiency, folic acid will not correct the neurologic manifestations. Therefore, folic acid supplementation alone may mask underlying cyanocobalamin deficiency resulting in further complications [142, 143]. High dose (400 µg/day) is well tolerated and generally without side effects [144].

Other Vitamins

Vitamin D

Vitamin D is involved in calcium metabolism. Vitamin D is a lipid soluble steroidal group of compounds that have endocrine activity. The primary action of vitamin D is to enhance the absorption of calcium from the gastrointestinal tract [145]. Vitamin D can be formed from the photo-conversion of 7-dehydrocholesterol in the skin. Dietary sources of vitamin D are converted from 25-hydroxychlecalciferol (25-hydroxyvitamin D$_3$) to 1,25-dihydroxychoecalciferol (1,25-dihydroxyvitamin D$_3$; calcitriol) in the kidney. The conversion to the active form is facilitated by the presence of parathyroid hormone (PTH).

Low intake and reduced serum levels of 25-hydroxychelcalciferol or reduced sun exposure [146, 147] can lead to lower levels of calcitriol and compensatory increases in PTH levels and activity. This compensatory increase in PTH is an attempt to increase production of calcitriol [148, 149]. Therefore, decreases in vitamin D status can result in secondary-hyerparathyroidism, which may lead to osteoclast-mediated bone resorption.

Reduced serum vitamin D levels and the compensatory increase may affect bone metabolism in PTH activity. Framingham Heart Study [150] data showed that a low vitamin D status has been associated with osteopenia and osteoarthritis of the knee. Supplementation with vitamin D has been demonstrated to increase bone density. This is likely as a result of reduced bone resorption and decreased PTH activity [151, 152].

While there was no decrease in hip fractures in healthy, independently-living elders, vitamin D supplementation was demonstrated to decrease hip and non-vertebral fractures in nursing home residents [153]. Therefore, vitamin D supplementation should be considered in elderly nursing-home residents [154].

Most vitamin D is formed from exposure to sunlight. During the winter months, with reduced sun exposure, elderly people may be prone to a seasonal reduction in vitamin D [155]. This is notably evident in those who are homebound [156] or in a nursing home [148, 157]. Nearly 95% of nursing home residents may have serum vitamin D levels below the normal range [157]. Moreover, this can also occur in those that are independently living [158]. The current RDA for vitamin D is 200 IU/day [62]. Normal vitamin D levels and seasonal variations in PTH levels can be avoided with vitamin D supplementation of 200 IU/day [147]. However, supplementation in healthy postmenopausal women with ≥800 IU/day has been demonstrated to reduce bone loss more so than in individuals supplemented with 200 IU/day. This then suggests that the current RDA is insufficient to reduce bone loss in the elderly [159].

The optimal means to supplement vitamin D is via fortified milk [157]. Lactose intolerance prohibits this practice. The incidence of lactose intolerance increases with age. Nearly 70% of elderly African-Americans and 20% of elderly Caucasians have clinical signs of lactose intolerance [160]. Supplementation with oral vitamin D (400 IU/day) is a safe means to reduce the incidence of vitamin D deficiency and the subsequent bone loss [161]. Vitamin D supplementation at this dose has been shown to effectively increase serum vitamin D levels and reduce PTH levels without causing hypercalcemia [148].

Vitamin K

Vitamin K is essential for the α-carboxylation of glutamic acid residues in many proteins particularly those involved in blood coagulation. Vitamin K is a lipid soluble vitamin derived from dietary sources such as green-leafy vegetables [phytomenadione (vitamin K_1)] or synthesized by gastrointestinal flora [menatetrenone (vitamin K_2)]. Serum vitamin K levels are a good indicator of overall nutritional status as they are unaffected by age and gender [162]. Vitamin K deficiency is rare in health independently living adults [163]. However, vitamin K deficiency can occur without signs of blood coagulopathy in persons with reduced intake [164].

Vitamin K may also play an important role in calcium metabolism, bone metabolism and potentially atherosclerosis [165]. Glutamic acid residues that have been α-carboxylated via vitamin K are capable of binding calcium and may be involved in calcium transport [162]. Bone formation may be impaired if osteocalcin (a protein released by osteoblasts) is not α-carboxylated due to decreased due to vitamin K deficiency. This may result in reduced bone formation due to its impaired ability to bind to hydroxyapatite [166]. Elderly patients with hip fractures have been found to have reduced circulating vitamin K levels, therefore reduced serum vitamin K levels may be a risk factor for osteoporosis [167] and bone fracture.

While vitamin K is lipid soluble, it is stored primarily in the liver. However, a significant amount is stored in the extra matrix lipids of bone. As one ages, vitamin K stores may be sequestered in the osteoblasts reducing circulating levels [168]. Vitamin

K may play a role in bone loss in the elderly. Supplementation with vitamin K may be a future therapy for osteoporosis as it may reduce urinary calcium losses particularly in postmenopausal women with high urinary calcium excretion [169]. Before vitamin K supplementation can be an acceptable treatment for the treatment and prevention of osteoporosis, long-term prospective trials are necessary [170].

Conclusions

It is generally well accepted in the United States that over-the-counter preparations are "safe". Since these are not under the jurisdiction of the Federal Drug Administration (FDA) of the United States, they may be considered by the general public as without side effect. High dose vitamin therapy is increasing at an alarming rate. In fact the elderly are now three times as likely to use high dose vitamin therapy as compared to 15 years ago [5]. This is further encouraged by claims that high doses of vitamins may prevent, halt, or slow the aging process in the general media. Often, over-the-counter vitamin preparations are ingested without regulation or consideration for possible toxicity.

It is important to consider that elderly persons are at risk for developing vitamin deficiency. Often, elders do not consume the current RDA for many vitamins. This may lead to further progression of disease states if not preventing morbidity associated with vitamin deficiency. Many institutionalized senior citizens are unable to consume the RDA of many vitamins because of dietary restrictions or for economic reasons. Optimally, a well-balanced meal containing fresh fruits and vegetables would suffice. Certainly, supplementation with vitamin preparations will be of benefit. An ideal vitamin supplement would provide the RDA of each vitamin plus 400 µg folic acid, 1 mg cyanocobalamin, 100 IU of vitamin E and elemental calcium 1000 mg [33]. Modest supplementation of these vitamins in combination with an adequate diet will be beneficial without the risk of toxicity.

At this time, with the exception of nicotinic acid therapy in hypercholesterolemia, there is no legitimate benefit from the use of large-dose vitamin therapy with the exception of overt deficient states or in concurrent use of some medications (Table 7.1). An argument can be made for a short-term trial of thiamine 50 mg/day or pyridoxine 50 mg/day for patients with peripheral neuropathy, or ascorbic acid 1000 mg/day in those with vascular fragility and poorly healing wounds. Likewise, the combination of folic acid (400 µg/day) and cyanocobalamin (1 mg/day) can be considered. While vitamin E therapy is controversial, supplementation with 100–200 IU/day is save and well tolerated [33].

It is essential to note that the recurring theme herein is that further, long-term studies are necessary before high-dose supplementation with over-the-counter vitamin preparations is an acceptable medical practice. It is the role of the medical caregive to enforce these recommendations pending further evidence.

Table 7.1. Vitamins that may be effected by commonly used medications [33]. (Adapted from Campbell and Thom [117])

Drug/drug class	Vitamins Depleted
Anti-convulsants	Riboflavin, cyanocobalamin, ascorbic acid, vitamin D, vitamin K, folic acid
Aspirin (Acetylsalicylic acid)	Ascorbic acid, pyridoxine, cyanocobalamin, vitamin K, vitamin K, folic acid
Cholestyramine	Retinol, cyanocobalamin, ascorbic acid, vitamin E, vitamin K, folic acid
Cholchicine	Cyanocobalamin
Corticosteroids	Riboflavin, ascorbic acid, vitamin D, folic acid
Digitalis	Riboflavin
Diuretics	Riboflavin, cyanocobalamin, vitamin D, folic acid
Isoniazid	Pyridoxine, nicotinic acid
Laxatives	Retinol, riboflavin, cyanocobalamin, vitamin D, folic acid
Metformin	Cyanocobalamin
Methotrexate	Folic acid
Triamterene	Folic acid

References

1. Blumberg J. Nutrient requirements of the healthy elderly: should there be specific RDAs? Nutr Rev 1994; 52 (8 Suppl.): S15–8
2. Rudman D, Abbasi AA, Isaacson K, et al. Observations on the nutrient intakes of eating-dependent nursing home residents: underutilization of micronutrient supplements. J Am Coll Nutr 1995; 14(6): 604–13.
3. Posner BM, Jette A, Smigelski C, et al. Nutritional risk in New England elders. J Gerontol1994; 49 (3 Suppl.) " M123-32
4. Shock NW, Grenlich RC, Andres R, et al. for the National In- stitute of Health (NIH). Normal human aging: the Baltimore Longitudinal Study of Aging. NIH Publication No.84-2450. Baltimore (MD): US Department of Health and Human services, 1984 Nov: 105-12
5. Jylha M. Ten-year change in the use of medical drugs among the elderly: a longitudinal study and cohort compari- son. J Clin Epidemiol 1994; 47 (1): 69–79
6. Mant A, Whicker S, Sook Kwok Y. Over-the-counter self- medication: the issues. Drugs Aging 1992; 2 (4): 257–61
7. Alfin-Slater RB. Vitamin use and abuse in elderly persons. Ann Intern Med 1988; 109: 896–9
8. Pitt HA, Costrini AM. Vitamin C prophylaxis in marine recruits. JAMA 1979; 241(9): 908–11.
9. Gray GE, Paganini-Hill A, Ross RK. Dietary intake and nutrient supplement use in a Southern California retire- ment community. Am J Clin Nutr 1983; 38: 122–8.
10. Schectman G. Estimating ascorbic acid requirements for cigarette smokers. Ann N Y Acad Sci 1993; 686: 335–45.
11. Schectman G, Byrd JC, Hoffmann R. Ascorbic acid requirements for smokers: analysis of a population study. Am J Clin Nutr 1991; 53: 1466–70.
12. Dawson EB, Harris WA, Teter MC, et al. Effect of ascorbic acid supplementation on the sperm quality of smokers. Fertil Steril 1992; 58(5): 1034–9
13. Levine M, Dhariwal KR, Welch RW, et al. Determination of optimal vitamin C requirements in humans. Am J Clin Nutr 1995; 62 Suppl.: 1347S–56S.
14. van der Wielen RPJ, van Heereveld HAEM, de Groot CPGM, et al. Nutritional status of elderly female nursing home residents: the effect of supplementation with a physiological dose of water-soluble vitamins. Eur J Clin Nutr 1995; 49: 665–74.
15. Flagg EW, Coates RJ, Greenberg RS. Epidemiologic studies of antioxidants and cancer in humans. J Am Coll Nutr 1995; 14 (5): 419–27.
16. Paolisso G, D'Amore A, Balbi V, et al. Plasma vitamin C affects glucose homeostasis in healthy subjects and in non-insulin-dependent diabetics. Am J Physiol 1994; 266: E261–8.
17. Stankova L, Riddle M, Larned J, et al. Plasma ascorbate concentrations and blood cell dehydroascorbate transport in patents with diabetes mellitus. Metabolsim 1984; 33(4): 347–53.
18. Paolisso G, Balbi V, Volpe C, et al. Metabolic benefits deriving from chronic vitamin C supplementation in aged non-insulin dependent diabetics. J Am Coll Nutr 1995; 14(4): 387–92.

19. Breslow R. Nutritional status and dietary intake of patients with pressure ulcers: review of research literature 1943 to 1989. Decubitus 1991; 4(1): 16–21.

20. Klaassen CD. Principles of toxicology and treatment of poisoning. In: Hardman JG, Limbird LE, eds. Goodman and Gilman's The Pharmacological Basis of Therapeutics. 9th ed. New York: McGraw-Hill, 1996: 63–75.

21. Gosh SK, Ekpo EB, Shah IU, et al. A double-blind, placebo-controlled parallel trial of vitamin C treatment in elderly patients with hypertension. Gerontology 1994; 40(5): 268–72.

22. Lovat LB, Lu U, Palmer AJ, et al. Double-blind trial of vitamin C in elderly hypertensives. J Hum Hypertens 1993; 7: 403–5.

23. Sherman DL, Keaney, Jr. JF, Biegelsen ES, et al. Pharmacological concentrations of ascorbic acid are required for the beneficial effect on endothelial vasomotor function in hypertension. Hypertension 2000; 35: 936–41.

24. Schorah CJ, Tormey WP, Brooks GH, et al. The effect of vitamin C supplements on body weight, serum proteins, and general health of an elderly population. Am J Clin Nutr 1994; 34: 871–6.

25. Bendich A. Safety issues regarding the use of vitamin supplements. Ann N y Acad Sci 1992; 669: 300-10.

26. Bendich A, Langseth L. Safety of vitamin A. Am J Clin Nutr 1989; 49: 358–71.

27. Jacob RA. Vitamin C. In: Shils ME, Olson JA, Shike M, editors. Modern nutrition in health and disease. 8th ed. Philadelphia: Lea and Febiger, 1994: 432–48.

28. Rees DC, Kelsey H, Richards JDM. Acute haemolysis induced by high dose ascorbic acid in glucose-6-phosphate dehydrogenase deficiency. BMJ 1993; 306: 841–2.

29. Wandzilak TR, D' Andre SD, Davis PA, et al. Effect of high dose vitamin C on urinary oxalate levels. J Urol 1994; 151: 834–7.

30. Strijdom JG, Marais BJ, Koeslag JH. Ascorbic acid causes spuriously low blood glucose measurements. S Afr Med J 1993; 83: 64–5.

31. Herbert V, Jacob E. Destruction of vitamin BI2 by ascorbic acid. JAMA 1974; 230: 241–2.

32. Herbert V, Jacob E, Wong KTJ, et al. Low serum BI2 1evels in patients receiving ascorbic acid in megadoses: studies concerning the effect of ascorbate on radioisotope vitamin BI2 assay. Am J Clin Nutr 1978; 31: 253–8.

33. Thurman JE, and Mooradian AD. Vitamin supplementation therapy in the elderly. Drugs and Aging 1997; 11(6): 433–49.

34. Vatassery GT, Johnson GJ, Krezowski AM. Changes in vitamin E concentrations in human plasma and platelets with age. J Am Coll Nutr 1983; 4: 369–75.

35. Kilic F, Milton K, Dzialoszynski T, et al. Modeling cortical cataractogenesis. 14. Reduction in lens damage in diabetic rats by a dietary regimen combining vitamins C and E and (-carotene. Dev Ophthalmol 1994; 26: 63–71

36. Augustin AJ, Briepohl W, Boker T, et al. Evidence for the prevention of oxidative tissue damage in the inner eye by vitamins E and C. Ger J Ophthalmol 1992; I: 394–8

37. Farrell PM, Roberts RJ. Vitamin E. In: Shils ME, Olson JA, Shike M, editors. Modern nutrition in health and disease. 8th ed. Philadelphia: Lea and Febiger, 1994: 326–41

38. Boyle P, Zaridze DG, Smans M. Descriptive epidemiology of colorectal cancer. Int J Cancer 1985; 36 (1): 9–18.

39. Sandier RS, Lyles CM, Peipins LA, et al. Diet and risk of colorectal adenomas: macronutrients, cholesterol, and fiber. J Natl Cancer Inst 1993; 85 (11): 884–91

40. Byers T, Perry G. Dietary carotenes, vitamin C and vitamin E as protective antioxidants in human cancers. Annu Rev Nutr 1992; 12: 139–59

41. Greenberg ER, Baron JA, Karagas MR, et al. Mortality associated with low plasma concentration of -carotene and the effect of oral supplementation. JAMA 1996; 275 (9): 699–703

42. The (-Tocopherol, (-Carotene Cancer Prevention Study Group. The effect of vitamin E and (-carotene on the incidence of lung cancer and other cancers in male smokers. N Engl J Med 1994; 330 (15): 1029–35

43. Kushi LH, Fee RM, Sellers TA, et al. Intake of vitamins A, C, and E and postmenopausal breast cancer: the Iowa Women's Health Study. Am J Epidemiol 1996; 144 (2): 165–74

44. Bursell S, Schlossman DK, Clermont AC, et al. High dose vitamin E supplementation normalized retinal blood flow and creatine clearance in patients with type 1 diabetes. Diabetes Care 1999; 22: 1245–51.

45. Meydani SN, Wu D, Santos MS, et al. Antioxidants and immune response in aged persons: overview of present evidence. Am J Clin Nutr 1995; 62 Suppl.: 14625–765

46. Sano M, Ernesto C, Thomas RG, et al. A controlled trial of selegiline, (-tocopherol, or both as treatment for Alzheimer's disease. N Engl J Med 1997; 336 (17): 1216–22

47. Rapola JM, Virtamo J, Haukka JK, et al. Effect of vitamin E and (-carotene on the incidence of angina pectoris: a randomized, double-blind, controlled trial. JAMA 1996; 275 (9): 693–8

48. Rimm EB, Stampfer MJ, Ascherio A, et al. Vitamin E consumption and the risk of coronary heart disease in men. N Engl J Med 1993; 328 (20): 1450–6

49. Kushi LH, Folsom AR, Prineas RJ, et al. Dietary antioxidant vitamins and death from coronary heart disease in postmenopausal women. NEJM 1996; 334 (18): 1156–62

50. Rudman D,. Abbasi AA, Isaacson K, et al. Observations on the nutrient intakes of eating-dependent nursing home residents: underutilisation of miicronutrient supplements. J Am Coll Nutr 1995; 14 (6): 604–13

51. Dieber-Rotheneder M, Puhl H, Waeg G, et al. Effect of oral supplementation with D-alpha-tocopherol on the vitamin E content of human low density lipoproteins and resistance to oxidation. J Lipid Res 1991; 32: 1325–32

52. Reaven PD, Herold DA, Barnett J, et al. Effects of vitamin E on susceptibility of low-density lipoprotein and low-density lipoprotein subfractions to oxidation and on protein glycation in NIDDM. Diabetes Care 1995; 18 (6): 807–16

53. Hodis HN, Mack WJ, LaBree L, et al. Serial coronary angiographic evidence that antioxidant vitamin intake reduces progression of coronary artery atherosclerosis. JAMA 1995; 273 (23): 1849–54

54. Tardif JC, Cote G, Lesperance J, et al. Probucol and multivitamins in the prevention of restenosis after coronary angioplasty. N Engl J Med 1997; 337 (6): 365–72
55. Stephens NG, Parsons A, Schofield PM, et al. Randomized controlled trial of vitamin E in patients with coronary disease: Cambridge Heart Antioxidant Study (CHAOS). Lancet 1996; 347: 781–6
56. Virtamo J, Rapola JM, Ripatti S, et al. Effect of vitamin E and beta carotene on the incidence of primary nonfatal myocardial infarction and fatal coronary heart disease. Arch Intern Med 1998; 158: 668–75
57. Brown BG, Zhao XQ, Chait A, et al. Simvastatin and niacin, antioxidant vitamins, or the combination for the prevention of coronary disease. New Engl J of Med 2001; 345(22): 1583–1592
58. Freedman JE. Anitoxidant versus lipid altering therapy - some answers, more questions. New Engl J of Med 2001; 345(22): 1636–37
59. The Heart Outcomes Prevention Evaluation Study Investigators, Vitamin E supplementation and cardiovascular evens in high-risk patents. NEJM 2000; 342: 154–60
60. Corrigan JJ. The effect of vitamin E on warfarin-induced vitamin K deficiency. Ann N Y Acad Sci 1982; 393: 361-8
61. Farrell PM, Roberts RJ. Vitamin E. In: Shils ME, Olson JA, Shike M, editors. Modern nutrition in health and disease. 8th ed. Philadelphia: Lea and Febiger, 1994: 326–41
62. National Research Council. Recommended dietary allowances. 10th ed. Washington, DC. National Academy Press, 1989 National Research Council. Recommended dietary allowances. lOth ed. Washington, DC. National Academy Press, 1989
63. Basu TK, Donald FA, Gargreaves JA, et al. Seasonal variation of vitamin A (retinol) status in older men and women. J Am Coll Nutr 1994; 13 (6): 641–5
64. Marcus R, Coulston AM. Water-soluble vitamins: the vitamin B complex and ascorbic acid. In: Wonsiewecz M, McCurdy P, editors. Goodman and Gilman's the pharmacological basis of therapeutics. 9th ed. New York: McGraw-Hill,1996: 1535–72
65. Bendich A, Langseth L. Safety of vitamin A. Am J Clin Nutr 1989; 49: 358-71
66. Shimizu H, Nagata C, Komatsu S, et al. Decreased serum retinol levels in women with cervical dysplasia. Br J Cancer 1996; 73 (12): 1600–4
67. Greenberg ER, Baron JA, Karagas MR, et al. Mortality associated with low plasma concentration of (-carotene and the effect of oral supplementation. JAMA 1996; 275 (9): 699–703
68. Wang XD. Review: absorption and metabolism of (-carotene. J Am Coll Nutr 1994; 13 (4): 314–25
69. Burton GW, Ingold KU. (-Carotene: an unusual type of lipid antioxidant. Science 1984; 224: 569–73
70. Zheng W, Sellers TA, Doyle TJ, et al. Retinol, antioxidant vitamins and cancers of the upper digestive tract in a prospective cohort study of postmenopausal women. Am J Epidemiol 1995; 142 (9): 955–60
71. Kushi LH, Fee RM, Sellers TA, et al. Intake of vitamins A, C, and E and postmenopausal breast cancer: the Iowa Women's Health Study. Am J Epidemiol1996; 144 (2): 165–74
72. Hennekens CH, Buring JE, Manson JE, et al. Lack of effect of long-term supplementation with (-carotene on the incidence of malignant neoplasms and cardiovascular disease. NEJM 1996; 334 (18): 1145–9
73. Christen WG, JM Gaziano, and CH Hennekens. Design of Physicians' Health Study II - a randomized trial of beta-carotene, vitamins E and C, and multivitamins, in prevention of cancer, cardiovascular disease, and eye disease, and review of results of completed trials. Ann Epidemiol 2000; 10: 125–134
74. Omenn GS, Goodman GE, Thornquist MD, et al. Effects of a combination of (-carotene and vitamin A on lung cancer and cardiovascular disease. NEJM 1996; 334 (18): 1150–5
75. Greenberg ER, Baron JA, Tosteson TD, et al. A clinical trial of antioxidant vitamins to prevent colorectal adenoma. N Engl J Med 1994; 331 (3): 141–7
76. Marwick C. Trials reveal no benefit, possible harm of (-carotene and vitamin A for lung cancer prevention. JAMA 1996; 275 (6): 422–3
77. Hathcock IN, Hattan DG, Jenkins MY, et al. Evaluation of vitamin A toxicity. Am J Clin Nutr 1990; 52 (2): 183–202
78. Olson JA. Vitamin A. retinoids. and carotenoids. In: Shils ME, Olson JA, Shike M, editors. Modern nutrition in health and disease. 8th ed. Philadelphia: Lea and Febiger, 1994: 287–307
79. Garewal HS, Diplock AT. How 'safe' are antioxidant vitamins? Drug Saf 1995; 13 (1): 8–14
80. Marcus R, Coulston AM. Water-soluble vitamins: the vitamin B complex and ascorbic acid. In: Wonsiewecz M, McCurdy P, editors. Goodman and Gilman's the pharmacological basis of therapeutics. 9thed. New York: McGraw-Hill,1996: 1535–72
81. Bettendorff L, Mastrogiacomo F, Kish SJ, et al. Thiamine, thiamine phosphates, and their metabolizing enzymes in human brain. J Neurochem 1996; 66 (1): 250–8
82. Reed RL, Mooradian AD. Nutritional status and dietary management of elderly diabetic patients. Clin Geriatr Med 1990; 6 (4): 883–901
83. Tanphaichitr V. Thiamin. In: Shils ME, Olson JA, Shike M, editors. Modem nutrition in health and disease. 8th ed. Philadelphia: Lea and Febiger, 1994: 359–65
84. Kwok T, Falconer-Smith JF, Potter JF, et al. Thiamine status of elderly patients with cardiac failure. Age Ageing 1992; 2 I (I): 67–71
85. Boisvert WA, Castaneda C, Mendoza I, et al. Prevalence of riboflavin deficiency among Guatemalan elderly people and its relationship to milk intake. Am J Clin Nutr 1993; 58 (1): 85–90
86. Bates CJ. Human riboflavin requirements and metabolic consequences of deficiency in man and animals. World Rev Nutr Diet 1987; 50: 215–65
87. Lowik MR, van den Berg H, Kistemaker C, et al. Interrelationships between riboflavin and vitamin B6 among elderly people (Dutch Nutrition Surveillance System). Int J Vitam Nutr Res 1994; 64 (3): 198–203

88. Boisvert WA, Mendoza 1, Castaneda C, et al. Riboflavin requirement of healthy elderly humans and its relationship to macro-nutrient composition of the diet. I Nutr 1993; 123 (5); 915–25

89. Winters LR, Yoon JS, Kalkwarf HJ, et al. Riboflavin requirements and exercise adaptation in older women. Am J Clin Nutr 1992; 56 (3): 526–32

90. McCormick OB. Riboflavin. In: Shils ME, Olson JA, Shike M, editors. Modem nutrition in health and disease. 8th ed. Philadelphia: Lea and Febiger, 1994: 366–75

91. Riggs KM, Spiro III A, Tucker K, et al. Relations of vitamin B-12, vitamin B-6, folate and homocysteine to cognitive performance in the Normative Aging Study. Am Clin Nutr 1996; 63 (3): 306–14

92. Deijen JB, van der Beck E, Orlebeke JF, et al. Vitamin B6 supplementation in elderly men: effects on mood, memory, performance and mental effort. Psychopharmacology 1992; 109: 489–96

93. van der Beek El, van Dokkum W, Wedel M, et al. Thiamin, riboflavin and vitamin B6: impact of restricted intake on physical performance in man. Am Coll Nutr 1994; 13 (6): 629–40

94. Ubbink JB, van der Merwe A, Delport R, et al. The effect of a subnormal vitamin B-6 status on homocysteine metabolism. Clin Invest 1996; 98 (1): 177–84

95. Ellis JM, McCully KS. Prevention of myocardial infarction by vitamin B6. Res Commun Mol Pathol Pharmacol 1995; 89 (2): 208–20

96. Nygard O, JE Nordrehaug, H Refsum, PM Ueland, M Farstad, SE Vollset. Plasma homocysteine levels and mortality in patients with coronary artery disease. NEJM 1997; 337: 230–6

97. Eikelboom JW, E Lonn, J Genest Jr., G Hankey, S Yusuf. Homocysteine and cardiovascular disease: a critical review of the epidemiologic evidence. Ann Intern Med. 1999; 131: 363–75

98. Oakshinamurti K, Paulsoe CS, Viswanathan M. Vitamin B6 and hypertension. Ann YAcad Sci 1990; 585: 241–9

99. Lal KJ, Oakshinamurti K. Calcium channels in vitamin B6 deficiency-induced hypertension. J Hypertens 1993; 11 (12): 1357–62

100. Meydani SN, Hayek M, Coleman L. Influence of vitamins E and B6 on immune response. Ann NY Acad Sci 1992; 669: 125–39

101. Meydani SN, Hayek M, Coleman L. Influence of vitamins E and B6 on immune response. Ann N y Acad Sci 1992; 669: 125–39

102. Ellis JM, Folkers K. Clinical aspects of treatment of carpal tunnel syndrome with vitamin B6. Ann N y Acad Sci 1990; 585: 302–20

103. Reynolds TM, Marshall PO, Brain AM. Hip fracture patients may be vitamin B6 deficient: controlled study of serum pyridoxal-5'-phosphate. Acta Orthop Scand 1992; 63 (6): 635–8

104. Bemstein AL. Vitamin B6 in clinical neurology. Ann N y Acad Sci 1990; 585: 250–60

105. Leklem IE. Vitamin B6. In: Shils ME, Olson JA, Shike M, editors. Modem nutrition in health and disease. 8th ed. Philadelphia: Lea and Febiger, 1994: 383–94

106. Joosten E, van den Berg A, Riezler R, etal. Metabolic evidence that deficiencies of vitamin B-12 (cobalamin), folate, and vitamin B-6 occur commonly in elderly people. Am J Clin Nutr 1993; 58 (4): 468–76

107. Leklem IE. Vitamin B6 reservoirs, receptors and red-cell reactions. Ann N y Acad Sci 1992; 669: 34–41

108. Bemstein AL. Vitamin B6 in clinical neurology. Ann N y Acad Sci 1990; 585: 250–60

109. Schaumburg H, Kaplan J, Windebank A, et al. Sensory neuropathy from pyridoxine abuse: a new megavitamin syndrome. N Engl J Med 1983; 309 (8): 445–8

110. Morimoto K, KawadaA, HirumaM, etal. Photosensitivity from pyridoxine hydrochloride (vitamin B6). J Am Acad Oermatol 1996; 35 (Pt 2): 304–5

111. Berger AR, Schaumburg HH, Schroeder C, et al. Dose response, coasting, and differential fiber vulnerability in human toxic neuropathy: a prospective study of pyridoxine neurotoxicity. Neurology 1992; 42 (7): 1367–70

112. Wilson JD. Vitamin deficiency and excess. In: Isselbacher KJ, Martin JB, Braunwald E, et al., editors. Harrison's principles of internal medicine. 13th ed. New York: McGraw-Hill, 1994: 472–80

113. Durrington PN. Drug therapy of hyperlipidaemia. In: Hyperlipidaemia: diagnosis and management. 2nd ed. Cambridge: Cambridge University Press, 1995: 258–90

114. Illingworth DR, Stein EA, Mitchel YB, et al. Comparative effects of lovastatin and niacin in primary hypercholesterolemia: a prospective trial. Arch Intern Med 1994; 154 (14): 1586–95

115. Miller NE. Pharmacological intervention for altering lipid metabolism. Drugs 1990; 40 Suppl. I: 26–31

116. Durrington PN. Drug therapy of hyperlipidaemia. In: Hyperlipidemia: diagnosis and management. 2nd ed. Cambridge: Cambridge University Press, 1995: 258–90

117. Coronary Drug Project Research Group. Clofibrate and niacin in coronary heart disease. JAMA 1975; 231:360–381

118. Carlson LA, Rosenhamer G. Reduction of mortality in the Stockholm Ischemic Heart Disease Study by combined treatment with clofibrate and nicotinic acid. Acta Med Scand 1988; 223:405–418

119. Dalton TA, Berry RS. Hepatotoxicity associated with sustained- release niacin. Am J Med 1992; 93 (I): 102–4

120. Wahlberg G, Walldius G, Efendic S. Effects of nicotinic acid on glucose tolerance and glucose incorporation into adipose tissue in hypertriglyceridaemia. Scand J Clin Lab Invest 1992; 52 (6): 537–45

121. Lipman TO. Vitamins: hormonal and metabolic interrelationships. In: Becker KL, editor. Principles and practice of endocrinology and metabolism. 2nd ed. Philadelphia: J.B. Lippincott, 1995: 50–6

122. Lindenbaum J, Rosenberg IH, Wilson PWF, et al. Prevalence of cobalamin deficiency in the Framingham elderly population. Am J Clin Nutr 1994; 60: 2–11

123. Pennypacker LC, Allen RH, Kelly JP, et al. High prevalence of cobalamin deficiency in elderly outpatients. J Am Geriatr Soc 1992; 40 (12): 1197–204

124. Cunha UG, RochaFL, Peixoto JM, etal. Vitamin B12 deficiency and dementia. Int Psychogeriatr 1995; 7 (I): 85–8

125. Crystal HA, Ortof E, Frishman WH, et al. Serum vitamin BI2 levels and incidence of dementia in a healthy elderly population: a report from the Bronx Longitudinal Aging Study. J Am Geriatr Soc 1994; 42 (9): 933–6
126. Carmel R. Subtle and atypical cobalamin deficiency states. Am J Hematol 1990; 34: 108–14
127. Allen RH, Stabler SP, Savage DG, et al. Metabolic abnormal ties in cobalamin (vitamin B12) and folate deficiency. FASEB J 1993; 7: 1344–53
128. Beck WS. Diagnosis of megaloblastic anemia. Annu Rev Med 1991; 42: 311–22
129. Fairbanks VF. Tests for pernicious anemia: the 'Schilling test'. Mayo Clin Proc 1983; 58: 541–4
130. Carmel R. Approach to a low vitamin B12 level [letter]. JAMA 1994; 272 (16): 1233
131. Carmel R. Subtle and atypical cobalamin deficiency states. Am J Hematol 1990; 34: 108–14
132. Rosenberg IH, Miller IW. Nutritional factors in physical and cognitive functions of elderly people. Am J Clin Nutr 1992; 55: 1237S–43S
133. Allen LH, Casterline J. Vitamin B-12 deficiency in elderly individuals: diagnosis and requirements. Am J Nutr 1994; 60: 12–14
134. Boushey CJ, Beresford SAA, Omenn GS, et al. A quantitative assessment of plasma homocysteine as a risk factor for vascular disease: probable benefits of increasing folic acid intakes. JAMA 1995; 274 (13): 1049–57
135. Selhub J, Jacques PF, Bostom AG, et al. Association between plasma homocysteine concentrations and extracranial carotid artery stenosis. N Engl J Med 1995; 332 (5): 286–91
136. Mudd SH, Skovby F, Levy HI, et al. The natural history of homocysteinuria due to cystathionine (-syntase deficiency. Am J Hum Genet 1985; 37:1–31
137. McCully KS. Vascular pathology of homocysteinemia: implications for the pathogenesis of arteriosclerosis. Am J Pathol 1969; 56:111–128
138. Schnyder G, Roffi M, Pin R, et al. Decreased rate of coronary restenosis after lowering of plasma homocysteine levels. New Engl J of Med 2001; 345(22): 1593–1600
139. Stampfer MJ, Willett WC. Homocysteine and marginal vitamin deficiency: the importance of adequate vitamin intake. JAMA 1993; 270 (22): 2726–7
140. Selhub J, Jacques PF, Wilson PWF, et al. Vitamin status and intake as primary determinants of homocysteinemia in an elderly population. JAMA 1993; 270 (22): 2693–91
141. Drinka PJ, Langer EH, Voeks SK, et al. Low serum folic acid levels in a nursing home population: a clinical experience. J Am Coll Nutr 1993; 12 (2): 186–9
142. Ubbink JB, Vermaak WJ, vander Merwe A, et al. Vitamin requirements for the treatment of hyperhomocysteinemia in humans. J Nutr 1994; 124 (10): 1927–33
143. Stampfer MJ, Malinow MR. Can lowering homocysteine levels reduce cardiovascular risk? N Engl J Med 1995; 332 (5): 328–9
144. Oakley GP, Adams MJ, Dickinson CM. More folic acid for everyone, now. J Nutr 1996; 126 Suppl.: 751S–5S
145. Waiters MR. Newly identified actions of the vitamin D endocrine system. Endocr Rev 1992; 13 (4): 719–64
146. Lips P, Hackeng WHL, Jongen MJM, et al. Seasonal variation in serum concentrations of parathyroid hormone in elderly people. J Clin Endocrinol Metab 1983; 57 (I): 204–6
147. Krall EA, Sahyoun N, Tannenbaum S, et al. Effect of vitamin D intake on seasonal variation in parathyroid hormone secretion in postmenopausal women. N Engl J Med 1989; 321 (26): 1777–83
148. Lips P, Wiersinga A, van Ginkel FC, et al. The effect of vitamin D supplementation on vitamin D status and parathyroid function in elderly subjects. J ClinEndocrinol Metab 1988; 67 (4): 644–50
149. Quesada JM, Coopmans W, Ruiz B, et al. Influence of vitamin D on parathyroid function in the elderly. J Clin Endocrinol Metab 1992; 75 (2): 494–501
150. McAlindon TE, Felson DT, Zhang Y, et al. Relation of dietary intake and serum levels of vitamin D to progression of osteoarthritis of the knee among participants in the Framingham study. Ann Intern Med 1996; 125 (5): 353–9
151. Ooms ME, Roos JC, Bezemer PD, et al. Prevention of bone loss by vitamin D supplementation in elderly women: a randomized double-blind trial. J Clin Endocrinol Metab 1995; 80 (4): 1052–8
152. Prestwood KM, Pannullo AM, Denny AM, et al. The effect of a short course of calcium and vitamin D on bone turnover in older women. Osteoporos Int 1996; 6.314–9
153. Chapuy MC, Arlot ME, Duboeuf F, et al. Vitamin D3 and calcium to prevent hip fractures in elderly women. N Engl J Med 1992; 327 (23): 1637–42
154. Lips P, Graafmans WC, Ooms ME, et al. Vitamin D supplementation and fracture incidence in elderly persons: a randomized, placebo-controlled clinical trial. Ann Intern Med 1996; 124 (4): 400–6
155. Salamone LM, Dallal GE, Zantos D, et al. Contributions of vitamin D intake and seasonal sunlight exposure to plasma 25-hydroxyvitamin D concentration in elderly women. Am J Clin Nutr 1994; 59 (1): 80–6
156. Gloth FM, Gundberg CM, Hollis BW, et al. Vitamin D deficiency in homebound elderly persons. JAMA 1995; 274(21): 1683–6
157. Keane EM, Rochfort A, Cox J, et al. Vitamin-D-fortified liquid milk: a highly effective method of vitamin D administration for house-bound and institutionalized elderly. Gerontology 1992; 38 (5): 280–4
158. van der Wielen RP, Lowik MR, van den Berg H, et al. Serum vitamin D concentrations among elderly people in Europe. Lancet 1995; 346: 207–10
159. Dawson-Hughes B, Harris SS, Krall EA, et al. Rates of bone loss in postmenopausal women randomly assigned to one of two dosages of vitamin D. Am J Clin Nutr 1995; 61 (5): 1140–5
160. Rao DR, Bello H, Warren AP, et al. Prevalence of lactose maldigestion: influence and interaction of age, race and sex. Dig Dis Sci 1994; 39 (7): 1519–24

161. McKenna MJ. Differences in vitamin D status between countries in young adults and the elderly. Am J Med 1992; 93 (1): 69-77
162. Heaney RP. Bone mass, nutrition and other lifestyle factors. Am J Med 1993; 95 Suppl. 5A: 29S-33S
163. Sokoll LJ, Sadowski JA. Comparison of biochemical indexes for assessing vitamin K nutritional status in a healthy adult population. Am J Clin Nutr 1996; 63 (4): 566-73
164. Ferland G, Sadoski JA, O'Brien ME. Dietary induced subclinical vitamin K deficiency in normal human subjects. J Clin Invest 1993; 91 (4): 1761-8
165. Jie KS, Bots ML, Vermeer C, et al. Vitamin K intake and osteocalcin levels in women with and without aortic atherosclerosis: a population-based study. Atherosclerosis 1995; 116 (I): 117-23
166. Szulc P, Chapuy MC, Meunier PJ, et al. Serum under-carboxylated osteocalcin is a marker of the risk of hip fracture in elderly women. J Clin Invest 1993; 91 (4): 1769-74
167. Hodges SJ, Akesson K, Vergnaud P, et al. Circulating levels of vitamins K1 and K2 decreased in elderly women with hip fracture. J Bone Miner Res 1993; 8 (10): 1241-5
168. Hodges SJ, Bejui J, Leclercq M, et al. Detection and measurement of vitamins K1 and K2 in human cortical and trabecular bone. J Bone Miner Res 1993; 8 (8): 1005-8
169. Knapen MH, Jie KS, Hamulyak K, et al. Vitamin K-induced changes in markers for osteoblast activity and urinary calcium loss. Calcif Tissue Int 1993; 53 (2): 81-5
170. Binkley NC, Suttie JW. Vitamin K nutrition and osteoporosis. J Nutr 1995; 125: 1812-21

8 Herbal Therapy and the Elderly

B.A. Bauer

Introduction

Just as the definition of what constitutes elderly seems to have many interpretations, so does the definition of what constitutes an herb. From a strict botanical perspective, an herb is "a seed-producing annual, biennial, or perennial that does not develop persistent woody tissue but dies down at the end of a growing season" [1]. Yet one of the most popular "herbs" worldwide (Gingko biloba) is in fact not an "herb" but a tree. Obviously strictly adhering to the classical botanical definition serves only to confuse the issue, both for medical professionals as well as for patients. The common or vernacular use generally means any plant or plant product, used for medicinal purposes. Some use the term "phytochemicals" to indicate those plant-derived products used for medicinal purposes. Often times, even substances that are not of plant-origin (e.g. glucosamine and chondroitin) are lumped into the general category of "herbal therapy". For the most part, for the purposes of this chapter, we will primarily focus on those therapeutics that are truly plant in origin.

It is important to realize that the regulatory environment regarding the manufacture and sale of botanicals varies greatly from country. In Germany, for example, phytomedicines are licensed, standardized and covered by the German Health Insurance if prescribed by a physician. Germany began to address the issue of growing herbal popularity over twenty years ago, when the German Commission E was established in 1978. The Commission was charged to bring some sense of order to the growing use of herbs and to develop a one or two page monograph on each of the approximately 300 herbs that were being commonly used. These monographs provide the framework for the integration of herbal medicines into the German health care system. Further, both German medical professionals and the German public generally have some familiarity with the proper and safe use of herbs, recognizing their potential for both harm and good.

This contrasts sharply with the state of affairs in the United States. Here, the regulatory oversight is provided largely under the auspices of the Dietary Supplement Health Education Act of 1994 [2]. Interestingly, this act came about as a result of increasing concerns about the quality of herbal and other dietary supplements. In particular, the eosinophilia myalgia syndrome, triggered by a tainted batch of L-tryptophan from a Japanese manufacturer, helped to coalesce growing concerns regarding such products. The Food and Drug Administration (FDA) announced a Proposal for Rule Making as a preliminary step to begin to develop tighter restrictions on the quality, safety and sale of herbs. However, this triggered a massive and well-organized campaign, largely coordinated by herbal manufacturers and health food storeowners. Customers of such stores were encouraged to write or call their congressional representatives and urge them not to let the FDA "take away my herbal supplements". The campaign was extremely effective, flooding Congress with mail and messages. In response, DSHEA was passed. Rather than granting the FDA greater regulatory oversight of the herbal market, in many respects, it did just the opposite. The Act specifically identified "dietary supplements" as a classification separate from food and drugs, clearly bypassing the safeguards associated with each of those classes. For the first time, manufacturers were allowed to issue dosage recommendations on their products' labels. Even more concerning, the Act specifically exempts manufacturers from demonstrating safety or efficacy of their product prior to marketing.

The act does preclude manufacturers from making specific medical claims, but does permit so-called "structure and function" claims. Thus a claim that a saw palmetto preparation decreases nocturia associated with BPH would not be permitted. However, a claim that the product "promotes men's prostate health" would be acceptable. Finally the Act requires the following disclaimer appear on all dietary supplement labels: "This product has not been approved by the FDA. It is not intended to treat, diagnose, cure or prevent any disease". Although supposedly intended to serve as a warning to the consumer, the disclaimer seems to receive as little attention as the disclaimers associated with tobacco or alcohol products.

Further complicating the issue in the United States is the fact that relatively few conventionally trained physicians or pharmacists receive much, if any, training in herbal therapies. These limitations, combined with an apparently insatiable public appetite for all therapies "natural" have proven to be a difficult and sometimes dangerous combination. Americans tend to view "natural" as equivalent with "safe". There also seems to be a significant proportion of the population that follows the maxim "If a little is good, a lot must be better". Both of these misconceptions combine to yield a potentially dangerous situation. In fact, all of these factors combined (physician and pharmacist unfamiliarity, consumer enthusiasm, and erroneous assumptions about the safety of herbs) may explain in part the relatively frequent reporting of herb toxicities or herb-drug interactions observed in the past five years.

All of these concerns are heightened even further when one considers specifically the aged portion of the population. Every potential concern and risk that is inherent in the use of herbs in general is amplified in the elderly. Comorbid conditions (e.g. hypertension, coronary artery disease, arthritis, diabetes, etc.) increase the likelihood of side effects or toxic effects. For example, ephedra-containing products have been reported to cause hypertension, strokes and even death. An obese, hypertensive elderly patient, searching for a "natural" treatment for obesity, may unwittingly choose a product with ephedra. Uncontrolled hypertension, stroke, rupture of an abdominal aortic aneurysm – all could be potential consequences.

Polypharmacy is also common in the elderly, heightening the risk of drug-herb interactions. The study of such interactions is still in its infancy but recognition is growing that many herbs can and do interact with many pharmaceutical drugs. For example, herbs can alter the metabolism of a drug, either speeding its clearance or delaying its metabolism. An example of the former is St. John's wort, an herb that is now recognized as increasing the activity of the cytochrome P450 enzyme system, and the CYP3A4 subsystem in particular. The latter enzyme system plays an important role in the metabolism of many different drugs. Thus, it is not surprising that there are now several reports in the literature of cases where drug levels were significantly reduced by the co-administration of St. John's wort. These include anti-retrovirals [3], digoxin [4], and cyclosporin [5].

These reports clearly highlight the potential risks of a casual approach to the use of herbs. SJW has been used for centuries, with a long track record of safety. That it is only within the last 2–3 years that its tremendous potential impact on a number of prescription medications is being recognized, documents all too clearly the need for increased knowledge, research and vigilance in this realm.

Herbs can also have an enhancing effect on pharmaceuticals if they slow the metabolism of a particular agent. For example, a proprietary brand of ginseng (Gin-sana) has been reported to cause a rise in the INR of a patient on a stable dose of coumadin [6]. Potentiation of the effects of warfarin, a common pharmaceutical in the elderly, and one with a narrow therapeutic index, can occur with multiple herbs via multiple mechanisms. Platelet inhibition occurs with ginkgo, ginger, garlic and feverfew.

It is also possible for herbs to interfere with the absorption of prescription products, as in the case of plantain (a source of psyllium) or to accelerate transit through the gut (e.g. laxative herbs such as senna), again resulting in a lower blood level of the drug. Constipation is a common and chronic problem for many of the elderly, and the likelihood of many of them trying an herbal product at some point in their lives is high. Recognizing and understanding the potential risks and benefits should allow for safer use of the herbs that a patient does decide to use.

Drug metabolism changes with age and the same is undoubtedly true for the metabolism of chemical constituents of herbal products as well. Thus, while we are just beginning to understand herbal pharmacology in the general population, we have yet to scratch the surface of what occurs in the elderly. There are undoubtedly unique challenges to the safe use of herbs in the elderly which are yet unknown.

However, the risks of herbal therapies are generally under-appreciated and the elderly, plagued with multiple chronic conditions, may be susceptible to their appeal. Most studies suggest that people are more likely to turn to alternative therapies when they are dealing with a chronic, incurable condition (e.g. arthritis) for which conventional medicine has not been able to provide a cure.

Finally, the purity of many herbal products is suspect in countries such as the United States, where the regulatory oversight is limited. Thus, toxicity has occurred when an herb was misidentified. For example, digitalis poisoning in a young woman occurred when foxglove was substituted for plantain [7]. Intentional substitution of herbs has also occurred, especially when the real herb is rare or expensive to produce (e.g. mandrake has been substituted for ginseng, resulting in scopolamine poisoning). Adulteration and contamination are also real concerns. Some herbs are harvested in countries with heavy industrial pollution. Plants harvested near such industrial sites often contain high amounts of lead, cadmium, arsenic or other heavy metals. Even more worrisome, lead is sometimes used as an active ingredient in some Ayurvedic medications.

All of which is not intended as an indictment of herbs in general. In fact, herbs have been used successfully as a mainstay of medical therapy around the world. The World Health Organization has estimated that 80% of the world's population uses some form of herbal therapy as part of their primary health care [8]. Thus, as one considers the growing ease of international travel, globalization of economies, and the rapid spread of information via the Internet, it is clear that herbs will continue to play a prominent role in healthcare for years to come.

And there are a growing number of herbs that have been studied (or are being studied) in large, randomized controlled studies. This data, combined with the knowledge gained from historical use and smaller prior studies, is allowing an evidence-based approach to the use of herbs. Thus, where such data exists, it is important for physicians and patients to incorporate that knowledge and apply it to the decision-making process regarding use of herbs. The following brief review of herbal therapies associated with specific ailments peculiar to the elderly is not meant to be exhaustive. Rather, it is intended to demonstrate that evidence-based decision making is possible and will hopefully serve as a framework for future decision making and education of patients.

Dementia

Ginkgo (*Ginkgo biloba*)

Background. Ginkgo is purportedly one of the oldest surviving plant species, making it somehow seem appropriate as a possible treatment for the elderly. While it has many purported beneficial effects on a variety of ailments (peripheral vascular disorders, vertigo, tinnitus and impotence) it is best known as a treatment for dementia. With little recent progress in developing an effective treatment (or preventative) for dementia, it is little wonder that interest in ginkgo has been growing.

Biochemistry. Ginkgo consists of multiple active constituents, the principal ones being flavonoids and terpene lactones (including bilobalide and several ginkgolides) [9]. Numerous studies, primarily involving a standardized *Ginkgo biloba* extract (GBE), have been performed, primarily in Europe. These studies demonstrate the GBE does cross the blood brain barrier, acts as a cerebral antioxidant, and increases vasodilation of cerebral vessels. Also, ginkgolide B inhibits binding of platelet-activating factor (PAF) [10]. Rat studies have also suggested increased survivability to hypoxic challenge in those animals pre-treated with ginkgo. All of these findings do not prove that the plant's constituents will have a positive effect on dementia but lend plausibility to the hypothesis.

Clinical Studies. One of the most frequently referenced studies is that of LeBars et al. [11]. Sponsored by Willmar Schwabe Pharm (patent holder for a specific extract of ginkgo – EGb761), this study randomized 202 patients with Alzheimer's disease to either

EGb761 or placebo. The study was performed in a randomized, double-blind fashion. Specific endpoints were changes in the Alzheimer's Disease Assessment Scale-Cognitive subscale (ADAS-Cog), the Geriatric Evaluation of Relative's Rating Instrument (GERRI), and the Clinical Global Impression of Change (CGIC). The latter scale showed no difference between groups. However, both the ADAS-Cog and GERRI scale values showed a statistically significant improvement in those patients treated with Egb761. Efficacy was also supported in a review by Ernst et al. [12] in 1999. Though only 9 of 18 reviewed studies were considered to be scientifically rigorous enough for inclusion, those that were reviewed did reveal statistically significant benefits. This generally favorable clinical evidence must be balanced against a recent negative study [13] that was methodologically sound and failed to demonstrate any benefit in 63 elderly patients with dementia.

Safety. Millions of doses of Ginkgo biloba are consumed on an annual basis worldwide. Reports of toxicity have been generally rare. However, there have been several reports of bleeding complications in the US literature [14–16].

Recommendations. Ginkgo as a treatment for dementia appears to have some scientific support, though the effect size is probably small. It appears to be generally safe with the caveat that bleeding may be an issue, probably secondary to PAF inhibition. Hence, if patients wish to use ginkgo, it is prudent to counsel them regarding this risk and to suggest avoiding concomitant use of anticoagulant medication.

Depression

St. John's Wort (*Hypericum perforatum*)

Background. The later years of life bring unique challenges: declining mobility, reduced vision and hearing, loss of friends and family members, etc. Especially in societies that value youth and disregard the aged, the aged may be faced with depression. Since many patients, regardless of age, find it difficult to discuss their symptoms of depression with family members or their physician, pharmaceutical treatment is often not made available. Thus, patients struggling with what they believe to be depressive symptoms are particularly likely to self-diagnose and self-prescribe treatment, when it is known and available. St. John's wort provides just such an opportunity.

One of the top 10 selling herbs in America for several years, it has proven to be tremendously popular and highly regarded. However, recent reports of adverse events, primarily in the realm of drug-herb interactions, must sound a cautionary note to those contemplating its use.

Biochemistry. There continues to be a great deal of controversy surrounding the biochemical effects of St. John's wort. Even questions regarding the active ingredient remain unsettled. Hypericin has long been considered the active ingredient by many researchers and as a result, many St. John's wort products are standardized to the content of hypericin. However, more recent studies suggest that the efficacy as an antidepressant is more closely tied to the content of hyperforin [17, 18].

Disregarding the controversy over which constituent plays the major role in activity of the product, the biochemistry remains still elusive. Studies suggest inhibition of reuptake of serotonin, norepinephrine, and dopamine [19, 20].

Clinical Studies. There seems little doubt that St. John's wort is effective for mild to moderate depression [21–23]. In regards to severe depression, the evidence is less supportive. In fact, a very recent study suggested that St. John's wort did not have efficacy in patients with severe depression [24].

Safety. Like many herbal products, St. John's wort has a long history of safe use, dating back hundreds of years. It is well recognized to cause photo toxicity in grazing animals (cows, sheep, and horses) when consumed in large amounts. This risk in humans seems to be minimal but still present, perhaps more so in patients using concentrated extracts. Reasonable precautions regarding avoiding excessive ultraviolet exposure can be recommended to patients who do choose to try the herb.

Of greater import is the increasingly recognized risk of interactions between St. John's Wort and pharmaceutical medications. It is clear now that St. John's Wort is an effective inducer of the cytochrome P450 enzyme system, and specifically the CYP3A4 subsystem. The induction of these enzyme systems would be expected to increase the metabolism of a number of drugs, and a growing list of published reports confirms this. Decreased levels of amitriptyline [25], cyclosprin [5], digoxin [4] and anti-retrovirals [3] have all been reported. Perhaps most illustrative of the potentially life-threatening potential of such interactions, two cardiac transplant patients both experienced acute rejection episodes after initiating St. John's Wort therapy. The herb dramatically decreased the baseline cyclosporin level in both patients, allowing rejection to occur.

Recommendations. The diagnosis of depression can be difficult, even for experienced clinicians. Thus, a patient who attempts to self-diagnose such a condition may or may not be correct. Assuming that any organic cause for the symptoms has been ruled out, the patient who wishes to try St. John's wort can be encouraged to do so, in partnership with their physician, following these caveats:

▶ The patient should be directed to a reliable and standardized preparation
▶ Warn the patient about the potential for photo toxicity and recommend appropriate precautions
▶ Avoid combining St. John's wort with ANY pharmaceutical medications. Until the full range of metabolic changes that can occur with St. John's wort therapy are fully characterized, it is best to assume that all drugs can have their blood levels significantly affected by St. John's wort.

Anxiety

Kava (*Piper methysticum*)

Background. Anxiety is another symptom complex that is very common but difficult for many patients to discuss. As a result, it is probably under-treated in general and probably more so in the elderly, where fears of side effects may limit physicians' willingness to prescribe medication. Again, aging and the isolation it may bring can make the elderly particularly susceptible to anxiety. Thus, the growing popularity of kava in the general public, and its subsequent increased availability, has led a growing number of elderly to experiment with kava.

Biochemistry. Unlike many other herbs, the active ingredients of kava have been fairly well characterized and designated kava lactones (or kava pyrones). These include, kawain, dihydrokawain, methysticin,and dihydromethysticin. While the dried herb typically yields 3.5% kava lactones [26] commercial extracts are usually standardized to yield 30–70% kava-lactones. The lactones possess sedative, muscle relaxant, and anticonvulsant activities [27]. The mechanism(s) of action for these various effects are not fully understood.

Clinical Studies. There have been numerous studies that suggest that kava is effective for the short-term treatment of anxiety. Six randomized, double-blind, placebo-controlled trials, using commercial kava preparations containing 70% kava-lactones were reviewed in 2000 [28]. This review confirmed that kava demonstrated superiority to placebo in the treatment of anxiety. One study comparing low dose benzodiazepines with a kava extract showed comparable efficacy between the treatments [29]. Of particular note to elderly women, one study [30] suggested benefit in treatment of anxiety symptoms in menopause.

Safety. Kava has a long history of use in the South Pacific Islands, but experience with the more concentrated commercial extracts is still emerging. Stomach upset, restlessness and drowsiness have been reported sporadically. Studies with follow-up extending to six months suggest that extracts are probably safe [28, 29, 31, 32]. However, recent reports suggest that hepatotoxicity is possible even after 1–3 months of treatment [33, 34]. These reports have caused Germany (and other countries) to suspend sales of kava products, pending more complete review. Finally, kava dermopathy is often written about but rarely seen. Yellowing of the skin along with an ichthyosis picture has been seen in users consuming high doses for extended periods of time [35].

Recommendations. Prior to the recent concerns regarding possible hepatotoxicty, kava seemed to be a welcome addition to the armamentarium of treatments for anxiety. However, until greater clarification regarding its potential hepatotoxicity is available, it is prudent to recommend that patients not consume kava for more than one month. If patients choose to use kava for an extended period of time, monitoring of LFT's is a reasonable precaution. Counsel patients to watch for signs of hepatitis and to seek medical advice should these occur.

Post-Menopausal Symptoms

Phytoestrogens (Soy - *Glycine max*)

Background. The proven and/or potential benefits of estrogen replacement therapy (ERT) include reduced risk of osteoporosis, cardiovascular disease, memory loss and amelioration of menopausal symptoms. Menopausal symptoms range from hot flashes to emotional lability and vaginal dryness. Severity can range from mild to debilitating. Yet the choice to pursue ERT is not a straightforward one. ERT can have side effects of its own (breast tenderness, erratic vaginal bleeding, weight gain, etc.).

But perhaps most troubling to the majority of potential users is the possible increased risk of breast cancer. While it is still the subject of much debate, the risk of breast cancer is a very real threat to many women contemplating the use of ERT. In the United States, only 35–40% of menopausal women ever start ERT, and only 15% continue it for an extended period of time [36]. With the aging of the population, more women will be living longer with the symptoms associated with menopause. Until the issue of breast cancer risk is definitively addressed, women are going to continue seek alternative treatments.

Attention has been increasingly focused on phytoestrogens because of a number of differences observed in women from areas with high soy consumption (e.g. Japan) compared with those from areas of low soy consumption (e.g. Unites States). For example, cardiovascular disease and several cancers (colon, prostate and breast) occur much less frequently in Japan compared with the United States. And apropos to the symptoms of menopause, the incidence of hot flashes in Asian women is dramatically lower than that of American women [37]. This epidemiological data combined with the fact that phytoestrogens are "natural", has led many women to consider them to be safe and therefore a good substitute for ERT.

Biochemistry. Phytoestrogens are naturally occurring plant estrogens, a diverse group of nonsteroidal compounds. Most interest has focused on one particular type of phytoestrogens, the isoflavones. Of these, the most important appear to be genistein and daidzen, and soy appears to be one of the richest sources for these particular phytoestrogens. Structurally, they are similar to human estrogen and can bind effectively to estrogen receptors [38]. However, the estrogenic effect of these compounds is substantially less than human estrogens and there is evidence of both estrogenic and anti-estrogenic effects [39, 40].

Clinical Studies. Studies evaluating the role of phytoestrogens and breast cancer are difficult to interpret. Some studies have suggested that phytoestrogens may actually promote breast cancer growth. But this appears to be in contradistinction to the observational studies that suggest women from regions with high soy intake have lower incidence of breast cancer. One postulation is that phytoestrogens have a predominant estrogenic effect in a low estrogen environment and predominant anti-estrogenic activity in a high-estrogen environment [41]. Until further evidence accumulates one way or the other, it remains unclear what effect supplemental levels of soy will have on the risk of breast cancer in post-menopausal women.

Yet apart from the question of its effect on risk of breast cancer, there remains the question of whether soy is effective as a treatment for menopausal symptoms. Studies that have specifically looked at this question [42–44] have generally shown a statistically significant reduction in the number of hot flashes and a more variable effect on other symptoms (such as mood swings).

Safety. As mentioned above, there remain several unanswered questions regarding the safety of soy supplementation in post-menopausal women. The chief of these concerns is whether soy has any potential to increase the risk of breast cancer when taken chronically as a supplement. While the risk is probably minimal at levels typically found in the diet, the level of risk associated with supra-dietary levels is unknown.

Recommendations. A woman who chooses to avoid ERT because of concerns related to the possible risk of breast cancer and instead chooses to treat her postmenopausal symptoms with soy may be trading one unknown for another. It is clear that in most regards, soy is not as effective at ameliorating postmenopausal symptoms as is ERT. And until further evidence is presented, it is difficult to know whether choosing soy will truly be less risky than ERT in terms of developing breast cancer. Because of the multiple unknowns regarding soy supplementation (safety, appropriate dose, etc.), it appears to be premature to recommend women to forego ERT and use phytoestrogens.

Evening Primrose Oil *(Oenothera biennis)*

Background. Evening primrose is an interesting plant with the habit of opening its flowers at night. Its history of use is less extensive than many herbs although Native Americans used it for numerous medicinal purposes. Research in the past two decades has helped to focus interest on some of the unique medicinal uses, one of these being the treatment of menopause.

Biochemistry. Evening primrose oil, which is derived from the seeds of the plant, generally contains 2–16% gamma-linolenic acid (GLA), 65–80% linoleic acid, and vitamin E [45]. GLA is a precursor of prostaglandins E1 and E2 and is thought to help improve the balance between inflammatory and noninflammatory prostaglandins and leukotrienes [45]. Patients with premenstrual syndrome are thought to have lower levels of GLA, possibly explaining some of Evening primrose oil's benefit in this condition [46]. By what mechanism it might reduce symptoms of hot flashes is not clear.

Clinical Studies. While there is some evidence to support the effectiveness of Evening primrose oil as a treatment for cyclic mastalgia (and to a lesser extent, non-cyclic mastalgia) [46, 47], there is little available evidence to support its use as a treatment for hot flashes [48].

Safety. In general, Evening primrose oil is well tolerated. Some patients have experienced indigestion, nausea, soft stools or diarrhea, and headache [49]. Theoretically, GLA could inhibit platelet aggregation [50] though clinical reports of bleeding problems are not found in the literature.

Recommendations. There appears to be little support for the use of Evening primrose oil by elderly women as a treatment for hot flashes. While generally safe, there is potential concern about the platelet inhibitory effects, especially when combined with other platelet inhibitors or anticoagulant medicines. Thus, if an elderly patient still wishes to try this herb, caution her about the need to avoid simultaneous use of other agents that may effect bleeding.

Black cohosh (*Cimicifuga racemosa*)

Background. Black cohosh has many interesting common names. Bugbane and bugwort both reflect its historical use as a means to eliminating bedbugs. Rattle Root reflects the noise the seeds make within the dried pods. It has a long history of use by Native Americans and became popular in Germany in the late 1800's. Its main historical use has been in the treatment of menopausal symptoms

Biochemistry. The exact mechanism of action of black cohosh is uncertain. Studies have been conflicting, with some early studies suggesting that it suppresses LH secretion. However, other studies suggest that there is no effect on LH, FSH, prolactin or estradiol in postmenopausal women [51–53]. Because of the presence of estrogen like-effects, concern has been raised about the safety of black cohosh in women with breast cancer. Laboratory evidence [54, 55] suggests that black cohosh does not stimulate proliferation of estrogen receptor-positive breast cancer cells. However, no long term, large-scale trials have specifically addressed the risks associated with long-term use, especially in breast cancer patients. One recent study [56] followed breast cancer survivors who took black cohosh to treat hot flashes. No negative effects with regards to breast cancer were observed, though the study was a short-term intervention.

Clinical Studies. There is a small body of literature that suggests black cohosh may be an effective treatment for hot flashes associated with menopause [52, 53, 57]. A very recent study [56] actually found no benefit on hot flashes in breast cancer survivors.

Safety. Black cohosh has traditionally been a well-tolerated herbal therapy, with minimal side effects. Some women do complain of mild nausea [54] but this generally seems to be a transient effect. Other infrequent side effects include headache, cramps and weight gain.

Recommendations. Black cohosh has a relatively long history of use, with minimal significant side effects reported. The evidence is at least supportive to suggest it can reduce hot flashes. However, there is no evidence to suggest what effect, if any, black cohosh has on bone density, cardiac mortality etc.

Dong quai (*Angelica sinensis, Angelica polymorpha*)

Background. Dong quai (also known as dang gui, tang-kuei or "female ginseng") has gained some popularity in the United States as a treatment for both premenstrual syndrome as well as for menopausal symptoms. It is a common component in many traditional Chinese preparations but it is not typically used for menopausal symptoms in that medical tradition.

Biochemistry. The root of the dong quai contains a rich variety of biochemicals, including numerous coumarins [58] some of which have vasodilating properties. In one study, an extract of dong quai was found to competitively inhibit estradiol binding to estrogen receptors [59].

Clinical Studies. There is a relative paucity of studies on dong quai as it relates to the treatment of menopause. Hirata et.al. [60] found no benefit on menopausal symptoms. There have been some studies of herbal blends containing dong quai having some benefit [61], but such findings are difficult to interpret clinically.

Safety. At recommended doses, dong quai is a well-tolerated herb, with side effects comparable to placebo in most studies. Reports of significant photodermatitis have occurred when individuals consumed high doses of dong quai. There is a case report of an interaction with warfarin [62].

Recommendations. Interest in dong quai has been spurred in part by the belief that it has a tradition of use in Chinese medicine for treating menopausal symptoms. Yet this is not a classical indication and dong quai is rarely used as a single herb but more commonly as part of a compound of herbs. There is no supporting literature to recommend it as a solitary herb to treat menopausal symptoms, it may carry some risk and thus elderly women should generally be discouraged from using it.

Benign Prostate Hypertrophy

Saw palmetto (*Serenoa repens*)

Background. The aging male is subject to a number of physiologic changes, but one of the most common and most distressing is benign prostatic hyperplasia (BPH) and its associated symptoms. Approximately 40% of men aged 70 years or older have symptoms (frequency, nocturia, weak stream, hesitancy) consistent with the diagnosis of BPH [63]. Current conventional therapeutics include pharmaceutical medications, procedures (such as microwave ablation) and surgery. Each of these choices has potentially significant serious side-effects (including impotence and incontinence). Once again, the twin pressures of an aging population and a condition that does not have a cure proffered from conventional medicine are leading an ever-increasing number of men to explore the herbal alternatives. The chief of these is saw palmetto, a dwarf palm common to the southeastern United States.

Biochemistry. The medicinal portion of the plant is extracted from the dried berries. The extracts have been characterized and include fatty acids and sterols. The sterols (e.g. beta-sitosterol) are thought to be responsible for the therapeutic effects.

Clinical Studies. A systematic review [64] of 18 randomized controlled trials (with a total of 2939 men enrolled) showed positive effects for saw palmetto. Compared to placebo, saw palmetto improved nocturia by 25%, peak urine flow by 28% and residual urine volume by 43%.

Safety. Saw palmetto appears to be safe. Side effects are mild and often did not exceed those associated with placebo in many trials. Importantly, saw palmetto does not appear to cause erectile dysfunction [64, 65].

Recommendations. An elderly male seeking relief from mild to moderate symptoms of BPH might find benefit from a quality saw palmetto product. The likelihood of significant side effects is small and may be less than with some conventional pharmaceuticals. It can be used as an alternative to conventional medical therapy or in conjunction with such treatment.

Circulatory Problems: Claudication

Ginkgo (*Ginkgo biloba*)

Background. Another common usage for ginkgo is in the treatment of claudication.

Biochemistry. Certain constituents of ginkgo may contribute to an improvement in peripheral circulations. Ginkgolide B acts as platelet activating factor inhibitor, resulting in decreased platelet aggregation [66]. Ginkgolides may also decrease smooth muscle contraction [67, 68].

Clinical Studies. There are several studies that document a statistically significant (but clinically modest) improvement in walking distance in patients with claudication who take ginkgo [69, 70]. A meta-analysis [71] of double-blind, randomized, and controlled trials included eight studies, of which seven favored ginkgo.

Safety. The safety issues are the same as discussed previously in the discussion of ginkgo and dementia.

Recommendations. Ginkgo extracts have been shown to modestly increase walking distance in patients with peripheral vascular disease and claudication. It is a reasonable therapeutic agent, as long as caution is exercised regarding its potential bleeding risks, especially when combined with other anti-platelet agents or anticoagulants.

Circulatory Problems: Venous Insufficiency

Horse chestnut (*Aesculus hippocastanum*)

Background. The use of horse chestnut as a treatment for venous insufficiency seems to be gaining popularity in the United States. It is touted as reducing varicose veins, relieving swelling and tiredness in legs, and reducing pruritis. Again, chronic venous insufficiency will continue to increase in incidence as the Baby Boom generation reaches its latter years. Conventional treatment (e.g. elevation, compression stockings) may not be palatable to a generation that seems intent on pursuing lifelong activities. Horse chestnut seems therefore destined to receive increased attention in the coming years.

Biochemistry. Horse chestnut seed contains aescin (escin) and the toxic glycoside aesculin (esculin) [72]. Thus, unprocessed seeds are toxic (and should not be confused with the fruit of the sweet chestnut, *Castanea sativa*, which is edible [73]). Aescin decreases venous capillary permeability and increases venous tone and flow [74].

Clinical Studies. Most of the published literature supports the efficacy of horse-chestnut seed extract (HCSE) (generally standardized to 16–20% aescin) in the treatment of the symptoms of venous insufficiency [75–78]. A comprehensive review of the literature [79] showed that oral HCSE reduced symptoms of venous insufficiency (leg pain, pruritus, and leg fatigue) as well as objective measures (leg volume and circumference at the ankle).

Safety. Horse chestnut extracts that have been properly produced to eliminate the aesculin component are generally safe. Minor pruritus and GI upset are reported but are generally self-limited [80]. Most studies have found an incidence of side effects comparable to placebo.

Recommendations. The symptoms associated with venous insufficiency can range from distracting to disabling. Conventional therapy can often be helpful but may not always relieve symptoms completely.

A trial of a standardized horse-chestnut seed extract, procured from a reliable manufacturer to exclude the potential toxicity of aesculin, appears to be a reasonable therapeutic option.

Energy Enhancers

Ginseng (*Panax ginseng*)

Background. Though not unique to the elderly, decreased energy is a particularly common complaint in this population. Ginseng is frequently tried because of its folklore reputation for enhancing athletic and/or sexual performance. In fact, it is classically viewed as an adaptogen, an agent that helps restore balance to the body and its systems. The idea that it can act as an energy "booster" is fairly recent and not well supported with studies.

Biochemistry. The various species of ginseng contain an interesting array of chemical constituents, the chief being a group of saponins called ginsenosides. There are several different ginsenosides, each with different pharmacological activity. In regards to energy, Panax ginseng saponins may increase serum cortisol concentrations [81, 82]. Adrenal function may also be affected [83, 84].

Clinical Studies. One intriguing study performed in Mexico looked at the effect of ginseng in a "highly stressed" population and found significant improvement in several quality of life factors [85]. There are surprisingly few scientifically sound studies (in English language journals) that evaluate ginseng as an athletic enhancer. Those that are available suggest little if any improvement in athletic performance [86, 87].

Safety. Side effects are generally minimal. Insomnia can occur [88] as well as tachycardia [89]. Both hypertension and hypotension have been reported, probably reflecting different compositions of extracts and varying proportions of specific ginsensodies [90]. There have also been reports of estrogen-like activity in postmenopausal women, who experienced mastalgia [91] and vaginal bleeding [92, 93].

Recommendations. Ginseng is one of the best selling herbs worldwide. It has achieved an almost legendary mystique and claims seem to attribute every manner of excellent effect to it. But the evidence at this point regarding its ability to influence fatigue is limited. It does seem to have some modest capability to improve resistance to stress and its side-effects appear to be limited.

Ma huang (*Ephedra sinica*)

Background. The discussion of the use of ma huang as an energy enhancer can be relatively brief as it is an herb with significant pharmacological activity and of such a nature to render it unsafe for consideration, especially in the elderly population. However, it is an herb that seems to find its way into a bewildering array of products, most advertised as energy enhancers, "fat burners" etc. As it may have potentially serious side effects, clinicians must have some familiarity with this agent.

Biochemistry. There are numerous species of ephedra but the commonly encountered one in diet aids and energy boosters is *Ephedra sinica*. The branches contain alkaloids, including ephedrine, pseudoephedrine, and sometimes small amounts of phenylpropanolamine. Reported effects include sympathetic nervous system stimulation [80], increased blood pressure [94] and central nervous system stimulation [89].

Clinical Studies. While ma huang may modestly increase weight loss [95] when combined with conventional approaches (i.e. low fat diet and exercise), the slight benefit is outweighed by the risks. Specific studies of ma huang as an energy enhancer are lacking, but anecdotal reports suggest it can be effective.

Safety. Beginning in the mid-90's, a growing number of adverse events were reported in association with ma huang [96]. These include CNS events (strokes, seizures) and cardiovascular events (myocardial infarction, arrhythmia, hypertension).

Recommendations. Whether they are seeking an aid in the battle to lose weight, or want a "pick-me-up", elderly patients need to know that any possible benefit of ma huang is outweighed by the potential risk.

Osteoarthritis

Glucosamine and Chondroitin

Background. Though not herbal in nature, glucosamine and chondroitin are dietary supplements and are being used by an ever-increasing number of patients seeking relief from the symptoms of osteoarthritis.

Biochemistry. Glucosamine is used for the synthesis of glycoproteins, glycolipids, and glycosaminoglycans, important elements in the cartilaginous structures of the body. Glucosamine sulfate is 90% absorbed after oral administration. The bioavailability is approximately 26% after first pass metabolism [97].

Chondroitin, a glucosaminoglycan, is derived from bovine cartilage. It serves as a substrate for the formation of the joint matrix structure [98]. Early studies suggested that chondroitin was not absorbed after oral administration but more recent studies [99] have refuted this, showing 8–18% absorption.

Clinical Studies. Glucosamine has been shown to be efficacious in a variety of clinical studies when used orally for osteoarthritis. These benefits have been consistently demonstrated in studies lasting from a few weeks to 3 years [100–103]. There is also data to suggest that glucosamine may actually slow joint space narrowing [104]. One study with negative implications for elderly patients showed that adding glucosamine to an existing analgesic regimen did not yield additional benefit [105].

Chondroitin also has supportive studies to suggest efficacy in treating osteoarthritis [100, 106, 107]. Treatment with chondroitin sulfate for 2–4 months may be required before significant improvement is experienced [107].

Safety. Both chondroitin and glucosamine appear to be very safe. Side effects include mild GI upset and headaches and have been comparable to placebo in most studies. Diarrhea and constipation have also been reported. One current concern is the risk that bovine cartilage sources for the manufacture of chondroitin could transmit bovine spongiform encephalopathy (BSE or "mad cow disease"). There have been no cases reported and bovine trachea is not felt to be likely to carry significant risk. However, some caution is still prudent.

Recommendations. Taken singly or (more frequently) in combination, glucosamine and chondroitin seem to have something to offer the elderly patient with osteoarthritis, at least of the knee and low back. Whether it has much benefit on smaller joints remains to be seen. The risks seem to be negligible and patients can be encouraged to try this supplement. The only potential worrisome caveat is the possibility that chondroitin might carry some risk of BSE – which is probably very limited. However, it is prudent to inquire into the manufacturing practices of a company and see what safeguards are in place before embarking on a chronic course of medication.

Ginger (*Zingiber officiale*)

Background. Ginger is most widely used as a treatment for nausea. Interest in it as a possible aid to the treatment of osteoarthritis has developed recently.

Biochemistry. The root and the rhizome of the ginger plant are generally used for medicinal purposes. The active constituents are collectively known as gingerols and have several well-characterized activities. Individually, various gingerols may possess antipyretic, analgesic, antitussive, cardiac inotropic, and sedative properties [90]. The anti-nausea effect may reside in the 6-gingerol component, which is thought to increase gastrointestinal motility [108]. In regards to its use as an aid in the treatment of arthritis, less is well known about potential mechanisms of action. There may be inhibition of cyclooxygenase and lipoxygenase pathways [109] but this mostly speculative at this point in time.

Clinical Studies. Studies regarding the efficacy of ginger in treating arthritis pain have been conflicting. Altman [110] found that ginger was superior to placebo in treating patients with knee pain. However, Bliddall [111] found that a ginger extract was comparable to placebo when compared against ibuprofen.

Safety. Ginger is very commonly used safely in cooking. When taken in larger amounts or in concentrated formulations for medicinal effect, the literature is a bit less clear. When used as a treatment for nausea in various clinical settings, it generally appears to be safe [112, 113]. Studies looking at its use for osteoarthritis, especially long-term use studies, are lacking. Very high doses (greater than 4 grams/day) might affect platelet function, and therefore caution should be exercised if combining high doses of the herb with other anticoagulant medications.

Recommendations. At this point in time, there is an intriguing body of literature that suggests ginger may have some salutary effect on arthritis symptoms. However, until long-term studies are available to more fully assess its safety when used chronically, use should probably be discouraged.

Discussing Herbs with Patients

Two concurrent trends seem to be likely to continue – the aging of the population and the fascination with "natural" therapies. An aging population, complete with all of the foibles inherent to the elderly state, will increasingly seek solutions and relief from a variety of sources. While pharmaceutical drugs continue to be faulted on the nightly news as a source of morbidity and expense, and while herbs are frequently touted as safe and natural, the physician or healthcare provider caring for the aged will increasingly encounter patients using (or interested in using) a natural plant medicine to treat themselves. Physicians can follow an often-tried technique – the "head in the sand" approach. When confronted with a patient that is using an herbal therapy, the physician simply labels all such substances as "snake oil", encourages the patient to "throw it in the trash" and moves on to "more important" issues. Unfortunately, the patient is quite likely to continue to use the substance(s) in question. Only from that point forward, the patient knows not to discuss the issue with their physician. This means the patient will have to rely on information obtained from family and friends, and increasingly, the Internet.

Another, and more favorable approach, is to listen carefully to the patient's concerns and begin an open dialogue. The use of herbs may represent the patient's attempt at meeting some need that conventional therapy has not yet fulfilled. Certainly, the elderly patient encounters a number of physical changes and challenges that are often not amenable to easy fixes by conventional medicine (e.g. arthritis, dementia). A patient's inquiry about a specific herb may be an opportunity to learn more about what is truly concerning to the patient. It also may simply be that the patient is curious and needs education about the pros and cons of trying herbal therapies. Any opportunity to teach is important to the healing professional and should not be missed. Spending time to make sure the seeking individual has basic knowledge about the herbal landscape can set the stage for a collaborative approach. Then, whether a patient chooses to continue (or start) an herbal therapy, the health care provider is part of the process and can partner with the patient to watch for adverse effects, monitor responses and re-evaluate the use of a particular therapy over time. This collaborative partnership seems to be the best approach to balancing the information patients receive from other sources, while still respecting patient autonomy and choice. Hopefully, with increased education of both patients and health care providers, herbs can assume an evidence-based position in the armamentarium of medicine for the elderly in the twenty-first century.

Information Sources

The above discussion of commonly encountered herbs in the elderly is of necessity focused and abbreviated. In actual practice, the clinician counseling an elderly patient could be faced with having to address any of hundreds of different herbs. Fortunately, there is an expanding repertoire of texts and Internet resources where a busy clinician can find critical information quickly. Following is a brief list of texts and Web sites that can provide rapid access to answers to questions regarding most commonly encountered herbs.

Texts

- ▶ Complete German Commission E Monographs, Therapeutic Guide to Herbal Medicines. Editor: Mark Blumenthal, American Botanical Council, 1998
- ▶ Herbal Medicine-Expanded Commission E Monographs. Mark Blumenthal (Editor) Integrative Medicine Communication, 1999
- ▶ PDR for Herbal Medicines, First Edition, Medical Economics Company, Inc. Montvale, NJ, 1998
- ▶ Schulz, V, Hansel R, Tyler V Rational Phytotherapy: A Physician's Guide to Herbal Medicine, Springer-Verlag, Berlin 1998
- ▶ Rotblatt M, Ziment I. Evidence-based Herbal Medicine, Hanley& Belfus, Philadelphia, 2001

Internet Sites

- ▶ Government sites:
  - ▸ http://dietary-supplements.info.nih.gov/
  - ▸ http://www.cfsan.fda.gov/~dms/supplmnt.html
- ▶ Proprietary sites:
  - ▸ http://www.naturaldatabase.com/
  - ▸ http://www.tnp.com/
  - ▸ http://www.herbmed.org/

References

1. Merriam-Webster's Collegiate Dictionary. 10th ed. Springfield, Mass: Merriam-Webster: 542, 1993.
2. USFDA, Center for Food Safety and Applied Nutrition: http://vm.cfsan.fda.gov/~dms/dietsupp.html
3. Piscitelli, SC, Burstein, AH, Chaitt, D, et al: Indinavir Concentrations and St. John's wort. Lancet, 355(9203), 547–8, 2000.
4. Johne A, Brockmoller J, Bauer S, et al: Pharmacokinetic interaction of digoxin with an herbal extract from St John's wort (Hypericum perforatum). Clin Pharmacol Ther, 66(4), 338–45, 1999.
5. Ruschitzka F, et al: Acute heart transplant rejection due to Saint John's wort [letter]. Lancet, 355(9203), 548–9, 2000.
6. Janetzky K, et al: Probable interaction between warfarin and ginseng. Am J Health Syst Pharmacy, 54, 692–693, 1997.
7. Slifman, NR, et al: Brief Report: Contamination of Botanical Dietary Supplements by Digitalis lanata. NEJM, Volume 339(12), 806–811, 1998.
8. Farnsworth N, et al: Medicinal plants in therapy. Bull World Health Org, 63, 965–81, 1985.
9. Chavez, ML, Chavez, PI: Ginkgo (Part 1): History, use, and pharmacologic properties. Hosp Pharm, 33, 658–672, 1998.
10. Smith, PF, Maclennan, K, and Darlington, CL: The Neuroprotective Properties of Ginkgo biloba Leaf: A Review of the Possible Relationship to Platelet-Activating Factor. J. Ethnopharmacol, 50, 131–139, 1996.
11. Le Bars, PL, Katz, MM, Berman, N, et al (North American EGb Study Group): A placebo-controlled trial of an extract of Ginkgo biloba for dementia. JAMA, 278, 1327–1332, 1997.
12. Ernst, E, Pittler, MH.: Ginkgo biloba for dementia: A systematic review of double-blind, placebo-controlled trials. Clin Drug Invest, 17, 301–308, 1999.
13. van Dongen, MCJM, van Rossum, E, Kessels, AGH, et al: The efficacy of Ginkgo for elderly people with dementia and age-associated memory impairment: New results of a randomized clinical trial. L Am Geriatr Soc. 48, 1183–1194, 2000.
14. Matthews, MJ Jr. Association of Ginkgo biloba with intracerebral hemorrhage. Neurology, 50, 1933–4, 1998.
15. Rosenblatt, M, Mindel, J.: Spontaneous hyphema associated with ingestion of Ginkgo biloba extract (letter). NEJM, 336, 1108, 1997.
16. Rowin, J, Lewis, SL.: Spontaneous bilateral subdural hematomas associated with chronic Ginkgo biloba ingestion. Neurology, 46. 1775–6, 1996.
17. Laakmann, G, Schüle, C, Baghai, T, Kieser, M.: St. John's wort in mild to moderate depression: The relevance of hyperforin for the clinical efficacy. Pharmacopsychiatry, 31(Suppl), 54–59, 1998.
18. Chatterjee, SS, Bhattacharya, SD, Wonnemann, M, et al.: Hyperforin as a possible antidepressant component of hypericum extracts. Life Sciences, 63, 499–510, 1998.
19. Nathan, PJ.: The experimental and clinical pharmacology of St. John's wort (Hypericum perforatum L.). Molec Psych, 4, 333–338, 1999.
20. Müller, WE, Rolli, M, Schäfer, C, Hafner, U.: Effects of hypericum extract (LI 160) in biochemical models of antidepressant activity. Pharmacopsychiatry, 30(Suppl), 102–107, 1997.
21. Linde, K, Ramirez, G, Mulrow, CD, et al.: St. John's wort for depression – An overview and meta-analysis of randomized clinical trials. BMJ, 313, 253–258, 1996.
22. Philipp, M, Kohnen, R, Hiller, K-O.: Hypericum extract versus imipramine or placebo in patients with moderate depression: Randomized multicentre study of treatment for eight weeks. BMJ, 319, 1534–1538, 1999.
23. Schrader, E, on behalf of the Study Group.: Equivalence of St. John's wort extract (ZE 117) and fluoxetine: a randomized, controlled study in mild-moderate depression. Int Clin Psychopharmacol, 15, 61–68, 2000.
24. Shelton, RC, Keller, MB, Gelenberg, A, et al.: Effectiveness of St John's wort in major depression. JAMA, 285, 1978–1986, 2001.
25. Roots, I, Johne, A, Schmider, Brockmoller, J, et al.: Interaction of an herbal extract from St. John's wort with amitriptyline and its metabolites. Clin Pharmacol Ther, 67(2), 159 (abstract PIII-69), 2000.
26. Schulz, V, Hansel, R, Tyler, VE.: Rational Phytotherapy: A Physician's Guide to Herbal Medicine. Terry C. Telger, transl. 3rd ed. Berlin, GER: Springer, 1998.
27. Singh, YN, Blumenthal, M. Kava.: An overview. HerbalGram, 39, 33–44, 46–55, 1997.
28. Pittler, MH, Ernst, E.: Efficacy of kava extract for treating anxiety: systematic review and meta-analysis. J Clin Psychopharmacol, 20(1), 84–9, 2000.
29. Woelk, H, Kapoula, O, Lehrl, S, et al.: [Comparison of kava special extract WS 1490 and benzodiazepines in patients with anxiety]. [Article in German]. Z Allg Med, 69, 271–7, 1993.
30. Warnecke, G.: [Psychosomatic dysfunctions in the female climacteric. Clinical effectiveness and tolerance of Kava extract WS 1490]. [Article in German]. Fortschr Med, 109(4), 119–22, 1991.
31. Volz, HP, Kieser, M.: Kava-kava extract WS 1490 versus placebo in anxiety disorders–a randomized placebo-controlled 25-week outpatient trial. Pharmacopsychiatry, 30(1), 1–5, 1997.
32. Malsch, U, Kieser, M.: Efficacy of kava-kava in the treatment of non-psychotic anxiety, following pretreatment with benzodiazepines. Psychopharmacology (Berl), 157, 277–83, 2001.
33. Escher, M, Desmeules, J.: Hepatitis associated with kava, an herbal remedy for anxiety. BMJ, 322, 139, 2001.
34. Russmann, S, Lauterberg, BH, Hebling, A.: Kava hepatotoxicity [letter]. Ann Intern Med, 135, 68, 2001.
35. Brinker, F.: Herb Contraindications and Drug Interactions. 2nd ed. Sandy, OR: Eclectic Medical Publications, 1998.

36. Keating, NL, Cleary, PD, Rossi, AS, Zaslavsky, AM, Ayanian, JZ: Use of hormone replacement therapy by postmeno-pausal women in the United States. Ann Intern Med, 130, 545–553, 1999.
37. Boulet, MJ, Oddens, BJ, Lehert, P, Vemer, HM, Visser, A.: Climacteric and menopause in seven southeast Asian coun-tries. Maturitas, 19, 157–176, 1994.
38. Setchell, KD.: Phytoestrogens: the biochemistry, physiology, and implications for human health of soy isoflavones. Am J Clin Nutr, 68(Suppl), 1333S-1346S, 1998.
39. Price, KR, Fenwick, GR.: Naturally occurring estrogens in foods – a review. Food Addit Contam, 2, 73–106, 1985.
40. Cassidy, A, Bingham, S, Setchell, KD.: Biological effects of a diet of soy protein rich in isoflavones on the menstrual cycle of pre-menopausal women. Am J Clin Nutr, 60, 333–340, 1994.
41. Glazier, MG, Bowman, MA.: A review of the evidence for the use of phytoestrogens as a replacement for traditional estrogen replacement therapy. Arch Intern Med, 161, 1161–1172, 2001.
42. Washburn, S, Burke, GL, Morgan, T, Anthony, M.: Effect of soy protein supplementation on serum lipoproteins, blood pressure, and menopausal symptoms in peri-menopausal women. Menopause, 6, 7–13, 1999.
43. Albertazzi, P, Pansini, F, Bonaccorsi, G, Zanotti, L, Forini, E, De Aloysio, D.: The effect of dietary soy supplementa-tion on hot flushes. Obstet Gynecol, 91, 6–11, 1998.
44. Murkies, AL, Lombard, C, Strauss, BJG.: Dietary flour supplementation decreases postmenopausal hot flushes: effects of soy and wheat. Maturitas, 21, 189–825, 1995.
45. Belch, J, Hill, A.: Evening primrose oil and borage oil in rheumatologic conditions. Am J Clin Nutr, 71(1), 352S-6S, 2000; Kleijnen, J.: Evening primrose oil. BMJ, 309, 824–825, 1994.
46. Hardy, ML.: Herbs of special interest to women. J Am Pharm Assoc, 40, 234–42, 2000.
47. Pye, JK, Mansel, RE, Hughes, LE.: Clinical experience of drug treatments for mastalgia. Lancet, 2(8451), 373–7, 1985.
48. Chenoy, R, et al.: Effect of oral gamolenic acid from evening primrose oil on menopausal flushing. BMJ, 308(6927), 501–3, 19 Feb 1994.
49. Newall, CA, Anderson, LA, Philpson, JD.: Herbal Medicine: A Guide for Healthcare Professionals. London, UK: The Pharmaceutical Press, 1996.
50. Guivernau, M, Meza, N, Barja, P, Roman, O.: Clinical and experimental study on the long-term effect of dietary gamma-linolenic acid on plasma lipids, platelet aggregation, thromboxane formation, and prostacyclin produc-tion. Prostaglandins Leukot Essent Fatty Acids, 51(5), 311–16, November 1994.
51. Robbers, JE, Tyler, VE.: Tyler's Herbs of Choice: The Therapeutic Use of Phytomedicinals. New York, NY: The Haworth Herbal Press, 1999
52. Foster, S.: Black cohosh (Cimicifuga racemosa): a literature review. Herbalgram, 45, 35–49, 1999.
53. Liske, E, Wustenberg, P.: Therapy of climacteric complaints with Cimicifuga racemosa: herbal medicine with clini-cally proven evidence. Menopause, 5, 250, 1998.
54. Liske, E. Therapeutic efficacy and safety of Cimicifuga racemosa for gynecologic disorders. Adv Ther, 15, 45–53, 1998.
55. Gruenwald, J.: Standardized black cohosh (Cimicifuga) extract clinical monograph. Q Rev Nat Med, 3, 117–25, 1998.
56. Jacobson, JS, Troxel, AB, Evans, J, et al.: Randomized trial of black cohosh for the treatment of hot flashes among women with a history of breast cancer. J Clin Oncol, 19, 2739–45, 2001.
57. Lieberman, S.: A Review of the effectiveness of Cimicifuga racemosa (Black Cohosh) for the symptoms of meno-pause. J Womens Health, 7(5), 525–9, 1998.
58. Foster, S, Tyler, VE.: Tyler's Honest Herbal: A Sensible Guide to the Use of Herbs and Related Remedies. 3rd ed., Binghamton, NY: Haworth Herbal Press, 1993.
59. Eagon, PK, Elm, MS, Hunter, DS, et al.: Medicinal herbs: modulation of estrogen action. Era of Hope Mtg, Dept Defense; Breast Cancer Res Prog, Atlanta, GA, June 8–11, 2000.
60. Hirata, JD, et al.: Does dong quai have estrogenic effects in postmenopausal women? A double-blind, placebo-con-trolled trial. Fertil Steril, 68(6), 981–6, 1997.
61. Hudson, TS, Standish, L, Breed, C, et al.: Clinical and endocrinological effects of a menopausal botanical formula. J Naturopathic Med, 7, 73–77, 1998.
62. Page, RL II, Lawrence, JD.: Potentiation of warfarin by dong quai. Pharmacotherapy, 19(7), 870–6, 1999.
63. Berry, SL, Coffey, DS, Walsh, PC, Ewing, LL.: The development of human benign prostatic hyperplasia with age. J Urol, 132, 474–479, 1984.
64. Wilt, TJ, Ishani, A, Stark, G, MacDonald, R, Lau, J, Mulrow, C.: Saw palmetto extracts for treatment of benign pro-static hyperplasia: a systematic review. JAMA, 280(18), 1604–1609, 1998.
65. Carraro, JC, Raynaud, JP, Koch, G, et al.: Comparison of phytotherapy (Permixon) with finasteride in the treatment of benign prostate hyperplasia: a randomized international study of 1,098 patients. Prostate, 29, 231–40, 1996.
66. Brautigam, MR, Blommaert, FA, Verleye, G, et al.: Treatment of age-related memory complaints with Gingko biloba extract: a randomized double blind placebo-controlled study. Phytomedicine, 5(6), 425–34, 1998.
67. Oken, BS, et al.: The efficacy of Ginkgo biloba on cognitive function in Alzheimer disease. Arch Neurol, 55(11), 1409–15, November 1998.
68. Paick, J, Lee, J.: An experimental study of the effect of ginkgo biloba extract on the human and rabbit corpus cavernosum tissue. J Urol, 156, 1876–80, 1996.
69. Schweizer, J, Hautmann, C.: Comparison of two dosages of Ginkgo biloba extract EGb 761 in patients with periph-eral arterial occlusive disease Fontain's stage IIb / a randomised, double-blind, multicentric clinical trial. Arzneimittelforchung, 49(11), 900–4, 1999.

70. Peters, H, Kieser, M, Holscher, U.: Demonstration of the efficacy of ginkgo biloba special extract EGb 761 on intermittent claudication – a placebo-controlled, double-blind multicenter trial. Vasa, 27, 106–10, 1998.

71. Pittler, MH, Ernst, E.: Ginkgo biloba extract for the treatment of intermittent claudication: a meta-analysis of randomized trials. Am J Med, 108, 276–81, 2000.

72. Leung, AY, Foster, S.: Encyclopedia of Common Natural Ingredients Used in Food, Drugs and Cosmetics. 2nd ed. New York, NY: John Wiley & Sons, 1996

73. Rotblatt, M, Ziment, I.: Evidence-based Herbal Medicine, Hanley& Belfus, Philadelphia, 238, 2001.

74. The Review of Natural Products by Facts and Comparisons. St. Louis, MO: Wolters Kluwer Co., 1999.

75. Greeske, K, Pohlmann, BK.: Horse chestnut seed extract-an effective therapy principle in general practice. Drug therapy of chronic venous insufficiency. Fortschr Med, 114(15), 196–200, 1996.

76. Diehm, C, et al.: Comparison of leg compression stocking and oral horse-chestnut seed extract in patients with chronic venous insufficiency. Lancet, 347(8997), 292–4, 1996.

77. Diehm, C, et al.: Medical edema protection-clinical benefit in patients with chronic deep vein incompetence. Vasa, 21(2), 188–92, 1992.

78. Bisler, H, et al.: Effects of horse-chestnut seed on transcapillary filtration in chronic venous insufficiency. Dtsch Med Wochenschr, 111(35), 1321–9, 1986.

79. Pittler, MH, Ernst, E.: Horse-chestnut seed extract for chronic venous insufficiency. A criteria-based systematic review. Arch Dermatol, 134(11), 1356–60, 1998.

80. Blumenthal, M, et al. ed.: The Complete German Commission E Monographs: Therapeutic Guide to Herbal Medicines. Trans. S. Klein. Boston, MA: American Botanical Council, 1998

81. Hiai, S, Yokoyama, H, Oura, H, et al.: Stimulation of pituitary-adrenocortical system by ginseng saponin. Endocrinol Jpn, 26, 661–5, 1979.

82. Kase, Y, Saitoh, K, Ishige, A, et al.: Mechanisms by which Hange-shashin-to reduces prostaglandin E2 levels. Biol Pharm Bull, 21, 1277–81, 1998.

83. The Review of Natural Products by Facts and Comparisons. St. Louis, MO: Wolters Kluwer Co., 1999

84. Robbers, JE, Speedie, MK, Tyler, VE.: Pharmacognosy and Pharmacobiotechnology. Baltimore, MD: Williams & Wilkins, 1996

85. Caso, MA, Vargas, RR, Salas, VA, Begona, IC.: Double-blind study of a multivitamin complex supplemented with ginseng extract. Drugs Exp Clin Res, 22, 323–9, 1996.

86. Allen, JD, McLung, J, Nelson, AG, Welsch, M.: Ginseng supplementation does not enhance healthy young adult's peak aerobic exercise performance. J Am Coll Nutr, 17(5), 462–6, 1998.

87. Engels, HJ, Wirth, JC.: No ergogenic effects of ginseng (Panax ginseng C.A. Meyer) during grades maximal aerobic exercise. J Am Diet Assoc, 97(10), 1110–5, 1997.

88. Scaglione, F, et al.: Efficacy and safety of the standardized Ginseng extract G115 for potentiating vaccination against the influenza syndrome and protection against the common cold. Drugs Exp Clin Res, 22, 65–72, 1996.

89. Schulz, V, Hansel, R, Tyler, VE.: Rational Phytotherapy: A Physician's Guide to Herbal Medicine. Terry C. Telger, transl. 3rd ed. Berlin, GER:Springer, 1998.

90. Foster, S, Tyler, VE.: Tyler's Honest Herbal: A Sensible Guide to the Use of Herbs and Related Remedies. 3rd ed., Binghamton, NY: Haworth Herbal Press, 1993.

91. Palmer, BV, et al.: Gin Seng and mastalgia. BMJ, 1, 1284, 1978.

92. Hopkins, MP, et al.: Ginseng face cream and unexplained vaginal bleeding. Am J Obstet Gynecol, 159, 1121–2, 1988.

93. Palop-Larrea, V, Gonzalvez-Perales, JL, Catalan-Oliver, C, et al.: Metrorrhagia and ginseng. Ann Pharmacother, 34, 1347–8, 2000.

94. Gruenwald, J, et al.: PDR for Herbal Medicines. 1st ed. Montvale, NJ: Medical Economics Company, Inc., 1998.

95. Boozer, CN, Nasser, JA, Heymsfield, SB, et al.: An herbal supplement containing Ma Huang-Guarana for weight loss: a randomized, double-blind trial. Int J Obes Relat Metab Disord, 25, 316–324, 2001.

96. Haller, CA, Benowitz, NL.: Adverse cardiovascular and central nervous system events associated with dietary supplements containing ephedra alkaloids. N Eng J Med, 343(25), 1833–8, 2000.

97. Barclay, TS, Tsourounis, C, McCart, GM.: Glucosamine. Ann Pharmacother, 32, 574–9, 1998.

98. Bucsi, L, Poor, G.: Efficacy and tolerability of oral chondroitin sulfate as a symptomatic slow-acting drug for osteoarthritis (SYSADOA) in the treatment of knee osteoarthritis. Osteoarthritis Cartilage, 6(Suppl A), 31–6, May 1998.

99. Silvestro, L, Lanzarotti, E, Marchi, E, et al.: Human pharmacokinetics of glycosaminoglycans using deuterium-labeled and unlabeled substances: evidence for oral absorption. Semin Thromb Hemost, 20(3), 281–92, 1994.

100. McAlindon, TE, LaValley, MP, Gulin, JP, Felson, DT.: Glucosamine and Chondroitin for Treatment of Osteoarthritis A Systematic Quality Assessment and Meta-analysis. JAMA, 283, 1469–75, 2000.

101. Lopes Vaz, AL.: Double-blind, clinical evaluation of the relative efficacy of ibuprofen and glucosamine sulphate in the management of osteoarthrosis of the knee in out-patients. Curr Med Res Opin, 8, 145–9, 1982.

102. Qiu, GX, et al.: Efficacy and safety of glucosamine sulfate versus ibuprofen in patients with knee osteoarthritis. Arzneimittelforschung, 48, 469–74, 1998.

103. Reginster, JY, Deroisy, R, Rovati, LC, et al.: Long-term effects of glucosamine sulfate on osteoarthritis progression: a randomized, placebo-controlled trial. Lancet, 357, 251–6, 2001.

104. Pavelka, K, Gatterova, J, Olejarova, M, et al.: Glucosamine sulfate decreases progression of knee osteoarthritis in a long-term, randomized, placebo-controlled, independent, confirmatory trial. ACR Abstract Concurrent Session. OA- Advances in Management. November 1, 2000. Page S384, Abstract 1908.

105. Rindone, JP, Hiller, D, Collacott, E, et al.: Randomized, controlled trial of glucosamine for treating osteoarthritis of the knee. West J Med, 172(2), 91–4, 2000.

106. Morreale, P, Manopulo, R, Galati, M, et al.: Comparison of the anti-inflammatory efficacy of chondroitin sulfate and diclofenac sodium in patients with knee osteoarthritis. J Rheumatol, 23(8), 1385–91, 1996.

107. Leeb, BF, Schweitzer, H, Montag, K, Smolen, JS.: A meta-analysis of chondroitin sulfate in the treatment of osteoarthritis. J Rheumatol, 27(1), 205–11, 2000.

108. Micklefield, GH, Redeker, Y, Meister, V, et al.: Effects of ginger on gastroduodenal motility. Int J Clin Pharmacol, Ther, 37(7), 341–6, 1999.

109. Srivastava, KC, Mustafa, T.: Ginger (Zingiber officinale) and rheumatic disorders. Medical Hypotheses, 29, 25–8, 1989.

110. Altman, RD, Marcussen, KC.: Effects of ginger extract on knee pain in patients with osteoarthritis. Arthritis Rheum, 44, 2531–38, 2001.

111. Bliddal, H, Rosetzsky, A, Schlichting, P, et al.: A randomized, placebo-controlled, cross-over study of ginger extracts and ibuprofen in osteoarthritis. Osteoarth Cartilage, 8, 9–12, 2000.

112. Fischer-Rasmussen, W, Kjaer, SK, Dahl, C, Asping, U.: Ginger treatment of hyperemesis gravidarum. Eur J Obstet Gynecol Reprod Biol, 38(1), 19–24, 1991.

113. Phillips, S, Ruggier, R, Hutchinson, SE.: Zingiber officinale (ginger)-an antiemetic for day case surgery. Anaesthesia, 48(8), 715–7, 1993.

9 The Use of Green Tea by the Elderly

F. Afaq, V.M. Adhami, H. Mukhtar

What one eats should serve as one's remedy (Hippocrates)

Introduction

The major issue of health importance for the young population, which will ultimately become elderly, is how to age healthy and remain disease free. To achieve this goal a concept has been around that "a healthy life style that includes good food, plenty of exercise and minimum mental stress" is the elixir for old age. The word "good" needs clarification. In the context of health it means the food which possesses health promoting effects by preventing the occurrence of disease. Thus, whatever good we eat and drink during our lifetime influences our life span and translates into a healthy old age. The subject of nutrition has, therefore, been an area of intense investigation during the past few decades. In spite of advances in research there is still significant number of premature deaths from debilitating diseases like cardiovascular disorders, many type of cancers, and neurological problems associated with aging, such as Alzheimer's disease, Parkinson's disease and other mental and psychiatric disorders. Many of these chronic diseases have been found to have some association with nutritional traditions, eating habits, and life-style. For example cigarette smoking, tobacco chewing and excessive alcohol use increases the risk for many diseases including cancer. On the other hand, some foods and beverages have a beneficial and protective effect. This understanding is based on differences in disease incidence as a function of locally prevailing nutritional habits.

At present, coronary heart disease is a major health problem in the West, but cerebrovascular diseases and stroke occur less frequently in Asia and, in particular, in parts of Japan and China. People in the Western world suffer from cancer of the breast, colon, prostate, ovary, whereas in the Far East the incidence of these cancers is comparatively lower, but cancers of the stomach and esophagus are major problems. Coordinated international efforts have provided leads and factual information on the causes of major diseases and have provided recommendations for prevention through avoidance of these causes. Populations with a high total fat intake have a risk of nutritionally linked cancers, such as those in the colon, breast, and prostate. In contrast, olive oil and canola oil do not increase the risk of the nutritionally linked cancers and of heart disease and therefore, are recommended as important dietary fats.

Tea has been consumed as a beverage since thousands of years. Anecdotal evidence indicated that tea, especially green tea consumption is associated with lower incidence of certain diseases. In recent years this has sparked the interest of many laboratories to examine health promoting and therapeutic benefits of green tea consumption. This academic interest is infact a fresh look to grandma's concept "if you are sick drink tea". An unresolved and often overstated issue is that this could be a universal solution to the problem of providing humanity with a safe beverage. Accumulating research is indicating that there are many benefits of green tea. Recent research shows that much of the beneficial effects of tea are mediated by a group of chemicals known as polyphenols present therein. Tea polyphenols are potent antioxidants, chemicals which have the ability to counteract oxidant radicals consistently produced in the body. It has become clear that oxidant radicals are responsible for many chronic diseases. Their formation in the body is widespread. While you are reading the article, as a result of environmental stress and metabolic imbalance, oxidant radicals are being produced and if they are not counteracted they will damage cellular macromolecular structures. Ordinarily humans have an elaborate defense system to counteract against oxidant radicals produced. However, at times, their formation is overwhelmed and the normal defense is unable to destroy them. Supplemental antioxidants in the body can counteract the oxidant radicals. Antioxidants in tea show many beneficial effects. For example these chemical agents can decrease the oxidation of low density lipoprotein-cholesterol, a risk factor for coronary heart disease. They can reduce the oxidation of DNA, consequent to the action of carcinogens and in addition, they induce enzymes in the liver and other tissue sites that help detoxify harmful chemicals. By virtue of this property green tea polyphenols can help reduce environmentally induced diseases. Tea polyphenols also decrease the rate of cell division, especially of transformed or damaged cells involved in cancer development. This property slows the growth of early cancer cells and may even be beneficial as adjuvant therapy for some cancer types. There are also some indications that regular intake of green tea modifies the intestinal bacterial flora, enhancing the growth of beneficial bacteria and eliminating those with possibly harmful attributes. Tea consumption has been found to be associated with both lifestyle and nutritional habit and was introduced all over the world by traders and travelers. One thing which makes tea attractive is that without a doubt it is the most widely consumed beverage, is cheap, and comes in a variety of flavors.

Tea and Its Constituents

Tea from the leaves of the plant Camellia sinensis, a species of the Theaceae family, is consumed by more than two thirds of the world's population and is the most popular beverage next only to water [1, 2]. Approximately 2.5 million metric tons of dried tea is manufactured annually. Tea leaves are processed differentially and are commercially available as black (78%), green (20%) and oolong tea (2%).

All teas are derived from the plant Camellia sinensis and the manufacture involves a series of drying and fermentation steps (Fig. 9.1). There are a lot of products sold in the market as herbal tea which are not derived from the plant Camellia sinensis. It must be clear that they are herbal extracts rather that tea. Green tea manufacture involves steaming fresh leaves at elevated temperatures followed by a series of drying and rolling steps so that the chemical composition essentially remains similar to that of the fresh leaves. Black tea production involves withering of plucked leaves followed

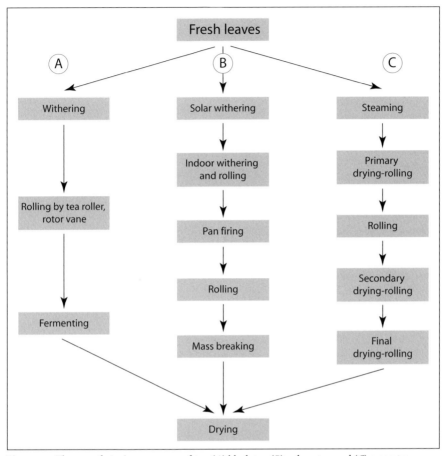

Figure 9.1. The manufactoring processes of tea: (A) black tea, (B) oolong tea, and (C) green tea

by extended fermentation. Thus, depending upon the extent of fermentation, the chemical composition of most black teas is different. Oolong tea is made by solar withering of tea leaves followed by partial fermentation.

Major green tea catechins are (–)-epigallocatechin-3-gallate (EGCG), (–)-epigallocatechin (EGC), (–)-epicatechin gallate (ECG), (–)-epicatechin (EC), (+) – gallocatechin, and (+) – catechins [1]. Tea is the best dietary source of catechins. EGCG is the major polyphenolic constituent present in green tea and a nicely brewed cup of green tea contains upto 300 mg of this chemical. Tea leaves are also a rich source of theanine and caffeine and these are soluble in hot water and impart flavor and taste to tea beverage. Quercetin, kaempferol and rutin are the most important flavonols in tea. Tea contains phenolic acids mainly caffeic, quinic and gallic acids. Theanine is an amino acid found only in tea leaves. Tea contains upto one-third of dry weight of catechins and other polyphenols like quercitin, myricitin and kaempferol [3] (Table 9.1).

Table 9.1. Composition of Tea

| | Amount [% dry weight] | |
	Green Tea	Black Tea
Catechins	30–42	10–12
epigallocatechin gallate	11	
epicatechin gallate	2	
gallocatechin gallate		
epicatechin	2	
epigallocatechin	10	
gallocatechin		
catechin		
Flavins		3–6
theaflavin-3-gallate		
theaflavin-3'-gallate		
theaflavin-3,3'-digallate		
Flavonols	5–10	6–8
quercetin		
kaempferol		
rutin		12–18
Thearubigens		
Theogallin	2–3	
Proanthoocyanin		
Methylxanthines	7–9	8–11
Caffeine	3–5	
Theobromine	0.1	
Theophylline	0.02	
Aminoacids		
Theanine	4–6	
Organic Acids		
Caffeine acid		
Quinine acid	2	
Gallic acid		

Tea and Its Biochemical Properties

According to traditional unscientific claims, some populations drank green tea to improve blood flow, to fight against cancer and cardiovascular disease, eliminate various toxins, and also to improve resistance to various diseases [4]. In recent years scientific basis for these beliefs is emerging because of new health claims about the benefits of green tea, its consumption among the human population is increasing. A lot of emphasis is being placed on events at the cellular level due to its strong antioxidant activity.

Several studies have suggested that polyphenols especially the flavonoids present in green tea possess a high antioxidant activity which in turn protects cells against the adverse effects of damaging reactive oxygen species (ROS) that are constantly produced in the body. Catechins, because of their phenolic properties can act as scavengers of radicals caused by ROS and prevent radical induced damage to cellular macromolecules and control the balance of many metabolic pathways [5, 6]. ROS such as superoxide radical, hydroxyl radical, singlet oxygen, hydrogen peroxide, peroxynitrite and alkoxyradicals cause cellular injury and cellular dysfunction by damaging lipids protein and nucleic acids, and cellular components such as ion channels, membranes and chromatin. The scavenging activity of different catechin molecules is related to the number of o-dihydroxy and o-hydroxyketo groups, C2-C3 double bonds, solubility, concentration, the accessibility of the active group to the oxidant and stability of the reaction product [7]. EGCG may also influence cellular mechanisms that are related to induction of mutagenesis such as DNA synthesis and repair processes [8]. The effects of green tea polyphenols may also be due to the chelation of metal ions. Polyphenols in all types tea chelate copper ions and this mechanism is suggested to protect low density lipoproteins from peroxidation [9]. Because of its chelating properties tea may also protect against toxicity due to heavy metals [10]. Catechins effects may involve alterations in signal transduction pathways, may modulate many endocrine systems and alter hormones and other physiological properties [11].

Tea, Disease Control and Prevention

Tea and Cancer

Numerous epidemiological studies have suggested the ability of green tea and its associated compounds to prevent some cancers but not all. This is understandable as cancer is a complex disease with multiple etiologies, even for one body site. Thus, it is a false hope that any nutritional or synthetic agent can prevent or treat all types of cancer. Based on a large volume of cell culture, animal and human observational studies, there is a hope that green tea consumption can retard cancer development at selected sites in some populations. The challenge is to find in what population what cancer site can be prevented by consuming green tea. This requires extensive undertaking for which considerable resources are required. Green tea catechins act as antioxidants and ROS scavengers, inhibit the growth of cancer in experimental animal models that raise the possibility that consumption of green tea and its associated catechins may lower cancer risk in humans. A study conducted in China it was found that humans that consume green tea more than two cups a day lower the risk of esophageal cancer by 50% [12]. In another study from Shanghai, China it was found that green tea users had a nearly 50% reduction in stomach cancer incidence [13]. An increased consumption of green tea was closely associated with a decreased number of axillary lymph node metastases among premenopausal patients with stage I and II breast cancer [14]. Increased consumption of green tea also correlated with decreased recurrence of stage

I and II breast cancer and the recurrence rate was 17% for individuals drinking more than five cups and 24% for those drinking less than four cups. Inhabitants of tea producing districts in Japan have a lower mortality due to stomach cancer, perhaps due to increased consumption of green tea [15, 16]. In addition to regular drinking this population consumes green tea in all types of products that include candy, gums, bread, shampoo, lotion, toothpaste etc. Thus, many studies are suggesting increased health benefits among populations consuming green tea.

Procarcinogens activated by phase I drug metabolizing enzymes such as cytochrome P450 enzyme system are able to modify genomic DNA and induce tumor formation. EGCG, a major constituent of green tea polyphenol, inhibits the action of phase I enzymes preventing the activation of procarcinogens, and induces phase II enzymes that conjugate active carcinogens, and results in inactivation, and excretion [17, 18]. Tea flavonoids can directly neutralize the procarcinogens by their strong ROS scavenging property before cell damage occurs. In Ames tests that assess DNA damage assays, and in scavenging superoxides tests EGCG was found to protect against DNA scissions, mutations, and in non-enzymatic interception of superoxide anions [19, 20]. Black, green and oolong teas was found to significantly decrease the reverse mutation induced by different mutagens in cell culture assays indicating its antimutagenic protection correlated with strong antioxidant properties that can prevent the development of cancer [21–23]. Studies have shown that EGCG and theaflavin-3–3-digallate block activated protein-1, a signal transducer initiating the development of skin carcinogenesis, and can also inhibit the mitotic signal transducers responsible for cell proliferation [24].

Oral consumption of green tea was found to reduce the risk of oral cancer in northern Italians and Chinese, esophageal cancer in Chinese women, gastric cancer in Swedish adolescents, pancreatic cancer in elderly Poles and residents of a retirement community in the U.S., and colon cancer amongst retired male self-defense officials in Japan. From this and other previous studies it is now generally believed that tea drinking has chemopreventive effects [25]. Cohort studies suggest a protective effect of green tea for colon [26], urinary bladder, stomach, pancreatic, and esophageal cancer [27]. In a Japanese population survey, an overall protection together with a slowdown in the increase of cancer incidence with age was reported [28]. The effects were found to be are more pronounced when the consumption was raised over 10 cups of tea per day.

In vitro studies revealed that catechin gallates selectively inhibit 5-α-reductase. This enzyme is responsible aganist the conversion of testosterone to 5-α dihydrotestosterone [29]. 5-α-dihydrotestosterone at high levels and has been implicated in the etiology of prostate cancer and male pattern baldness. Recently it has been suggested that regular consumption of green tea may prolong life expectancy and quality of life in prostate cancer patients. Consistent with this, our recent studies have shown that green tea polyphenols inhibit the growth and progression of prostate cancer in an animal model. Prostate cancer is an attractive target for prevention by green tea because this disease is typically diagnosed in older men and thus even a modest delay in disease development could produce substantial benefit to population which is at high risk of prostate cancer [30]. Green tea polyphenols have been shown to be antimutagenic, lowering the formation of heterocyclic amines and also have been shown to reduce the occurrence of chromosome aberrations during mutagen exposure [31, 32].

Tea and Cardiovascular Diseases

The onset of cardiovascular disease depends on numerous factors that can be modulated by diet. Green tea consumption by males above 49 years of age has been shown to be associated with decreased serum concentrations of total cholesterol and with concomitant decrease in proportion of low density lipoprotein [33]. In a study of an elderly group in the Netherlands suffering from coronary heart disease, tea consumption was found to reduce the risk of death from this condition [34]. Green tea was also found to lower the incidence of stroke in the elderly population [35]. Lipid peroxidation especially the oxidation of low density lipoprotein (LDL) has been implicated in the etiology of atherosclerosis. A recent cross-sectional study also revealed that in people consuming more than ten cups of green tea per day, there was a decrease in serum cholesterol levels, a decrease in LDL, very low density lipoprotein and triglycerides, a increase in high density lipoproteins, and a reduction in atherogenic index. In the same study, tea consumption was also found to decrease the levels of serum markers of liver damage [36].

Tea and Longevity

There is some evidence that tea drinking may also promote longevity. The best evidence for this is the low mortality rates amongst Japanese females who are traditional practitioners of the tea ceremony [37]. One way to slow aging is to prevent the production and accumulation of active oxygen and lipid peroxides in the body. It has been shown, for example, that the higher the concentration of the powerful antioxidants vitamins E and C in the bodies of animals, the longer they live. This suggests that active consumption of agents that are effective antioxidants may prolong the aging process. Green tea is rich in anti-oxidizing compounds. It has recently been demonstrated that catechins in green tea are far stronger antioxidants than vitamin E (about 20 times stronger in fact). Although there is no direct evidence that suggests a relationship between green tea consumption and aging, the very fact that green tea contains powerful antioxidants is a strong foundation for believing that it can help control and delay the process of aging. It is believed that in the near future, Japan will become a society with a large population of elderly people. The Saitama Cancer Center in Japan conducted an 8-year follow-up survey concerning the effects of green tea on the prolongation of human life using 8,500 participants in Saitama Prefecture. Those who had more than 3 cups of green tea every day had an average life span of 66 years for males and 68 years for females. However, those who had more than 10 cups of green tea per day had an average life span of 70 years for males and 74 years for females. In this study, a decreased relative risk of death from cardiovascular disease was also found for people consuming over 10 cups of green tea a day, and importantly green tea consumption also had life-prolonging effects [38].

Tea and Osteoporosis

Low bone-mineral density known as osteoporosis is the biggest cause of fractures among elderly women. Hormone deficiencies are the leading cause of this disease where bones and joints become thin and fragile. Tea is reported to protect against hip fractures [39]. A recent study suggests that drinking daily one to six cups of tea may significantly reduce the risk of bone fracture by increasing bone mineral density. Studies suggest that isoflavonoids in tea increase bone mineral density and help reduce the risk of fractures in old age. Flavonoids are brightly colored chemicals found in fruit, vegetables and herbs – are being credited with an increasing number of positive effects on health. Of the 1,256 women surveyed, aged between 65 and 76 years, 1,134 drank at least one cup of tea every day. Bone-mineral density at the base of the spine and at 2 hip regions was significantly higher in tea-drinkers when the data were adjusted to account for age and body weight [40]. Milky tea contains calcium, which could help to protect bones.

Tea and Neurological Effects

Tea components such as EGCG and ECG competitively inhibit tyrosinase, the rate-limiting enzyme in the synthesis of melanin, L-dihydroxyphenylalanine, norepinephrine, and epinephrine [41]. EGCG and EGC competitively inhibit catechol-o-methyltransferase (COMT), one of the major enzymes in the metabolism of catecholamines associated with Parkinson's disease [42]. Diminished COMT activity delays the metabolism of norepinephrine and epinephrine and may cause subsequent increases in sympathetic thermogenesis. This may explain why humans increase their 24-h energy expenditure after consuming EGCG-containing green tea extracts and why EGCG alone or synergistically with caffeine augments and prolongs sympathetic stimulation of thermogenesis in rat brown adipose tissues [43]. High activity of Prolylendopeptidase is found in patients with Alzheimers disease and other neuropathological disorders and some studies have shown that this enzyme could be inhibited by EGCG [44].

Tea, Arthritis and Inflammation

In an animal study we found that consumption of green tea polyphenols produce a significant reduction in arthritis incidence with a marked reduction of inflammatory mediators, of neutral endopeptidase activity, of IgG and type II collagen-specific IgG levels in arthritic joints in mice [45]. Many published studies have suggested that green tea has anti-inflammatory properties and new research is beginning to explain why. Previous animal studies and other laboratory researches have found that polyphenols in green tea are potent anti-inflammatory agents, but the mechanism behind this action is not well understood. EGCG inhibits the expression of the interleukin gene involved in the inflammatory response [46]. EGCG was found to block the expression of many biological parameters associated with enhanced inflammatory responses.

Tea and Its Miscellaneous Effects

Green tea polyphenols are believed to offer protection against tooth decay by
▶ killing the causative bacteria, such as Streptococcus mutans [47];
▶ inhibiting the collagenase activity of the bacteria resident below the gum line [48],
▶ increasing the resistance of tooth enamel to acid induced erosion [49].

All teas are a rich source of fluoride and thus can strengthen tooth enamel. Even a cup a day can provide a significant amount of fluoride. Tea can also reduce plaque formation on teeth that can lead to gum inflammation and bleeding and eventually lost teeth. On the negative side, tea compounds can discolor teeth.

In Japan, tea flavonoids given to elderly women on feeding tubes was found to reduce fecal odor and favorably altered the gut bacteria [50]. The study was repeated in bedridden elderly not on feeding tubes, and again green tea was shown to improve their gut bacteria [51]. These studies have also raised the possibility of using green tea in other settings where gut bacteria are disturbed, such as after taking antibiotics.

In the gastrointestinal tract tea polyphenols modulate the composition of the gut micro-flora. A high content of clostridia and a low percent of bifidobacteria have been observed in the intestinal microflora of patients with colon cancer. Tea polyphenols selectively inhibit the growth of clostridia and promote bifidobacteria colonisation contributing to a decrease in the pH value of feces [52]. Viruses, bacteria, and worms have been implicated in the development of cancers; hepatitis viruses, herpes viruses, Helicobacter pylori, and parasitic worms are some well-known causes of cancer [19]. Tea can play another role in the prevention of cancer through its antimicrobial activity [53]. It has been demonstrated that tea can inhibit the growth of Helicobacter pylori which is associated with gastric cancer [54]. The cellular process involved could be the generation of powerful oxidants to destroy the invaders and protect the cells. Bacteria can also synthesize nitrosating agents endogenously and activate macrophages [55]. Nitrosating agents that are potentially carcinogenic can be destroyed by polyphenols.

Conclusions

Studies with human population are complex. Due to diversity in food habits, lifestyle, heredity, age, gender and environment, unambiguous interpretation of the data becomes difficult. In epidemiological studies about effects of green tea consumption on health promotion, the confounding factors are generally more variable than the effect tested and the results are not conclusive. This is an issue in most studies where the beneficial or adverse effects of a single nutrient in a complex diet consumed by humans are examined. However, as elaborated in this chapter there is a reason to believe that the consumption of green tea may have health promoting effects in humans. Perhaps the most important reason to drink plenty of tea is that it also helps people to maintain enough water in their tissues. This is especially important during the hot summer-

time. Active, people, those who spend a lot of time outdoors and the elderly are particularly prone to dehydration if they are overly exposed to hot temperatures. Studies on
the health effects of green tea in humans are continuing, and scientists believe that
there is still a long road ahead to showing that tea helps prevent certain diseases. The
challenge for science is to predict for which diseases and which populations there
could be greater benefit by consuming green tea.

References

1. Katiyar SK and Mukhtar H (1996) Tea in chemoprevention of cancer: Epidemiological and experimental studies.
   Int J Oncol 8: 221–238
2. Yang CS, Wang ZY (1993) Tea and cancer. J Natl Cancer Inst 85: 1038–1049.
3. Dufresne CJ Farnworth ER (2001) A review of latest research findings on the health promotion properties of tea.
   J Nutr Biochem 12: 404–421
4. Balentine DA, Wiseman SA, Bouwens LC (1997) The chemistry of tea flavonoids. Crit Rev Food Sci Nutr 37:
   693–704
5. Rice-Evans CA, Diplock AT (1993) Current status of antioxidant therapy. Free Radic Biol Med 15: 77–96
6. Wei H, Zhang X, Zhao JF, Wang ZY, Bickers D, Lebwohl M (1996) Scavenging of hydrogen peroxide and inhibition
   of ultraviolet light-induced oxidative DNA damage by aqueous extracts from green and black teas. Free Radic Biol
   Med 26: 1427–1435
7. Sergediene E, Jonsson K, Szymusiak H, Tyrakowska B, Rietjens IM, Cenas N (1999) Prooxidant toxicity of polyphenolic antioxidants to HL-60 cells: description of quantitative structure-activity relationships. FEBS Lett 462:
   392–396
8. Hayatsu H, Inada N, Kakutani T, Arimoto S, Negishi T, Mori K, Okuda T, Sakata I (1992) Suppression of genotoxicity
   of carcinogens by (-)-epigallocatechin gallate. Prev Med 21: 370–376
9. Yokozawa T, Dong E, Liu ZW, Shibata T, Hasegawa M, Watanabe H, Oura H (1997) Magnesium lithospermate B
   ameliorates cephaloridine-induced renal injury. Exp Toxicol Pathol 49: 337–341
10. Kim MJ, Rhee SJ (1994) Effect of Korean green tea, oolong tea and black tea beverage on the removal of cadmium
    in rat. J Kor Soc Food Nutr 23: 784–791
11. Kao YH, Hiipakka RA, Liao S (2000) Modulation of endocrine systems and food intake by green tea epigallocatechin
    gallate. Endocrinology 141: 980–987
12. Gao YT, McLaughlin JK, Blot WJ, Ji BT, Dai Q, Fraumeni JF Jr (1994) Reduced risk of esophageal cancer associated
    with green tea consumption. J Natl Cancer Inst 86: 855–858
13. Yu GP, Hsieh CC, Wang LY, Yu SZ, Li XL, Jin TH (1995) Green-tea consumption and risk of stomach cancer: a popu-
    lation-based case-control study in Shanghai, China. Cancer Causes Control 6: 532–538
14. Nakachi K, Suemasu K, Suga K, Takeo T, Imai K, Higashi Y (1998) Influence of drinking green tea on breast can-
    cer malignancy among Japanese patients. Jpn J Cancer Res 89: 254–261
15. Kono S, Ikeda M, Tokudome S, Kuratsune M (1988) A case-control study of gastric cancer and diet in northern
    Kyushu, Japan. Jpn J Cancer Res 79: 1067–1074
16. Oguni I, Nasu K, Kanaya S, Ota Y, Yamamoto, S and Nomura T (1989) Epidemiological and experimental studies
    on the anti-tumor activity by green tea extracts. Jpn J Nutr 47: 93–102
17. Gordon MH (1996) Dietary anti-oxidants in disease prevention. Natural Prod Rep 13: 265–273
18. Lin JK, Liang YC, Lin-Shiau SY (1999) Cancer chemoprevention by tea polyphenols through mitotic signal trans-
    duction blockade. Biochem Pharmacol 58: 911–915
19. Pillai SP, Mitscher LA, Mennon SR, Pillai CA, Shankel DM (1999) Antimutagenic/antioxidant activity of green tea
    components and related compounds. J Envir Pathol Toxicol Oncol 18: 147–158
20. Yoshioka H, Akai G, Yoshinaga K, Hasegawa H, Yoshioka H (1996) Protecting effect of a green tea percolate and its
    main constituents against gamma ray-induced scission of DNA. Biosci Biotechnol Biochem 60: 117–119
21. Yamada J, Tonita Y (1994) Antimutagenic activity of water extract of black tea and oolong tea. Biosc Biotect Biochem
    12: 2197–2200
22. Kuroda Y, Hara Y (1999) Antimutagenic and anticarcinogenic activity of tea polyphenols. Mutat Res 436: 69–97
23. Steele VE, Kelloff GJ, Balentine D, Boone CW, Mehta R, Bagheri D, Sigman CC, Zhu S, Sharma S (2000) Compara-
    tive chemopreventive mechanisms of green tea, black tea and selected polyphenol extracts measured by in vitro
    bioassays. Carcinogenesis 21: 63–67
24. Chung JY, Huang C, Meng X, Dong Z, Yang CS (1999) Inhibition of activator protein 1 activity and cell growth by
    purified green tea and black tea polyphenols in H-ras-transformed cells: structure-activity relationship and mecha-
    nisms involved. Cancer Res 59: 4610–4617 25.

25. Schwarz B, Bischof HP, Kunze M (1994) Coffee, tea and lifestyle. Prev Med 23: 377–384
26. Landau JM, Wang ZY, Yang ZY, Ding W, Yang CS (1998) Inhibition of spontaneous formation of lung tumors and rhabdomyosarcomas in A/J mice by black and green tea. Carcinogenesis 19: 501–507
27. Bushman JL (1998) Green tea and cancer in humans: A review of the literature. Nutr Cancer 31: 151–159
28. Imai K, Suga K, Nakachi K (1997) Cancer-preventive effects of drinking green tea among a Japanese population. Prev Med 26: 769–775
29. Shatsung L, Hiipakka RA (1995) Selective inhibition of steroid 5-a-reductase isoenzymes by tea epicatechin 3-gallate and EGC3-gallate. Biochem Biophys Res Commun 214: 833–838
30. Gupta S, Hastak K, Ahmad N, Lewin JS, Mukhtar H (2001) Inhibition of prostate carcinogenesis in TRAMP mice by oral infusion of green tea polyphenols. Proc Natl Acad Sci 98: 10350–10355
31. Weisburger JH, Nagao M, Wakabayashi K, Oguri A (1994) Prevention of heterocyclic amine formation by tea and tea polyphenols. Cancer Lett 83: 143–147
32. Sasaki YF, Yamada H, Shimoi K, Kator K, Kinae N (1993) The aclastogen-suppressing effects of green tea, Po-lei tea and Rooi bos tea in CHO cells and mice. Mutat. Res 286: 221–232
33. Kono S, Shinchi K, Wakabayashi K, Honjo S, Todoroki I, Sakurai Y, Imanishi K, Nishikawa H, Ogawa S, Katsurada M (1996) Relation of green tea consumption to serum lipids and lipoproteins in Japanese men. J Epidemiol 6: 128–133
34. Hertog MG, Feskens EJ, Hollman PC, Katan MB, Kromhout D (1993) Dietary antioxidant flavonoids and risk of coronary heart disease: The Zutphen elderly study. Lancet 342: 1007–1011
35. Sato Y, Nakatsuka H, Watanabe T, Hisamichi S, Shimizu H, Fujisaku S, Ichinowatari Y, Ida Y, Suda S, Kato K (1989) Possible contribution of green tea drinking to the prevention of stroke. Tohoku J Exp Med 157: 337–343
36. Imai K, Nakachi K (1995) Cross-sectional study of the effects of drinking green tea on cardiovascular and liver diseases. Bt Med J 310: 693–696
37. Sadakata, S (1995) Mortality among female practitioners of Chanyou (Japanese tea ceremony). Tohoku J Exp Med 166: 475–477
38. Suganuma M, Okabe S, Komori A, Sueoka E, Sueoka N, Kozu T, Sakai Y (1996) Japanese green tea as a cancer preventive in humans. Nutr Rev 54: S67-S70
39. Kanis J, Johnell O, Gullberg B, Allander E, Elffors L, Ranstam J, Dequeker J, Dilsen G, Gennari C, Vaz AL, Lyritis G, Mazzuoli G, Miravet L, Passeri M, Perez Cano R, Rapado A, Ribot C (1999) Risk factors for hip fracture in men from Southern Europe: The MEDOS study. Osteoporosis Int 9: 45–55
40. Hegarty VM, May HM, Khaw KT (2000) Tea drinking and bone mineral density in older women. Am J Clin Nutr 71: 1003–1007
41. No JK, Soung DY, Kim YJ, Shim KH, Jun YS, Rhee SH, Yokozawa T, Chung HY (1999) Inhibition of tyrosinase by green tea components. Life Sci 65: L241-PL-246
42. Akiyama K, Shimizu Y, Yokoi I, Kabuto H, Mori A, Ozaki M (1989) Effects of epigallocatechin and epigallocatechin-3-O-gallate on catechol-o-methyltransferase. Neuroscience 15: 262–264
43. Dulloo AG, Seydoux J, Girardier L, Chantre P, Vandermander J (2000) Green tea and thermogenesis: Interactions between catechin-polyphenols, caffeine and sympathetic activity. Int J Obes Relat Metab Disord 24: 252–258
44. Fan W, Tezuka Y, Komatsu K, Namba T, Kadota S (1999) Prolyl endopeptidase inhibitors from the underground part of Rhodiola sacra S.H. Fu. Biol Pharm Bull 22: 157–161
45. Haqqi TM, Anthony DD, Gupta S, Ahmad N, Lee MS, Kumar GK, Mukhtar H (1999) Prevention of collagen-induced arthritis in mice by apolyphenolic fraction from green tea. Proc Natl Acad Sci 96: 4524–4529
46. Suganuma M, Sueoka E, Sueoka N, Okabe S, Fujiki H (2000) Mechanisms of cancer prevention by tea polyphenols based on inhibition of TNF-alpha expression. Biofactors 13: 67–72
47. Horiba N, Maekawa Y, Ito M, Matsumoto T, Nakamura H (1991) A pilot study of Japanese green tea as a medicament: Antibacterial and bactericidal effects. J Endod 17: 122–124
48. Makimura M, Hirasawa M, Kobayashi K, Indo J, Sakanaka S, Taguchi T, Otake S (1993) Inhibitory effect of tea catechins on collagenase activity. J Periodontol. 64: 630–636
49. Yu H, Oho T, Xu LX (1995) Effects of several tea components on acid resistance of human tooth enamel. J Dent 23: 101–105
50. Goto K, Kanaya S, Nishikawa T (1998) The influence of tea catechins on fecal flora of elderly residents in long-term care facilities. Ann Long-Term Care 6: 43–48
51. Goto K, Kanaya S, Ishigami T, Hara Y (1999) The effects of tea catechins on fecal conditions of elderly residents in a long-term care facility. J Nutr Sci Vitaminol 45: 135–141
52. Yamamoto Y, Juneja LR, Chu DC, Kim M (1997) Chemistry and applications of green tea. CRC Press LLC: Boca Raton USA.
53. Weisburger JH (1999) Tea and Health: the underlying mechanisms. Proc Soc Exper Biol Med 220: 271–275
54. Ernest P (1999) Review article: the role of inflammation in the pathogenesis of gastric cancer. Aliment Pharmacol Therapeutics 13 (Suppl 1): 13–18
55. Lampe JW (1999) Health effects of vegetables and fruits: assessing mechanisms of action in human experimental studies. Am J Clin Nutr 70 (Suppl.): 475S-490S

10 Chiropractic Spinal Manipulation for the Elderly?

E. Ernst

Introduction

A recent survey suggested that 58% of elderly Americans use some form of complementary/alternative medicine [1]. As chiropractic is one of the most popular types of complementary/alternative medicine [2], many elderly people are likely to try chiropractic at least occasionally. This chapter is aimed at reviewing the evidence for or against the use of chiropractic spinal manipulation (SM) in this particular population.

Definitions

There are numerous definitions of chiropractic: The American Chiropractic Association states the following on its web site [3]: "Chiropractic is a branch of the healing arts which is concerned with human health and disease processes. Doctors of Chiropractic are physicians who consider man as an integrated being and give special attention to the physiological and biochemical aspects including structural, spinal, musculoskeletal, neurological, vascular, nutritional emotional and environmental relationships. The practice and procedures which may be employed by Doctors of Chiropractic are based on the academic and clinical training received in and through accredited chiropractic colleges and include, but are not limited to, the use of current diagnostic and therapeutic procedures. Such procedures specifically include the adjustment and manipulation of the articulations and the adjacent tissues of the human body, particularly of the spinal column. Included is the treatment of intersegmental aberrations for alleviation of related functional disorders."

While this may constitute a sufficient definition, it should be noted that: "doctors" and "physicians" used to be individuals who studied medicine at a conventional medical school. The definition also leaves the question unanswered, why chiropractic SM might be expected to treat medical conditions in the first place. Essentially, chiropractors believe that most human illnesses are caused by a subluxation or malalignment of spinal joints and that SM will normalise this allowing the body to heal itself. Chiropractors use a range of techniques of which SM is probably the commonest. The American Chiropractic Association states that: "A manipulation is a passive manual maneuver during which the three-joint complex is carried beyond the normal physiological range of movement without exceeding the boundaries of anatomical integrity.

The essential characteristic is a thrust – a brief, sudden, and carefully administered 'impulsion' that is given at the end of the normal passive range of movement. The "dynamic thrust" is the defining factor, which distinguishes manipulation from other forms of manual therapy. The thrust technique can be low or high velocity. The most common characteristics of the adjustive dynamic thrust are a controlled force delivered with high velocity, in a specific direction or line of drive, at a regulated magnitude and depth. In short, manipulation is a passive dynamic thrust that causes an audible release (cavitation) and attempts to increase the manipulated joint's range of motion. [4]

Osteopaths also use SM but put more emphasis on soft tissue techniques. In the US, osteopaths have moved significantly towards mainstream medicine and many osteopaths use the full range of medical therapies much like conventional physicians.

Survey data suggest that chiropractors regularly use SM for elderly patients and complement it with a range of additional therapies, e.g. exercise, dietary advice, or dietary supplements [5]. Similar types of evidence also imply that, in the US, chiropractors treat a wide range of medical conditions including pain after injury, headache, musculoskeletal problems, abdominal pain, and other symptoms [6]. However, today back pain is by far the most common condition treated by chiropractors.

Effectiveness

The following section focuses on the effectiveness of chiropractic SM for various conditions. The emphasis will be put on elderly patients.

Back pain

Expert opinion is clearly in favour of SM for acute, uncomplicated and (to a lesser degree) other types of back pain [7]. Yet the data from rigorous clinical trials are far less clear cut. Several randomised clinical trials (RCTs) are available but their results are not uniform. A recent systematic review [8] concluded that there is moderate evidence of short-term efficacy for SM in the treatment of acute low back pain and for SM therapy combined with mobilisation for chronic low back pain. This moderate evidence of efficacy rests on a very small amount of RCTs. Although some RCTs and prospective studies show promising results, the data are insufficient to draw conclusions regarding the short-term efficacy of SM therapy for the treatment of lumbar radiculopathy. The evidence is also inconclusive for the long-term efficacy of SM for the treatment of any type of low back pain.

As some of the RCTs in this review were not of chiropractic SM, it is worth looking at this particular subset of studies. A systematic review identified 8 such RCTs [9]. All had serious flaws in their design, execution and reporting. Because of the great variety of outcome measures and follow-up timing, statistical pooling of the RCTs was not possible. A narrative review, however, did not provide convincing evidence for the effectiveness of chiropractic SM for acute or chronic low back pain [9].

Since the publication of these reviews, further RCTs of SM have become available (e.g. [10, 11, 12]). These trials are of good methodological quality and their results therefore attain a relatively high level of conclusiveness. None of these studies demonstrated the superiority of SM over control treatment. Most of these studies include patients older than 60 years but none was conducted specifically in populations of elderly patients. The bottom line therefore is that SM is not of proven benefit to elderly patients suffering from (any type of) low back pain.

Headache disorders

Computerized literature searches were carried out in 4 databases to identify all RCTs of SM for any type of headache [13]. Eight trials met our inclusion criteria. Three examined tension-type headaches, three migraine, one "cervicogenic" headache, and one "spondylogenic" chronic headache. In two studies, patients receiving SM showed comparable improvements in migraine and tension headaches compared to drug treatment. In the 4 studies employing some "sham" interventions (e.g. laser light therapy), results were less conclusive with two studies showing a benefit for SM and two studies failing to find such an effect. Considerable methodological limitations were observed in most trials, the principal one being inadequate control for non-specific (placebo) effects. The most frequently encountered methodological limitations in clinical trials of chiropractic spinal manipulation are listed in Table 10.1.

Despite claims to the contrary, the data available to date do not support the notion that SM is an effective treatment for headache. It is unclear to what extent the observed treatment effects can be explained by specific therapeutic effects of SM or by non-specific factors (e.g. of personal attention, expectation, demand characteristics).

Other conditions

We recently published a series of systematic reviews of complementary/alternative treatments in book form [14]. It included a range of medical conditions relevant to elderly patients. The evidence pertaining to SM is summarised in Table 10. 2. Promising evidence of adequate volume emerged only for neck pain. However, a recent study casts doubt on the notion that SM is the optimal treatment for neck pain [15]. In this three-armed study, 191 patients (aged 44.3 ± 10.6 years) with chronic mechanical neck pain were randomised to receive 20 sessions of SM or exercise, or SM combined with exercise. The results suggested that strengthening exercises, whether in combination with SM or as a sole treatment, were more beneficial than the use of SM alone.

There are numerous further conditions which are relevant to elderly individuals and for which SM has been tested, albeit not specifically in elderly patients. These conditions include fibromyalgia [16], Parkinson's disease [17], duodenal ulcer [18], and carpal tunnel syndrome [19]. The individual trials are burdened with serious methodological weaknesses. Moreover, for most studies there is an almost total lack of independent replication. For none of these conditions is the evidence sufficient to warrant recommendations for SM use.

Table 10.1. Frequent methodological limitations of clinical trials of chiropractic SM

Problem	Implication	Possible Solution
Small sample size	Danger of type II error	Determine sample size through power calculation
Complex interventions are not adequately described	Results are difficult to interpret, independent replication impossible	Define treatments in detail such that independent replication is possible
Statistical approach invalid or not optimal	Results are not reliable	Consult statistician during planning period of the study
Inadequate or no control of placebo effects	No distinction between specific and non-specific therapeutic effects possible	Introduce credible sham intervention
No patient-blinding	Result may be influenced by patient expectation	Use sham intervention and test for success of patient-blinding
No evaluator-blinding	Results may be influenced by evaluator expectation	Introduce evaluator-blinding (which is no major problem)
Primary research question not clear	Interpretation of results ambiguous	Define research question and interpret results accordingly
Follow-up too short	Results are not clinically meaningful	Introduce adequate follow-up period
Treatment provided by one therapist	Study does not test the intervention per se but the competence of the therapist	Use more than one therapist
No reporting of adverse events	Risk-benefit ratio not accessible	Insist on rigorous reporting of adverse events
No reporting of cost	Cost-effectiveness not accessible	Consult health economist during planning period of the trial

Table 10.2. Evidence of effectiveness for other indications

Indication	Weight of evidence	Direction of evidence
Anxiety	O	→
Asthma	OO	→
Chronic fatigue syndrome	O	↗
Menopause	O	→
Neck pain	OO	↗

O insufficient weight, OO moderate weight, OOO sufficient weight. "Weight" is used here as a complex measure composed of: 1) the volume, 2) the level (e.g. randomised clinical trial or meta-analysis), 3) the quality of the evidence (for more details see [14]).

SM more than a placebo?

Vis a vis the data summarised above, the question arises whether SM is more than a placebo. To investigate this question, a systematic review of the published literature was performed [20]. Literature searches were carried out in Medline, Embase and The Cochrane Library. All sham-controlled trials of SM were considered. Seven such studies were located. Their methodological quality was variable. Collectively these data did not show therapeutic effects beyond placebo. The three most rigorous studies were negative. The results available to date thus do not demonstrate that the perceived therapeutic success of SM is due to a specific therapeutic effect. This fact, it seems, is important when interpreting the results of clinical trials of SM.

Safety

Adverse effects

SM has repeatedly been associated with adverse effects and serious complications [21]. To summarise the evidence on the risks of SM, a further systematic review was conducted [22]. Papers were located through three electronic databases (Medline, Embase, The Cochrane Library), contacting experts, scanning reference lists of relevant articles and searching departmental files. Recent reports in any language containing data relating to risks associated with SM were included, irrespective of the profession of the therapist. Data from prospective investigations suggest that minor transient adverse events occur in approximately half of SM patients.

Minor Adverse Effects Frequently Associated With Spinal Manipulation

▶ Local discomfort
▶ Headache
▶ Fatigue
▶ Distant discomfort

Prospective studies show that these sensations are experienced by about 50% of chiropractic patients.

The most common serious adverse events reported in the literature are vertebrobasilar accidents, disk herniation and cauda equina syndrome. We therefore concluded that SM is not risk-free. Minor adverse events are common and largely inherent in the treatment modality. Serious complications appear to be rare but their incidence is currently not known. Table 10.3 summarises examples of adverse events recently reported in elderly patients [23–26].

Contra-indications

As with its indications, the contra-indications of SM have not been established beyond reasonable doubt. Some contra-indications which today are widely accepted are

▶ Abnormalities of blood coagulation
▶ Cervical spondylosis
▶ Hypermobility syndrome

Table 10.3. Serious adverse events of spinal manipulation in elderly patients – examples of recent case reports

First author (year)	Patient (age)	Indication	Therapist (therapy)	Adverse event	Outcome	Causality
Haldemann (1992)	woman (82)	Knee osteo-arthritis	Chiropractor and orthopaedic surgeon (manipulation)	Bone fracture	Not mentioned	Uncertain
	woman (72)	Pain	Chiropractor (23 treatment sessions within 6 weeks)	Multiple spinal compression fractures	Not mentioned	Possible
McPartland (1996)	woman (67)	Back pain	Massage therapist (craniosacral intraoral treatment)	Pain and swelling in temporomandibular joint for 1 month	Full recovery	Likely
Ruelle (1999)	woman (64)	Back pain	Chiropractor (manipulation of lumbar spine)	Thoracic epidural hematoma	Surgical evacuation of hematoma, full recovery	Likely
Stevinson (2001)	man (70)	Not known	Not known	Bilateral vertebral artery dissections, brain stem stroke	Full recovery	Likely
Stevinson (2001)	"woman in her 60's"	Not known	Not known	Myelopathy, parasthesias in all extremities	Permanent neurological deficit	Likely

- ▶ Inflammatory diseases of the spine
- ▶ Malignant diseases of the spine
- ▶ Myelopathy
- ▶ Osteoporosis
- ▶ Treatment with anticoagulants
- ▶ Vertebral bony abnormalities
- ▶ Vertebrobasilar insufficiency

In the context of this article, the most notable contra-indication is clearly osteoporosis. It is therefore conceivable that the risk of SM is higher for elderly individuals than for populations of lower ages.

Conclusion

Chiropractic spinal manipulation is popular and many elderly individuals use this therapeutic approach mostly (but not exclusively) for musculoskeletal complaints, e.g. back and neck pain. Even though numerous studies of SM have been carried out, few of them have been specifically performed with elderly patients. The evidence from rigorous clinical trials of SM for any condition is far from convincing at present. The data for acute back and neck pain are promising but unfortunately not fully convincing. The evidence for all other indications is even less compelling. Mild adverse effects after SM are common. Serious adverse effects are on record but their frequency is presently not known. Contra-indications for SM include osteoporosis which would seem to render SM contra-indicated for the majority of elderly individuals.

Given this state of affairs, it would seem unwise to recommend SM to elderly individuals. Those who try SM despite the lack of encouraging evidence should be informed about the lack of proven benefit and about the risk which may be higher in the elderly compared to younger patients.

References

1. Cherniack EP, Senzel RS, Pan CX (2001) Correlates use of alternative medicine by the elderly in an urban population. J Altern Comp Med 7: 277–280
2. Eisenberg D, David RB, Ettner SL et al (1998) Trends in alternative medicine use in the United States; 1990–1997. JAMA 280: 1569–1575
3. American Chiropractic Association (1999) About chiropractic. http://www amerchiro org/about_chiro/index html
4. American Chiropractic Association (1999) Policy statement on spinal manipulation. Aug: 1–12
5. Rupert RL, Manello D, Sandefur R (2000) Maintenance care: health promotion services administered to US chiropractic patients aged 65 and older, Part II. J Manipulative Physiol Ther 23: 10–19
6. Hurwitz EL, Coulter ID, Adams AH, Genovese BJ, Shekelle PG (1998) Use of chiropractic services from 1985 through 1991 in the United States and Canada. Amer J Public Health 88: 771–776
7. Ernst E, Pittler MH (1999) Experts" opinions on complementary/alternative therapies for low back pain. J Manip Phys Ther 22: 87–90
8. Bronfort G (1999) Spinal manipulation. Current state of research and its indications. Neurol Clinics North America 17: 91–111
9. Assendelft WJJ, Koes BW, van der Heijden GJMG, Bouter LM (1996) The effectiveness of chiropractic for treatment of low back pain: an update and attempt at statistical pooling. J Manipul Physiol Ther 19: 499–507
10. Skargren EI, Oberg BE, Carlsson PG, Gade M (1997) Cost and effectiveness analysis of chiropractic and physiotherapy treatment for low back and neck pain – six-month follow-up. Spine 22: 2167–2177
11. Cherkin DC, Deyo RA, Battie M, Street J, Barlow W (1998) A comparison of physical therapy, chiropractic manipulation, and provision of an educational booklet for the treatment of patients with low back pain. N Engl J Med 339: 1021–1029
12. Burton AK, Tillotson KM, Cleary J (2000) Single-blind randomised controlled trial of chemonucleolysis and manipulation in the treatment of symptomatic lumbar disc herniation. Eur Spine J 9: 202–207
13. Astin JA, Ernst E (2001) The effectiveness of spinal manipulation for the treatment of headache disorders: A systematic review of randomised clinical trials. Submitted for publication
14. Ernst E, Pittler MH, Stevinson C, White AR, Eisenberg D (2001) The desktop guide to complementary and alternative medicine. Edinburgh, Mosby.
15. Bronfort G, Evans R, Nelson B, Aker PD, Goldsmith CH, Vernon H (2001) A randomised clinical trial of exercise and spinal manipulation for patients with chronic neck pain. Spine 26: 788–799
16. Hains G, Hains F (2000) Combined ischemic compression and spinal manipulation in the treatment of fibromyalgia: a preliminary estimate of dose and efficacy. J Manip Physiol Ther 23: 225–230
17. Elster EL (2000) Upper cervical chiropractic management of a patient with Parkinson"s disease: a case report. J Manip Physiol Ther 23: 573–577
18. Pikalov AA, Kharin VV (1994) Use of spinal manipulative therapy in the treatment of duodenal ulcer: a pilot study. J Manip Physiol Ther 17: 310–313
19. Davis PT, Hulbert JR (1998) Carpal tunnel syndrome – conservative and nonconservative treatment – a chiropractic physicians perspective. J Manipulative & Physiological Therapeutics 21: 356–362

20. Ernst E, Harkness EF (2001) Spinal manipulation: a systematic review of sham-controlled, double-blind, randomised clinical trials. J Pain Sympt Man 24: 879–889
21. Di Fabio RP (1999) Manipulation of the cervical spine: risks and benefits. Physical Ther 79: 50–65
22. Stevinson C, Ernst E (2001) Risks associated with spinal manipulation. submitted for publication
23. Halderman S, Rubinstein SM (1992) Compression fractures in patients undergoing spinal manipulative therapy. J Manipulative Physiol Ther 15: 45–54
24. McPartland JM (1996) Craniosacral iatrogenesis. Side-effects from cranial-sacral treatment case reports and commentary. J Bodywork and Movement Therapies 1: 2–5
25. Ruelle A, Datti R, Pisani R (1999) Thoracic epidural hematoma after spinal manipulation therapy. J Spinal Disorders 12: 534–536
26. Stevinson C, Honan W, Cooke B, Ernst E (2001) Neurological complications of cervical spine manipulation. J Roy Soc Med 94: 107–110

11 Unconventional Western Medicine

R. McCarney, P. Fisher

Introduction

A number of forms of complementary or alternative medicine currently practised have their origins in the western intellectual tradition: Western Europe and North America. This chapter aims to outline some of the more common forms of CAM of western origin, particularly those supported by evidence of clinical effectiveness.

These therapies are diverse in form and origins but a number of common threads do exist, notably most of them are explicitly holistic in their approach and many are vitalistic. That is to say, they are founded on the idea of stimulating, facilitating or directing the body's own self-healing processes, repair and maintenance mechanisms. In unconventional western medicine the concept is most frequently termed "Vis medicatrix naturae" – the natural healing force.

Vitalism was generally abandoned by western medicine during the 19th century. As a consequence of the scientific revolution which transformed medicine, the vital force was perceived as metaphysical, referring to an abstract principle, intangible and difficult even to define, let alone measure. But recent insights deriving from complexity theory, particularly "emergent properties" (behaviour of a system which cannot be predicted from the properties of its component parts alone), offer new ways of thinking about vitalism [1, 2].

There are similarities and analogies between some western CAM therapies and traditional therapies of oriental origin, but care should be exercised in making comparisons. Vis medicatrix naturae is clearly a different concept from, say the qi (chi) of East Asian philosophy. Although on the practical level there are similarities and analogies between some western CAM therapies and traditional therapies of oriental origin, care should be exercised in making comparison. Because of the different cultural and philosophical backgrounds, simplistic attempts to reconcile theoretical explanations and terminology may be misleading.

Homeopathy

What is it?

Homeopathy is a therapeutic system based on the principle of treating like with like (often quoted in Latin "Similia similibus curentur", "let like be cured by like"). Secondary principles of homeopathy include holism, homeopaths often say that they "do not treat diseases, but sick people" and the use of the minimum dose. Thus, the homeo-path seeks a match between the syndrome presented by a patient and the syndrome produced by a medicinal substance. For instance the homeopathic medicine *Apis mellifica* is made from whole crushed bees. It may be used to treat a range of problems resembling the effects of a beesting, including angioedema, acute inflammatory ar-thritis and acute renal failure: hymenoptera (bees and wasps) stings can cause acute glomerulonephritis in susceptible individuals).

About 60% of homeopathic medicines are of plant origin, but they may be pro-duced from animal, vegetable or mineral sources, or from disease products (known as nosodes). Homeopathic medicines are manufactured according to a specialised phar-macopoeia (The Homeopathic Pharmacopoeia of the United States in the US, similar officially-recognised pharmacopoeias exist in other countries).

The starting point of a homeopathic remedy is the "mother tincture", produced by letting the specified ingredient stand in an ethanol water mixture for several weeks. Insoluble substances are first triturated with lactose before being suspended in the same medium. The mother tincture is then serially diluted with vigorous shaking (suc-cussion) at each stage, a process sometimes known as "potentisation". The most com-mon dilution scales are the decimal in which successive dilutions are 1:10 (usually denoted x in English-speaking countries, D or DH in most other countries) and centesimal scales (c, C, or CH), with dilutions in steps of 1:100. A number of other methods of dilution are in use, these include the 50 Millesimal (LM), and Korsakov methods. The resulting liquid dilution is usually absorbed onto pills of lactose and/or sucrose before packing, and administered by allowing the pills to dissolve in the mouth. Homeopathic medicines may also be left in liquid form.

Commonly used dilutions include 6 and 30 c, corresponding respectively to dilu-tions of 10^{-12} and 10^{-60} of the mother tincture. Avogadro's Constant (the number of atoms or molecules in a gram mole of a substance) is of the order of 10^{23}. The implica-tion is that, while a 6 c dilution may contain some molecules of the mother tincture, it is extremely unlikely that the 30 c dilution will do so. Such dilutions are known as "ultramolecular", and it is the claims made for their action which are the source of most of the controversy surrounding homeopathy.

History

Homeopathy was founded by the German physician Samuel Hahnemann (1755–1843) in 1796. He became disillusioned with the "heroic" (i.e. very large!) doses and gross bloodletting practised by his medical contemporaries. Hahnemann noticed by experi-menting on himself that quinine, effective in the treatment of malaria, could provoke symptoms similar to malaria. This lead him to propose the principle "let like be cured by like" (*similia similibus curentur*). This idea can be found in the writings of Para-celsus and in the Hippocratic Corpus, but Hahnemann was the first to develop it sys-tematically.

Hahnemann initially used large doses but gradually adopted smaller and smaller doses, culminating in the idea of "potentisation" used today. He originated the idea of "provings" (or homeopathic pathogenetic trials). These are a form of trial in which healthy volunteers take a substance and the symptoms, mapped to the type of person susceptible to the substance, are noted. The prescribing symptoms used in homeopathy derive from provings, toxicology and clinical experience. This information is compiled in materia medicas and indexed in repertories, which are available as computer software.

Homeopathy was widespread in 19th century North America. In the 1890's as many as 20% of American physicians considered themselves homeopaths and there were many homeopathic medical colleges. Most of the homeopathic medical colleges closed or converted to conventional medical education following the Flexner Report (1910) on Medical education. There was a steady decline in the number of homeopathic practitioners for most of the 20th century, but this trend has reversed in the last two decades.

Possible Indications with Evidence

To date there have been over 200 clinical trials of homeopathy. A number of systematic reviews show that homeopathic medicines (in general) have an effect over and above placebo. Kleijnen's et al.'s [3] criteria-based analysis found that of the 105 trials with interpretable results 77% were positive, with the more methodologically sound trials more likely to produce positive results. They concluded that the evidence presented would be sufficient to establish homeopathy as a regular treatment for a number of conditions. Linde et al.'s meta-analysis [4] of 89 trials found a combined odds ratio of 2.45 (95% C.I. 2.05, 2.93) in favour of homeopathy, and concluded that "the results of the meta-analysis are not compatible with the hypothesis that the effects of homeopathy are completely due to placebo". Cucherat et al, in a review commissioned by the European Commission, with strict inclusion criteria, reviewed 16 trials including 2617 patients. The combined P value was highly significant [5]. All three reviews call for further research in the area.

Possible indications for the elderly where homeopathy appears effective includes rheumatism, arthritis, influenza-like illnesses, varicose veins and allergy. A systematic review of homeopathic remedies for the treatment of osteoarthritis [6] included four randomised controlled trials and found they favoured homeopathic treatment. Their conclusion was that due to the small number of trials reviewed more research is warranted, although the results seemed promising. A comparative randomised, double-blind controlled trial of homeopathic gel against Piroxicam gel found that the homeopathic gel at least as effective, with a better safety profile [7]. Of the four randomised controlled trials of homeopathic treatments for rheumatoid arthritis reviewed by Linde and colleagues in his systematic review [4], all four were positive.

A Cochrane review of seven trials of Oscillococcinum [8] for treating influenza concluded that there is evidence for its effect in reducing the duration of illness, but a protective effect was not apparent. In an randomised placebo controlled trial of 61 patients, Poikiven, a combined homeopathic preparation, was found to be effective on a number of objective and subjective symptoms in treating primary varicosity [9]. There is also evidence that homeopathy can play a part in treating perennial allergic rhinitis [10]. This series of trials found a significant effect, over and above that of placebo, on objective as well as subjective measures.

Mechanism of Action

The mechanism of action of homeopathic high dilutions is currently unknown. Indeed the main reason for the controversy surrounding homeopathy is the implausibility of the claim that "ultra molecular" dilutions, diluted beyond the point at which any molecule of the mother tincture is unlikely to remain have any specific effects. The mechanism of action of such dilutions is not comprehensible in terms of current scientific concepts. Current theories center on the "Information Medicine Hypothesis" which proposes that water and perhaps other polar solvents are capable, under certain circumstances of storing information about substances with which they have been in contact and of transmitting this to sensitized biosystems. There is now a significant body of theoretical and experimental work in this area focusing on formation of sustained dynamic structures in aqueous solutions, capable of storing information [11].

A Typical Consultation

History taking and examination feature in a typical consultation in a manner similar to that found in conventional medicine, although consultations tend to be longer and more wide-ranging. Homeopaths may investigate for example personality traits, physical features, environmental influences, patterns of disease within families and relationships. The initial consultation usually lasts for 45 minutes to over an hour, generally less for subsequent interviews.

Safety Issues

The safety profile of homeopathy is very good. A comprehensive literature review [12] found 10 clinical trial reports of adverse effects (mostly mild and transient symptoms); 19 from case reports (3 of which were judged as "probably"attributable to homeopathic medicines); and 18 from "provings" between 1970 and 1995. It should be noted however that they found the quality of reporting to be generally poor and there was frequent confusion between herbal and homeopathic preparations. Underreporting is probable.

Training of Practitioners

Three US states (Arizona, Connecticut, Nevada) have state homeopathic boards which license MDs in the practise of homeopathy. Elsewhere MDs are regulated by the regular state medical board. A number of states also license NDs, who may practice homeopathy (see below). The North American Society of Homeopaths (NASH) registers practitioners who are not health professionals.

In the UK, the practice of homeopathy is essentially unregulated, there is no legal requirement for homeopathic practitioners to undertake training, or to be registered. The Faculty of Homeopathy is a statutory body which accredits the training of and registers homeopathic physicians and other health professionals (including veterinarians, dentists and pharmacists) who use homeopathy within their normal domains of competence.

How to Identify Practitioners

In US states without homeopathic licensing boards and which do not license NDs, it may be difficult to identify adequately trained practitioners. Lists are available from the National Center for Homeopathy in Alexandria, VA.

The Faculty of Homeopathy accredits health professionals at various levels LFHom (a basic qualification), DFHom (dentists and pharmacists) and MFHom (specialist qualifications). The Society of Homeopaths accredits non-medically qualified practitioners (RSHom and FSHom).

Naturopathy

What is it?

Naturopathy is an umbrella term rather than a specific form of medical practice. It emphasises prevention, treatment and the promotion of health through natural therapeutic methods which encourage self-healing and return to a harmonious state (homeostasis; absence of disease along with a sense of well-being).

The five main principles of Naturopathy are:

▶ *First Do No Harm (Primum non Nocere):* Naturopathic medicine avoids harming the patient by utilizing methods and medicinal substances which minimize the risk of harmful side effects; avoiding the suppression of symptoms; and acknowledging and respecting the individual's healing process, using the least force necessary to diagnose and treat.

▶ *The Healing Power of Nature (Vis Medicatrix Naturae):* Naturopathic medicine recognies the inherent self-healing capacity of the body. Naturopathics try to identify and remove obstacles to recovery and facilitate this healing ability.

▶ *Identify and Treat the Causes (Tolle Causam):* Naturopaths seeks to identify and remove the underlying causes of illness, rather than to suppress symptoms.

▶ *Doctor as Teacher (Docere):* Naturopaths educate the patient and encourage personal responsibility for health.

▶ *Treat the Whole Person:* Naturopaths treat each individual by taking into account physical, mental, emotional, genetic, environmental, social, spiritual and other factors.

▶ *Prevention:* Naturopaths emphasize disease prevention, assessment of risk factors and susceptibility to disease.

Naturopathy is a holistic system, treating the individual as a whole. Indeed the naturopathic triad of the structural aspects of the body (including for example posture, muscle and bone condition), the biochemical (stemming from nutrition), and mental or emotional aspects, are seen as being totally interrelated with dysfunction in one part leading to disruption of the other parts.

In practice the main therapeutic methods used by naturopaths are: clinical nutrition (including dietary exclusion, fasting and supplementation), homeopathy, phytotherapy (herbal medicine), hydrotherapy and physical medicine and counselling. Some naturopaths also practice acupuncture and other forms of complementary medicine. As naturopathy is a general approach to health care, rather than a specific therapy other treatments such as yoga, osteopathy or psychotherapy may form part of the regime.

History

Modern naturopathy has its origins in the 19th century in a number of individuals, notably the German priest Father Sebastian Kneipp (1821–1897). Kneipp advocated therapies such as balneotherapy (bathing therapy) and phytotherapy.

Benedict Lust (1872–1945), a student of Kneipp's, brought naturopathy to the United States and formed the American Institute of Naturopathy in 1902. The large number of dubious therapies which fell under the banner of naturopathy (many of which have now fallen by the wayside) made it the subject of severe criticism by the conventional medical establishment in the early 20th century. Many naturopathic medical schools were closed down as a consequence of the Flexner Report (1910) on Medical Education in the USA. Naturopathy remains controversial but Naturopathic Doctors (NDs) are licensed in twelve U.S. states.

Possible Indications with Evidence

Naturopathy is believed to help a large range of both acute and chronic problems common in the elderly, including arthritis and circulatory disorders. It is difficult however to comment on its effectiveness, because there is a paucity of good quality research on naturopathy as a whole, because naturopathy can potentially involve a large number of possible therapies. Research on phytotherapy, nutrition and balneotherapy among other methods might apply to naturopathy.

There is considerable evidence however that such modalities (as used by naturopaths) may be helpful. For instance fasting and vegetarian diets appears to confer long term benefit in rheumatoid arthritis [13], dietary supplementation with glycosaminoglycans appears to be effective in osteoarthritis [14] and herbal Gingko biloba effective for dementia and peripheral circulatory problems [15, 16]. A Cochrane review of balneotherapy for arthritis identified 10 trials with a total of 607 patients, and generally positive results, although there were many methodological problems with the included studies [17].

Mechanism of Action

Since naturopathy is an umbrella term, there is unlikely to be a single mechanism of action. But the various therapies subsumed under "naturopathy" are united by the idea of stimulating and directing the Vis medicatrix naturae – the innate maintenance and repair mechanisms of the human body. The existence and nature of this concept are woefully under-researched areas. As for the component therapies, plausibility varies considerably.

A Typical Consultation

In-depth first consultation lasting for up to one hour enquiring about many aspects of the patients life; including for example diet, relationships and job details. If an osteopathic examination is undertaken then it would include stripping to underwear. Length of treatment will depend on how established the condition being treated is, perhaps from 1 to 6 months of twice-monthly sessions. In some European countries, particularly Germany, naturopathy (Naturheilkunde in German) is well-established, with many spas that use various naturopathic treatments. Patients typically stay for periods of 1–3 weeks at a time, and costs may be reimbursed by health care insurers.

Safety Issues

Again due to the large number of possible treatment modalities involved it is difficult to comment on the safety of naturopathy. With some treatments used (such as osteopathy) there is the possibility of serious adverse events and with other (such as relaxation therapy) there are unlikely to be serious adverse events. The patient should remain under the care of a medically-qualified physician at all times and be carefully monitored.

Training of Practitioners

The following colleges in North America offer ND degree programmes which entitle recipients to sit a licensing exam in one of the states which have licensing boards for NDs:

▶ National College of Naturopathic Medicine (Portland, OR)
▶ Bastyr University (Seattle, WA)
▶ Southwest College of Naturopathic Medicine (Tempe, AZ)
▶ Canadian College of Naturopathic Medicine (Toronto, ONT, Canada)
▶ University of Bridgeport College of Naturopathic Medicine (Bridgeport, CT)

There are also several non-accredited correspondence schools operating in the U.S. In most European countries, Naturopathy is practised by doctors with specialist training.

How to Identify Practitioners

In the United States Naturopathic Physicians holding the degree of Doctor of Naturopathy (ND) Naturopathic practice is currently (as of October 2001) legally recognised in 12 US states (Alaska, Arizona, Connecticut, Florida, Hawaii, Maine, Montana, New Hampshire, Oregon, Utah, Vermont and Washington) and four Canadian Provinces (British Columbia, Saskatchewan, Manitoba and Ontario). The American Association of Naturopathic Physicians (AANP) is closely linked to the accredited colleges and membership is limited to those who are eligible for licenses in licensing states. The Homeopathic Academy of Naturopathic Physicians (HANP) requires an accredited degree for membership as well as additional homeopathic training.

In the UK, the practice of Naturopathy is essentially unregulated. In Germany Heilpraktikers, who receive a basic training but are registered, may use naturopathic methods.

Anthroposophical Medicine

What is it?

Anthroposophy is a philosophy founded by the Austrian Rudolph Steiner (1860–1925). Steiner described it as "a way of schooling oneself and gaining knowledge. It seeks to unite the spiritual element in us with the spiritual element in the natural world". Anthroposophy has implications for many aspects of human life including medicine. Anthroposophical medicine, like Naturopathy, has a number of elements. These include Eurythmy, a form of therapeutic exercise and Iscador, a fermented product of Mistletoe (*Viscum album*) used in the treatment of cancer. Most Anthroposophical doctors use homeopathy. Anthroposophical medicine is particularly popular in German-speaking countries.

Possible Indications with Evidence

A review of clinical trials of mistletoe preparations (mostly Iscador, but also the mistletoe preparations Helixor and Eurixor) for cancer identified 11 controlled trials in carcinoma of the breast, bowel, bronchus, female genital tract and stomach. Ten trials showed at least a positive trend, in terms of survival, but most suffered from methodological flaws [18]. There do not appear to be any controlled trials of anthroposophical medicine in other conditions. Guidance on prescribing of Iscador, produced by a British consensus group, is available [19].

Mechanism of Action

Mistletoe contains cytotoxic lectins, but these may not be the active principles.

Training of Practitioners

Anthroposophical doctors are generally conventionally trained doctors with additional training.

A Typical Consultation

Anthroposophical medical consultations are similar to those of physicians using homeopathy and naturopathy.

Safety Issues

Iscador often causes a mild local skin reaction, and may cause low grade pyrexia. These are considered favourable responses. Severe adverse reactions are rare.

How to Identify Practitioners

The Weleda company which manufactures homeopathic and anthroposophic medicines has affiliates in many countries and can supply lists of practitioners.

Alexander Technique

What is it?

A system of education rather than a therapy, designed to help "rediscover" natural posture, improve coordination and increase awareness of "unhealthy" motor and mental habits, which lead to tension and stress that adversely effects the functioning of the whole body.

The Alexander Technique is founded on three principles:

▶ The relationship between head, neck and spine is crucial to the body's ability to function optimally
▶ The organism functions as a whole
▶ Function is affected by use

The first principle, the idea of a "Primary Control" is central to the Technique and refers to the interrelation and harmonious working of the head, neck and back. The mind and body are seen as an integrated whole, the Technique works with both to address bad habits and achieve better posture and control. Although of Western origin there is overlap with some Eastern techniques, such as yoga and tai chi. For example in tai chi there is the idea of the suspended head-top, where back, neck and head are in alignment; in tai chi and yoga there is also the idea of the interrelatedness of mind and body or of posture and breathing. There are also similarities with other western methods including Feldenkrais, Rolfing and various forms of bodywork.

History

The technique is named after an Australian actor, Frederick Matthias Alexander (1869–1955) who developed it around 1900. Alexander suffered from recurrent loss of voice whilst performing. Through self-observation, he concluded that his vocal problems were due to the tense position in which he habitually held his head and neck. By correcting his posture, he was able to cure his vocal problems.

Possible Indications with Evidence

The Alexander Technique is purportedly useful for a number of musculo-skeletal problems, vocal problems, and mental problems such as anxiety and stress. There is limited evidence on its effectiveness. One small controlled trial found a significant effect on balance training in older adults [20]. A further uncontrolled trial with 7 patients found a significant improvement in depression and physical function in patients with Parkinson's disease [21]; the author of this, Stallibrass, is currently conducting a definitive trial. Another matched-control study [22] of 20 healthy subjects found a significant effect on respiratory function (lung capacity and peak expiratory flow rate) after a course of Alexander Technique training. A larger, uncontrolled study on 67 back-pain patients found a multi-disciplinary approach including Alexander Technique gave benefit lasting at least 6 months [23]. Although patients seemed to benefit, this was an uncontrolled study and it is difficult to identify the benefit of one therapy among the six interventions used.

Mechanism of Action

Alexander Technique is thought of as improving the efficiency of movement and posture, leading to reduction of muscular tension in the system and possibly improving circulation. There is some evidence for the benefit from employing the mind to reduce damaging habitual behaviour patterns [24].

A Typical Consultation

One-to-one sessions lasting 45–60 minutes, in a specially equipped studio with body-work table and mirror. Some teachers also work with groups. The Technique involves exercise and gentle hands-on guidance. Recommended number of treatments can be from 25–40, starting with two or three per week. The system requires daily practise away from the class.

Safety Issues

There are no reported major safety concerns with the technique.

Training of Practitioners

Typically, Alexander teachers will have completed a 3 year full-time study program at an accredited teacher training course involving 1500–1600 hours of instruction.

How to Identify Practitioners

Reputable practitioners should be members of one of the professional bodies. The main international bodies are the Society of Teachers of the Alexander Technique (STAT) and Alexander Technique International (ATI). In North America, teachers may be members of the North American Society of Teachers of the Alexander Technique (NASTAT) or the American Society of Teachers of the Alexander Technique (amSAT).

Aromatherapy

What is it?

Aromatherapy is the use of concentrated essential oils derived from the various parts of plants, flowers or trees, in a healing context. The commonest methods of therapeutic administration are inhalation and massage.

History

The use of essential oils has been an integral part of many healing traditions since ancient times, most notably the Ayurvedic tradition from India, Traditional Chinese Medicine and in Egypt and the Middle East. René-Maurice Gattefosse, a French Chemist working in the perfumery industry who became interested in the therapeutic use of oils from his own experiences, first coined the term "aromatherapy" in a paper written in 1928. The first book in English about aromatherapy, Robert Tisserand's "The Art of Aromatherapy" was published in 1977 [25] and sparked much of the current interest in the method.

Possible Indications with Evidence

Unfortunately there are many unsupported claims about aromatherapy based on anecdotal evidence [26, 27]. There is limited evidence however for an anxiolytic effect from aromatherapy. A systematic review found six controlled trials investigating aromatherapy in a variety of hospital settings [28]. Methodological quality varied (but was generally low), 5 were randomised (one partially randomised), only one was double-blinded. All but one study found a statistically significant difference on at least some measures from control. There is limited evidence for the use of tea-tree oil for some types of fungal infections; it is unclear whether this is symptomatic benefit or an anti-mycotic effect [26].

Mechanism of Action

It is possible that the smell from essential oils can directly stimulate the limbic system, the area of the brain that controls emotional response, motivation and non-verbal thought [29]. There is also some evidence that essential oils can be absorbed through the skin and have pharmacological effects [26].

A Typical Consultation

The first consultation will involve an in-depth interview about personal and medical history, followed by a treatment, that will last for 1–2 hours in total. Treatment will include a massage with a single or a blend of oils, always diluted with a carrier oil. Treatments repeated on perhaps a weekly or fortnightly basis. There is of course much scope for self-medication with aromatherapy.

Safety Issues

The likelihood of adverse reactions is low, although they have been reported and include allergic reactions, photosensitisation, nausea and headache [26]. There is the possibility of drug interaction; one reported case involving warfarin [26]. There are theoretical possibilities of interactions with other medications. Essential oils should always be applied diluted in a carrier oil, pregnancy, contagious disease, recent surgery or skin injury and local thrombophlebitis are contraindications.

Training of Practitioners

Current regulation of aromatherapy practitioners is poor [27]. The National Association for Holistic Aromatherapy (NAHA) requires at least 200 hours of training and practical tuition including modules in anatomy and physiology, with various assessments before graduation. Considerable numbers of nurses and other health professionals now use aromatherapy.

How to Identify Practitioners

Due to the unregulated nature of the profession it is difficult to recommend any particular school. As with other unregulated practitioners, health professionals should satisfy themselves that the practitioner is adequately trained, ethical and aware of the limits of her/his competence before referring or recommending patients.

Autogenic Training

What is it?

Autogenic training (literally "self origin", or training produced by oneself or through ones own resources) is a system of mental exercises designed to positively influence mental and physical function. It increases body awareness of changes occurring when we relax, and provides various techniques to cope with stress.

History

Developed in the early 20th century by the German psychiatrist and neurologist, Dr. Johannes H. Schultz (1884–1970), building on the work of his mentor Oskar Vogt. It was introduced to North America by the German physician Wolfgang Luthe, who emigrated to Montreal, Canada in the 1950's, and in the UK in the late 1970's by Dr. Malcolm Carruthers and psychotherapist Vera Diamond, who studied with Luthe.

Possible Indications with Evidence

There is evidence that autogenic training can help with hypertension [30], with four of the five trials reviewed having positive results, and anxiety [31], where seven out of the eight reviewed trials were positive; the methodological quality of all the reviewed studies however is low. Another review [32] as reported by Ernst [33] found a positive effect in hypertension, asthma, intestinal diseases, glaucoma and eczema.

Mechanism of Action

It is believed that the deep relaxation resulting from the training allows us to manually shift from the "fight and flight" response to the resting response with its accompanying benefits.

A Typical Consultation

Training is taught either individually or in small groups. Weekly sessions tend to last an hour or so and only require comfortable clothing, sitting or lying in a relaxed position. The system does require daily practise. A course of around eight sessions is normal, with a follow-up session to revise the technique perhaps two months following.

Safety Issues

Generally safe, not recommended for those with severe mental health problems. Recommended use alongside standard care, with careful monitoring of relevant condition (for example alteration of medication may be needed with hypertension).

Training of Practitioners

The techniques used in autogenic training are quite simple and in the public domain, so care must be taken in assessing a teachers credentials.

How to Identify Practitioners

Many practitioners are health care professionals, particularly in mental health, and integrate autogenic training into their practice. There is no regulation or restriction of who may practice. In some countries there are reputable professional associations, such as the British Autogenic Society.

Hypnotherapy

What is it?

Hypnotherapy is a method of inducing altered states of consciousness to bring about healing by suggestion. It is a blanket term and can involve many possible methods for inducing this state as well as therapeutic techniques. The altered state is seen as being similar to the trance-like states sometimes experienced between sleep and waking.

History

The Austrian physician, Franz Anton Mesmer (1734–1815), is considered the father of hypnosis. He developed the idea of "animal magnetism" (from his erroneous idea of controlling the magnetic flux in the body), whereby he induced a trance-like state in individuals. "Mesmerism" achieved widespread popularity in the late 18th and early 19th centuries, this was followed by disillusionment due to the many charlatans practising. The term hypnosis was coined in 1843 by the Scottish surgeon James Braid (1795–1860). Hypnosis has fallen in and out of favour; but there is significant current use by physicians, dentists and psychologists.

Possible Indications with Evidence

A meta analysis of 18 trials of hypnotherapy showed a significant analgesic effect [34]. There is also evidence for its role as an integral part of cognitive-behavioural psychotherapy for conditions such as anxiety, insomnia and hypertension [35]. Hypnotherapy may also be helpful in a range of conditions including asthma, preparation for surgery, dermatological conditions, irritable bowel syndrome, haemorrhagic disorders, nausea and vomiting in oncology [36]. It appears to be ineffective in smoking cessation [37].

Mechanism of Action

There is much debate over the mechanism of action of hypnotherapy. Some see it as allowing direct access to the unconscious mind, which will increase an individual's susceptibility to suggestion. It is possible however that hypnotherapy is nothing more than an advanced relaxation technique. There are observed physiological changes when in a hypnotic state, such as heart rate and digestive functioning, but it is unclear how these are triggered.

A Typical Consultation

A typical initial consultation may last an hour or more and may not involve hypnotherapy, as trust is an important factor to establish in the therapeutic relationship. As well as extensive history taking, a full explanation should be given of what the therapy will entail and what can reasonably be expected of it. Treatment of a dozen weekly sessions (of course depending on the condition being treated) is not uncommon, which may include training in self-hypnosis. Sometimes the therapy occurs in a group session.

Safety Issues

Generally safe in the hands of an experienced practitioner although recall of painful memories have been reported. It is contraindicated in severe mental health problems including psychosis and personality disorder.

Training of Practitioners

Accreditation and training standards of hypnotherapy practitioners vary widely, most practitioners are not members of health professions. However considerable numbers of doctors, clinical psychologists and dentist use hypnotherapy.

How to Identify Practitioners

It is safest to refer to practitioners who are registered health professionals with additional training in hypnosis. Before referring to a practitioner who is not an accredited health professional, health professionals should satisfy themselves that the practitioner is adequately trained, ethical and aware of the limits of her/his competence.

Massage

What is it?

The manipulation of soft tissue by a variety of techniques. It is sometimes used as a response to injury or imbalances in health to promote healing and sometimes simply to promote health and well-being. Massage is something that we are all familiar with, perhaps to the extent that it could be considered an instinctual reaction [26] to injury or anxiety.

History

Many types of massage are currently practised including (but not limited to) reflexology (massage of points on the feet that are believed to be linked to areas of the body); acupressure (massage involving the acupuncture points); shiatsu (a Japanese form of acupressure); connective tissue massage (where regions of the back are considered to be correspond to other parts of the body); and Swedish massage.

Swedish massage can be seen as the systematisation of Western traditions, developed in the mid-19th century by Per Henrik Ling. Ling believed in the stimulating effect of massage on circulation and other bodily processes. Swedish massage is a common form used today both in conventional practice (by physiotherapists) and other complementary practitioners.

Possible Indications with Evidence

Two reviews, assessing four controlled trials each, looked at abdominal massage for chronic constipation [38] and massage for treating lower back pain [39] and found some preliminary evidence in both cases. There is some evidence (although based on small, and in some cases uncontrolled studies) to suggest massage may be beneficial in treating anxiety in hospitalised or institutionalised patients [40–42]. A review of massage in the management of diabetes [43] found limited evidence of an effect of massage in insulin absorption, normalisation of blood glucose levels and relieving symptoms associated diabetic neuropathy.

Massage also may be useful in promoting psychological well-being in coronary artery bypass graft patients following surgery, based on the findings of a small, pragmatic controlled trial [44].

Mechanism of Action

Massage undoubtedly has physiological effects. There is good evidence that local and systemic effects on blood flow can occur from certain massage techniques, some evidence that lymph flow can be increased and it has also been found to reduce muscular tension in some cases [26].

A Typical Consultation

A medical history will be taken to establish possible contraindications followed by massage, which may include the use of essential oils in a relaxed atmosphere. The whole session typically lasts 30–60 minutes and depending on the area and type of massage is likely to involve the removal of at least some items of clothing.

Safety Issues

Serious adverse effects are unlikely. Possible contraindications include dermatological or musculoskeletal problems.

Training of Practitioners

Therapeutic massage is widely practised by health professionals, particularly physical therapists (physiotherapists) who integrate it into their normal practice.

How to Identify Practitioners

The most widely recognised qualifications are those awarded by the International Therapy Examinations Council (ITEC).

Conclusion

"Unconventional Western Medicine" refers to a diverse group of therapies, many of which share a commitment to holism and are vitalistic in philosophy. We have not attempted a comprehensive survey, but highlighted those which are supported by clinical trial evidence in conditions prevalent in the elderly. Adverse treatment reactions are particularly common in elderly patients, the therapies we have discussed are relatively safe and unlikely to cause adverse reactions. The holistic focus of many of these therapies means that they may improve general well-being and quality of life, in general these therapies are associated with good patient acceptance and compliance.

Specific indications particularly prevalent in older people in which various forms of unconventional Western Medicine may be helpful include a range of musculoskeletal, rheumatic and arthritic conditions, pain, anxiety, insomnia, depression, malignant disease and movement disorders.

In terms of research, although there is more evidence on these therapies than is often supposed, all of them need further research. There is little evidence specific to their use in older people. Vitalism, common to many of these therapies, is virtually a taboo subject in modern scientific discourse, associated with metaphysical and pre-scientific ideas. Yet at a minimum vitalism simply refers to the innate tendency of living organisms to self-heal and restore a dynamic equilibrium, a property almost so self-evident as to escape notice. Perhaps this is the reason why, although there is abundant research on the mechanisms involved: inflammation, immunity, homeostasis etc., very little research has been done on the broader pattern, the circumstances under which these mechanisms fail, and how they may be stimulated.

At the pragmatic level, one of the most difficult problems for health professionals wishing to refer for CAM treatments, or to train themselves, is to identify reputable practitioners and training programs. Regulation and accreditation vary widely between jurisdictions. The safest course is to refer to licensed or accredited health professionals, but this may not always be possible. If it is not possible, health professionals should remember that they are liable for the advice they give as well as the treatments they prescribe. They should satisfy themselves that any practitioner whom they recommend, or to whom they refer, is adequately trained, ethical and aware of the limits of his or her competence. If in doubt, health professionals should review patients at intervals while they are receiving treatment from a CAM practitioner who is not officially accredited.

References

1. Bellavite P, Signorini A (1995) Homeopathy: A Frontier in Medical Science. Berkeley, North Atlantic Books.
2. Milgrom LR (2002) Vitalism, complexity and the concept of spin. Homeopathy 91: 26–31.
3. Kleijnen J, Knipschild P, ter Reit G (1991) Clinical trials of homeopathy. British Medical Journal 302: 316–323.
4. Linde K, Clausius N, Ramirez G, et al. (1997) Are the clinical effects of homeopathy placebo effects? A meta-analysis of placebo-controlled trials. Lancet 350: 834–843.
5. Cucherat M, Haugh MC, Gooch M, Boissel JP (2000) Evidence of clinical efficacy of homeopathy. A meta-analysis of clinical trials. European Journal of Clinical Pharmacology 56:27–33.
6. Long L, Ernst E (2001) Homeopathic remedies in the treatment of osteoarthritis: a systematic review. British Homeopathic Journal 90: 37–43.
7. Van Haselen R, Fisher P (2000) A randomised controlled trial comparing topical Piroxicam gel with a homeopathic gel in osteoarthritis of the knee. Rheumatology 39:714–719
8. Vickers AJ, Smith C (2002) Homoeopathic Oscillococcinum for preventing and treating influenza and influenza-like syndromes (Cochrane Review). In: The Cochrane Library, Issue 1, 2002. Oxford: Update Software.
9. Ernst E, Saradeth T, Resch KL (1990) Complementary treatment of varicose veins – a randomized; placebo-controlled; double-blind trial. Phlebology 5(3);157–163.
10. Taylor M, Reilly D, Llewellyn-Jones RH, McSharry C, Aitchison TC (2000) Randomised controlled trial of homoeopathy versus placebo in perennial allergic rhinitis with overview of four trial series. British Medical Journal 321: 471–476.
11. Schulte J (1999) Effects of potentization in aqueous solutions. British Homeopathic Journal 88:155–160.
12. Dantas F, Rampes H (1999) Do homoeopathic medicines provoke adverse effects? Conference proceedings: Improving the success of homoeopathy. Royal London Homoeopathic Hospital, pp 70–74.
13. Muller H, de Toledo FW, Resch KL (2001) Fasting followed by vegetarian diet in patients with rheumatoid arthritis: a systematic review. Scandinavian Journal of Rheumatology 30:1–10.
14. McAlindon TE, LaValley MP, Gulin JP, Felson DT (2000) Glucosamine and chondroitin for treatment of osteoarthritis: a systematic quality assessment and meta-analysis. JAMA 283:1469–75.
15. Ernst E, Pittler MH (1999) Ginkgo biloba for dementia: A systematic review of double blind, placebo-controlled trials. Clin Drug Invest. 17(4): 301–308.
16. Pittler MH. Ernst E (2000) Ginkgo biloba extract for the treatment of intermittent claudication: a meta-analysis of randomized trials. American J Medicine 108:276–8.
17. Verhagen AP. de Vet HC. de Bie RA. Kessels AG. Boers M. Knipschild PG (2000) Balneotherapy for rheumatoid arthritis and osteoarthritis. Cochrane Database of Systematic Reviews, Issue 2.
18. Kleijnen J, Knipschild P (1994) Mistletoe treatment for cancer: review of controlled trials in humans. Phytomedicine 1:255–260.
19. Iscador Prescribing Guidance (2001). Weleda (UK), Ilkeston.
20. Dennis RJ (1999) Functional Reach Improvement in Normal Older Women After Alexander Technique Instruction. Journal of Gerontology: Medical Sciences 54(1): M8-M11.
21. Stallibrass C (1997) An Evaluation of the Alexander Technique for the Management of Disability in Parkinson's Disease – a Preliminary Study. Clinical Rehabilitation 11: 7–12.
22. Austin JHM, Ausubel P (1992) Enhanced Respiratory Muscular Function in Normal Adults after Lessons in Proprioceptive Musculoskeletal Education without Exercises. Chest 102: 486–490.
23. Elkayam O, Ben Itzhak S, Avrahami E, et al. (1996) Multidisciplinary approach to chronic back pain: prognostic elements of the outcome. Clinical & Experimental Rheumatology 14(3):281–8.
24. Alexander Technique (2001) in: Ernst E, Pittler M, Stevinson C, White A. The Desktop Guide to Complementary and Alternative Medicine: an Evidence-Based Approach, London. Pp31–33.
25. Tisserand R (1977) The Art of Aromatherapy. C.W. Daniel, Saffron Walden.
26. Vickers A (1996) Massage and Aromatherapy: A Guide for Health Professionals. Chapman and Hall, London.
27. Barrett S (2001) Aromatherapy: Making Dollars out of Scents. (http://www.quackwatch.com/01Quackery RelatedTopics/aroma.html)
28. Cooke B, Ernst E (2000) Aromatherapy: a systematic review. British Journal of General Practice 50: 493–496.

29. Van Toller S (1996) Introduction to the sense of smell. In: Vickers A, Massage and Aromatherapy: A Guide for Health Professionals. Chapman and Hall, London.
30. Kanji N, White A R, Ernst E (1999) Anti-hypertensive effects of Autogenic Training: A systematic review. Perfusion 12: 279–282.
31. Kanji N, Ernst E (2000) Autogenic Training for Stress and Anxiety: a systematic review. Complementary Therapies in Medicine 8: 106–110.
32. Stetter F, Kupper S (1998) Autogenic Training – Qualitative Meta-Analysis of Controlled Clinical Studies and Relation to Naturopathy [German]. Forschende Komplementärmedizin 5: 211–223.
33. Autogenic Training (2001) in: Ernst E, Pittler M, Stevinson C, White A. The Desktop Guide to Complementary and Alternative Medicine: an Evidence-Based Approach, London. pp35–38.
34. Montgomery GH, Du Hamel KN, Redd WH (2000) A meta-analysis of hypnotically induced analgesia: how effective is hypnosis? International Journal of Clinical and Experimental Hypnotherapy 48: 138–153.
35. Kirsch I, Mongomery G, Sapirstein G (1995) Hypnosis as an adjunct to cognitive-behavioural psychotherapy: a meta-analysis. J Consult Clin Psychol 63: 214–220.
36. Pinnell CM. Covino NA (2000) Empirical findings on the use of hypnosis in medicine: a critical review. International Journal of Clinical & Experimental Hypnosis 48:170–94.
37. Abbot NC, Stead LF, White AR, Barnes J, Ernst E (1999) Hypnotherapy for smoking cessation (Cochrane Review). In Cochrane Library, Oxford Update Software.
38. Ernst E (1999) Abdominal massage therapy for chronic constipation: a systematic review of controlled clinical trials. Forsch Komplementärmed 6: 149–151.
39. Ernst E (1999) Massage therapy for low back pain: a systematic review. Journal of Pain Symptoms and Management 17: 65–69.
40. Fraser J, Kerr JR (1993) Psychophysiological effects of back massage on elderly institutionalised patients. Journal of Advanced Nursing 18(20): 238–245.
41. Sims S (1986) Slow stroke back massage for cancer patients. Nurse Times 82(13): 47–50.
42. Ferrell-Torry AT, Glick OJ (1993) The use of therapeutic massage as a nursing intervention to modify anxiety and the perception of cancer pain. Cancer Nursing 16(2): 93–101.
43. Ezzo J, Donner T, Nickols D, Cox M (2001) Is massage useful in the management of diabetes? A systematic review. Diabetes Spectrum 14(4): 218–224.
44. Hattan J, King L, Griffiths P (2002) The impact of foot massage and guided relaxation following cardiac surgery: a randomized controlled trial. Journal Of Advanced Nursing 37 (2): 199–207.

12 The Use of Traditional Japanese and Chinese Medicine for the Elderly

K. Miyamoto
With a Preface by E.P. Cherniack

Preface

Traditional Chinese medicine (TCM) and traditional Japanese or "Kampo" medicine (TJM), unlike many other forms of complementary and alternative medicine (CAM), have a literature of use to treat disorders of aging. However, as with virtually all other forms of CAM, there is a exceedingly small number of investigations many of which have major methodological flaws, preventing one from drawing firm conclusions about any of their benefits. Virtually all of the studies were performed in the Far East. We will narrow the focus of the discussion to medications used in TCM and TJM and exclude the use of acupuncture, which is discussed in another chapter.

Some of these substances have been used to retard the aging process itself. In a controlled trial, close to 350 old rats were divided into two groups, one a control, and the other a group to which a Kampo compound of eight herbs, *Hachimi-jio-gan* was added to food [1]. The rats fed the supplement had a greater spontaneous rate of wheel turning in their cages and had a higher angle of posture than control rats.

Another compound used in treatment of circulatory disorders, *bi-zhong-yi-qi-tang* (BZYQT), was tested on cognition in normal and senescence-accelerated mice (SAM) [2]. There was dose-dependent improvement in memory in both strains, and augmentation of motor coordination and performance in the SAM mice, with elevated dopamine and noradrenaline levels of the cortex observed at higher doses of BZYQT.

TJ-960, another Kampo medication, and a placebo were given to different groups of young and aged SAM mice for five months [3]. Young mice given TJ-960 had greater levels of nitric oxide synthetase (NOS) than those given a placebo, but old mice given had lower NOS levels than placebo. The authors speculated that aging is accompanied by increased NOS levels, which might be ameliorated through TJ-960 administration.

The Japanese herbal compound *kami-untan-to* (KUT) and a control substance were given to aged mice for three months [4]. The KUT-treated mice had an increased survival, higher levels of acetylcholine and a higher density of choline acetyltransferase-reactive neurons of the brain in the medial septum, vertical limbs of the diagonal band of Broca, and the nucleus basalis Meynert. The augmentation of the acetylcholenergic system might imply potential for the medication in the treatment of Alzheimer's disease.

There have been clinical trials of Chinese medications. A Chinese memory-enhancing medicine, *NaO Li Su*, (a combination of bee pollen, radix polygoni multiflore, semen ziziphi spinosae, radix salviae multiorhize, fructus schisandrae, and fructus ligustris lucidae), was given to 100 elderly subjects in Denmark with complaints of memory disorders in a double-blind placebo controlled trial for three months [5]. Unfortunately, cognitive improvement was not found.

Another substance, the *da huang* (radix et rhizoma rhei) was noted to improve memory in a trial in China [6]. Another chinese medication increased Folstein Mini-Mental Status exam scores in a small unblinded uncontrolled trial of ten Alzheimer's Disease patients over three months [7]. The substance *banxia houpo tang* (BHT, or *hange koboku-to* in Japanese) was studied as an enhancer of the swallowing reflex in thirty-two elderly patients with a history of aspiration pneumonia in a placebo-controlled trial of one month [8]. There was a significant improvement in the reflex as measured by latency time of response in the intervention group. The latency time in the treated group was reduced by more than seventy percent.

Acupressure was investigated as a treatment for sleep disorders in a randomized placebo-controlled trial in eighty-four subjects [9]. Acupressure proved superior to a sham procedure in several parameters of sleep quality.

One of the best-known compound derived from Chinese herbs and extract is PC-SPES, which contains a combination of eight herbs (ginseng, saw palmetto, chrysanthemum, rabdosia, dyers woad, baikal skullcap, licorice, *reishi,* and *san-qi*) [10] and has been used as a treatment for prostate cancer. Its effect may be due its estrogenic activity [11].

While there have been reports of its improvement in measurements of chemical markers of prostate cancer, most of the trials of its use have been rather small [12]. PC-has produced dose-dependent tumor inhibition in studies on rats [13]. Eighty to one-hundred percent of patients with androgen-independent prostate cancer [10, 11] and forty percent of patients with androgen-independent cancer [14] in small retrospective surveys had a decline in PSA. In a prospective trial of seventy patients, fifty-four percent had a fifty percent decline in PSA, which was maintained for an average of sixteen weeks [15]. Slightly more than half of the patients in this investigation had androgen-dependent prostate cancer, and, of these, all experienced at least an eighty percent decline in PSA, which was maintained for an average of more than a year. Slightly less than ten percent had either allergic reactions or thromboembolic events. In a small study of subjects with advanced metastatic disease, there was significant improvement in pain, quality of life scales, and PSA [16]. There have been case reports of large increases in PSA after discontinuation of PC-SPES [17], disseminated intravascular coagulation [18], and pulmonary embolus [19].

There have been many trials of TCM and TJM to treat other illnesses not specific to age, some of which may be relevant to the elderly. A complete discussion of these trials is beyond the scope of this brief introduction to the topic. However the studied medications include: *fei xin ling* syrup for cor pulmonale [20], TJ-108 (a ginseng compound) for Hepatitis C [21], TJ-43 for ulcers in rats [22], *niaodujing*(NDJ) in 105 patients with chronic renal failure [23], *wen-pi-tang* for renal failure [24] another Chinese compound in the treatment of more than two hundred case of gastric carcinoma [25], *oren-gedoku-to* in colon cancer prevention in rats [26], *juzen-taiho* as an adjuvant to interferon-alpha in the treatment of lung metastates of renal cell carcinoma [27], *shi-quan-da-bu-tang* in immune function in mice [28], *daio-kanzo-to* on the inhibition of cholera toxin *in vitro* [29], *ganlingsan* liquid for chronic osteomyelitis in 300 patients [30], J-41 for herpes simplex-1 infection in mice [31], TJ-135 in experimentally-induced hepatitis in mice [32], TW-001 for seizures in rats [33], TJ-24 in anti-psychotic induced parkinsonism [34], *tone luo kai bi* in 180 patients in a randomized double-blind placebo controlled trial for rheumatoid arthritis [35], *shenqi fuzheng* as a chemo-therapy adjuvant in gastrointestinal tumors in almost 200 patients [36] and *bimikang* for allergic rhinitis [37].

There have been a number of *in vitro* studies of the medicinal properties of TCM and TJM substances. *Guan-mai-shu* inhibited tissue-type plasminogen activator [38], *megusurino-ki* causes tumor necrosis factor alpha release [39], *hong bei si chou* inhibited endothelin [40], *juzen-taiho-to* stimulated hematopoietic stem cells [41], and *sho-saiko-to* was immune-enhancing [42].

Many TCM or TJM medications have been known to interact with conventional medications, laboratory tests, or cause adverse reactions. While these will be discussed in greater detail in the chapter on adverse reactions of CAM, among these that have noted in the past decade include: alteration of digoxin [43] and warfarin [44] levels by *dan shen*, and causation of lung fibroblast apoptosis and interstitial pneumonia by *shosaiko-to* [45].

There have been several investigations about how patients choose between TCM/TJM and conventional medications. In the late 1980s, an epidemiologic survey of thirteen teaching hospitals in Taiwan observed that two-thirds of patients visited CAM clinics and one-third TCM clinics [46, 47]. Correlates of TCM use were place of birth, occupation, religion, overall health, severity of acute illness, and etiology of illness. Businessmen and farmers, practitioners of folk-religion, and patients with musculosketal, sensory organ, and skin diseases were more likely to use TCM. Lam interviewed residents of Hong Kong and was told that they view conventional medications as providing an immediate, but sometimes too strong a relief, and TCM as offering a slower treatment, but one that will address the cause of the disorder [48]. Forty-three percent of first and second generation Chinese immigrants seen in an US emergency room used TCM [49]. Among patients visiting practitioners in Canada, twenty-eight percent reported current use of TCM herbal medicines, most commonly for infections, rheumatologic and respiratory disorders [59].

References

1. Ninomiya H, Kato S, Okuda H (2001) Effects of hachimi-jio-gan in aged rats. Journal of Alternative and Complementary Medicine 7(4): 355–359.
2. Shih H, Chang K, Chen F et al. (2000) Anti-aging effects of the traditional Chinese medicine bu-zhong-yi-qi-tang in mice. American Journal of Chinese Medicine 28(1): 77–86.
3. Inada K, Yokoi I, Kabuto H et al. (1996) Age-related increase in nitric oxide synthetase activity in senescence accelerated mouse brain and the effect of long-term administration of superoxide radical scavenger. Mechanisms of Ageing and Development 89(2): 95–102.
4. Wang Q, Iwasaki K, Suzuki T et al. (2000) Potentiation of brain acetylcholine neurons by kami-untan-to (KUT) in aged mice: implications for a possible antidementia drug. Phytomedicine 7(4): 253–258.
5. Iversen T, Fiirgaard K, Schriver P et al. (1997) The effect of Nao LiSu on memory functions and blood chemistry in elderly people. Journal of Ethnopharmacology 56(2): 109–116.
6. Tian J, Du H, Yang H et al. (1997) A clinical study on compound da huang (radix et rhizoma rhei) preparations for improvement of senile persons' memory ability. Journal of Traditional Chnese Medicine 17(3): 168–173.
7. Oishi M, Mochizuki Y, Takasu T et al. (1998) Effectiveness of traditional Chinese medicine in Alzheimer disease. Alzheimer's Disease and Associated Disorders 12(3): 247–250.
8. Iwasaki K, Wang Q, Nakagawa T et al. (1999) The traditional Chinese medicine banxia houpo tang improves swallowing reflex. Phytomedicine 6(2): 103–106.
9. Chen M, Lin L, Wu S (1999) The effectiveness of acupressure in improving the quality of sleep in institutionalized patients. Journal of Gerontology A: Biological Sciences and Medical Sciences 54(8): M389–394.
10. Porterfield H (2000) UsToo PC-SPES surveys: review of studies and update of previous survey results. Molecular Urology 4(3): 289–291.

11. DiPaola R, Zhang H, Labert G et al. (1998) Clinical and biological activity of an estrogenic herbal combination (PC-SPES) in prostate cancer. New England Journal of Medicine 339(12): 785–791.
12. de lat Taille (2001) PC SPES in prostate cancer: a critical review of the literature. Progress in Urology 11(3): 428–432.
13. Tiwari R, Geliebter J, Garikapaty V et al. (1999) Anti-tumor effects of PC SPES, an herbal formulation in prostate cancer. International Journal of Oncology 14(4): 713–719.
14. Oh W, George D, Hackmann K et al. (2001) Activity of the herbal combination, PC-SPES, in the treatment of patients with androgen-independent prostate cancer. Urology 57(1): 122–126.
15. Small E, Frohlich M, Bok R et al. (2000) Prospective trial of the herbal supplement PC-SPES in patients with progressive prostate cancer. Journal of Clinical Oncology 18(21): 3595–3603.
16. Pfeifer B, Pirani J, Hamann S et al. (2000) PC-SPES, a dietary supplement for the treatment of hormone-refractory prostate cancer. British Journal of Urology International 85(4): 481–485.
17. Oh W, George D, Kantoff P (2002) Rapid rise of serum prostate specific antigen levels after discontinuation of the herbal therapy PC-SPES in patients with advanced prostate cancer. Cancer 94(3): 686–689.
18. Lock M, Loblaw D, Choo R et al. (2001) Disseminated intravascular coagulation and PC-SPES: a case report and literature review. Canadian Journal of Urology 8(4):1326–1329.
19. Schiff J, Ziecheck W, Choi B (2002) Pulmonary embolus related to PC-SPES use in a patient with PSA recurrence after radical prostatectomy. Urology 59(3): 444.
20. Liu W, Yang R (1997) Treatment of acute exacerbation of chronic cor pulmonale with fei xin ling syrup. Journal of Traditional Chinese Medicine 17(1): 21–25.
21. Cyong J, Ki S, Iijima K et al. (2000) Clincal and pharmacological studies on liver diseases treated with Kampo herbal medicine. American Journal of Chinese Medicine 28(3–4): 351–360.
22. Arakawa T, Higuchi K, Fujiwara Y et al. (1999) Gastroprotection by liu-jun-zi-tang (TJ-43): possible mediation of nitric oxide but not prostaglandins or sulfhydryls. Drugs Under Experimental and Clinical Research 25(5): 207–210.
23. Wang Y, Xu L, Cheng X (1996) Clinical study on niaodujing in treating chronic renal failure. Zhongguo Zhong XI Yi Jie He Za Zhi 16(11): 649–651.
24. Mitsuma T, Yokozawa Y, Oura H (1999) Clinical evaluation of kampo medication, mainly with wen-pi-tang, on the progression of chronic renal failure. 41(8): 769–777.
25. Lin C, Zhu X, Chai Z (1995) The treatment of gastric carcinoma in III stage. Zhongua Wai Ke Za Zhi 33(9): 548–550.
26. Fukutake M, Miura N, Yammamoto M et al. (2000) Suppressive effect of the herbal medicine oren-gedoku-to on cyclooxygenase-2 activity and azomethane-induced aberrant crypt foci development in rats. Cancer Letters 157(1): 9–14.
27. Muraishi Y, Mitani N, Yamaura T et al. (2000) Effect of interferon-alpha A/D in combination with the Japanese and Chinese traditional herbal medicine juzen-taiho-to on lung metastates of murine renal cell carcinoma. Anticancer Research 20(5A): 2931–2937.
28. Wu Y, Zhang Y, Wu et al. (1998) Effects of erkang, a modified formulation of Chinese folk medicine shi-quan-da-bu-tang on mice. Journal of Ethnopharmacology 61(2): 153–159.
29. Oi H, Matsuura D, Miyake M et al. (2002) Identification in traditional herbal medications and confirmation by synthesis of factors that inhibit cholera toxin-induced fluid accumulation. Proceedings of the National Academy of Sciences 99(5): 3042–3046.
30. Guo Z, Dong F, Chen (1999) 311 cases o chronic osteomyelitis treated by soaking with ganlingsan liquid. Journal of Traditional Chinese Medicine 19(2): 100–104.
31. Kido T, Mori K, Daikuhara H et al. (2000) The protective effect of hochu-ekki-to (TJ-41), a Japanese herbal medicine, against HSV-1 infection in mitomycin C-treated mice. Anticancer Research 20(6A): 4109–4113.
32. Yamashiki M, Mase A, Arai I et al. (2000) Effects of the Japanese herbal medicine "Inchinko-to" (TJ-135) on concavalin A-induced hepatitis in mice. Clinical Science 99(5): 421–431.
33. Wu H, Huang C, Li L et al. The Chinese herbal medicine Chai-Hu-Long-Ku-Mu-Li-Tan (TW-001) exerts anticonvulsant effects against different experimental models of seizure in rats. Japanese Journal of Pharmacology 82(3): 247–260.
34. Ishikawa T, Funahashi T, Kudo J (2000) Effectiveness of the Kampo kami-shoyo-san (TJ-24) for tremor of antipsychotic-induced parkinsonism. Psychiatry and Clinical Neuroscience. 54(5): 579–582.
35. Shi Y, Zhang H, Du X et al. (1999) A double blind observation for the therapeutic effects of tong luo kai bi tablets on rheumatoid arthritis. Journal of Traditional Chinese Medicine 19(3): 166–172.
36. Xin M, Wang J, Zhou C (1998) Clinical study on Shenqi Fuzheng injection combined with chemotherapy in treating malignant tumor of the digestive tract. Zhongguo Zhong Xi Yi Jie He Za Zhi 18(11): 658–661.
37. Bao L, Sun Q, Hu L (1997) Clinical and experimental study for allergic rhinits with treatment of bimikang mixture. Zhongguo Zhong Xi Yi Jie He Za Zhi 17(2): 70–72.
38. Xiong X, Mo S (1993) Effects of guan-mai-shu on tissue-type plasmniogen activator inhibitor in the plasma of patients with coronary heart disease. Zhongguo Zhong Xi Yi Jie He Za Zhi 13(12): 708–709, 727–729.
39. Okabe S. Suganuma M, Imayoshi Y et al. (2001) New TNF-alpha releasing inhibitors, geraniin and corilagin, in leaves of Acer nikoense, Megusurino-ki. Biological Pharmacology Bulletin 24(10): 1145–1148.

40. Yang L, Wang F, Liu M (1998) A study of an endothelin antagonist from a Chinese anti-snake venom medicinal herb. Journal of Cardiovascular Pharmacology 31(suppl 1): S249–250.
41. Hisha H, Yamada H, Sakurai M et al. (1997) Isolation and identification of hematopoietic stem cell-stimulating substances from Kampo (Japanese herbal) medicine, Juzen-taiho-to. Blood 90(3): 1002–1030.
42. Borchers A, Sakai S, Henderson G et al. (2000) Shosaiko-to and other Kampo (Japanese herbal) medicines: a review of their immunomodulatory activities. Journal of Ethnopharmacology 73(1–2): 1–13.
43. Wahed A, Dasgupta A (2001) Positive and negative in vitro interference of Chinese medicine dan shen in serum digoxin measurement. Elimination of interference by monitoring free digoxin concentration. American Journal of Clinical Pathology 116(3): 403–408.
44. Yu C, Chan J, Sanderson J (1997) Chinese herbs and warfarin potentiation by 'danshen'. Journal of Internal Medicine 241(4): 337–339.
45. Liu Z, Tanaka S, Horigome H et al. (2002) Induction of apoptosis in human lung fibroblast in vitro by shosaiko-to derived phenolic metabolites. Biological Pharmacology Bulletin 25(1): 37–41.
46. Kang J, Chen C, Chou P (1996) Factors related to the choice between traditional Chinese medicine and modern Western medicine among patients with two-method treatment. Zhonghua Yi Xue Za Zhi 57(6): 405–412.
47. Kang J, Lee C, Chen C et al. (1994) Factors related to the choice of clinic between Chinese traditional medicine and Western medicine. Journal of the Formosan Medical Association 93(suppl 1): S49–55.
48. Lam T (2001) Strengths and weakness of traditional Chinese medicine and Western medicine in the eyes of some Hong Kong Chinese. Journal of Epidemiology and Community Health 55(10):762–765.
49. Pearl W, Leo P, Tsang W (1995) Use of Chinese therapies among Chinese patients seeking emergency department care. Annals of Emergency Medicine 26(6): 735–738.
50. Wong L, Jue P, Lam A et al. (1998) Chinese herbal medicine and acupuncture. How do patients who consult family physicians use these therapies? Canadian Family Physician 44: 1009–1015.

Traditional Japanese and Chinese Medicine for the Elderly

In Asia, there are a lot of systematic traditional medicines, such as traditional Chinese medicine (TCM) in China, traditional Japanese medicine (TJM or Kampo medicine) in Japan, traditional Korean medicine (TKM) in Korea, and traditional Ayurvedic medicine in India. In this chapter, TCM and TJM will be mainly focused on according to the author's practical experiences with TJM, which is originally based on TCM.

For the basic understanding of TCM/TJM, readers need some knowledge about the system of TCM/TJM including its history. Acupuncture is also a very important method in TCM/TJM. However, due to the limitation of space for this chapter, the author can only introduce the minimum basic information of the system in TCM/TJM by explaining classic theories and concepts as simply and comprehensively as possible.

For further information on TCM/TJM, see the references cited in the last part.

TCM and TJM

Origins of TCM and its Development in China

The origin of TCM has not yet been clarified, but there have been some legendary masters such as Bian-Que, Shen-Nong or Huang-Di in ancient China approximately four to five thousands years ago. Living in an age when there were no scientific devices, they observed human body carefully, using their five senses. They travelled all over, and collected and tried every plant, animal, and mineral which might be useful as medicine. Due to their numerous experiences and efforts, medical knowledge had been accumulated.

Some aspects of early medical practice in China are described in "the Historical Memoirs" (Shi Ji), which is the first book in a series of dynastic records written about 2,500 years ago. In this book, various forms of diagnostic procedures, such as pulse examination, inspection of the tongue, and history-taking methods are described. Moreover, the therapeutic modalities of acupuncture, moxibustion, massage, remedial exercise and the use of plant medicines are also discussed.

The earliest extant text on medicine is "the Yellow Emperor's Inner Classic" (Huang Di Nei Jing) which was completed in the later era of the Warring States period (475–221 B.C.), based on the natural philosophy including the "*Yin-Yang*" theory and the "Five Element" doctrines. Numerous topics, including the explanation of disease, the physiology and pathology of the internal organs, and anatomy are covered in this book. The Inner Classic is still highly regarded as an important classic textbook and is being studied in all the colleges that teach traditional Chinese medicine in China today.

In the Han dynasty (206 B.C.–220 A.D.) era, subsequent important medical classics were published. The first is "Shen Nong's Materia Medica" (Shen Nong Ben Cao Jing) which records 365 different types of medicinal substances of plant, animal and mineral nature, noting their properties and effects. The second is "the Classic of Difficult Issues" (Nan Jing) which elaborated and clarified the theories of the Inner Classic, especially the discussions and uses of Five Element doctrine, and the use of the wrist pulse for diagnosis. The third is "the Discussion of Cold Induced Disorders" (Shan Han Za Bin Lung) which classified the stages of infectious and febrile diseases into six categories, and summarizes the treatments in each stage, listing 370 prescriptions.

"The Discussion of Cold Induced Disorders" was later separated into two books; one is "Shan Han Lung" which deals about acute disorders, and the other is "Jingui Yaolue" dealing with chronic disorders respectively. These two classic manuals for treating diseases are now also highly regarded as important textbooks both in China and in Japan. Based on "the Yellow Emperor's Inner Classic" and "the Discussion of Cold Induced Disorders", TCM was systematically completed and developed afterwards.

The golden age of Chinese medicine occurred between the 4th and 10th centuries, when public apothecaries and hospitals were founded, an official pharmacopeia was composed, foreign ideas studied, new methods developed, and new treatises written.

In the Jin dynasty and Yuan dynasty (960–1367 A.D.), four great masters, Liu Hejian, Zhang Zi-he, Li Dong-yuan and Zhu Dan-xi, developed new additional theories. Further, in the Ming dynasty (1540 A.D.–), Li Shi-zhen, who traveled everywhere to find medicinal herbs and to study about their growth, wrote a book "Ben Cao Gang Mu", a book in 52 volumes on the natural medicines including 1892 "Yao" (medicinal plants, animals and minerals) and is considered as the most complete book on Chinese medicinal products.

In Qing dynasty (1636 A.D.–), the "epidemic febrile disease theory" developed by Ye Tian-shi added more medications and a wider variety of ways to treat diseases. In the later period of Qing Dynasty, western medicine was imported into China and influenced TCM. Integrative medicine in recent China combines western and Chinese medicine partial collaboration, but TCM still exists.

Importation of TCM and Development in Japan as TJM

In Japan, the first importation of oriental medicine was from Korea at 414 A.D., though it was also influenced by Chinese medicine. Afterwards, Chinese medicine was directly imported between the 7th and 10th century. However, it was used only by aristocrats, not the general public. Sanki Tashiro (1465–1537 A.D.), the founder of TJM, brought TCM into Japan after 12 years of studying abroad in China during the Ming dynasty. His apprentice, Dosan Manase, developed TCM and established the *Gosei-ha Kampo* school based on *Jin* and *Yuan* TCM. *Gosei-ha Kampo* medicine had long been the mainstream of Japanese traditional medicine (TJM), usually called as Kampo medicine. However, Gen-i Nagoya (1638–1696 A.D.) criticized *Gosei-ha* medicine since it was too idealistic and theoretical. Nagoya and his colleague established *Koho-ha Kampo* medicine, which put a greater importance on TCM classics, like *Shan Han Lung*. After Todo Yoshimasu (1702–1773 A.D.) published two important textbooks, *Ruijuhou* (practical manual based on *Shan Han Lung*) and *Yakucho* (Planta Medica), their *Koho-ha Kampo* medicine became more and more accepted in Japan to the present day. Since TJM, Kampo medicine, has developed on the basis of TCM, it is very similar to TCM but different in some respects, especially in the abdominal examination designed originally by Yoshimasu. The abdominal examination is more important in Japan than in China.

Kampo medicine had also been influenced by the western medicine, and there once was a crisis about the abolition of Kampo medicine by the government in the beginning of 20th century. However, the merits of the natural materials are now being recognized once again, and Kampo medicine has survived. Kampo medicine and Kampo extract formulas had been officially approved in 1976 by the Japanese health insurance system, and they have taken a firm hold on the Japanese medical healthcare. Additionally, the recent progress in the scientific research on Kampo medicine has further confirmed that TCM and TJM will become more important in the 21st century.

Yin-Yang Theory, Five Elements, the Essential Substances and Six Stages

Yin-Yang Theory. All phenomena which occur around the world or in the entire universe consists of two innate opposing aspects. These opposing aspects are called *Yin* and *Yang*, corresponding to "negative" and "positive" respectively. Yin-Yang has its roots in ancient Chinese cosmology. The meaning of *Yin* and *Yang* originally comes from the dark side and the bright side of the mountains, or its contrasting shaded and sunlit slopes. The "*Yin*" also represents the female or the shaded aspect, the earth, darkness, the moon, and passivity. The "*Yang*", in contrast, represents the male, light, sun, heaven, and the active principle in nature. A simple comparison between *Yin* and *Yang* patterns is listed below (Table 12.1).

Table 12.1. Set of Yin and Yang patterns

	Cosmos				Temperature	Sex	Activity	
		Light						
Yang	Heaven	Sun	Day	Light	Heat	Male	Exterior	Active
Yin	Earth	Moon	Night	Shade	Cold	Female	Interior	Inactive

Table 12.2. *Ba gang* (four paired opposing factors)

Yin	Cold	Interior (deep)	Deficiency (weak)
Yang	Heat	Exterior (superficial)	Excess (strong)

In the study of TCM/TJM, the concept of *Yin* and *Yang* is indispensable. Even a disease itself is expressed as a *Yang* or a *Yin* (will be described later). The important opposing concepts corresponding *Yin* and *Yang* in TCM/TJM are the followings (Table 12.2). These four paired factors are called "eight principles" (*Ba gang* in Chinese).

When a person is regarded as "inclining to the *yang* state," the following symptoms occur: heat, fever, restlessness, hyperactivity, and exaltation. On the other hand, when "inclining to the *yin* state," the following symptoms occur: cold, inactivity, and lethargy.

To put in another way, *Yin* and *Yang* comprise all the body substances, including blood and metabolic energy. In other words, *Yin* and *Yang* can be described as "water" and "fire" respectively. Since the balance inside the human body is kept stable by the *Yin/Yang* balance, the principle in treating diseases can be simply described as the harmonization of *Yin* and *Yang*.

Body fluids and blood circulate inside the body, transferring metabolic products and producing energy, which is described in TCM/TJM as *Yin* producing *Yang*. Conversely, energy produces heat (fire) and many metabolic products, including blood and metabolic water, i.e., *Yang* producing *Yin*. Accordingly, *Yin* and *Yang* nurture each other and between *Yin* and *Yang* there exists a transformative potential. This relationship between *Yin* and *Yang* is well illustrated by a traditional diagram (Fig. 12.1).

The universe is symbolically composed of the primal forces of *Yin* and *Yang*, represented as black and white. However, each half contains a reverse colored spot, indicating that there are no absolutes. *Yin* and *Yang* form a unified circular whole, showing that both forces only exist in relation to each other. They are mutually interdependent

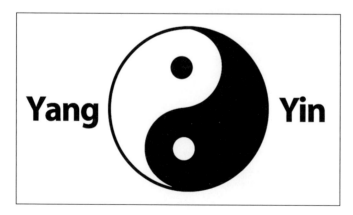

Figure 12.1. Diagram of Yin Yang

Table 12.3. Five Elements theory

Substance	Attribute
Wood	The process of germination and a tendency to spread outward
Fire	An emblem for heat and growth with an impulse for flaring upwards
Earth	Transformation and nourishment with a tendency towards containment
Metal	The maturing process and a concentrating influence
Water	Coolness, decay, transmutation, and storage, with a downward, flowing motion

partners, therefore one cannot exist without the other. The symbol also shows the tendency of *Yin* and *Yang* towards balance, for their overall appearance is one of equal strength.

Five Elements. In addition to *Yin-Yang* theory, the Five Elements theory is also an important system in TCM/TJM. The five substances: wood, fire, earth, metal, and water specifically symbolize the fundamental qualities and behavioral patterns intrinsic to the universe (Table 12.3).

The Five Elements apply to any phenomenon occurring in the universe and observations from clinical and practical experience have been added later.

Zou Yin (350–270 B.C.), a brilliant philosopher, combined the *Yin-Yang* doctrine with the Five Elements, and is credited with developing an original method of induction used to interpret and predict human and natural affairs in an orderly way.

There are two important patterning methods within the Five Element model known as the Generative and the Control cycles (*xiang sheng* and *xiang ke*). The Generative cycle is the inherent order of activity found amongst the elements, i.e. germination (wood), growth (fire), nourishment (earth), ripening (metal), and decay with the guarding and storage of the seed-essence (water), which allows the cycle to begin again at the germination stage. The other is the Control cycle of which relationship is the following; water quenching fire, fire melting metal, metal cutting wood, wood digging soil, and soil damming water.

The five elements also correspond to five organs (Fig. 12.2) and relate to emotions, sense organs and tissues (Table 12.4).

In Figure 12.2, each organ has a "tonifying" (enhancing) effect or a sedating effect on the next organ along with the generative cycle or the control cycle. For example, anger (excess state of liver, wood) enhances the activity of the nervous system (heart, fire) and sedates appetite (spleen, earth). Through these dynamics of organs and elements, ancient people provided a valuable framework in which to describe and understand many aspects of health and illness.

The essential substances. In addition to the five elements and organs, Chinese medicine identifies three substances circulating in our body that form the basis for the development and maintenance of the human body. They are: *qi* (energy), blood, and water (watery fluids). Blood and water are easy to understand even for the practitioners in the western medicine. However, although the classic texts take the concept of *qi* for granted, it is difficult for the occidental mind to grasp the idea.

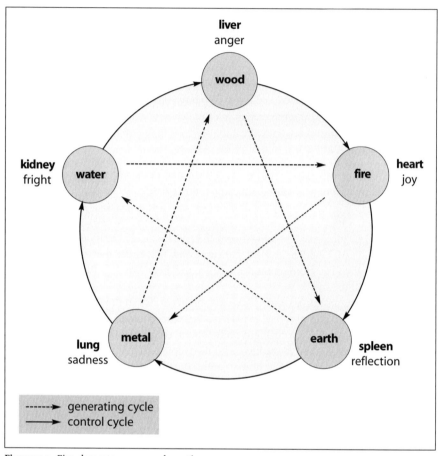

Figure 12.2. Five elements, organs and emotions

Table 12.4. Five Elements and their relationship to organs, emotions and tissues

	Wood	Fire	Earth	Metal	Water
Main organs	Liver	Heart	Spleen[a]	Lungs	Kidneys
	Gall	Small	Stomach	Colon	Bladder
	Bladder	Intestines			
Five emotions	Anger	Joy	Pensiveness	Grief	Fright
Five sense organs	Eyes	Tongue	Mouth	Nose	Ears
Tissues	Tendons and nails	Blood and the vascular system	Muscles	Hair and skin	Bones and marrow

[a] The concept of "spleen", which means the digestive function in TCM/TJM, is different from the anatomical organ in the modern medicine.

Qi represents the essential life energy within human beings which circulates throughout the body. Qi as a power source circulates and activates organic functioning, and appears in various forms.

According to the theory of Yin-Yang, metabolic energy is a part of Yang.

The energy for organ metabolism is called Yang-Qi, and Yang-Qi is responsible for warming, invigorating and protecting the body. Metabolism-controlling factors are the metabolic products are referred to as Yin fluids. These Yin fluids are represented in the living organism by blood and body fluids, their function being to control the production of Yang-Qi, preventing excessive Yang, and thus acting in a sedating manner on the Yang-Qi metabolism. Maintenance of the equilibrium between Yang-Qi and Yin-fluids is referred to as the Yang-Qi/Yin-fluid balance. As described previously, since the balance of the body is maintained by the fire/water balance, namely the Yang-Qi/Yin-fluid balance, disturbance of this balance results in various stages of disease.

Imbalance of Qi, Blood and Water. Imbalance of qi, blood and water can be diagnosed by "diagnostic score" designed by Terasawa. Imbalance of circulating substances and related symptoms is summarized in following Table 12.5.

Six Stages of Disease. Since every disease has its characteristic stage according to the degree of its progression, the proper medicines can be selected by identifying the particular stage of the disease. In TCM/TJM, the all of the stages of the disease are also divided into yang and yin stages. Healthy, positive power, the natural self-healing

Table 12.5. Imbalance of circulating substances

Qi	Deficiency Depression/Stasis Circulation disharmony	General fatigue, easy fatigability, lack of will power, appetite loss, daytime sleepiness, organ ptosis, weak abdominal tensionDepression, a sensation of "heaviness" in the head, the sensation of feeling a lump in the throat, costal pain, abdominal distension and "meteorism" simultaneous sensation of heat and cold, coughing attacks, irritability, erythema of the face, palpitations of the abdominal aorta, recurrent headaches, paroxysmal tachycardia, emesis without nausea
Blood	Deficiency Stasis	Paleness of the face, eye fatigue, muscular cramps, dry skin, dystrophy of the skin, vertigo, hair loss, alopecia "Livid" gingiva, "livid" tongue, dark-rimmed eyes, para umbilical tenderness, hemorrhoids, subcutaneous hemorrhage
Water fluid	Stasis	Tendency to develop edema, hydrothorax, ascites, watery diarrhea, swelling or stiffness of joints, a "water"-like sound on auscultation of the epigastric region, oligouria, polyuria

Table 12.6. Clinical manifestations in six stages

| | Yang stage | | | Yin stage | |
Tai Yang Bing	Shao Yang Bing	Yang Min Bing	Tai Yin Bing	Shao Yin Bing	Jue Yin Bing
Chills, fever, headache, stiff neck etc.	Bitter taste in the mouth, dry throat, dizziness, intermittent fever, chest discomfort, anorexia, nausea, etc.	Fever without chills, sweating, anxiety, thirst etc.	Diarrhea, vomiting, abdominal pain etc.	Chills, coldness of extremities, diarrhea etc.	Shock (terminal stage)

power, is superior in *yang* stage and invasive negative power is dominant in the *yin* stage. Furthermore, both *yang* and *yin* stages are divided into three stages each, *Tai Yang Bing*, *Shao Yang Bing* and *Yang Min Bing* for *Yang* stages and *Tai Yin Bing*, *Shao Yin Bing* and *Jue Yin Bing* for *yin* stages.

Clinical manifestations in each stage are listed in Table 12.6 and Fig. 12.3.

The most appropriate prescriptions for each stage should be used, and they are described in the classic treatment manual, "The Discussion of Cold-Induced Disorders".

Cause of Diseases

In TCM/TJM, there are three basic causes that generate imbalance in the living organism:

▶ Internal causes: the seven emotions: anger, joy, pensiveness, worry, grief, fear, fright;
▶ external causes: the six environmental excesses: wind, cold, heat, humidity, dryness, fire;
▶ other causes: lifestyle, trauma, hereditary.

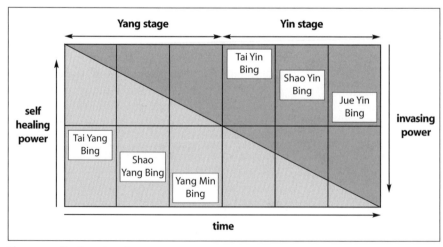

Figure 12.3. Six stages in a disease

Every organism has a self-healing potential, dependent on Qi, blood, and body fluids. If the organism is in a state of equilibrium, the subject will not acquire any disease, whereas if this balance is disturbed, the organism will acquire disease, showing symptoms which indicate the state of disorder.

Internal causes are emotional stress, which is represented in the classical terminology by the seven emotions. The relation between the seven emotions and the theory of the five organs and five elements has been previously outlined briefly.

The six external causes of disease are discussed as follows: Environmental conditions themselves are harmless if they are not excessive, and these conditions are called as the six *qi*. However, if these factors are in excess, they become the pathogenic six "evils", and cause disease. The relationship between the six *qi* and six "evils" is relative. If the condition of the organism is deficient, the six *qi* become "evils" resulting in disease. For example, during the exposure of the person to a certain degree of cold, such as through what many people would consider "comfortable" air conditioning, some individuals might catch cold. Geographical location and climate of a country affect the disposition to certain diseases of the people living there. For example, in regions where the cold season lasts longer, people frequently use mechanical heating systems, which often causes pathogenic dryness, and corresponding symptoms are frequently observed. Recent developments in technology have made our lives more comfortable, but, in some cases, have also increased pathogenic factors. Artificial changes of the temperature inside homes and workplaces by air conditioning systems have easily allowed pathogenic cold and humidity to develop, and cold-related diseases are more often seen in people using air conditioners if they are already in a state of *qi*-deficiency.

Another precipitant factor in diseases like diabetes mellitus or hypertension occurs when a person eats too much and becomes obese. Subsequently, if a person can change his lifestyle, the risk of developing such diseases could be minimized. In addition, according to the recent research about the genome, since the causes of many diseases are influenced by both heredity and lifestyle, the development of disease can be minimized by changing one's lifestyle, even if a person has a hereditary disease.

Diagnosis and Treatment

Conformation (*Zheng* in Chinese or *Sho* in Japanese) and Treatment (*Fang* in Chinese or *Ho* in Japanese):

In TCM/TJM, the determination of therapy (selection of the most appropriate prescription) is based on "the conformation of the patient". The "conformation", namely the clinical presentation of the patient, is at the same time the diagnosis for the patient based upon the pathophysiological concepts of TCM/TJM. The unique nature of these concepts and the means of their identification were discussed previously. Just as each person has his own personality and character, each TCM/TJM prescription has its own particular character.

Basically, the conformation of the patient dictates the medication given, and the names of the type of conformation and the corresponding treatment are the same. For example, if a patient who shows the *sho* of *ma huang tang* (*mao-to* in Japanese), the corresponding *ho* is also *ma huang tang,* and the medication of this name (*ma huang tang*) is deemed the most appropriate treatment for the disease. Accordingly, if patients

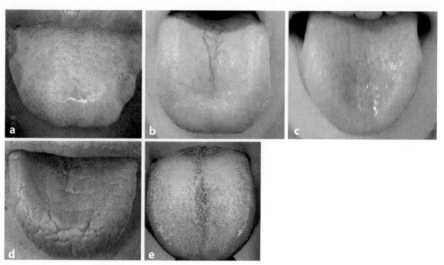

Figure 12.4. Water and fire balance of the tongue

have different diseases in their initial stages, such as the common cold or hepatitis, but the patients show the same conformation, the same prescription is selected for both patients. This is called as *yi bing dong zhi* (treating different diseases by the same medicine). On the contrary, the reverse relationship is called as *dong bing yi zhi* (treating one disease by different medicines). For example, suppose there are two patients, one showing initial signs of common cold and the other treated with interferon for his chronic hepatitis. Both show fever, chill, headaches, and arthralgia, among other similar symptoms, and they are diagnosed both in the *tai yang bing* stage from the aspect of TCM/TJM. Then, the medicine known as *ma huang tang* is selected for both. In this case, the latter is considered to be in the stage of drug-induced *tai yang bing*.

In TCM/TJM, four diagnostic methods are necessary to determine the conformation of the patient. Four diagnosis methods are

▶ observation,
▶ auscultation and olfaction,
▶ history-taking, and
▶ palpation.

Visual observation includes tongue inspection which is very informative. The tongue is examined for mobility, shape, color, and coating. The tongue reflects the state of the organs, essential substances, and the presence of any pernicious influences with great accuracy. Simply said, the tongue reflects "water/fire" balance. The following set of photographs (Fig. 12.4) shows the water/fire balance. The central one (C) is the tongue of a healthy balance. The left two are edematous (A) and with a thick white coating (B) implying a overly hydrated state, and the other two are dry (D) and with a yellow coating (E) implying a state dominated by "fire". When qi is deficient, water becomes dominant and the tongue also becomes edematous. Furthermore, toothmarks around the tongue are often observed. In addition to the "water/fire" balance, the "blood balance" is also recognizable, and dark color of the tongue shows blood "stasis".

Listening to the quality and strength of the voice and the rhythm, strength, and depth of the breathing for any abnormal sounds, smelling halitosis or other odors exuded from the body, urine, and stool, and taking history from the patient is also important to obtain clinical information. In inquiring, one asks many questions about a variety of subjects from food preferences and emotions to the regularity of bowel movements. The patient is observed as a "holistic" being. An illness is not considered an isolated part of the person, and a patient is regarded in his entirety as a living being. To regard a patient "holistically", which tends to be often neglected by the modern western medicine, is one of the most important perspectives of TCM/TJM.

Among many questions, one inquires about "fire/water" balance by asking about one's sensation of heat, thirst, or cold, among other things, which Western medicine does not consider very important, but are very informative in guiding the parameters of TCM/TJM treatment of patients.

Palpation, i.e. pulse and abdominal examinations, are particularly important to determine the conformation of the patient. However, these specific examinations requires much refined practice and extensive experience to master. Furthermore, these skills are often regarded as art, and they have not been fully evaluated enough yet scientifically. Due to the limitations of space in this chapter, the author cannot introduce pulse examination in TCM/TJM in its entirety, but only describe it in brief. In TCM/TJM, there are 28 kinds of pulses, related to pathological or physiological status of the patient. The information from the wrist pulse, such as the rate, strength, tension, smoothness, thickness, depth, among others, are obtained using three fingers of both the examiner's hands.

The wrist pulse of the radial artery is divided into three positions, and five organs correspond to each position (Fig. 12.5, Table 12.7).

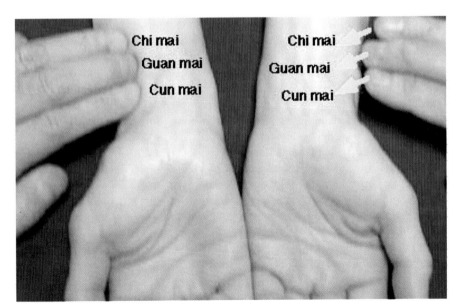

Figure 12.5. Pulse diagnosis by three fingers

Table 12.7. Pulse and organ related position

Pulse and its position	Right	Left
Cun mai (peripheral)	Lung	Heart
Guan mai (gate)	Spleen	Liver
Chi mai (root)	Kidney	Kidney

Table 12.8. Relationship between abdominal signs and imbalance in the body

Diagnosis	Sign of	Susceptible to
Sub-navel hyposthenia (reduced tension in lower abdominal region)	Kidney deficiency	Medications which "tonify" the kidney
Hypochondoric discomfort or tenderness	*Shao yang bing*	Medications including *Bupleuri*
Epigastric discomfort or tenderness	*Shao yang bing* or *Tai yin bing*	Medications "tonifying" stomach or intestine
Epigastric "water-like" sounds	Water imbalance (excess)	Medications regulating water or "tonifying" the spleen
Palpitation of abdominal aorta	*Qi* imbalance	Medications including *Cinnamomum* and *Glycyrhiza*
Periumbilical tenderness	"Blood stasis"	Medications eliminating "blood stasis"

For example, both right and left *chi mai* correspond to the kidneys and a weak pulse of *chi mai* is often a sign of kidney deficiency, if the other kidney related signs like sub-navel hyposthenia in the abdominal examination and symptoms such as lumbago, nocturia, or difficulty in hearing are observed at the same time.

Comparing palpation between in China, Korea, and Japan, pulse examination is regarded as more important in China and Korea. Abdominal examination is regarded as more important in Japan. Using the abdominal examination, an imbalance in the patient's condition can be detected. Table 12.8 summarizes some abdominal signs of imbalances of the body.

Utilizing the four diagnostic methods, clinical information about the patient can be obtained. Then, the collected information is analyzed, and the conformation is eventually diagnosed by using TCM/TJM parameters – *yin* and *yang*, the five organs related to five elements, the essential substances (Qi, blood and body fluids) and the six stages of the disease, leading to the selection of the appropriate medication. This is the process of diagnosis and the determination of treatment. Conformation is diagnosed at a certain point in time, representing only a static situation. However, the process of disease is dynamic and always changeable. Therefore, to keep track of consequent changes, repeated diagnoses are required during the course of illness, and if necessary, therapeutic regimens may have to be altered.

As previously described, since the principle of treatment is the harmonization of *yin-yang* balance, the rule of treatment is simply stated as "to restore the balance of the body, remove or decrease any excess, and to supply, increase, or tonify to correct any deficiency". According to this rule, and by analyzing TCM/TJM parameters, the most appropriate medication is selected for the patient.

Use of TCM and TJM for the Elderly

In ancient China, most of the Emperors in many dynasties longed for eternal life and sought drugs of natural origin from the whole country for their longevity. Korea was well known to foreigners as a land with plenty of famous traditional drugs, such as ginseng, or herbs of "eternal youth". This was one of the reasons that the origin of natural traditional medicine developed in China and Korea.

There is a difference between normal aging and successful (healthy) aging. Normal aging often brings about diseases and impairments which are characteristically seen among the elderly. However, some elderly people seem to escape from specific diseases altogether, and are said to have died simply because of "old age". The latter may maintain an active, healthy life until death. Healthy aging, which everyone hopes to have, refers to a process by which deleterious effects are minimized, preserving function until senescence makes continued life impossible.

Since the elderly, in general, have multiple diseases, they often visit many departments in a hospital, and the medications they use to treat those diseases will increase as well as the costs of those medicines. Both annual national medical expenses, and the population of elderly people in Japan are increasing year by year as well as in many other countries, which is become more dramatic in this century. In addition, many of the diseases among elderly people are chronic, and they need long-term administration of multiple drugs. However, the synergistic effects of drugs have not been fully investigated, and multiple and longer-term administration tends to produce harmful side effects of drugs.

On the other hand, from the aspect of TCM/TJM, the cause of their diseases seems to be one or a few. Therefore, if they are treated by one or a few prescriptions in TCM/TJM, the final cost in the treatment could be reduced.

All formulas in TCM/TJM are made in a harmonious form. Each constituent has its own role independently and, at the same time, cooperatively. The constituent is designated four roles, called "principle", "associate", "adjuvant", and "messenger". These medicines (*yao* in Chinese) are also called as the "emperor" *yao*, the "minister" *yao*, the "assistant" *yao* and the "messenger" *yao*

▶ The "emperor" *yao* has strong therapeutic effects, and sometimes shows a toxic effect. It needs to be controlled to make sure no side effects would arise when combined with other *yao*.

▶ The "minister "*yao* assists or enhances the effect of the "emperor" *yao*.

▶ The "assistant "*yao* leads the effects of the superior *yao* to the proper regions with the help of the "messenger" *yao*.

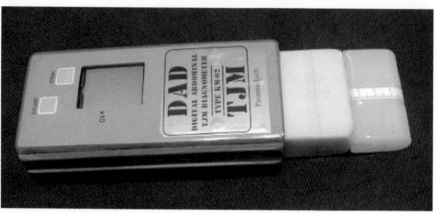

Figure 12.6. Digital abdominal diagnometer

▶ The "messenger" *yao* reduces the toxicity of powerful *yao* and enhance the synergistic effect with the help of the "assistant" yao.

This harmonizing and cooperative action of four groups of *yao* is called as *jun chen zuo shi* (*kun-shin-sa-shi* in Japanese) of TCM/TJM, and some medications show unexpected drastic effects, even if the action of each constituent is individually mild or weak. Accordingly, medicines in TCM/TJM are less harmful and are more suitable if taken over a long period of time. Moreover, since many of the medicines in TCM/TJM have usually multiple actions corresponding to the conformation of the patient, multiple complaints and symptoms of the patient can be improved by using only one medication or a few.

Among the five organs, aging begins earliest in the kidneys, according to the description of "The Yellow Emperor's Inner Classic". Aging of kidneys manifests itself in a variety of symptoms such as lumbago, cataracts, a cold sensation of the lower extremities, nocturia, hearing loss , impotence, and xerosis of the skin, among others. According to the description in "The Yellow Emperor's Inner Classic", aging, accompanied by kidney deficiency, begins from the age of 40 in male and 35 in female.

As previously described, kidney deficiency is diagnosed by weak pulse of *chi mai* and sub-navel hyposthenia (SNH), which is reduced tension in lower abdominal region of the patient. If the patient has these signs, and/or kidney related complaints listed above, his conformation is diagnosed as the *sho* of *ba-wei-di-huang-wan* or *liu-wei-wan*, among others, and a corresponding medication will be selected. These medications which "tonify" kidneys might be effective in improving the patient's complaints. One of the necessary conditions for kidney deficiency is SNH on abdominal examination. However, the diagnosis of SNH depends on the skill of an examiner with extensive experience, and the degree of SNH is expressed as strong, moderate, slight or none. This diagnosis is not scientific and is difficult to validate scientifically. One of the ways that TCM/TJM will be accepted and integrated into conventional medicine, is through the use of an evidence-based analysis. Accordingly, the author has designed a new device (Fig. 12.6) which can easily measure and analyze the abdominal information. Using this device, the abdominal information, especially SNH, can be measured digitally. The new device is known as a "Digital TJM Abdominal Diagnometer."

The device has a probe with a length scale, which is the substitute for the fingers of examiner on the mobile part, and a recording apparatus with a digital scale on the other side. When examiner places this device on the abdomen of the patient and maneuvers the device until the probe sinks in 2 cm depth as to replicate the placement of the hands or fingers on the abdomen and subsequent release of the hands from the abdomen of a TJM examination, the peak pressure is automatically recorded.

To analyze the degree of SNH, SNH index is designed and calculated as the following equation:

SNH index = pressure in the upper abdomen (kg)/pressure in the lower abdomen (kg)

In our clinical study, the SNH index was measured using the Diagnometer and the presence of SNH was diagnosed by two experts in TJM for 109 patients. According to the examiner's diagnosis, SNH was observed in the patients whose SNH index was more than 1.5 and there was high rate of correlation between the diagnosis and the SNH index (80–90%), indicating that it is possible to diagnose SNH by the SNH index.

Furthermore, the SNH index between the young and the elderly was compared. The patients were divided into two groups, young and elderly. "Elderly" was defined as above age 40 for males and 35 for females, based on the description of "the Yellow Emperor's Inner Classic". The characteristics of the groups were for males ($n = 37$, age 51.5 ± 19.4) and for females ($n = 72$, age 44.2 ± 15.7). The SNH index was larger in the elderly group and smaller in the young group both in males and females, suggesting that the description of "the Yellow Emperor's Inner Classic" was correct that age-related changes in the SNH begin at 40 and 35 years old in males and females, respectively.

Many of the cases in which the SNH index was more than 2.5 were diagnosed as having strong SNH and "tonifying" kidney prescriptions, such as *ba wei di huang wan* or *niu che shen qi wan* were prescribed.

These prescriptions were regarded as highly effective and at the same time immediate. Three cases are shown below:

Case 1. Age 55, female:
▶ Chief complaint: orthopedic-treatment resistant lumbago and numbness of the lower extremities.
▶ SNH index: 2.92
▶ Prescription: Niu Che Shen Qi Wan
▶ Progress:
  ▸ 2 weeks later: pain decreased
  ▸ 4 weeks later: pain further diminished and numbness is much improved.
  ▸ 6 weeks later: both complaints have almost completely resolved

Case 2. Age 63, female:
▶ Chief complaint: antibiotics resistant repeated cystitis.
▶ SNH index: 2.69

▶ Prescription: Ba Wei Di Huang Wan
▶ Progress: 3 months later: General status has been improved, and in no need of antibiotics

Case 3. Age 42, female:
▶ Chief complaint: uncomfortable and abnormally increased bowel movements and sounds
▶ SNH index: 3.06
▶ Prescription: Ba Wei Di Huang Wan
▶ Progress:
  ▸ 2 weeks later: bowel sounds decreased
  ▸ 4 weeks later: further resolution of symptoms

Usually, kidney "tonifying" medications are used for the patients who have kidney-related complaints. However, unusual complaints such as the cases listed above can be improved by an SNH-index directed "tonifying" kidney medication, suggesting that the SNH index can be used to help select medications which "tonify" the kidney.

The "five organs theory" can be used to explain the progress of the third case. As described before, the relation between spleen (gastrointestinal function) and kidneys belongs to the "control cycle" and when kidney is relatively deficient, function of spleen becomes dominant and intestinal activity will be increased. "Tonifying" the kidney restores the imbalance between the spleen and kidneys, which leads to improvement through the increased intestinal activity of the patient.

Treatment of Other Symptoms and Signs Often Seen Among the Elderly

In addition to kidney deficiency, the conformations in the elderly tend to be in the *yin* stage. Thus, the important strategy for the treatment of diseases among the elderly is to supply, increase, or "tonify" to correct the lack or deficiency. There are many *ho-zai* (supplying and tonifying prescriptions) in TCM/TJM, e.g., *bu zhong yi qi tang, shi quan*

Table 12.9. Prescriptions(*Ho-zai*) "tonifying" the Yin state and their indications

Ho-zai	Indications and symptoms seen in the subjects
Bu Zhong Yi Qi Tang	*Qi* deficiency, dysfunction of digestive system, fatigue, appetite loss, weakness of muscles, "ptotic" tendency in the viscera, hemorrhoids
Shi Quan Da Bu Tang	Excessive fatigue after surgical operation or with chronic diseases, fatigue, appetite loss, night sweat, anemia, coolness of extremities
Ren Shen Yang Rong Tang	Excessive fatigue with chronic diseases, dysfunction of digestive system after surgery, fatigue, appetite loss, night sweat, anemia, coolness of extremities

da bu tang, ren shen yang rong tang, among others Most of these prescriptions include ginseng (*ren shen*) and astragalus (*huang qi*), thus they are also called *shen qi* medications. A representative three medications and their indications are listed in the following Table 12.9.

Concluding Remarks

From the viewpoint of the author of this chapter, the use of every medicine should be evidence-based and, at the same time, history-based. TCM has at least four to five thousands years' history, numerable clinical trials in ancient times, and accomplished classic medical textbooks, i.e. "the Yellow Emperor's Inner Classic " or "Shen Nong's Materia Medica", which are still regarded as important today, though no meta-analyses of treatment outcomes, nor statistically-based research to clarify the mechanisms of the medicines has been performed on TCM.

On the other hand, although it is true that Western medicine is based on "science", it has only a few hundreds years' history. Come to think of it, what is science? Is TCM/TJM just mystic or superstitious?

Although the TCM/TJM is considered as a complementary or alternative medicine, and difficult to grasp for the occidental mind, those who read this chapter might have realized that TCM/TJM is not just complementary and alternative, but it is one of a number of complete systems of medicine which is different from Western medicine.

TCM/TJM is a complete medical system with both a holistic approach to the patient and a long history; it is a treasure for all mankind. Accordingly, what I want to stress most is that TCM/TJM should be more frequently utilized to promote health and a better life. Every system is not perfect, and different systems should aid, encourage, and stimulate one another.

References

1. Kampo: Japanese-oriental medicine, insights from clinical cases. Katsutoshi Terasawa. K.K. Standard McIntyre, Tokyo, Japan, 1993
2. Synopsis of prescriptions of the Golden Chamber. Zhang Zhong-jin. New World Press, Beijing, China, 1987
3. Tao and Dharma: Chinese medicine and Ayurveda. Robert Svoboda and Arnie lade. Eastland Press, CA, USA, 1995
4. Shoyaku Handbook (in Japanese). Terutane Yamada and Munetetsu Tei. Tsumura Co. Tokyo, Japan, 1994
5. Chinese-English Chinese English Medical Word-Ocean Dictionary. Shan Xi Ren Min Publisher, Shan Xi, China, 1995
6. Complementary/Alternative Medicine: An Evidence-Based Approach. John W. Spencer and Joseph J. Jacobs. Mosby inc., St. Louis, USA, 1999
7. The Base of kampo Medicine (in Japanese). Kosei Takayama. Tsumura Co., fukuoka, Japan, 1994
8. Japamese-English Dictionary of Oriental medicine (in Japanese and English). Munetetsu Tei Isei Co. Tokyo, Japan, 1987
9. New Scientific Diagnosis for Abdominal Examination by Digital. Abdominal TJM (Traditional Japanese Medicine) Diagnometer.
10. Koji Miyamoto and Kiwamu Okita. Abstract, 11th International Congress of Oriental medicine, Seoul, 2001

13 Acupuncture in the Context of Traditional Chinese Medicine

N.S. Cherniack, E.P Cherniack

Acupuncture is a method of treatment that involves the insertion of fine needles in the skin at crucial points believed to be of health significance [1–4]. The term acupuncture is European and was invented by Willem Ten Rhyne a Dutch physician in the early part of the seventeenth century. Acupuncture originated in China more than 4000 years ago as part of system of medicine that involves not just the insertion of needles, but in addition employs in addition therapeutic approaches such as moxibustion, cupping, herbal products, tuina and qiquong [3]. The first complete summary of Chinese medicine The Yellow Emperor's Cannon of Medicine appeared about 300 B.C., the time of the Warring States period in China [1, 3–5]. It deals not just with medical matters but also with philosophical concepts of the operation of the universe that melded Taoism with concepts of Confucianism. The Taoist concept is that health is the attainment of a harmony between opposing forces that exist in the natural world. Confucianism considers the body to be sacred and that it should remain intact in life and death. This latter concept hindered the development of surgery and promoted the use of non-invasive treatments of disease such as acupuncture [1, 4, 5]. The twelve volume Classic of Acupuncture and Moxibustion or Zhen Jiu Yi Jung was written almost 1800 years ago. With continued observation the description of acupuncture continued to evolve in China and grew more detailed. With the passage of time, additional acupuncture points and the connecting pathways between them were mapped. In the eleventh century Wei-Yi redefined the acupuncture points and compiled an Illustrated Manual on the Points for Acupuncture and Moxibustion on the New Bronze Model [1, 4]. Li Shih-Chen in the sixteenth century wrote the classical Chinese Materia Medica and wrote a paper on Eight Extra Channels for acupuncture describing their course and indications for their use [1, 4]. With the arrival of Europeans acupuncture began to decline in prestige and many acupuncturist seemed to be no more than "pavement physicians" and Chinese medicine tended to concentrate more on massage and herbal preparations [1, 4, 5]. After the Communists took power in China there was a resurgence of national interest in acupuncture and it was proposed that traditional medicines be "scientized". New research institutes were established which have led to the development of new ways of using and giving acupuncture [1, 4]. Acupuncture has even been used for anesthesia during surgery. In part because it is better during surgery to apply acupuncture away from the site of the incision, the idea that there were areas of the body in which there were homunculi like the ear which existed in ancient China and in other cultures like Egypt was refined and expanded [1, 4–7].

Chinese Medicine and acupuncture were probably introduced into the United States around the time of the California gold rush when large numbers of Chinese immigrated [1, 4]. They have been used for every kind of disease but probably most often in this country among the aged for musculo-skletal disorders and also for breathlessness and for the chronic pain with cancer for example (see chapters on respiratory disease and cancer) and [8–26]. Its been estimated that Americans make 5 to 12 million visits to acupuncturists annually and spend 50 million dollars on acupuncture treatments.

Traditional Chinese Medicine

Traditional Chinese Medicine is based on a kind of homeostatic concept that there are male or positive and female or negative forces in the universe that oppose and at the same time complement each other and must be maintained in balance [1–4]. Negative (Yin) forces are dark, cold, female, and passive; while the positive (Yang) forces are light, warm, positive and male. The material world consists of five elements: metal, wood, fire, water and earth. These elements like the positive and negative forces are interdependent. Yin processes are either energy conserving or Yin; or energy using Yang. Personality can reflect the balance of Yin and Yang with Yin people being inward and shy, while yang people are more outward and aggressive. Health results when Yang and Yin forces are in balance and disease occurs, when either one is deficient. Yin deficiency causes illnesses such as insomnia while Yang deficiency leads to problems such as cold feet. Similarly disease can occur when the elements that make up an organ are out of kilter. The organs of the body according to traditional Chinese medicine are the Zhang Fu and consist of five solid Yin and six hollow Yang organs [3]. These only roughly correspond to the organs of Western medicine. For example in Chinese medicine the "liver" which is considered to have the quality of wood and is susceptible to being set aflame by fire, plays a major role in emotional state and is responsible for the smooth flow of qi and blood around the body [1, 4].

According to Taoism qi is one of the three treasures that affect health. The other two are jing and shen. Jing is a kind or regenerative essence or stored energy. There is no exact translation for these terms but they are often translated as essence, vitality and spirit. Qi is the most familiar term and is the energy that allows the body to move and think. Jing is burned in the body and used up by excessive behavior or overwork be it physical, mental or emotional. Shen is a kind of combination of qi and jing [4, 5].

Treatment begins in Chinese Medicine by diagnosing the nature of the imbalance that is responsible for ill health and then applying appropriate measures to restore it. Which of the several modalities of Chinese medicine and the mix with which they are used and in terms of acupuncture the specific procedures and points to needle can vary among patients even those who appear to have identical symptoms. This is because of perceived differences in their internal states and because of such differences in the external environment such as season and living conditions [4, 5].

The traditional Chinese practitioner uses four diagnostic approaches that closely resemble those use by Western physicians and include observing, listening, smelling, inquiring, and palpating. Feeling the pulse is a major part of the examination. The urine is also examined [4, 5].

Chinese herbs have Yin and Yang characteristics. Persons with a Yang personality may benefit from Yin drugs and vice versa. In addition tonics can be characterized as jing, qi or shen promoting. Applying the principles of the three treasures to the prescribing of herbals is called in China, Superior Herbalism. More than eighteen hundred drugs, mainly natural substances are used in Chinese medicine. In ancient China, drugs were chewed or given in decoction or tinctures or as powders. Ointments and pastes were also used for skin conditions and boils. Currently many Chinese medicines now are available as capsules, pills and some by injection. Various herbal remedies used in traditional Chinese Medicine are described in the chapter on herbal medicines and in the chapters dealing with specific diseases.

Traditional Chinese Medicine also includes physical training and massage therapy. Qigong is a system of physical training combining aerobic conditioning, isometrics, isotonics, meditation, and relaxation [4, 5]. There are 5 major schools of qigong; Taoist, Buddhist, Confucian, martial arts and medical. Medical qigong is the cultivation and control of vital energy. It includes breathing exercises to help induce relaxation and meditation. It has been used to treat chronic pain, to overcome addictions and cure diseases often considered psychosomatic in the West. Practicing qigong according to Traditional Chinese Medicine improves the circulation of qi. It makes one who practices it more sensitive to imbalances in the body of yin and yang. There are some risks associated with qigong and the acutely ill, pregnant women, and the mentally deranged should not use it.

Tuina uses massage and manipulation techniques to establish a harmonious flow of Qi [4, 5]. Tuina methods include massage of muscles and tendons, and manipulation to improve muscle and tendon alignment. Tuina is particularly used to treat musculoskeletal disorders but is also used for sedation and relaxation. Tuina has been used in China for over 2000 years. External compresses, liniments, and herbal poultices are used to enhance the manipulations. Tuina sessions last from thirty-minutes to an hour. In a typical session the patient who wears loose fitting clothing and is barefoot is massaged while lying on a floor mat. Phlebitis, infections and fractures are considered contraindications to tuina.

Acupuncture

Acupuncture is the most widely used in the West of the various physical, mental, and chemical modalities of traditional Chinese medicine [1, 5]. It aims to maintain energy flow in the body. Qi is the essence of life and is seen as the potential energy that traverses the universe and each person. Stagnation in the flow of qi can cause pain, vomiting etc. The internal organs and limbs are linked by meridians i.e. pathways that conduct qi. Meridians do not correspond to nerve or circulation pathways. There are two kinds of pathways: jing, main channels that course longitudinally and laterally running channels called luo which regulate, spiritual, mental, emotional and physical health and in turn are influenced by the Yin-Yang balance. There are 12 major and

8 extra channels near the surface of the body through which qi flows [4]. Along these channels are 365 acupuncture points and over 1500 additional points, which can be needled, to reduce symptoms and restore qi flow. In addition there exist ashi or pain points and microsystems of points, which contain that can be needled to reduce symptoms. These microsystems are situated in the ear, hand, and scalp [4, 5].

Diseases treatable by acupuncture fall into two categories: those which affect the channels and due to blockage of qi and those, which are more complex and affect the Zhang and Fu organs [3]. Some illnesses such as migraine are thought to combine both kinds of disorder. Diseases of the channels are treated by penetrating both local acupuncture points a distal point on the channel that crosses the painful area. In diseases of the organs particular points on channels are selected to sedate or stimulate that organ. While there are no hard and fast rules for selecting points there are groups of special points that represent particular organs. These are divided into back shu and the front mu points. If the zhang organs are diseased (yin organs) back points are selected while the front points are chosen for afflictions of the Fu (yang) organs. Each channel has a point that represents one of the five elements that can be used to excite or depress particular organs. In cases of pain tender points are called Asa hi points and are always used along with local acupuncture points [4].

The first acupuncture needles were made of stone (Bian stones) but gradually metallic needles made of gold, silver, and bronze and currently of steel replaced these. The needles originally had different shapes e.g. round, blunt, arrow shaped and filform [1, 4]. Currently filiform needles are almost exclusively used [9].

In order to obtain a therapeutic effect the acupuncturist needs considerable training since success depends on the speed with which the needle is inserted, the depth of penetration, the angle of insertion, and the length of time its left in the skin as well as the number of needles and their positioning. Often the needles are flicked, rotated, or otherwise manipulated after they are in place. Sometimes burning moxa leaves are placed at the site of stimulation (moxabustion) [4]. Moxa can be used in different ways. Loose moxa can be fashioned into a cone and burnt on the skin or it may be burnt on ginger or garlic or on a stick kept a few centimeters from the skin.

Acupressure that is applying stimulation to skin points with the hands rather than needles has been used particularly in the treatment of nausea and vomiting [6]. For example in a recent study in 17 women undergoing chemotherapy acupressure performed by applying pressure to the forearm and below the knee for 3 minutes was evaluated in nausea prevention. Significant differences between control and treated groups occurred only in the first 10 days [6]. Pressure producing wristbands, which may work in a similar manner to acupressure, are commonly offered as a remedy for seasickness. One form of acupressure is one finger pushing to treat internal diseases.

New techniques of acupuncture have been devised. A variety of appliances have been invented to apply weak electrical currents to the acupuncture needle [7]. Some measure the electrical resistance and conductance over different skin points and can be used to select sites for penetration or are used in diagnosis. Low-level lasers may be used instead of needles to stimulate specific points on the skin. Usually wavelengths in the red (600–700 nm) and in the near infrared range (800–1000 nm) are used [7]. The infrared beams penetrate more deeply. Attempts have also been made to combine acupuncture and magnetic therapy. Acupuncture confined to the ear has become quite popular and at least 40 points have on the ear have been described. Ear acupuncture is based on the idea that the external ear is a homunculus in which all the organs and parts of the body are represented. Penetration of specific points in the ear allows diseases of the body to be treated. Ear acupuncture has been developed by the French and by especially the Chinese as a method of anesthesia used during surgery. The French doctor Paul Nogier developed a detailed map of acupuncture points, which is still in use [4].

In the last thirty years scalp acupuncture has been developed to treat brain injuries such as stroke. It has little or nothing to do with traditional Chinese medicine theory [7]. It is based on the idea that stimulation of the scalp over damaged areas of the cortex will hasten recovery. All points on the scalp are considered to be representations of functional areas of the brain. Motor, sensory, optic, speech etc points have been mapped on the scalp. A 2 or 3-inch needles are used and inserted down into the subcutaneous tissue. The needles are rotated at rates of about 200 times a minute for about five minutes or are stimulated electrically. It is purported to be particularly useful in reducing muscle spasm.

There are very few side effects of acupuncture treatment. Rarely infection has been reported or puncture of organs. In 1996 the FDA approved the use of acupuncture needles by licensed practitioners [8, 9].

Each state has it own requirements for acupuncturists. As of the year 2000, 38 states required licensure and often 3 years of training. Treatments usually consist of the placement of three and often considerably more needles, which remain in place about 20 minutes. Some common conditions in which acupuncture has been used are listed below [10–26]:

▶ Migraine
▶ Low back pain
▶ Asthma
▶ Cancer
▶ Angina
▶ Indigestion
▶ Constipation
▶ Smoking cessation
▶ Fibromyalgia
▶ Carpal tunnel syndrome
▶ Tennis elbow
▶ Osteoarthritis
▶ Endometriosis
▶ Menstrual cramps
▶ Depression
▶ Dental pain

Acupuncture is increasing used together with other forms of complementary medicine as well as an adjunct to standard Western medicine therapies. Some studies report a decrease in the need for pain-killing drugs when acupuncture is used [22–23, 26, 27].

There are currently several on-going studies of the efficacy of acupuncture. Some are federally funded. Most have been inconclusive. An NIH panel in 1997 concluded that because of the then paucity of research that was adequately controlled it was difficult to comment definitively on the effectiveness of acupuncture [25]. However there is support for the use of acupuncture in the treatment of post-operative nausea and in nausea induced by pregnancy or chemotherapy [25]. Also the panel stated that acupuncture might be useful in fibromyalgia, treating dental pain, low back pain, tennis elbow, carpal tunnel syndrome, and osteoarthritis and myofascial pain. Current federally funded research deals with the use of electroacupuncture in osteoarthritis of the knee, mapping area of the brain involved in opiod dependence using electro-acupuncture, the effects of acupuncture in hypertension, and the usefulness of acupuncture in heart failure through the reduction of sympathetic activity.

Back problems are one of the more common reasons for using alternative care. In 1997, one-third of patients suffering with back pain used alternative care usually chiropractic. Although acupuncture has been used extensively in the treatment of low back pain there have been relatively few studies of its efficacy.

Fifty patients with low back pain were studied in Lund [26]. These patients with low back pain were divided into three groups: manual acupuncture, electroacupuncture, and placebo treatment with mock electroacupuncture. Treatment was given weekly for eight weeks. Patients kept records of pain intensity, activity, sleep, and medication use. At the end of treatment 14 of 34 patients receiving acupuncture were improved but only 2 of the 16 control patients.

In another study of 262 patients with low back pain acupuncture was found to be relatively ineffective; while massage was more effective than either acupuncture or self-education [27]. The massage group used the least medication and had the lowest costs of subsequent care.

It is of interest that a study at the University of Maryland found that older people with osteoarthritis who used acupuncture plus conventional therapy had more pain than those who used conventional treatment alone. A small study of 11 women with a major depressive disorder found that half became significantly better with acupuncture (NCCAM web site).

In addition to efficacy research in animal models is examining the cellular and molecular basis of acupuncture. Current ideas are that acupuncture causes the release of enkephalins, opiods, or other chemicals such as cytokines into muscles, the spinal cord and/or the brain, or that it blocks transmission up nerve fibers. Stimulating acupuncture points has been shown to facilitate the rate at which electromagnetic signals are transmitted. These signals could somehow be involved in the release of chemicals. Animal studies have also shown that opiods and other neurotransmitters can be released in the brain as a result of acupuncture [28, 29].

As in other areas of alternative medicine there are obstacles to the fair evaluation of efficacy using western scientific methods. Acupuncture traditionally takes place within a system that also uses a number of other non-western approaches to medicine, which in a sense can result in a sense to its use "out of context". The large number of acupuncture points makes it difficult to select "control" points when the effects of acupuncture in a specific disease are being evaluated. While sham needles have been developed which appear to penetrate the skin but do not actually do so, acupuncture needling produces distinctive sensations that are not reproduced by the sham needles [30].

References

1. Hoizey D., Hoizey M. A history of Chinese Medicine Vancouver, UBC Press, 1993
2. Veith I. The Yellow Emperor's Classic of Medicine. Univ. of California Press, 1949
3. Ross J, Zang Fu. The organ systems of traditional Chinese medicine. Edinburgh: Churchill Livingston.1985
4. Pockert M, Ullmann C (1988) Chinese Medicine (Howson M, translator) (1st US edition) (NewYork: Morrow)
5. Dong P, Esser AH. Chi Gong: The Ancient Chinese Way to Health. New York Paragon House
6. Dibble SL, Chapman J, Mack KA, Shih, A. Acupressure for nausea: results of a pilot study. Oncology Nursing Forum 2000. 27:41–47
7. Naeser MA. Acupuncture and laser acupuncture in the treatment of paralysis of stroke patients, carpal tunnel syndrome and alopecia areata. Frontier Perspectives 5:8–15, 1996
8. Yamashita H, Tsukayama H, Hiroshi BA, Tanno Y, Nishijo K. Adverse events related to acupuncture. J Amer Med Assoc 1998; 280: 1563–1564.
9. Ernst E, White AR. Prospective studies of the safety of acupuncture: a systematic review. Am J Med 2001; 110: 481–485.
10. Jobst KA. A critical analysis of acupuncture in pulmonary disease; efficacy and safety of the acupuncture needle. J Alternat Comp Med 1995 1 57–85
11. Ballegard S, Norelund S, Smidt DF (1996) Cost-benefit ratio of combined use of acupuncture, shiatsu, and life-style adjustment for treatment of patients with severe angina pectoris. Acupuncture and Electro-therapeutic Research 21: 187–97
12. Ballegard S, Jensen G, Pedersen F, Nissen VH. Acupuncture in severe, stable angina pectoris: a randomized trial. Acta Med Scand. 220: 307–13,(1986)
13. Tashkin DP, Bresler DE et al. Comparison of real and simulated acupuncture and isoproterenol in the methacholine-induced asthma. Ann Allergy 1997; 76: 855–863
14. Linde K, Jobst K, Panton J. Acupuncture for chronic asthma. The Cochrane database of systemic reviews 2000(2) CD000008
15. Davies A, Lewith G, Goddard J, Howarth P. The effect of acupuncture on non- allergic rhinitis; a controlled pilot study. Alternative Therapies in Health and Medicine 4: 70–74, 1998
16. Jobst K, McPherson K, Brown V, Flethcher HJ, Mole P, Chen JH, Arrowsmith J, Efthimiou J, Maciocia G, Shifrin K, Lane DJ. Controlled trial of acupuncture for disabling breathlessness. Lancet 1986; Dec 20–27; 2(8521–22): 1416–1419
17. Tandon MK, Soh PFT, Wood AT. Acupuncture for bronchial asthma? A double-blind cross over study. Med J Aust. 154: 409, 1991
18. Dias PLR, Subramaniam S, Lionel NDW. Effects of acupuncture in bronchial asthma. J R Soc Med 1982; 75: 245–8.
19. Kleijnen J, Ter Riet G, Knipschild P. Acupuncture and asthma: review of controlled trials. Thorax 1991; 46: 799–802.
20. Alimi D, Rubino C, Leandri EP, Brule SF. Analgesic effects of auricular acupuncture for cancer pain. J Pain Symptom Management 2000; 19: 81–82.
22. Xu S, Liu Z, Li Y (1995) Treatment of cancerous abdominal pain by acupuncture in Zuslani: a report of 92 cases. J Tradit. Chin. Med. 15: 189–191
23. Gadsby JG, Franks P, Jarvis P, et al. (1997) Acupuncture-like transcutaneous electrical nerve stimulation within palliative care: a pilot study. Complement Ther Med. 5: 13–18
24. Allen JJB An acupuncture treatment study for unipolar depression. Psychological Science 1998. 9: 397–401
25. Acupuncture. NIH consensus statement. NIH vol. 15: Nov 3–5, 1997
26. Carlsson CP, Sjolund BH. Acupuncture for chronic low back pain: a randomized placebo-controlled study with long term follow-up. Clin J Pain 2001; 17: 296–305
27. Cherkin DC, Eisenberg D, Sherman KJ, Barlow W, Kaptchuk TJ, Street J, Deyo RA. Randomized trial comparing traditional Chinese medical acupuncture, therapeutic massage, and self-care education for chronic low back pain. Arch Int Med 2001; 161:1081–8
28. Wu, B, Zhou RX, Zhou MS. Effect of Acupuncture on Interleukin-2 level and NK cell immonoactivity of peripheral blood of malignant tumor patients. Chung Kuo Chung His I Chieh Ho Tsa Chich 1994; 14: 537–9
29. Cheng XD, Wu GC, He QZ and Cao XD. Effect of electroacupuncture on the activities of tyrosine protein kinase in subcellular fractions of activated T lymphocytes from traumatized rats. Acupuncture & Electrotherapeutics Res 1998, 23: 161–170
30. Vincent C, Lewith G, Placebo controls for acupuncture studies. J Roy Soc Med 1995; 88:199–202

14 Current Practice of Acupuncture – Use in Common Diseases of the Elderly

Xiao Chun Yu, Jiang Hong Ye, Wen Hsien Wu

Acupuncture is an easily practiced and effective therapy for the prevention and treatment of various diseases, through the use of needles stimulating the human body by trained practitioners with special manipulating skills, based on theories of "meridian" and "acupoint" of Traditional Chinese Medicine (TCM). In clinical practice, acupuncturists proceed as follows: first a precise diagnosis is made based on an overall analysis of the signs and syndromes of patients, and then, appropriate acupoints of "channels" are chosen for stimulation by needling methods using established therapeutic principles.

The Meridians

The meridian system, composed of channels and collaterals, is a specific network of conduits in which "*qi*" i.e., energy and blood, are circulated and transported to all parts of the body. The channels are the main structures, which can be likened to the trunks of trees, and are located deep in the body. The collaterals are the thin branches of the meridian system which are situated superficially and connect with channels. The collaterals form a network distributed over all the body. The meridian system also connects physiologically the "*zangfu*" i.e., internal organs and limbs, and communicates with all tissues and organs of the body, including the upper, lower, interior and exterior ones(See chapter on Traditional Chinese Medicine and Acupuncture)

The Organization of Meridian System

Regular Channels

There are 12 regular channels, 8 extra channels, and 3 types of subordinate channels: 12 divergent channels, 12 muscle regions and 12 cutaneous regions. There are 15 collaterals in addition to superficial collaterals and the minute collaterals. This is shown in Figure 14.1.

The twelve regular channels are the main trunks of the meridian system. They are named according to several factors including their properties in the classification of *yin* and *yang*, the viscera they connect to, and the regions they pass through. Since each of the twelve channels directly connects to one organ, its name includes the organ's name, the location of the region through which the channel passes, such as hand or

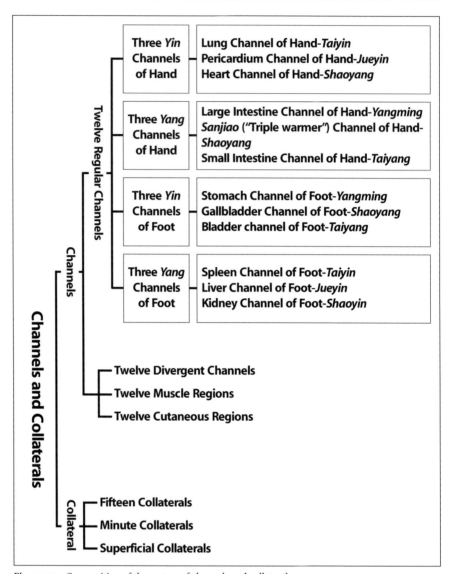

Figure 14.1. Composition of the system of channels and collaterals

foot, and whether it is interior, exterior, anterior, middle, or posterior. *Yin* and *Yang* properties are another important factor in naming the channels. Each of the six *zang* organs (interior) are connected to their corresponding exterior regions by six inter-linked (*Yin*) channels, three each of hand and foot, and by collaterals to the *fu* organ which are linked by six channels (*Yang*), again three each of hand and foot. *Yang* channels belong to *fu* organs and link to *zang* organs and *Yin* channels by their branches and collaterals. For example, the heart channel of hand-*shaoyin* pertains to the heart and links to the small intestine; while the small intestine channel of "hand-*taiyang*" belongs to the small intestine and links "vital energy" to heart. The whole system of meridians is a ring-like, endless transportation system in which *qi* and blood circle from one channel to another linked through the collaterals between them. The order for the circulation of *qi* and blood in the regular channels system is shown in Figure 14.2.

The twelve divergent channels are the branches by which the regular channels can join or separate to reach various areas of the body and can emerge from or enter deeply into the body.

The twelve muscle regions refer to branches of regular channels, which distribute the *qi* and blood of regular channels to the muscles, tendons and joints, especially to those of the limbs. The function of muscle regions is to keep the joints flexing and extending normally. The twelve cutaneous regions are the superficial parts of the body, where the twelve regular channels distribute the *qi*.

Eight extraordinary channels (*Du, Ren, Chong, Dai, Yinqiao, Yangqiao, Yinwei and Yangwei* channels) pass through the body by ways different from the regular channels. They do not connect with any *zangfu* organ and have no the interior and exterior relation to each other. The function of the eight extra channels is to strengthen the communication between the regular channels and adjust the storage, permeation and pouring of the *qi* and blood of the regular channels.

The fifteen collaterals include the twelve collaterals from the twelve regular channels, the collaterals of *Ren* and *Du* channels and the major collaterals of the spleen. The names of the fifteen collaterals come from the points, which they separate. The function of the fifteen collaterals is to reinforce the connection between the *Yin* and *Yang* channels as well as the external-internal channels on the body surface. Superficial collaterals refer to those distributing on the surface of the body. Minute collaterals are the smallest branches that transport *qi* and blood to the all parts of the body and nourish them.

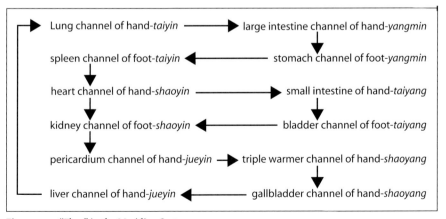

Figure 14.2. "Flow" in the Meridian System

Distribution of the Fourteen Channels on the Body Surface (12 Regular and Ren and Du)

The 14 channels refer to the 12 regular channels plus *Ren* and *Du* channels. The *Yin* channels spread to the thoracic and abdominal regions and the medial aspects of limbs. There are three *yin* channels of the hand on the upper limbs and three *yin* channels of the foot on the lower limbs. The *Yang* channels spread on the head, face, the lumbar region, the back and the lateral aspects of the limbs. Like the *Yin* channels, the 3 *Yang* channels of the hand are located on the upper limbs and 3 *Yang* channels of the foot on the lower limbs. For the *Yang* channels on the limb, the *Yangmin* channels are the anterior ones; the *Shaoyang* the medium ones, and the *Taiyang* the posterior ones. For the six *Yin* channels, *Taiyin* channels are the anterior ones, *Jueyin* channels the medium ones, and the *Shaoyin*, the posterior ones. Both *Jueyin* channels of foot are anterior and *Taiyin* ones are medium. *Ren* and *Du* channels feed respectively the anterior and posterior aspects of the midline of the trunk, the neck, the head and the face. The *Ren* channel regulates the functions of all *Yin* channels and *Du*, the functions of all *Yang* channels.

In summary, channels and collaterals, connect with the all the tissues and organs and transport *qi* and blood to form an organic whole.

The system of channels and collaterals is also a way by which the pathogens invade and leave the body. The symptoms caused by abnormalities in the system can suggest syndromes of pathology of related internal organs, aiding in the diagnosis of diseases. Finally, according to the theory, channels and collaterals allow treatment, because the acupoints are the points on channels where *qi* and "information" produced by needling can be distributed.

Current Theories on the Nature of the Meridian System

There are three major ideas on the essential components of the "channels" that comprise the meridian system:
- *Jingluo* (channels and collaterals) are mainly composed of nervous, vascular, and lymphatic systems. This idea is based on the following facts:
  - Clinically, when the acupoints are infiltrated by local anesthetic, no sensations can be felt upon needling. The sensation is essential to the effect of acupuncture.
  - Experimentally, no acupuncture response can be produced after cutting the dorsal roots containing afferents from the sensory field of the acupoints stimulated.
  - Some distributing areas of channels described by the ancient literature of TCM are almost the same as anatomical neural pathways. For example, the distributing lines of Lung channels of "hand-*Taiyin*" follow the pathway of lateral bundle of muscular and cutaneous nerves on the upper limb; the transportation "traces" of heart channels of "Hand-*Shaoyin*" follow the pathways of the ulnar nerves; and those of pericardium channels of "hand-*jueyin*" are consistent with the pathways of the median nerves.
- Blood vessels are the major component of the meridian system. According to ancient Chinese literature, channels are filled and nourished by the blood. *Canon of Eleven Channels and Moxibustion*, written in the Han dynasty, is generally consid-

ered the first book to record the channel system before *Canon of Medicine*. In this book, each channel is designated with only one Chinese character, *MAI*, which refers to blood vessel, indicating that in TCM, blood vessels are the original components of meridians.

▸ The "*Cunkou*" area where the physicians of TCM detect the pulse is actually at the *taiyuan* point of lung channel of hand-*taiyin*.
▸ In the theory of TCM, one of the major function of channel is to transport *qi* and blood. However the blood is known to be circulated by vessels according to the theories of western medicine.
▸ In the clinical practice of acupuncture, stimulating blood vessels to produce bleeding is frequently used to treat certain diseases.
▸ Anatomically, both the vessel system and channel system have network-like structures.

▶ (Some scholars consider the lymphatic system one of the components of meridian system because the lymphatic system also has a network-like structure.

▶ According to Z.W. Meng, because the transmission speeds along channels of about 0.1 m/min are much lower than the transmission speeds of 80–120 m/min of the somatic nervous system, and 0.5–2 m/min of the autonomic nervous system, the meridian system is a "third equilibrating system" that is involved in physiological regulation [14].

Acupoints

TCM considers acupoints points on the body surface where *qi* of meridians distribute. Besides the primary function of mediating the curative effect of acupuncture, acupoints can also reflect pathological changes in meridian and internal organs. All the acupoints are classified into three types as follows:

▶ Regular acupoints: These acupoints are on the 12 regular channels and *Ren* and *Du* channels. They have their own names, locations, and pertain to one of the above 14 channels.
▶ Extra acupoints: Extra acupoints are not located on the regular channels, but have their own well-defined locations and names.
▶ "*Ashi*" acupoints: *Ashi* points refer to tender points which reflect the pathological changes of corresponding internal organs.

Stimulation of acupoints has following therapeutic objectives:
▶ To treat pathological changes of nearby tissues or organ.
▶ To treat disorders of distant tissues or organs.
▶ To cause particular curative effects in certain disorders.

The acupuncturist generally uses following methods to locate the acupoint:
▶ Bone-length measurement: uses bone segments as markers to measure the distance of various parts of the body so as to finally locate the acupoints.
▶ Anatomical landmarks on the surface of the body

▶ Simple measurement
▶ Finger measurement: in this measurement, the acupoints are located utilizing the length or width of a patient's finger as a ruler.

Experimental studies suggest that acupoints have relatively special structures. Most acupoints are close to nervous bundles [1]. There is also evidence indicating that regions around the acupoints are innervated by much richer nerve endings, bundles, and plexi than non-acupoints [2, 3, 4], postulating a close relationship between acupoints and the nervous system. Following blockage or cutting of the innervation of the acupoint, the effect of acupuncture completely disappeared [5, 6], further supporting the close relation between acupoints and nervous system. In addition, earlier studies on the somato-sympathetic reflex found that activating different sensory receptors induced different physiological responses [7, 8, 9].

General Principles of Acupuncture

In clinical practice, acupuncturists usually select more than one acupoint targeting the symptoms and pathogenesis of diseases, according to the theory of meridians. There are five commonly used methods to select the acupoints as follows:
▶ Selecting acupoints on channels pertaining to the diseased viscera
▶ Selecting both exterior-interior acupoints simultaneously
▶ Selecting both anterior-posterior acupoints simultaneously
▶ Selecting both remote-local acupoint simultaneously
▶ Selecting both left and right acupoints simultaneously.

The following are three major principles of acupuncture treatment:

Balancing Yin and Yang. TCM teaches that a relative imbalance between *yin* and *yang* is the cause of all disease and pain. Thus, regulating *yin* and *yang* is the basic principle for the use of acupuncture.

Correcting the Deficiency of Qi, "Vital Energy", and Discharging the Pathogens. Another basic principle is that all diseases result from either deficiency of vital energy or excess of pathogenic factors. Therefore, strengthening any insufficiency in the resistance of the body and reducing the excess of pathogens in the body are very important in treatment by acupuncture.

Treating Both Primary and Secondary Factors Simultaneously. The primary and secondary factors causing disorders are interrelated. The original disease is primary, while the complications are secondary. If a treatment of the secondary is urgent, it should be treated first. If the disease is a chronic one, the amount of "vital energy" should be considered the primary problem.

Needling Manipulations

Acupuncture is stimulation by needling of acupoints with many manipulating techniques. Experience suggests that if sensations, namely, "*De Qi*" (arrival of *qi*) in Chinese, including soreness, numbness, distention and heaviness are induced during treatment, the greater the effect. Therefore, most acupuncturists try to produce these sensations using many different techniques of needle manipulation in their clinical practice, such as pushing, pulling, rotating, and twirling the needles. Lin et al. reported that the points in which such sensations can be induced contain small vessels intertwined with small nerve bundles, nerve endings, and even nerve thick trunks or branches [10]. Stimulating skeletal muscle produces mostly the sensation of distention, stimulating the nervous trunk or a main branch usually creates soreness and numbness, stimulating blood vessels usually induces pain, and stimulating tendon or periosteum leads to a feeling of soreness.

It is interesting that different needling manipulations [11], for instance, pulling-pushing and rotating or twirling, were demonstrated to activate different types of somatic sensory receptors. Even the primary afferent fibers activated by the various manipulations are also different from one another [12]. It is well known that the physiological responses produced by the activation of different kinds of primary afferent fibers [13] are clearly different.

There are several methods of needle insertion, such as perpendicular, oblique, and horizontal insertions. The three methods of insertion differ in what is stimulated by each. For example, perpendicular insertion stimulates the receptors in both skin and muscle; while horizontal insertion stimulates only cutaneous sensory receptors. Therefore, it is possible that different results will be achieved by a given inserting method.

References

1. The college of TCM, The review of current literatures on the research of meridians. Page 51–81. 1979.
2. Zhou PH, Qian PD, Huang DK, Gu HY, Wang HR. The relationship between acupoints on channels and peripheral nerves. Symposium 1 of National Conference on Acupuncture and Moxibustion and Acupunctural Analgesia. Page 233, 1979.
3. Hu PR and Zhao ZY. A topographically anatomic study on the main acupoints of triple warmer channel of Hand-shaoyang. Learned journal of Jinzhou College of Medicine. (3): 1–10, 1980.
4. Yang f, Ren SZ. The regularity of the relationship between acupoints and innvertion. Research on acupuncture and moxibustion and acupunctural analgesia. Scientific Press (China), page 441–445, 1986.
5. Dept. of Physiology of Zunyi College of Medicine. Symposium 2 of National Cofference on Acupuncture and Moxibustion and Acupunctural Analgesia. Press of People's Health, 165, 1979.
6. Shanghai Second College of Medcine et al. Symposium 1 of National Cofference on Acupuncture and Moxibustion and Acupunctural Analgesia. Page 236, 1979.
7. Leem JW et al. Cutanious sensory receptors in the rat foot. J of Neurophysiol. 69(5): 1993.
8. Coote JH et al. The reflex nature of the pressor response to muscular exercise. J Physiol.(London) 215: 789–804, 1970.
9. Horeyseck G and Janig W. Activation and inhibition of vasoconstrictors in skin and muscle nerves upon stimulation of skin receptors. Proc. Intern. Congr. Physiol. Sci. Munich (9): 26, 1971.
10. Lin WZ, Xu HM, Wang ZY, Dai JC, Chen GM, Shen JY. Observation on the structures of needling sensations of acupoints and their afferent pathway in the human body. Research on acupuncture and moxibustion and acupunctural analgesia. Scientific Press (China), page 323–330, 1986.
11. Dong QS, Dong XM, Li HM, Chen D, Xian MQ. The relations between acupuncture manipulations and responsive discharges of deep receptors. Acupuncture Research (1): 75–82, 1993

12. Dong QS, Dong XM. Relation between acupuncture manipulations and afferent fibers of muscular nerves. Shanghai Journal of Acupuncture (1): 37–41, 1989
13. Fussey I et al. Evoked activity in afferent sympath nerves in response to peripheral nerve stimulation in the dog. J Physiol.(London) 200: 77P-78P, 1969.
14. Meng ZW, Origination and formation of theory of meridian system and its prospects. Chinese Acupuncture (5): 25–28, 1982)

Application of Acupuncture in the Treatment of Diseases of the Elderly

TCM attributes the pathological changes in older persons to the impaired *zangfu* organs resulting from insufficiency of *qi*, blood, "vital energy", and "resistant factors" with age. Therefore, the old people are physiologically different from other adults and manifest a specific pathophysiology of disease development as described below:
▶ Insidious onset of disease due to deficiency of *qi* and blood
▶ Simultaneous attack by several diseases, of which most are chronic
▶ Tendency to become suddenly worse based on imbalance of *yin* and *yang*
▶ Tendency to be invaded by pathogens, manifested as tendency to develop both excessive and insufficient TCM physiologic properties

Health and longevity have been the foremost desires of all people since antiquity. People have been continuously seeking methods to prolong life and prevent diseases and aging. For the elderly, disease is the major cause of death. In ancient times, the Chinese developed many methods of treating and preventing diseases of the elderly, of which acupuncture is both effective and simple. In the following sections, we will discuss the treatment and the prevention of diseases of older individuals by acupuncture.

Coronary Heart Disease

Coronary heart disease (CHD) is characterized by myocardial ischemia, hypoxia or necrosis induced mainly by coronary atherosclerosis. In TCM, CHD belongs the categories of obstruction of *qi* in the chest, angina pectoris, and precordial pain with cold limbs. The major clinical manifestations are angina pectoris and myocardial infarction.
There are mainly four causes of the disease according to TCM described below:
▶ Pathogenic "cold invasion" plus essential deficiency of *yang* in the chest, which lead to coronary vasoconstriction and, finally, obstruction of the heart channel.
▶ Internal damage due to seven modes of emotions.
▶ Improper diet including excessive consumption of fatty foods with sweet and heavy flavors, resulting in stagnation of "phlegm" and "turbid fluid".
▶ Insufficient *yang* in both kidney and heart due to impaired physiological function with age.

Etiology and Symptomatology of CHD According to TCM

▶ Obstruction of *yang* in the chest: palpitations and cardiac pain with an "oppressive" feeling in the chest or chest pain radiating to the back which is worse with cold, cold limbs, a pale, thick tongue, and a deep, slow pulse.
▶ Stagnation of *qi* and blood stasis: a fixed stabbing pain in the chest, depression, dark lips, a dark-red tongue with petechiae, and a "taut" and uneven pulse.
▶ Internal stagnation of "phlegm" and "turbid fluid": a sensation of fullness in the chest, dyspnea, sputum production, anorexia, abdominal distention, a pale tongue with a white, sticky coating, and a "slippery" pulse.

Treatment

▶ Main acupoints are divided into two groups which are stimulated alternately.
  ▶ *Xinshu* (B15), *Jujue* (), *Xinping* (2 cun above *shaohai* [])
  ▶ *Neiguan* (P6), *Juejinshu* (), *Tanzhong* (R).
▶ Supplementary acupoints:
  ▶ for the deficiency of *yang*, *Guanyuan* or *Dazhui*
  ▶ for the stagnation of "phlegm", *Fenglong* or *Feishu*
  ▶ for the stagnation of qi and blood, *Geshu* or *Xuehai*, *Qihai*, or *Zusanli*.
▶ Manipulations: Gentle stimulation, for patients with these deficiencies cold moxibustion can be used. After the arrival of *qi*, the needles are scraped at the points on the back for 2 minutes and retained at the limb points for about twenty minutes.
▶ The course of treatment: once a day for a total of ten treatments, which is followed by another course of treatment after a 3–5 day interval.

Brief Review

There is much evidence for the treatment of coronary heart diseases(CHD) by acupuncture in China. Wang et al. [1] treated 1300 cases of CHD by puncturing at several major points, such as *shenmen*, and *laogong*. A good response was obtained in 798 cases, some response in 430 cases, and no effect in 92 cases. Liu et al. [2] selected the *xinshu*, *jueyinshu*, *neiguan* and *tanzhong* acupuncture points. They used an "even reinforcing-reducing" method once a day for ten treatments. After total two courses, the cure rates were 92.31%, 62.50% and 62.51% for angina pectoris, arrhythmias and other EKG disorders respectively. Using the *xinshu*, *jueyinshu*, *neiguan*, *xishang*, *yanglingquan*, and *sanyinjiao* as major points, Xu et al. [3] treated 160 cases of CHD with two courses each, which consisted of 15 treatments given once a day. Angina symptom improvement was obtained in 89.4%, cure in 87.9%, and disappearance of arrhythmias occurred in 64.3%. Furthermore, many studies on the underlying mechanism of the treatment of CHD by acupuncture have also been performed in mainland China in the past several decades. Many factors, including SOD [4], norepinephrine, epinephrine [5], cAMP[6], myocardial consumption of oxygen, free fatty acid, glucose [7], and the sympathetic nervous system[8] were shown to be involved in the improvement caused by acupuncture or electric acupuncture in cardiac function in animals with myocardial ischemia or infarction.

References

1. Wang ZH. Treating 1300 cases of angina pectoris in the patients with CHD by needling mainly at *shenmen, laogong* and *houxi* points. Liaoning Journal of TCM (3): 39, 1992
2. Xu GG, Li XD, Lou FX, Wang J, Wang RH, Wu GR, Wen Y and Xue XP. Clinical investigation on the treatment of 32 cases of CHD by acupuncture. Anhui Clinical Journal of TCM 7(1): 1–3, 1995
3. Liu FQ. Analysis of clinical curative effects on the treatment of 160 cases of CHD by acupuncture. Clinical Journal of Acupuncture and Moxibustion 13(6):20–21, 1997
4. Yu XC, Fu WX, Song LM and Meng JB. Investigation on acupuncture-induced change of SOD in blood of coronary sinus in the dogs with experimental myocardial ischemia. Chinese Journal of Pathophysiology 7(2): 206–207, 1991
5. Liu JL, Zhang ZL, Liu JL and Chen SP. Effect of acupuncture on plasma monoaminal neurotransmitter in the rabbits with acute myocardial ischmemia. Chinese Acupuncture and Moxibustion (10): 604–605, 1997
6. Wu XP, Huang EM, Wang YW, Liu YX, Yan SX and Hu P. Effect of acupuncture on levels of myocardial cAMP and cGMP in the rabbits with acute myocardial ischemia. Shanghai Journal of Acupuncture and Moxibustion 15(1): 36–37, 1996
7. Gao CH, Meng JB, Fu WX and Song LM. Effects of electric acupuncture at "Neiguan" points on the metabolism of glucose and free fatty acid in the dogs with myocardial ischemia and angina pectoris. Acupuncture Research 15(1): 66–69, 1991
8. Zhang JL, Cao QS, Chen SP and Liu JL. Regulating role played by sympathetic neurons of upper thoracic segment in the relation between "Neiguan" and heart. Chinese Journal of Traditional Medical Science and Technology (1): 6–9, 1996

Essential Hypertension

Hypertension is a common disease in older people. It is characterized by a high arterial pressure (systolic pressure ≥140 or diastolic pressure ≥90 mmHg) and which is also implicated in other disorders. The major symptoms are headache, dizziness, palpitation, dysphoria, insomnia, and lassitude. In later stages, various symptoms may occur based on the degree of damage to organs such as heart, brain, and kidney.

Etiology and Symptomatology of Hypertension According to TCM

▶ Excess of "liver-*yang*": Symptoms: dizziness, headache, tinnitus, distention of the head, tendency to easily lose one's temper, insomnia, erythema of the face and conjunctivae, constipation, erythematous tongue with a yellow coating, and a "taut", rapid, and "forceful" pulse.
▶ Stagnation of "phlegm" due to deficiency of "spleen": Symptoms: dizziness, headache, sensation of "heaviness" and distention of the head, lassitude, sensation of fullness in the chest, sputum production, anorexia, somnolence, a thick and pale tongue with a white, sticky coating, and a "taut and slippery" pulse.
▶ Insufficiency of *yin* of the kidney and liver: Symptoms: dizziness, headache, tinnitus, blurry vision, sensations of excessive warmth in palms and soles, sensations of weakness in the loins and legs, a red tongue with loss of coating, and a "taut", "thin" and rapid pulse.

Treatment

▶ Main points: *quchi, taichong,* and *zusanli.* Supplementary points: For excess of "liver-*yang*", *fengchi, taiyang* plus ear-points: "groove" for the lowering of blood pressure, hypo-cortex, Liver point, Subcortex point.
▶ For stagnation of "phlegm", *fenglong, pishu* plus ear-points: "groove" for the lowering blood pressure, Spleen point.

▶ For "insufficiency" of the kidney and liver, *sanyinjiao, shenshu, ganshu* plus ear-points: the "groove" for the lowering of blood pressure, Kidney, Liver. and Adrenal gland points.

The main (basic) points and supplementary points are stimulated simultaneously with medium intensity "pulling-pushing" and "rotating-twirling" manipulations once every other day or twice weekly, for a total of four treatments. Three continuous courses can be administered.

Brief Review

Acupuncture has often been suggested to be effective in the treatment of essential hypertension in China by both clinical experience and experimental studies. Zhang et al. [1] reported that the systolic and diastolic pressures of patients with essential hypertension were significantly reduced by acupuncture only at bilateral *quchi* points. By stimulating *Zanzhu* points with even-reinforcing-reducing manipulation, Yao et al. [2] satisfactory treated hypertensive patients. In another study, 83 hypertensive patients were punctured at *xin* ear points. Of the 83 cases, 98% were successfully treated [3]. Needling bilateral *shugu* was also shown to be satisfactory in the treatment of hypertension. In addition, modalities such as ear-acupuncture [4], capping [5], moxibustion [6] and scalp acupuncture [7] were also shown to be useful. Further studies on the mechanisms underlying acupuncture suggest that acupuncture effectively treats hypertension by improving blood rheology and microcirculation[8], reducing total pressure resistance[3] and the level of plasma angiotensin II [9].

References

1. Zhang SJ, Ji QS and Li J. The observation on curative effect and changes of rheoencephalogram in the patient with hypertension by acupuncture at quchi points. Zhejiang Journal of TCM 25(12): 559–560, 1990
2. Yao WH, and Liu HX. Clinical observation on the immediate reduction of blood pressure by needling at *Zanzhu* points. Journal of TCM 35(6): 340, 1994
3. Yan J, Li WL, Yi SX, Wang JJ, Wang LH, Yao XX and Chen AP. The observation of the curative effect of activation of propagation of sensation on 85 cases of hypertension. Hubei Journal of TCM (3): 41, 1987
4. Huang HQ and Liang SZ. Chinese Journal of integrated Traditional and Western Medicine 11(11): 654–656, 1991
5. Zhang C, Zhao N, Wang QM, Liu W and Li J. The preliminary observation on the effect of fire-capping on the blood pressure. Chinese Acupuncture and Moxibustion 10(3): 46, 1990
6. Chen Q. The treatment of 132 cases of hypertension by the combination of moxibustion at baihui point and Compressing ear-points. Chinese Acupuncture and Moxibustion 11(1): 6, 1991
7. Fang YP, Fang BZ and DU MX. The observation on the curative effect of hypertension induced by scalp-acupuncture. Chinese Acupuncture and Moxibustion 8(4): 2–5, 1988
8. Chen Q and Zhou YP. The effect of acupuncture on nail microcirculation in the patients with hypertension. Journal of Anhui College of TCM 9(3): 49–51, 1990
9. Wang T, Lu YM, Cheng KM and Wang L. Change of angiotensin II in the regulation of blood pressure by acupuncture. Acupuncture Research (4): 285–291, 1982

Diabetes Mellitus

Diabetes mellitus can be divided into 2 types: essential and secondary. Essential is more commonly seen in the elderly, and most are non-insulin-dependent. Diabetes mellitus is similar to the syndrome "*xiaoke*" in TCM. The disease is characterized by the symptoms of polydipsia, polyphagia, polyuria and "*magersucht*"(pathologic leanness).

Etiology and Symptomatology of Diabetes Mellitus According to TCM

► Excessive "heat" due to deficiency of *yin*: Thirst, preference for cold drinks,, excessive hunger and overeating, irascibility, polyuria, a red or yellow urine, constipation, a red dry tongue with a yellow coating, and a fast and "slippery" pulse.
► Deficiency of both *qi* and *yin*: Thirst with dry mouth, weakness of the loins and legs, palpitations, excessive perspiration, dizziness, tinnitus, blurry vision, a thick tongue with teeth-marks on the edges and a white coating, and a "deep, thin" pulse.
► Insufficiency of *yin* and *yang*: Cold limbs, cold intolerance, pallor, tinnitus, mid-abdominal pain, occasionally fever and night sweats, thirst, impotence, polyuria with a turbid urine, a pallid tongue with a white, dry coating, and a "deep", "thin" and weak pulse.

Treatment

► Main acupoints: *zusanli, qihai, shenshu, pishu*
► Supplementary acupoints: for heavy thirst, *zhigou*; and excessive hunger and polyphagia, *zhongwan* and *tianshu*; for polyuria, *guanyuan*;
► Manipulations: "even reinforcing and reducing" at the main acupoints until the arrival of *qi*, followed by retention needles for 30 minutes; "reducing" at the supplementary acupoints
► Course of treatment: once every other day or twice per week. One course includes seven treatments, and three continuous courses can be administered.

Brief Review

In China, treatment of diabetes mellitus by acupuncture can be traced back to ancient times. The first case of treatment mentioned in an academic journal was described in the 1950s. During the 1960s and 70s, reports gradually increased. Since the 1980s, an increasing number of articles detailing both clinical practice and experimental investigation exploring mechanisms underlying treatment of diabetes mellitus by acupuncture have been published. Zhou et al. [1] demonstrated through levels of blood and urine glucose that acupuncture can be used as a first-line therapy for diabetes. Other symptoms in 178 patients with type II of diabetes were improved after acupuncture. The cure rate was 94.9%. Additional studies [2–4] achieved similar results using *Sanyinjiao* points. Experimental [5, 6] and clinical investigation [2] suggested that the effects of acupuncture were mediated by the biphasic regulation of pancreatic α-cell function.

References

1. Zhou C, Li XZ and Chang BZ. Treatment of 178 cases of type II of diabetes mellitus by the combination of pressed needles with body acupuncture. Chinese Acupuncture and Moxibustion (1): 38, 1998
2. Zhu XF. Clinical study on the treatment of 246 cases of diabetes by acupuncture. Chinese Acupuncture and Moxibustion (1): 5–6, 1991
3. Hou AL. observation on the change of blood glucose in the diabetes patients after acupuncture at sanyinjiao points. Zhejiang Journal of TCM 28(9): 411, 1993
4. Guo GZ, Xu GL and Li DL. Clinical study on the effect of acupuncture on blood glucose. Jilin Journal of Traditional Chinese Medicine (3): 19, 1990

5. Kang SY, Xiong XH and Lin J. Effect of acupuncture at different time on the sugar tolerance of normal rats. Shanghai Journal of Acupuncture and Moxibustion 15(4): 33–34, 1996
6. Guo SC, Du FT, Wang JY and Zhang TQ. Observation on thee curative effect of acupuncture on diabetes. Shannxi Journal of Chinese Traditional Medicine 13(10): 460–461, 1992

Paralysis Agitans (Parkinson's Disease)

Paralysis agitans or Parkinson's disease is characterized by tremor, muscular rigidity, slow motion, and loss of postural reflexes. Slow onset, gradual progression, and long duration are the main clinical features of the disease. Most patients suffering from the disease are 50 to 65 years of age. *Paralysis agitans* is categorized in TCM by a "tremor syndrome" which is induced, in TCM theory, by liver dysfunction, and pathogenic "wind" and "dampness". Symptoms:

▶ Tremor: a tremor occurs in one upper limb initially and gradually develops in other limbs, the lips, tongue, and finally the head in the most severe cases. The tremor becomes more severe with rest and stress.
▶ Muscle rigidity leading to postural deficits including: antiverted head, flexion of the trunk, elbow, and metacarpophalangeal joints, and muscular hypertonia resulting in "lead-pipe rigidity".
▶ Bradykinesia and loss of attitudinal reflex, loss of voluntary motion, hypomimia ("mask-like faces") and loss of nictitation (ability to wink). Difficulty in initiating movement and "festinating gait".

Etiology and Symptomatology of Parkinson's Disease According to TCM

▶ "Wind stirring" due to "phlegm-heat": tremor, hypomimia, and decreasased motion, a sensation of "fullness" and "oppression" in the chest, cough, yellow sputum, dry feces, yellow urine, a red tongue with a yellow, greasy coating, and a taut and "greasy" pulse.
▶ Deficiency of *qi* and blood: tremor: flexion of the limbs, dizziness, palpitationd, lassitude, a thick tongue with teeth-marks at the edge, and a "deep", "thin", and weak pulse.
▶ Insufficient "vital essence" of liver and kidney: tremor, bradykinesia, dizziness, tinnitus, weakness of the loins and legs, a pallid, red tongue with decreased coating, a "taut and thin" or a "thin and rapid" pulse.

Treatment

▶ Main acupoints: *hegu, waiguan, fengchi, quchi, waigua, yangliquan*, and scalp acupuncture to the "chorea-trembling-controlling area".
▶ Supplementary points: for "wind stirring" due to "phlegm-heat", *fenglong, pishu, taichong*; for deficiency of *qi* and blood, *qihai, xuehai, geshu, pishu*; for insufficient "vital essence" of liver and kidney: *taixi, ganshu, yongquan, taichong*.
▶ Manipulations: for "wind stirring" due to "phlegm-heat": administering primarily a "reducing manipulation" method; and for the other twor syndromes, primarily a "reinforcing" method. Four continuous courses of ten treatments each, once or twice a day.

Brief Review

A satisfactory effect of acupuncture on 30 cases of Parkinson's disease was reported by Qin et al. In their study, *sishencong, fengchi, hegu, yanglingquan*, and *taichong* were the main acupoints. The treatment was performed once every other day. After 30 treatments, symptoms were improved to varying degrees in 24 cases. No improvement was achieved in only 6 cases following acupuncture [1].

Another investigation of 42 cases of *paralysis agitans* treated by electric acupuncture plus acupoint injection of vitamin B_1 and B_{12} was performed by Tao and Zhang. Improvement was achieved in 93% (39 of 42 cases) [2]. Liu et al. reported that *paralysis agitans* can also be treated by the combination of body acupuncture with scalp acupuncture, achieving symptomatic improvement in 79.9% of 159 cases [3]. A comparable result was demonstrated by Xie and Jiang in 56 patients treated similarly with body and scalp acupuncture [4].

Data from other studies [5] further support the results of clinical trials. Acupuncture may achieve its curative effect through improvement of cerebral circulation [6], regulation of the activity of SOD [7] and alteration of levels of neurotransmitters, such as DA and NE [8], and TH [9].

References

1. Qin LF and Qian DH. The treatment of *paralysis agitans* by acupuncture. Chinese Acupuncture and Moxibustion 9(6): 16, 1989
2. Tao HY and Zhang M. Treatment of *paralysis agitans* by electric acupuncture and point-injection. Chinese Acupuncture and Moxibustion 9(5): 17, 1989
3. Liu JY, Ren XQ, Liu AH, Yu MJ, Yang JH, Chen GP, Zhang LX and Jiang DS. Observation on the curative effect of acupuncture on *paralysis agitans*. Clinical Journal of Acupuncture and Moxibustion 9(5): 10–11, 1993
4. Xie YF, Jiang DS. Clinical investigation on the treatment 56 cases of Parkinson's disease by TCM. Chinese Journal of Integrated Traditional and Western Medicine 13(8): 490, 1993
5. Luo MF and Wang P. Experimental study on the treatment of *paralysis agitans* by electric acupuncture. Chinese Acupuncture and Moxibustion 14(5): 39–49, 1994
6. Wang LL, He C, Zhao M, Liu YG, Zhuang XL. Effect of aucpuncture on the cerebral blood flow in the patients with Parkinson's disease. Chinese Acupuncture and Moxibustion 19(2): 115–117, 1999
7. Zhang L, Xi GF, Yu HZ. Effect of the combined acupuncture with herbal drugs on the level of plasma SOD in the patients with Parkinson's disease. Shanghai Journal of Acupuncture and Moxibustion 15(6): 3–4, 1996
8. He C, Wang LL, Dong HT, Wang JM, Ma P. Effect of acupuncture on cerebral level of monoaminal neurotransmitters in the rats with experimental Parkinson's disease. Acupuncture Research 23(1): 44–48, 1998
9. Luo MF, Wang ZY, Wang P. Effect of electric acupuncture on TH of nigral substance and marrow of adrenal gland in the rats with experimental paralysis agitans. Acupuncture Research 22(4): 292–294, 1997

Sequelae of Cerebrovascular Accidents

"Sequelae" refer to symptoms such as hemiplegia, slurred speech, and deviation of the mouth and eyes following an acute cerebrovascular accident, which are divided into two types, ischemic and hemorrhagic. In TCM, these are considered the result of a "stroke of wind".

Clinical symptoms include hemiplegia, numbness of the muscles and skin, slurred speech or aphasia, deviation of the mouth and eyes, numbness, weakness, and atrophy or apraxia of the limbs.

Etiology and Symptomatology of Stroke According to TCM

▶ Sudden asthenia of "liver-*yang*" and disturbing "upward" effect of "wind-heat" on the brain: hemiplegia, deviation of the month and tongue, rigidity of the tongue, slurred speech, dizziness, headache, bitter taste, a pharyngeal sensation of dryness, dysphoria, and irascibility, a red tongue with a thin yellow coating, and a "taut, forceful" pulse.

▶ Obstruction of channels by "wind-phlegm" and "blood stasis": hemiplegia, deviation of the mouth and tongue, rigidity of the tongue, slurred speech, dizziness, hemianesthesia, discoloration of the tongue with a white coating, and a "taut and slippery" pulse.

▶ Deficiency of *qi* with "blood stasis": hemiplegia, deviation of the mouth and tongue, rigidity of the tongue, slurred speech, hemianesthesia, a pale face, palpitations, dyspnea, loose stool, distention of the limbs, a pale and discolored tongue with a white coating, and a "thin, deep" pulse.

▶ "Stirring of wind" due to deficiency of *yin*: hemiplegia, deviation of month and tongue, rigidity of the tongue, slurred speech, dizziness, hemianesthesia, insomnia, warmth of the palms and soles, erythema or loss of color and loss of coating of the tongue, and a "taut and thin" pulse.

Treatment

▶ Main acupoints: *Baihui, fengfu, zusanli, yanglingquan* plus scalp acupuncture areas such as the contralateral motor area, sensory area, foot motor and sensory areas, and speech area.

▶ Supplementary points: for paralysis of the upper limbs, *jianyu, quchi, waiguan hegu*; for paralysis of lower limbs*: huantiao, zusanlli*, and yanglingquan; for the deviation of month, *dicang, jiache*; for slurred speech: *yamen, lianquan*; for dizziness: *fengchi, fenglong, taichong*.

▶ Manipulation: "even reinforcing-reducing "manipulation, stimulating unaffected limbs and/or diseased limbs, with retention of needles for 30 minutes, once a day for a total of 30 sessions as a course of treatment.

Brief Review

It is well known that acupuncture has been frequently used to treat the sequelae of stroke for many years in China. The results are very satisfactory, especially in the treatment of hemiplegia and the slurred speech. Using acupuncture, Luo showed significant improvements of hemiplegia, facial paralysis, slurred speech, muscle strength, and activities of daily living in 157 stroke patients lasting from 2–270 days [1]. It is interesting that "great" acupuncture produced a much better curative effect than "tan-puncturing" [2]. Moreover, *ziwuliuzhu*, a special point-selecting method, was shown to be helpful in reinforcing the curative effect of acupuncture on the sequelae of stroke [3]. Even in the treatment of acute stroke, acupuncture may also be beneficial [4, 5]. Acupuncture may produce its effect by altering TXA2/PGI2 [6], SOD [7], NO [8] and cAMP

[9], improving micro-circulation [6]. Further studies indicated that the effects may depend on temporal factors, such as time of onset of treatment, duration of treatment, intervals between courses of treatment, and needle retention time [10].

References

1. Luo XG. Treatment of 73 cases of hemiplegia in the patients attacked by stroke by the combination of acupuncture and movement. Journal of Guiyang College of TCM 19(3): 53–54, 1997
2. Liu GT and Xiao YJ. The influence of electric needling "*JUCI*" on nail-bed microcirculation of apoplectic patients. Acupuncture Research 15(1): 40, 1990
3. Zhang R, Pang LD, Xia YL and Yao JH. Effect of method of "*zi-wu-liu-zhu-na-jia-fa*" on the nail-bed microcirculation in 68 cases of stroke with hemiparalysis. Shanghai Journal of Acupuncture and Moxibustion (1):10–11, 1992
4. Hu GQ and Shi XM. Basic research on the treatment of stroke by the manipulation of "dredging and waking brain". Chinese Acupuncture and Moxibustion (2): 33–35, 1992
5. Zhou CS, Wu XL, Kong DQ, Wang RJ, Liu YM and Song QZ. The clinical observation on acupuncture-induced changes of activity of SOD in the patients with ischemic stroke. Chinese Acupuncture and Moxibustion (6): 19–20, 1993
6. Li F, Dong JY, Guo CJ, Jiao XM and Yin KJ. Effect of electric acupuncture on TXB2, 6-keto-PGFIa in the rats with acute ischemic cerebral apoplexy(cerebral infarction). Journal of Fourth University of Military Medicine 18(3): 228–230, 1997
7. Zhao YG, Li P, Zhao LR, Gao X and Qian GQ. Changes of circulating endothelia cells of blood in the rabbits with cerebral infarction followed by reperfusion and the effect of acupuncture. Journal of Micro-circulation 6(2): 5–6, 1996
8. Xu GN, Xu GS, Zhong P, Wang LF Zhu SL and Chen QZ. Effect of electric acupuncture at *Du* meridian on content of nitric oxide and endothelin in the rats with acute cerebral ischemia. Acupuncture Research 21(3): 18–21, 1996
9. Yang J, Li HX, Wu YS and Xu LT. Effect of electric acupuncture on cAMP/cGMP and angiotensin II in the rabbits with acute cerebral ischemia. Chinese Acupuncture and Moxibustion (5): 38–40, 1996
10. He SM, Zhu CJ, Ma XL, Yang M. Discussion on the correlation between the curative effects and "time"-related factors during the treatment of stroke by acupuncture. Chinese Acupuncture and Moxibustion (12): 757, 1999

Dementia

Dementia is characterized by decreased abilities of memory, judgment, calculation, and speech, often accompanied by emotional disturbance. Symptoms include short-term memory loss, confusion, wandering, getting lost in familiar places, urinary or fecal incontinence, behavioral disturbance, such as laughing or crying inappropriately, dysphasia, dyspraxia, and difficulty in handling finances and following directions. There are two common causes of dementia in older people, Alzheimer's disease and multi-infarct dementia. Alzheimer's disease is the most common cause of dementia in older persons. Alzheimer's disease develops when nerve cells in the brain die. Symptoms begin slowly and become steadily worse. At this time, no one knows what causes the nerve cells to die, and there is no cure for the disease. The second most common cause of dementia in older people is multi-infarct dementia. Multi-infarct dementia usually affects people between the ages of 60 and 75. Multi-infarct dementia is caused by a series of strokes that damage or destroy brain tissue. Symptoms that begin suddenly may suggest multi-infarct dementia.

Etiology and Symptomatology of Dementia According to TCM

According to TCM dementia is divided into following types:
▶ Deficiency of "vital essence" of kidney: Apathy, depression, decreased intelligence, gait disorder, a sensation lack of warmth of the limbs, flushing of the face, impotence, urinary and fecal incontinence, pallor of the tongue with loss of coating, and a "deep," "thin," or weak pulse.

▶ Deficiency of both *qi* and blood: Depression, loss of speech, reduction of intelligence, apathy, retardation, daytime sleepiness and nighttime insomnia, anxiety, a sallow complexion, pallor of the nails and tongue, and a "thin" and weak pulse.

▶ Obstruction of brain by "phlegm": A "trance-like" state, weight gain, apathy, loss of intelligence, cough and sputum production, snoring, slurred speech, rigidity of the tongue, increase in thickness and pallor of the tongue with a white greasy coating, and a "deep" and "slippery" pulse.

▶ Hyperactivity of "liver-*yang*": Dizziness, distention of the head, erythema and flushing of the face, forgetfulness, dysphoria, and irascibility, tinnitus, distention of the eyes, numbness of the limbs and difficulty with movement, erythema of the tongue with a thin yellow coating, and a "taut" and "forceful" pulse.

▶ Hyperactivity of *yang* due to deficiency of *yin*: Dizziness, a sensation of excessive warmth in five areas(both palms, soles, and heart), forgetfulness, sleep disturbance, thirst but aversion to drinking, numbness, atrophic muscles, weakness of the loins and legs, an erythematous tongue with a decreased coating, and a "taut" and "thin" pulse.

Treatment

▶ Main acupoints: *neiguan, shenmen, baihui, dazhui, fengfu, xuanzhong*
▶ Supplementary acupoints:
  ▸ For deficiency of "vital essence" of kidney: *shenshu, juegu, zusanli*; using mainly the "reinforcing" method.
  ▸ For deficiency of both qi and blood: *ganshu, tangzhong, geshu, qihai*; using mainly the "reinforcing" method.
  ▸ For obstruction by "phlegm": *fenglong, laogong*; using mainly the "reducing" method.
  ▸ For hyperactivity of "liver-*yang*", *taichong, fengchi;* using mainly the "reducing" method.
  ▸ For excessive "liver-*yang*" due to deficiency of *yin*: *taixi, ganshu, sanyingjiao*, using both the "reinforcing" and "reducing" methods, with retention of the needles for 20 minutes, once a day, for 30 sessions of treatment.

Brief Review

In the past few decades, an increasing number of studies have investigated the use of acupuncture in dementia. Many acupuncture-related therapeutic methods including body acupuncture, electric acupuncture, acupoint-injection, capping and the combination of acupuncture with herbal drugs. etc. have been utilized. Stimulating *zhongwan, fenglong, neiguan* and *fengchi* points with a "rotating-twirling" and "even reinforcing-reducing" manipulation, Liu et al. showed symptomatic improvement by about 90% in a total of 50 cases [1]. Electrical acupuncture was also shown to cure 68.3% of a total of 60 cases [2]. Twenty-three of 25 cases were significantly improved by injection of cytidine diphosphocholine at acupoints including *shenting, touwei, meishong* etc. [3]. In another study, 16 of a total 18 patients were improved by "capping" along the *Du* and "bladder" channels of "foot-*taiyang*" [4]. Acupuncture, together with herbal medicines, were also an effective therapeutic method [5]. Modulating cholinergic receptors [6], promoting the cerebral circulation [1], and regulating the cerebral ratio of cAMP/cGMP [7] and TX2/PGI2 [8] may be important factors in the effect of acupuncture.

References

1. Liu HA, Hou DF, Diao ZY and Wang Y. Clinical observation and study of mechanism on the treatment of vascular dementia by acupuncture with manipulation of resolving turbidity and enhancing intelligence. Chinese Acupuncture and Moxibustion 17(9): 521–525, 1997
2. Liu J, Peng XH, Lin DD, Li CD, Jiang ZY, Zeng L, Jia SJ, Liao SL and Li YK. Clinical investigation of the treatment of vascular dementia by scalp-acupuncture. Chinese Acupuncture and Moxibustion 18(4): 197, 1998
3. Yang YH and Zhang JF. Treatment of 25 cases of vascular dementia by injection at scalp acupoints. Hubei Journal of TCM 19(5): 43, 1997
4. Yang ZZ. Treatment of 18 cases of senile dementia by moved capping at the points of back *shu*. New Journal of Traditional Chinese Medicine 28(12): 31, 1996
5. Liang Z, Wu TQ and Hu L. Treatment of senile dementia by the combination of acupuncture with herbal medicine. Chinese Acupuncture and Moxibustion 18(12): 712–714, 1998
6. Mo QZ, Gong B, Fang J, Li JP, Huang JT, Chen KH, Kuang XW and Wang JM. Influence of acupuncture at zusanli on function of 5-HT and M-receptor at rat's brain and spleen. Acupuncture Research 19(1): 33–36, 1994
7. Fang J, Gong B, Mo QZ, Li JD, Kuang XW and Xu WD. influence of acupuncture at zusanli on cyclic necleotide contents of plasma, and different brain regions and spleen in rats. Acupuncture Research 19(1): 42–45, 1994
8. Li YH, Zhuang XL Zheng Q and Yang WH. Clinical investigation on the treatment of vascular dementia. Chinese Acupuncture and Moxibustion 18(11): 645–647, 1998

Benign Prostatic Hypertrophy (BPH)

BPH, a common disease in older male people, is clinically manifested as polyuria, hesitancy, incontinence, hematuria, and urinary retention(uroschesis). This is similar to the category of dysuria and incontinence in TCM. According to the western medicine, BPH may be induced primarily by reduction of the level of testosterone in the elderly. In TCM theory, there are several mechanisms mediating the development of the disease: excessive lung "heat", caudal flow of pathogenic "damp-heat", sinking of *qi* in the "middle warmer, reduced *yin* of kidney, and deficiency of "kidney-*yang*".

Etiology and Symptomatology of BPH According to TCM

▶ Excessive "heat" of the lung: Tenesmus of the bladder, dysuria, anuria, dry throat and mouth, thirst, polydipsia, cough with sticky sputum, shallow, rapid respiration, a red tongue with a thin yellow coating, and a rapid pulse.
▶ Caudal flow of pathogenic "damp-heat": Distension of the lower abdomen, hematuria, oliguria, anuria, dysuria, urethral pain, a sensation of a bitter and sticky taste, thirst but aversion to drinking, a erythematous tongue with a yellow and greasy coating, and a rapid pulse.
▶ "Sinking" of *qi* in the "middle warmer": Caudal distention of the lower abdomen, polyuria, hesitancy, incontinence, lassitude, anorexia, dyspenea, a pale tongue with a thin coating, and a "thin" and weak pulse.
▶ Impaired or "consumed" "kidney-*yin*": Poluyuria, dysuria, oliguria or anuria, dry throat, sensation of excessive warmth in the palms and soles, dizziness, insomnia, constipation, lassitude of the loins and legs, an erythematous tongue, decreased salivation, and a "thin" and rapid pulse.

▶ Insufficiency of "kidney-*yang*": Dysuria, dribbling, anuria, incontinence, pallor, dysphoria, lassitude of the loins and legs, cold intolerance, pallor of the tongue with a white coating, a "deep, thin" and weak pulse.

Treatment

▶ Main acupoints: *zusanli, zhongji, sanyinjiao, ba liao,* (for the puncturing *zhongji* point, it will be best to strongly and repeatedly stimulate the point, producing paresthesias radiating to the perineal region or the penis).
▶ For excessive lung "heat": *shaoshang, yuji,* using the "reducing" method. For downwards flow of damp-heat, *taichong, quchi, fenglong,* using the reducing method
▶ For "sinking" of *qi* in the "middle warmer": *tanzhong qihai, pishu,* through the "reinforcing" method
▶ For impaired or depleted "kidney-*yin*": *shenshu, taixi, sanyinjiao,* using primarily the "reducing" method
▶ For insufficiency of "kidney-*yang*": using the "reducing" method plus moxibustion

The treatments are once a day or every other day. Each course consists of 14 treatments. Three course are given with a 3–5 day interval between each course.

Brief Review

The treatments of both BPH and chronic prostatitis by acupuncture have been frequently reported together, as many patients suffer from both disorders. It was demonstrated by Ma that alleviating symptoms of chronic prostatitis by needling the relieves BPH symptoms [1]. Similar result were also achieved by Lin in 68 cases of chronic prostatitis [2]. Hu and Wang effectively treated 87.17% of 39 patients with BPH by needling and moxibustion [3]. Wu et al. significantly improved 27 of 30 cases of BPH by a combination of needling and drugs. In this study, only three cases did not show improvement [4].

References

1. Ma S. Analysis on the treatment of chronic prostatitis by needling and moxibustion with drugs. Chinese Acupuncture and Moxibustion (6): 339–340, 1999
2. Lin YP. Observation on the treatment of 68 cases of chronic prostasis by acupuncture. Chinese Acupuncture and Moxibustion (8): 465–466, 1999
3. Hu JF and Wang GM. The treatment of prostatic hyperplasia by acupuncture and moxibustion. Clinical Journal of Acupuncture and Moxibustion 16(11): 7–8, 2000
4. Wu CH, Shi SW and Zhang ZS. The treatment of 30 cases of prostatic hyperplasia by the combination of needling and herbal medicine. Clinical Journal of Acupuncture and Moxibustion 14(9): 15, 2000

Osteoporosis

Essential osteoporosis is a common metabolic osteopathy in post-menopausal women and men over age 70. The main symptoms are bone pain, fracture, reduced body height and kyphosis, which are induced by the hypomineralization(reduced ratio of mineral substances to bone matrix) in the bone with age or after menopause. TCM theory states that "kidney controls bone and nourishes the bone marrow" and "kidney stores 'congenital essence'". Therefore, according to TCM, essential osteoporosis is primarily the result of a deficiency of "vital *qi*" of the kidney.

Etiology and Symptomatology of Osteoporosis According to TCM

▶ Deficiency of "kidney-*yang*": Pain in the loins and back which are worse at night, a sensation of distension of the muscles on the back, fracture or kyphosis in severe cases, weakness of the lower limbs, pain in the heels with a sensation of cold on the skin around the painful area, loss of warmth of the limbs, shortness of breath, lassitude, polyuria, clear urine, pallor, pallor of the tongue with a white coating, and a "deep, thin" and weak pulse.

▶ Insufficiency of "kidney-*yin*": Soreness and pain of the flanks and back, occasional bone pain, arthralgias, sensation of excessive warmth of the pelvis and back, sensation of excessive warmth of the palms and soles, palpitations, irritability, dizziness, tinnitus, weakness of the lower limbs, erythema of the tongue with loss of coating, and a "taut, thin" and rapid pulse.

Treatment

▶ Main acupoints: *shenshu, ganshu, zusanli, hegu, dazhu*
▶ Supplementary acupoints: for deficiency of kidney-yang, dazhui, shenjue, guanyuan, minmen plus moxibustion
▶ For dificiency of "kidney-*yang*": *sanyinjiao, zhiyin, geshu, taixi*
▶ Manipulations using the "reinforcing" method, retention of needles for 20 minutes.

Treatments are once every other day for the first 3 weeks. One course is 9 treatments, and a total of four courses are administered with a 5 day interval between courses.

Brief Review

Treatment utilizing acupuncture and moxibustion targeting the kidney has used as a major therapeutic approach against osteoporosis. In China, moxibustion has been used slightly more frequently than acupuncture. Both acupuncture and moxibustion have been reported to be effective. Puncturing at *shenshu, pishu, zusanli, taibai* and *taixi* with "reinforcing" manipulation significantly improved the symptoms of osteoporosis in the elderly [1]. Lassitude, and pain in the loins and legs in patients with osteoporosis were significantly attenuated after drug-moxibustion [2]. Bone density in patients (average age =63) years was enhanced by moxibustion, possibly through its effect on the kidney [3]. Wang et al. three years later obtained similar results [4]. Acupuncture and moxibution treated osteoporosis in an animal model in which osteoporosis was induced by dexamethasone [5] and bilateral oophorectomy [6]. Some studies suggest the effect of acupuncture on osteoporosis may be mediated by alteration of hypothalamus-pituitary-adrenal gland axis function [7].

References

1. Liu Y, Wang WJ. Clinical investigation on the treatment of osteoporosis by acupuncture with the method of reinforcing kidney and strengthening spleen. Clinical Journal of Acupuncture and Moxibustion 12(7): 24–25, 1996
2. Zhang L. Study on the regulation of bone density in elderly patients by drug-moxibustion. Correspondence Journal of TCM 16(1): 35, 1997
3. Ju SS, Ding JY, Wang CH. Discussion on the regulation of bone density in senile patients by moxibustion. Clinical Journal of Acupuncture and Moxibustion 11(9): 37–38, 1995
4. Wang CH, Zhang ZH, Li F and Zhou AP. Clinical investigation on the effect of acupuncture to the density of bone in the patients with deficiency of kidney-yang. Chinese Acupuncture and Moxibustion 18(5): 270, 1998
5. Wu MS, Li E, Lin FS. Regulation of the transportation pathway of neural hormone in the rats with osteoporosis by kanggusong point-sticking agent. Journal of Hebei Univerisity of Medicine 20(1): 33–34, 1999
6. Zhao YX, Yan ZG, Shao SJ and Yu AS. Effect of acupuncture on the experimental osteoporosis. Chinese Acupuncture and Moxibustion 19(5): 301–303, 1999
7. Zhao YX, Shao SJ, Yu AS and Yan ZG. A preliminary investigation of the segmental distribution of the afferent fibers in acupoint DU-4, ovary and adrenal gland wit HRP method. Acupuncture Research 24(4): 294–296, 1999

Periarthritis of Shoulder (Scalpulohumeral Periarthritis)

Periarthritis of shoulder is an aseptic inflammation of the soft tissue around the joint of shoulder. It is manifested as progressive pain of shoulder joint accompanied by dyskinesis. The exact cause is not well understood. It may be caused by immunologic, anatomical, and hormonal factors. In TCM, it is classified as a *bi* syndrome (rheumatic pain). Moreover, the TCM theory proposes that the disease is the result of a renal disorder.

Symptoms: The patients feel pain in the anterior exterior aspect of shoulder which can radiate to the elbow, hand and scapular, and is worse at night. The abduction of the shoulder joint is limited in early stages, and there is limitation of movement of the shoulder in all directions in severe disease.

Treatment

▶ Main acupoints: *jianyu, jianfeng, jianliao, quchi, tiaokou.*
▶ For tenderness at the acromion: *yinlingquan, chize, taiyuan*
▶ For difficulty with adduction: *yanglingquan, waiguan*

Treatment consists of retention of the needles for 20 minutes or including moxibustion after arrival of the *qi*. The "even reinforcing-reducing" method is used for one minute, once every other day. A course consists of twelve treatments, and three courses are given with a 5 days interval between courses.

Brief Review

Various acupuncture and acupuncture-related therapeutic methods have been used to treat periarthritis of shoulder, including single point stimulation [1], multi-point stimulation [2], moxibustion [3], electric acupuncture [4], injection at points [5], and fire-needling [6] No one set of acupoints were used; most studies used local points around the shoulder, neck, nape and upper arms [7]. A "point-penetrating" manipulation was reported to be most effective [8].

References

1. Jiang DQ and Liu WA. The treatment of 246 cases of periarthritis of shoulder by acupuncture. Shanghai Journal of Acupuncture and Moxibustion (3): 24, 1987
2. Xin QM. The treatment of 30 cases of chronic prostasis by combination or acupuncture and radiation with TDp. Journal of Acupuncture and Moxibustion 6(1): 11, 1990
3. Chen LP. Clinical observation of the treatment of 135 cases of periarthritis of shoulder by the warming moxibustion with simple rack. Chinese Acupuncture and Moxibustion 10(4): 27–28, 1990
4. Gao XG. The observation on the treatment of periarthritis of shoulder by electric acupuncture. Jiangxi Journal of TCM (3): 37, 1987
5. Li HQ, Wang ZY, Hou DY, Wang ML and Sang RX. The observation on the treatment of 74 cases of periarthritis of shoulder by the injection with antongding at Zusanli points. Chinese Journal of Integrated Traditional and Western Medicine 10(6): 350, 1990
6. Xia XC. The treatment of 50 cases of periarthritis of shoulder by cui-puncturing at Rushu point. Hubei Journal of TCM (2): 32, 1988
7. Zou YP. The clinical observation on the treatment of periarthritis of shoulder by the moxibustion with Musk rope. Journal of Acupuncture and Moxibustion 5(4): 33, 1989
8. Li YF and Zhu W. The treatment of 200 cases or periarthritis of shoulder by needling and fire-capping at Sitou points. Journal of Acupuncture and Moxibustion 6 (3): 12, 1990

Cervical Spondylopathy

Cervical spondylosis is characterized by a series of symptoms resulting from the stimulation or compression of cervical nerve roots, spinal cord, cervical spinal meninges, cervical sympathetic nerves, and autonomic innervation of the vertebral arteries and esophagus, which may be the result of trauma, aging, and metabolic disorders, among other causes. In TCM, it is classified as a type of *bi* or *wei* syndrome, which is manifested by headache, dizziness, stiffness or pain in the neck or shoulder. The main causes include impaired or deficient *qi* and blood and insufficiency of "vital *qi*" of the liver and kidney.

Etiology and Symptomatology of Cervical Spondylopathy According to TCM

▶ Obstruction of the channel of *taiyang*: Neck and shoulder pain radiating to the upper limbs, difficulty in rotation or movement of the head, stiffness of cervical muscles and trunk, loss of strength and numbness of the hands, dizziness, slight erythema of the tongue with a white coating, and a "superficial and distending" pulse.

▶ *Bi* syndrome: Pain in the neck, shoulder, and back which may radiate to upper limbs, cold intolerance, neck stiffness, a cord-like area of stiffness and pain in the nape of the neck, numbness and weakness of the hands, anorexia, whole body pain, a pallid and distended tongue, and a "deep," slow pulse.

▶ Obstruction by "phlegm" and "blood stasis": Dizziness, decreased vision and hearing, palpitations, nausea, vomiting, a sensation of obstruction of the pharynx, a sensation of chest pressure, a sensation of pain and heaviness of the limbs, lassitude, numbness, loss of warmth and edema of the limbs, syncope, coma, pallor of the tongue with a cloudy coating, and an uneven, slow, and irregular pulse.

▶ Deficiency of "vital *qi*" in kidney and liver: Dizziness, blurry vision, tinnitus, loss of hearing, headache, insomnia, forgetfulness, weak and atrophic limbs, dyskinesia, stiffness, clonus, tremor, abnormalities of balance and gait, paralysis, urinary and fecal incontinence, loss of tongue mass and coating, and a "thin" and uneven pulse.

Treatment

▶ Main acupoints: *dazhui, fengfu, tianzhu, juegu*
▶ Supplementary acupoints:
  ▶ For obstruction of the *taiyang* channel: *houxi, tianzong, jianzhongshu*
  ▶ For *Bi* syndrome: *pishu, jianyu, fenglong* plus moxibustion
  ▶ For obstruction by "phlegm" and "blood stasis": *fenglong, pishu, yinlingquan, xuehai, geshu*
  ▶ For deficiency of "vital *qi*" in the kidney and liver: *shenshu, ganshu, sanyinjiao, zusanli, geshu, taixi*
▶ Manipulations: For type the first three types, a "reducing" method should be performed and "reinforcing puncture" is used to treat the fourth type. A "warmly-capping" method may be used on the main acupoints (capping of short duration or retention until the region of the capped skin becomes red).

Treatments are given once every other day; a course consists of seven treatments. Four courses are used with a 5 days interval between courses.

Brief Review

In recent years, the incidence of the cervical spondylopathy has increased, including among the young. In China it was shown that both acupuncture and moxibustion were curative therapeutic methods to the disease [1]. Acupuncture and acupuncture-related therapeutic methods have been used to treat the disease, including hand-needling [2], electric needling [3], water-needling [4] ear-needling [5] and laser-radiation on acupoints [6]. All methods were reported to be effective. In addition, the cervical *Jiaji* points were often used for body-acupuncture [1, 3, 7].

References

1. Li BQ and Zhan Y. The situation of the treatment of cervical spondylopathy by acupuncture in the recent 10 years. Clinical Journal of Acpuncture and Moxibustion 14(12): 46–49, 1998
2. Peng JX et al. The treatment of 85 cases of cervical spondylopathy by needling at *Jiaji* points. Chinese Acupuncture and Moxibustion (1): 22, 1996
3. Wang CY. The treatment on 144 cases of nervous root type of cervical spondylopathy by electric needling at Jiaji points. Clinical Journal of Acpuncture and Moxibustion 14(5): 23–24, 1998
4. Guan Q and Zhang WM. Clinical observation on the treatment of 518 cases of cervical spondylopathy by the injection at acupoints. Chinese Acupuncture and Moxibustion 10(1): 10–11, 1990
5. Mu QX, Chen GS and Zhong YM. The observation on the immediate effect induced by electric ear-needling at sensitive points of cervical region in the patients with cervical spondylopathy. Jiangsu Journal of TCM. 16(11): 29–30, 1995
6. Xie KY, Zhao GF and Lu JM. The treatment of neck-shoulder syndrome by the radiation of Helium-Neon laser. Shanghai Journal of Acupuncture and Moxibustion 7(3): 16–17, 1988
7. Wang WL, Chen XD and Li YC. The treatment of 883 cases of cervical spondylopathy by acupuncture at cervical Jiaji points. Chinese Acupuncture and Moxibustion 18(7): 412, 1998

15 Tai Chi Use and the Elderly

S.J. Farrell

Complimentary medicine use in western societies continues to increase. Part of this gaining acceptance includes the use of eastern movement theories. Eastern movement therapies have been practiced for many hundreds of years in order to enhance physical and emotional well being as well as for prevention and treatment of disease. These theories have been especially helpful to the elderly due to ease of program development and enactment, lack of significant side effects, and generally low cost. Tai chi is such a program that will be discussed here. The following is a summated review of the concepts of tai chi including applicable published reports of the benefits to the elderly.

General

Tai Chi is also known as T'ai ch' uan, Tai chi chuan, Tai chi quan, and Taijiquan [1, 2]. Tai chi carries the meaning of "supreme ultimate" while chuan carries the meaning of "fist". The exact origin of tai chi is unclear but most believe it was developed as a martial art. Many reports declare that the origin lies in the Ming dynasty greater than 300 years ago. One legend attributes the origin to a Taoist priest named Chang San Feng. Reportedly he developed tai chi after viewing an altercation between a snake and a crane [1]. Others have said the movements of tai chi are based on similar movements exhibited by the snake, crane, tiger, and dragon [3].

Irrespective of the origin, most agree that tai chi began as a martial art that continues today. One report states that tai chi was originally considered a form of shadow boxing and later evolved into a way to combat enemies [2]. Nowadays, the practice of tai chi is also used in prevention and treatment of health disorders. The principle of tai chi lies in a source of internal energy called the chi. The chi originates in the dan tien or tan tien [1, 3]. This area is located a few inches below the umbilicus [1]. The energy flows throughout the body in channels in a harmonious way. The alteration of this energy flow is the basis for the use of tai chi in health concerns and martial arts practice. By practicing tai chi movements, the chi is stimulated and redirected to promote health and well being as well as to help prevent disease. With regard to martial arts practice, the movements also stimulate the chi, which in turn is translated into effective pushes and kicks.

Tai chi has been practiced for many hundreds of years according to many schools of thought such as the Chen, Yang, Yin, and Sun approaches [2]. Many of these approaches utilize sets or forms of low impact routines. In 1956, the tai chi masters met in China and adopted a simplified and condensed form of tai chi that brought together many of the principles of the approaches mentioned previously. Although the short form of tai chi remains quite popular today, many practitioners still adhere to the original long form tenets.

The routines, also called sets or forms, involve coordinated movements of such body parts as the head, neck and spine, hands, wrists, knees, hips, and ankles [3]. The practitioner attempts to remain relaxed throughout the routines. They must be conscious of body position and trunk alignment [2]. Deep breathing also helps create a relaxed state. The mind must remain alert and calm to enhance propioceptive feedback relating to body position and movement. Once these criteria are met, the practitioner can then perform the coordinated and sequenced movements that are inherent to tai chi. In order to gain expertise in tai chi many years of practice is needed.

Tai chi has been prominent in Asian culture for many decades. Even today it is included in many martial arts organized competitions [1]. Not all use is in such an organized environment. Across Western cultures, tai chi is gaining momentum in popularity. The elderly have in many ways been in the forefront of the increase in popularity. As chronic disease persists in an ever-increasing population, individuals are looking to less traditional methods in addressing health care needs. Tai chi is an excellent way to address these needs from perspectives of prevention and treatment of chronic illness and disability. The following is a review of the literature with regard to the benefit and uses of tai chi in the elderly.

Cardiopulmonary System

Cardiopulmonary disease is known to be quite prevalent in the older population. From coronary artery disease to cerebrovascular disease, cardiopulmonary illness and disability have a great effect on healthcare costs both direct and indirect. Tai chi has been shown to exhibit a positive influence on the cardiopulmonary system via a number of studies. While these studies vary somewhat in opinion as to whether tai chi provides for a level of light or moderate exercise intensity, little debate is present when discussing the benefits of tai chi.

Brown et al. wanted to examine the effects of the long form of tai chi on certain pulmonary parameters [4]. Experienced tai chi practitioners were tested using tai chi methods compared to cycle ergometry. Similar exertion levels were maintained by monitoring oxygen consumption. Results showed that under tai chi conditions, subjects had both lower ventilatory frequency and ventilatory equivalent. The ratio of dead space ventilation to tidal volume was more favorable. Schneider et al. found similar results in comparing tai chi practitioners to another martial art wing chun [5]. Wing chun reports a greater level of exercise intensity based on metabolic equivalents. Yet, results of each test group after treadmill testing did not show appreciable differences in maximum oxygen consumption or heart rate. The ventilatory equivalent was also lower in the tai chi group.

Other cardiopulmonary effects have been reported in the medical literature. Tai chi has been shown to be effective in lowering blood pressure. Young et al. examined the effect of tai chi compared to other randomized subjects that were involved in a 12-week moderate intensity aerobic exercise program of walking and low-impact aerobic dance. The study participants were at least sixty years old and had been sedentary prior to the study. None were considered to be hypertensive prior to the study. Results revealed a comparable reduction in blood pressure in both the tai chi group as well as the aerobic exercise group. Channer also looked at tai chi and blood pressure effects in patients that had experienced myocardial infarction [6]. Participants were randomized to tai chi, aerobic exercise, and support control groups. Both the tai chi and exercise groups showed decrease in systolic blood pressure. Therefore, a conclusion could be drawn that tai chi is as effective as moderate intensity exercise in lowering blood pressure.

According to the American Heart Association, greater than 4.7 millions Americans are now alive with heart failure [7]. In 1997 alone, $3.7 billion dollars were paid to Medicare beneficiaries for costs incurred attributable to heart failure. Extrapolation of these numbers worldwide would indicate global cause for concern. Tai chi though may be used to address this concern in the geriatric population. Fontana et al. wanted to investigate the effects of tai chi on the heart failure population [8]. Prior to their study, the safety of tai chi in this population was assessed by comparing metabolic equivalents in healthy adults [9]. They found that the energy expenditure for tai chi was similar to that of many activities of daily living. Subsequently they studied tai chi and the effects in heart failure patients. Pertinent variables measured included heart failure symptom scores, dyspnea scores, and exercise tolerance. Subjects were placed in a biweekly class of tai chi. Results showed decreases in heart failure symptom scores and dyspnea scores. An increase in distance walked over six minutes after tai chi was shown. While this study did not only include elderly participants, it may indicate yet another method to combat heart failure and the associated disability in older individuals.

Aging has been shown to be associated with a decline in body function related to exercise capacity and thermoregulatory response to environmental conditions [10, 11]. At times this can ultimately affect mortality rates. Tai chi may have a positive effect in these areas. Lai et al. examined the two-year trends of exercise capacity after participation in tai chi exercise [10]. This study focused on older subjects (mean age 64 +/- 9 years) with no major co-morbidities in the areas of cardiovascular, pulmonary, or musculoskeletal disease. The test group performed tai chi on the average five times per week compared to sedentary activity of the control group. Results showed the tai chi group had a reduction in maximal oxygen consumption during cycle ergometry by 2.8–2.9% compared to 6.6–7.4% in the sedentary control group. Thus a conclusion was drawn that tai chi may help delay the decline in cardiorespiratory function in older populations. Wang et al. evaluated the effect of tai chi on the response of microcirculation in healthy geriatric men [11]. Test subjects were placed in tai chi protocols at least three times were week and were then assessed against sedentary controls that were age matched and body size matched. Outcome measures revealed improvement in skin blood flow, cutaneous vascular conductance, and skin temperature during exercise. Thus tai chi may help in supporting the thermoregulatory response that is needed by older individuals in response to heat stress.

Balance

Balance issues and falls in the elderly continue to be major health concern as the general geriatric population increases in number [12]. Significant sequelae of falls, most notably hip and wrist fractures, have placed great financial hardship on the healthcare industry [13]. Sheldon has shown that standing sway increases and one-legged standing ability decreases with age [14]. Wolson et al. has reported that up to fifty percent of the elderly may exhibit loss of balance due to decrease in visual, ankle, and foot inputs [15].

Many studies have examined the effect of tai chi on balance and falls. Tse et al. compared a test group of experienced elderly tai chi practitioners to elderly nonpractitioners. Results of five balance tests showed that the tai chi group attained significantly better scores indicating superior balance ability [16]. Twenty-two persons with mild balance disorders were studied by Hain et al. [17]. Three objective tests involving posturography, Romberg testing, and reach testing as well as two questionnaires focusing on dizziness and general health were utilized. Participants underwent eight one-hour sessions of tai chi by a trained instructor. They were then to practice daily for at least thirty minutes. Support materials such as videotapes and written illustrations were provided. After eight weeks subjects were retested and found to have improvements in performance on the posturography and dizziness survey. Less significant improvement was noted in the Romberg test and general health survey. Reach testing showed no improvement. A more recent study by Wong et al. also showed an improvement in postural stability with tai chi [18]. Elderly subjects who had practiced tai chi for two to thirty five years were compared to controls using six progressively more difficult balance tests. In more simple balance tasks no difference in the groups existed. With more difficult tasks of balance such as simultaneously altering visual and proprioceptive conditions, the tai chi group tested to a much better degree.

Not all literature though is as convincing in supporting the use of tai chi for balance enhancement and prevention of falls. In the Atlanta Frailty and Injuries: Cooperative study of Intervention Techniques (FISCIT) trials, subjects were randomized to 15 weeks of tai chi training, computerized balance training, or educational classes [2, 19, 20]. While results showed that the tai chi group did experience fewer falls and that there was a delay in time before falls occurred, only the computerized balance training group exhibited actual improvement in postural stability. Conclusions drawn from this study indicate that the elderly test subjects did show less fear of falling compared to other test groups. Therefore, the overall improvement with regard to falls may be due to altered confidence and not directly to tai chi effects and postural stability.

Other studies also show mixed results regarding the effects of tai chi training and practice in relation to balance and falls. Wolfson et al. wanted to determine if tai chi had an effect on maintenance of balance gains [21]. In this study, elderly subjects of mean age 80 were placed in balance and strengthening programs. These programs included equilibrium control exercises, biofeedback, and lower extremity weight lifting. Results over three months showed an improvement in all balance measures. Subjects tested at levels that placed them at levels comparable to individuals three to ten years younger. After this initial improvement in balance measures, participants were then placed in a six-month tai chi program. After six months of tai chi, significant continued but decreased gains were noted in test subjects. Therefore one could draw the conclusion that tai chi was responsible for the continued gains in balance. One cannot state though that the gains were not attributable to the initial exercise and balance programs and not the tai chi. A less encouraging report was published recently by Nowalk et al. [22]. This study encompassed two years and looked at older individuals in long term care facilities. Participants were randomized to a resistance and endurance exercise group, a tai chi exercise group, or to a control group. Exercise classes were held three times per week over a two-year period. All subjects were monitored periodically for cognitive and physical functioning. Fall reports within the long-term care facility reporting system were also monitored. Outcomes measured included time to first fall, time to death, number of days hospitalized, and incidence of falls. Overall, no statistical significance was noted between the exercise groups and the control groups.

Musculoskeletal System

Surprisingly, limited work is available concerning tai chi effects on the musculoskeletal system. Much anecdotal evidence abounds but the literature lacks peer reviewed publications [23]. Lan et al. has produced evidence that tai chi may improve flexibility and strength in separate studies [24–26]. Both elderly men and women were compared to control groups in looking at thoracolumbar spine flexibility as measured by inclinometer and knee extensor and flexor strength as measured by peak torque dynamometer readings. Results showed test groups had overall better spine flexibility and muscle strength.

Movement force variability of the upper extremities was examined by Yan [27]. Previous studies have shown that the ability to perform arm movements decreases with age [28–32]. These movements tend to become less coordinated, slower, and more variable. Yan enrolled elderly subjects into a tai chi group or into a walking and jogging group. At the conclusion of the eight-week study, measurements were taken as to force variability of upper extremity movements. The tai chi group showed significant improvement in force variability compared to the other test group that only performed walking or jogging.

Arthritis of varying types can affect older individuals causing great disability and secondary health problems due to lack of mobility [3]. Although the medical literature is limited on this topic, a few reports are available. With regard to rheumatoid arthritis, Kirsteins et al. wanted to investigate as to whether tai chi would be harmful to patients [33]. Over a ten-week period, a tai chi group that practiced one to two times per week was compared to controls. Results revealed no major difference between the groups with regard to increasing pain. Improvements were noted in joint edema, joint pain, walking time, and grip strength. The authors thus concluded that tai chi would safe as a weight bearing exercise for patients with rheumatoid arthritis. Van Deusen et al. compared a control group to dance group that incorporated tenets of tai chi [34]. Patients were randomized. The tai chi based dance group also incorporated elements of relaxation technique and group discussion. Results showed the tai chi test group possessed greater range of motion at the shoulder with greater perceived benefits while statistical benefit was noted with wrist and lower extremity range of motion. A more recent report looked at the effects of tai chi in conjunction with osteoarthritis. Hartman et al. conducted a randomized, prospective study that compared a tai chi group to controls [35]. Mean age was 68 years. The tai chi group had tai chi sessions twice per week for twelve weeks. At the conclusion, the tai chi group exhibited significant improvements in self-efficacy for arthritis symptoms, level of tension and general satisfaction with health status. No significant changes were noted for one-leg balance, walking speed over fifty feet, and sit-to stand transfers.

Other Health Benefits

Few other reports are available regarding the benefits of tai chi. Kutner et al. participated in the previously mentioned Atlanta FISCIT trials [36]. They reported after questioning participants that tai chi and balance training both increased confidence in balance and movement. Only the tai chi group though reported greater satisfaction with activities of daily living and overall general life satisfaction. Jin reported that tai chi showed comparable benefit in reducing emotional stress to brisk walking [37]. Outcome measures included cortisol levels and mood testing.

Summary

Currently, the general population continues to grow. Along with this growth come a greater percentage of older individuals. This fact may be attributable to longer lifespan due to improvements and advancements in medical treatment, and better prevention techniques of disease and disability. In the past Western medical practitioners have embraced fairly rigid ideas regarding this prevention and treatment of disease. Only more recently have Eastern thoughts and ideas made inroads into medical doctrine. Included in the category of complementary medicine is Eastern movement theory which is inclusive of tai chi. Tai chi utilizes the "mind-body" approach to health and well-being.

Tai chi was originally practiced in China but now practitioners can be found worldwide in many environments from parks to formal classes. Tai chi has become especially popular with older generations for a number of reasons. Tai chi can be taught easily and relatively inexpensively. No major equipment is needed and almost any place can accommodate tai chi practice. The movements involved in tai chi are slow and coordinated and not ballistic in nature. This limits the impact on senior practitioners who may not able to tolerate high impact activities.

The medical evidence that generally supports the use of tai chi in the elderly is presented here. While the information is somewhat limited, as the popularity of tai chi continues to grow so will the medical evidence that will likely advocate it's use for personal health and well-being.

References

1. Farrell S, Ross A, Sehgal K (1999) Eastern Movement Therapies. In: Schulman R, Cotter A, Harmon R (eds) Physical Medicine and Rehabilitation Clinics of North America Vol. 10, No. 3: 617–629
2. Wolf S, Coogler C, Xu T (1997) Exploring the basis for Tai Chi Chuan as a therapeutic exercise approach. Archives of Physical Medicine and Rehabilitation 78: 886–892
3. Lumsden D, Baccala A, Martire J (1998) T'ai chi for osteoarthritis: an introduction for primary care physicians. Geriatrics 98: 84
4. Brown D, Mucci W, Hetzler R (1985) Cardiovascular and ventilatory responses during formalized T'ai Chi Ch'uan exercise. Research Quarterly for Exercise and Sport 60: 246–250
5. Schneider D, Leung R (1991) Metabolic and cardiorespiratory responses to the performance of wing chun and t'ai chi ch'uan exercise. International Journal of Sports Medicine 12: 319–323
6. Channer K, Barrow D, Barrow R (1996) Changes in haemodynamic parameters following T'ai Chi Ch'uan and aerobic exercise in patients recovering from acute myocardial infarction. Postgraduate Medicine 72:349–351.
7. American Heart Association (2001) http://www.americanheart.org
8. Fontana J, Colella C, Baas L, Ghazi F (2000) T'ai Chi Chih as an intervention for heart failure. Nursing Clinics of North America 35: 1031–1046
9. Fontana J, Colella C, Wilson B (2000) The energy costs of a modified form of T'ai chi exercise. Nursing Research 49: 91–96
10. Lai JS, Lan C, Wong MK, Teng SH (1995) Two-year trends in cardiorespiratory function among older Tai Chi Chuan practitioners and sedentary subjects. Journal of the American Geriatrics Society 43: 1222–1227
11. Wang JS, Lan C, Wong MK (2001) Tai Chi Chuan training to enhance microcirculatory function in healthy elderly men. Archives of Physical Medicine and Rehabilitation 82: 1176–1180
12. Kessenich C (1998) Tai Chi as a method of fall prevention in the elderly. Orthopaedic Nursing 17: 27–30
13. Ross M, Presswalla J (1998) The therapeutic effects of Tai Chi for the elderly. Journal of Gerontological Nursing 24: 45–47
14. Sheldon J (1963) The effects of age on the control of sway. Gerontology Clinics 5: 129–138
15. Wolson L, Whipple R, Judge J, Amerman P, Derby C, King M (1993) Training balance and strength in the elderly to improve function. Journal of the American Geriatrics Society 41: 341–343
16. Tse SK, Bailey D (1992) T'ai chi and postural control in the elderly. American Journal of Occupational Therapy 46: 295–300
17. Hain T, Fuller L, Weil L, Kotsias J (1999) Effects of T'ai Chi on balance. Archives of Otolaryngology-Head and Neck Surgery 125: 1191–1195
18. Wong A, Lin YC, Chou SW, Tang FT, Wong PY (2001) Coordination exercise and postural stability in elderly people: effect of Tai Chi Chuan. Archives of Physical Medicine and Rehabilitation 82: 608–612
19. Wolf S, Barnhart H, Kutner N, McNeely E, Coogler C, Xu T (1996) Reducing frailty and falls in older persons: an investigation of Tai Chi and computerized balance training. Journal of the American Geriatrics Society 44: 489–497
20. Wolf S, Barnhart H, Ellison G, Coogler C (1997) The effect of tai chi quan and computerized balance training on postural stability in older subjects. Physical Therapy 77: 371–381
21. Wolfson L, Whipple R, Derby C, Judge J, King M, Amerman P, Schmidt J, Smyers D (1996) Balance and strength training in older adults: intervention gains and Tai Chi maintenance. Journal of the American Geriatrics Society 44: 498–506
22. Nowalk M (2001) A randomized trial of exercise programs among older individuals living in two long-term care facilities: the FallsFREE program. Journal of the American Geriatrics Society 49: 859–865
23. Luskin F, Newell K, Griffith M, Holmes M, Telles S, DiNucci E, Marvasti F, Hill M, Pelletier K, Haskell W (2000) A review of mind/body therapies in the treatment of musculoskeletal disorders with implications for the elderly. Alternative Therapies In Health and Medicine 6: 46–56
24. Lan C, Lai JS, Chen SY, Wong MK (2000) Tai Chi Chuan to improve muscular strength and endurance in elderly individuals: a pilot study. Archives of Physical Medicine and Rehabilitation 81: 604–607
25. Lan C, Lai JS, Wong MK, Yu ML (1996) Cardiorespiratory function, flexibility, and body composition among geriatric Tai Chi Chuan practitioners. Archives of Physical Medicine and Rehabilitation 77: 612–616
26. Lan C, Lai JS, Chen SY, Wong MK (1998) 12-month Tai Chi training in the elderly: its effect on health and fitness. Medicine and Science in Sports and Exercise 30: 345–351
27. Yan J (1999) Tai Chi practice reduces movement force variability for seniors. The Journals of Gerontology 54: 629–634

28. Goggin N, Meeuwsen H (1992) Age-related differences in the control of spatial aiming movements. Research Quarterly for Exercise and Sport 63: 366–372

29. Yan J (1998) Aging and rapid aiming arm control. Experimental Aging Research 24: 55–69

30. Spirduso W (1975) Reaction time and movement time as a function of age and activity level. Journal of Gerontology 30: 435–440

31. Welford A (1984) Between bodily changes and performance: some possible reasons for slowing with age. Experimental Aging Research 2: 73–88

32. Cole K (1991) Grip force control in older adults. Journal of Motor Behavior 23: 251–258

33. Kirsteins A, Dietz F, Hwang S (1991) Evaluating the safety and potential use of a weightbearing exercise, t'ai ch'uan, for rheumatoid arthritis patients. American Journal of Physical Medicine and Rehabilitation 70: 136–141

34. Van Deusen J, Harlowe D (1987) Efficacy of the ROM dance program for adults with rheumatoid arthritis. American Journal of Occupational Therapy 40: 90–95

35. Hartman C, Manos T, Winter C, Hartman D, Li B, Smith J (2000) Effects of T'ai Chi training on function and quality of life indicators in older adults with osteoarthritis. Journal of the American Geriatrics Society 48: 1553–1559

36. Kutner N, Barnhart H, Wolf S (1997) Self-report benefits of t'ai chi practice by older adults. Journal of Gerontology 52: 242–246

37. Jin P (1992) Efficacy of t'ai chi, brisk walking, meditation, and reading in reducing mental and emotional stress. Journal of Psychosomatic Research 36: 361–370

16 Ayurveda – The Ancient Scientific Medicine with Natural Healing

I. Ramakrishna Krishna
With a Preface by E.P. Cherniack

Preface

In India and Sri Lanka, individuals have the option of using either Ayurveda or conventional medication. A study was done in which more than 700 "pseudo-patients" were sent to both types of practitioners in Sri Lanka [1]. It was observed that the majority of patients sent to both types of medical care providers received Western medications.

However, there have been a number of medications used in ayurveda that have been tested in formal scientific investigations. Khan and Balick noted that 166 different plant species had been described in the literature as used in Ayurvedic medicine [2]. Close to half had been tested in humans and almost two third had been tested in animals. However, many of the trials suffer from methodologic deficiencies such as inadequate sample size, lack of randomizations, and inappropriate controls.

These trials were not specifically performed on the elderly, but many of the disorders that were the subjects of the studies are prevalent among the elderly. Although many of the trials are small, they may suggest therapies that may be important in the future.

As mentioned in the chapter on rheumatology and alternative medicine Kulkarni et al. performed a double-blinded placebo-controlled trial on the use of articulin, an Ayurvedic formulation of several herbs an minerals on forty-two subjects with osteoarthritis for three months. There were improvements on joint pain and disability scores, although no radiologic change was noted [3].

Chopra et al. tested RA-1, an ayurvedic plant abstract in a sixteen-week double blind placebo controlled trial in almost 200 patients with rheumatoid arthritis [4]. Subjects were evaluated by American College of Rheumatology criteria for disease manifestations. RA-1 induced a 50% reduction in swollen joint count and approximately 25% more patients using RA-1 had a lower rheumatoid factor than those who received a placebo. Side effects were not severe, nor were there any difference in adverse reactions between the two groups.

HP-200, a compound from an Ayurvedic medication was tested in an unblinded study against sinemet in the treatment of Parkinson's disease [5]. Both groups resulted in statistically significant improvements in Parkinson's disease rating scales from baseline in this twelve week trial.

In another small and unblinded trial, the resin of an Ayurvedic medical plant Boswellia serrata, was tested as a treatment for chronic colitis in India [6]. Twenty percent more subjects who received the plant resin improved over placebo in one of several criteria including histopathology and electrolytes.

What follows is a discussion of Ayurvedic medicine by a practitioner. It is intended to provide insight into the complexities of Ayurveda.

References

1. Waxler-Morrison N (1988) Plural medicine in Sri-Lanka: do Ayurvedic and Western medical practices differ? Social Science and Medicine 27(5): 531–544.
2. Khan S, Balick M (2001) Therapeutic plants of Ayurveda: a review of selected clinical and other studies for 166 species. Journal of Alternative and Complementary Medicine 7(5): 405–515.
3. Kulkarni R, Patki P, Jog V (1991) Treatment of osteoarthritis with a herbomineral formulation: a double-blind, placebo-controlled, cross-over study. Journal Ethnopharmacol 33(1–2): 91–95
4. Chopra A, Lavin P, Patwardhan B (2000) Randomized double blind trial of an ayurvedic plant derived formulation for treatment of rheumatoid arthritis. Journal of Rheumatology 27(6): 1365–1372.
5. Parkinson's Disease Study Group (2001) An alternative medicine treatment for Parkinson's disease: results of a multicenter clinical trial. HP-200 in Parkinson's Disease Study Group. Journal of Alternative and Complementary Medicine 1(3): 249–255.
6. Gupta I, Parihar A, Malhotra P et al. (2001) Effects of gum resin of Boswellia serrata in patients with chronic colitis. Planta Medica 67(5): 391–395.

Ayurveda – The Ancient Scientific Medicine with Natural Healing

At the beginning of this Chapter on Ayurveda, I offer my profuse gratitude to the great profession of medicine and its scholars who have given us eternal relief from suffering. My sincere *pranams* (acknowledgements of gratitude) to the ancient scholars of ayurveda, from Lord Dhanwantari to Lords Aswins, who visualized the deepest roots of sufferings of the Creation and who know the micro-therapeutic values of each minute part of plants, and minerals, and to Panchabhutas, Acharya Charaka, Susrutha, Kasyapa, Vagbhata, commentators such as Chakrapani, and the scholars of our times, including the young intelligensia. My sincere gratitude is due to my *guruji*, my wife, my daughter, and my beloved friend Murthy and family for the inspiration and help extended.

Ayurveda "A Science"

Ayurveda is a science of life. It deals with life in all its details, namely, causes of benefit and injury (*Hita* and *Ahita*), happiness and unhappiness (*Sukha* and *Dukkha*), pleasant duration of life, *Ayu* (i.e., a healthy life span) and *Veda*, the complete knowledge of its *indriyas* (i.e., senses). It was narrated by the Creator Himself (i.e., Brahman). It consists of all branches of human life: *Atshanga* Ayurveda. Life is defined by ancient scholars as a pleasant state of body, mind and soul. A life is a real life where one lives without a psychological and physical suffering. The advent of scientific and research and development is making life safer day by day and increasing the life span. However, the modern drugs, if not administered properly, are proving ineffective or even harmful at a later stage. A powerful drug like an antibiotic or a life saving drug like a steroid today may become harmful tomorrow. So, there is every need to select a system which is harmless. Ayurveda, the ancient system of Indian medicine offers a more safe and natural therapy for every ailment which a human being encounters with.

We shall first discuss Ayurveda as a science, give a brief explanation of important terms, their scopes and effects on "seasons" of human life, approaches for diagnosis, and therapies suggested in the system. The yoga and meditations are also a part of this science. In this concise chapter, it is difficult to give a complete discussion.

Origin of Ayurveda

The Ayurveda, the *Veda* of long life and of therapeutics, was first known from Brahman, the Creator of Universe. From Brahman to Prajapati and later to Aswins, the divine twins (medical doctors of the heaven). According to Susruta, Indra taught Ayurveda to Dhanvantari (the God of surgery and medicine), and finally passed by the devine to the mankind through sages. Ancient scholars like Charaka, Susruta, Vagbhata, agree that the original Ayurveda is an *Upanga* of *Atharveda* which consisted of:

▶ *Kaya* (General medicine);
▶ *Graha* (Demonology);
▶ *Bala* (Paediatrics);
▶ *Agadhantra* (Toxicology);
▶ *Salya* (Surgery);
▶ *Salakya* (E.N.T.);
▶ *Rasayana* (Rejuvenation therapy);
▶ *Vajikaranam* (Aprodisiac). Charaka, and Vagbhata mainly concentrated on *Kaya Chikitsa* and Susruta on *Salya*.

The Chinese traveller Huan-Tsang (671–695 AD) knew those eight parts of Indian medicine in the order in which they are mentioned in Susruta's writings and says that these eight parts existed originally in eight books, but were later condensed by a man. This remark can be taken as based on the above Indian account, especially because he mentions Sakra (Indra) as the first author. In earlier days all these branches were compiled into one book known as *Samahitha* (i.e., a collection of various topics). The ancient writers like Charaka, Susrutha, Vagbhatha, Kasyapa made their own *Samhithas*. But in recent times, the Council of Indian Medicine made subject wise text books which are collected from all the *Samhithas*.

A science or a pursuit has always an objective (*prayojana*) before it. The objective of ayurveda is maintenance of the metabolic equilibrium of the human psychosomatic machine, and restoration to normality if the homeostasis is upset or disturbed by undesirable factors. The maximum life span of an individual in this *Kaliyuga* is stated to be 100 years. During this period, an individual should have a harmonious and coordinated pursuit of the three objectives of life:

▶ *Dharma* – the acquisition of religious merit,
▶ *Artha* – the acquisition of wealth,
▶ *Kama* – the satisfaction of desires.

There are three stages of life:
▶ *Balyavastha* – childhood
▶ *Yuvastha* – youth, and
▶ *Vridhavastha* – old age.

Health (*swasthya*) is defined as:
▶ well balanced metabolism (*dhatusamya*) and
▶ a happy state of the being, the senses, and the mind (*prasanna-atma-indiriya-manas*).

"Senses" here means the five organs of perception (smell, taste, sight, touch and hearing) coupled with the five organs of action namely, mouth, hands, feet, and organs of speech, excretion and reproduction.

A Disease (*vyadhi*) is defined as *dukkha-samyoga* (i.g., contact with unpleasantness-physical or mental) *Dukkha* has no exact equivalent in the English language; it stands for physical discomfort, pain, or suffering, as well as for mental anguish including the pangs of jealousy, anger, fear, avarice, greed, hate passion, harshness, cruelty, sorrow etc. It describes all that is unpleasant to the body and the mind.

Diseases are fourfold:
- adventitious (*agantuka*),
- physical (*shaariraka*),
- mental (*manasika*), and
- natural (*svabhavika*).

The adventitious disease results from external factors: cuts, bites, stings, injuries, accidents etc.

The physical disease consists of internal ailments, nutritional and metabolic imbalances, growth and inflammations, diseases of infection, tissue degeneration, etc. Infectious diseases, in ayurveda, even though of external origin, are included in the physical diseases, as no infection takes place in the presence of immunity: an internal trait.

Mental disease, in ayurveda, differs from the mental disorders as understood by the modern medicine. Diseases like insanity, schizophrenia, hypochondria, melancholia, paranoia etc., which are partly mental and partly physical, and which do respond to tranquilising drug treatments to a certain degree, do not represent the true ayurvedic concept of the mental disease which is represented by states of anger and wrath, pride and vanity, greed, avarice, treachery, falsehood, indiscipline, uncurbed desires, hate, fear, cruelty, distress, sorrow, anxiety, unhappiness etc.

Natural diseases cover birth, natural old age, death, natural hunger, natural thirst, and natural sleep, as these phenomena do not fall outside the definition of disease, i.e., *Dukkha-samyoga* (contact with unpleasantness) given above.

Generally speaking, the adventitious disease is treated surgically, the physical disease medically, the mental disease psychologically, and the natural disease spiritually. This is ayurveda in a nutshell.

This covers all the principles of allopathy, homeopathy and naturopathy. There are 42 alternate therapeutic approaches arising out of the permutations and combinations offered by this definition. This explains why the ayurvedic system is not in a position to disapprove of any of these 'pathies' and also why it is called the mother of medical sciences. Homeopathy (treatment by similars) and allopathy (treatment by contraries) can be regarded, in the words of the founder of the former Hahnemann, as "the exact opposite" of each other. But to ayurveda, both are acceptable alternate approaches. Thus, the homeopathic opium which cures constipation and the allopathic opium which causes it, both fall within the ayurvedic therapeutic measures.

The definition of medicine in Ayurveda is even wider: "Nothing exists in the realm of thought or experience that cannot be used as a medicine (i.e., a therapeutic agent). What it really means is that all existing phenomena, physical, physiological, psychic, or emotional, e.g., anger, tranquility, joy, sorrow, fear, confidence, love, hate, food, drinks, drugs (of mineral, vegetable or animal origin), fasts, massages, postures and exercises, desirable or undesirable experiences, situations, social, climatic or geo-graphical conditions, laudatory or adverse comments, abuse, praise, good, bad, or indifferent thoughts, etc., have a bearing on the body chemistry. There is nothing that can be experienced or conceived of that does not influence the body or the mind of the individual to a lesser or greater extent. Merely hearing the name or thinking of a friend or foe can affect the metabolism for better or worse. Since anything that effects the constitution one way or the other can be utilsed as a therapeutic agent, there is no-thing that is not a medicine.

Concept of Tridoshas. In ayurveda the *tridoshic* concept is the pivotal principle. What does it really mean? There are three basic constituent complexes in the physiological system, called *Doshas* or the *Dhatus*. We can treat these two words as synonymous. The *doshas* or *dhatus* are the irreducible ultimate basic metabolic principles governing the entire psychosomatic structure of the living organisms. They are classified into *Vayu* (or *Vata*), *Pitta* and *Kapha* (or *sleshma*). These terms cannot be easily translated into modern medical terms. In litteral translation they can be called "wind", "bile", and "phlegm". But this is highly misleading. Actually, the terms embrace much more be-tween them. They sustain the whole body metabolism. Or to put in another way, the whole physiological system can be somatotyped according to these three *doshas*.

No true mono-*doshic* individual exists. Matter, in order to be animate, has to be tri-*doshic*. Life is inconceivable in the absence of even one of the *doshas*. An ideal balance between the activities and structure of the three respective *doshic* factors constitutes the "absolute normality" of the constitution, i.e., a perfectly normal state of health form the metabolic viewpoint. In reality, however, such a norm does not exist as the psycho-somatic and metabolic structure is not fixed and rigid. It fluctuates, not only from individual to individual, but within the individual himself. Therefore, it is the predomi-nance of a particular *dosha* which decides the individual' type, and not the absence of the other *doshas*. Even where a *dosha* is predominant, the activities of the non-predominant ones cannot fall below a certain minimum. There are limits within which the minimum tri-*doshic* equilibrium must be maintained; outside these limits, the organism will cease to live. Between this lowest limit and the "absolute" normal, there exist innumerable permutations and combinations of the tri-*doshic* activities which represent deviations from the normal. Once the disturbances in the equilibrium cross the limits of the wide latitude provided for the concept of health, the *prakriti* (normal health) changes into *vikriti* (disease).

People were divided into three types, namely, the *Vata-prakriti*, the *Pitta-prakriti*, and the *Kapha-prakriti*. It is interesting to note that Dr. W. H. Sheldon, in his modern classics on somatotyping, "the varieties of human physique" and "the varieties of tem-perament" has divided humans into three basic types – ectomorphs, mesomorphs and endomorphs. Compared with the ayurvedic classification, Sheldon's classification appears almost too simplistic, based on inadequate knowledge of the total human organism: its internal and external mechanisms, how they interact apart from the in-fluences exerted by the environment.

It is impossible to offer an exposition of the "tri-*doshic*" concept within the limited scope of this article, since "medicine" in ayurveda covers every thought, action, word, experience, and substance that exists in the world. One can not think of anything which shall not fall into anyone of the three categories of the *vatic, paittic* and *kaphaic* kingdoms. Thus, the sun is *paittic* and the shade *kaphaic* or *vata-kaphaic* in nature. A stimulant is a *paittic* drug and a sedative a *kaphaic* drug. An alchoholic drink being *paittic,* will increase the *paittic* activity in the body, and the *anti-paittic,* or *kaphaic,* coconut water will counter the action. Similarly, anger will intensify the *paittic* activity in the body, and cheerfulness the *kaphaic* and *anti-paittic* activity.

No thought, word, action, experience, occurrence, or substance, coming into physical of psychic contact with the living organisms, fails to exert an influence, howsoever small, on its *doshic* equilibrium. The *pitta-prakriti* individual, for example, when subjected to the use of purely physical substances, such as *makaradhwaja* (a heating ayurvedic stimulant), musk, *asafoetida*, ginger, chillies, *brinjals*, or their modern counterparts such as adrenalin, thyroid hormones, hydrochloric acid, fish, pistachios, cashews, walnuts, stimulants and 'hot' spices, or emotional factors, like an upsurge of courage, or anger, will find them acting adversely on his constitution as all of them, being *paittic,* will aggravate his aleady *pitta-prakriti* nature, as they will promote his tendency to *kaphaic* disorders.

Since all physical, physiological, and/or psychological phenomena influence these ultimate irreducible basic psychosomatic constituents of the living matter, the tri-*doshic* complex has been aptly interpreted as the "physico-physio-psychological organismal phenomena" complex.

The imbalance of the *doshic* equilibrium constitutes disease. Restoration of the constitution to a balanced metabolism constitutes cure. Maintenance of the normal metabolism, and its protection against invasion by anything that disturbs the equilibrium of emotional, dietetic, external, epidemic or any other factors, constitutes hygiene.

Conducts of Seasons (*ritu-charya*)

As per ayurveda, the year is divided into six seasons (*ritus*). The northward movement of the sun and its act of dehydration bring out three seasons, beginning from the late winter (*shishira*) to summer (*grishma*). The southward movement of sun, and its act of hydration, give rise to the other three seasons, beginning with the rainy (varsha) to early winter (*hemanta*). Keeping in view the predominance of taste and strength, the first classification seasons is shown in Table 16.1.

Ayurveda suggests the observation of *Ritu Charya* and *Dina charya* and "do"s and "do not"s of the changes of a season (*ritu charya*) and daily living of ideal life (*dina-charya*), makes the human body and mind resistive, and has kept it in a state of pleasantness for centuries. The sages who observed this lived a long span of life with a highly pleasant state of body and mind.

The three *doshas* go through three stages during the year, i.e., *pitta* is accumulated in *varsha* (rainy season), provoked in Sharad (autumn) and is automatically pacified in *hemantha* (early winter). *Kapha* is accumulated in *hemantha* (early winter), provoked in *Vasantha* (spring), and is automatically pacified in *grishma* (summer). *Vata* is accumulated in *grishma* (summer), provoked in *pravrit* (early rainy season), and is automatically pacified in *sharad* (autumn). The *Doshas* are eliminated during their

Table 16.1. Classification seasons

Ayana	Ritu
Uttarayana (adana kala) or period of dehydration (debilitating period)	1. Shishira (late winter) 2. Vasantha (spring) 3. Grishma (summer)
Dakshinayana (visarga kala) or the period of hydration (strengthening period)	1. Varsha (rainy season) 2. Sharad (autumn) 3. Hemantha (early winter)

"provoked" or "vitiated" states, i.e., *pitta* is eliminated by purgative in *sharad* (autumn), *kapha* is eliminated by vomiting in *vasanta* (spring), and the *vata* is eliminated by enemas (*basti*) in *pravrit* (early rainy season), The vitiated stage of particular *dosha* produces particular diseases pertaining to it. The preventive measure, if properly followed, does not allow the *doshas* to produce the disease.

We shall now expand the chapter on *Ritucharya* and the seasonal regimen:

Uttarayana. Because of the nature of the path, both the sun and wind become very strong (powerful) and dry during this *ayana* (*uttarayana*), and take away all the cooling qualities of the earth; *tikta* (bitter), kasaya (astringent) and (pungent) tastes are more powerful respectively in the three successive *ritus*, hence this *adanakala* is *agneya* (predominantly fire-like in nature).

Dakshinayana. The three *ritus* commencing with *varsa*. *Varsa, sarat* and *hemantha* form the *dakshinayana* (southern solostice) and *visarga kala* (the period in which the sun releases the strength of people), because the moon is more powerful and the sun loses its strength. The earth becomes cooled of the heat of sunlight by the effect of clouds, rain, and cold wind. The unctuous tastes – *amla* (sour), *lavana* (salt) and *madhura* (sweet) – are powerful (respectively) during this period.

Regimen During Each Season

Hemantha Ritucharya. In *hemantha,* people are strong. The *amla* ("fire" in the elementary tract vis a vis digestive activity) becomes powerful, because it gets obstructed (from spreading out) by the cold in the atmosphere. It begins to digest the tissues of the body and is supported (helped) by *vayu* (*vata* in the body). In this *hemantha* (winter), use of (substances of) sweet, sour and salt tastes should be made.

As the nights are longer, people feel hungry in the (early) morning, so after attending to ablutions, they should resort to the regimen as enumerated in an *abhyanga* (oil-bath over the head and body) procedure, using medicated oil with "vata" alleviating property; *murdha-taila* (bathing the head with more of oil), mild massaging of the body, wrestling with skilled (wrestlers) of half their strength, and judicious use of "trampling" exercise of the body (by experts in that art).

After these, the oil (covering the head and body) should be removed by washing with an astringent (decoctions, powders etc.,) and bathing. Then, a fine paste/powder of *kumkuma* (*kesara*) and *darpa* (*kasturi*) should be applied, and the body exposed to the fumes of *aguru* (meat soup mixed with fats), meat of fattened, i.e., well nourished, animals, wine prepared with *jaggery* (molasses), and the supernatant portion of *sura*. *Sura* should be made of food prepared from the flour of wheat, black grain products, sugarcane, and milk. Food prepared from freshly harvested corn, muscle, fat, and edible oils should be partaken, warm water should be used for ablutions, thick sheets made of cotton, leather, silk, wool or bark of trees which are light in weight should be used during sleep, exposure to sunlight and fire should be resorted to judiciously, and footwear should always be warm. Women who have well-developed breasts and buttocks, who are enchanting and made exhilarating by the use of fragrant fumes, scents, and youthfulness, and who are thus well-liked, drive away the cold (by their embrace etc.).

People who spend their time residing in houses kept warm by fire, in inner-most apartments, encircled with others, or in underground chambers, will not be effected by the disorders (diseases) due to cold and dryness. Even in *sisira* (cold, dewy season), the same regimen (as described above) should be adopted more intensely, for during this period cold and dryness are more severe, being the effects of *adana kala* (the forthcoming semester).

Vasantha Ritu-Charya. *Kapha*, which has undergone increase in *sisira* (winter season), becomes liquified by the heat of the sun in *vasantha* (spring). This diminishes the *agni* (digestive activity in the alimantary tract), and gives rise to many diseases. Hence, *kapha* should be controlled quickly, by resorting to strong emesis, nasal medication and other therapies, foods which are easily digestible, dry (moisture-free, fat-free) physical exercises, (dry) massage and mild "trampling". Having thus vanquished (mitigated) the *kapha*, the person should take a bath, anoint the body with the paste of *karpura, chandana, aguru, and kumkuma*, make use of old *yava* (barley), *godhuma* (wheat), *ksaudra* (honey), eat meat of desert animals and meat roasted in fire, and drink the juice of mango fruit mixed with fragrant substances in the company of friends, served by the beloved (women), made more pleasant by the sweet scent of their bodies and the grace of their lily-like eyes, producing satisfaction to the mind and heart. One should also make use of unspoiled beverages, such as *asava* (a fermented infusion), *arista* (a fermented decoction), *sidhu* (fermented sugarcane juice), *mardvika* (fermented grape juice) *madhava* (honey water), water boiled with *sragavera* or *sa-ramba* (extract of trees such as asana, kanada etc.) or water mixed with honey, or plain water.

The person should spend his midday happily in the company of friends engaged in pleasant games, pastimes, story telling etc., in forests (or gardens) with little sunlight which have cool breezes from the south, and are surrounded by reservoirs of water, with trees of different kinds of beautiful and sweet smelling flowers and cuckoos everywhere, making pleasant sounds and engaging in love-play. Foods which are hard to digest or fatty, sour or sweet, exposure to cold, and sleeping at daytime and exposure to the eastern breeze, should be avoided.

Grishma Ritucharya. In *grishma* (summer) the sun's rays become powerful, day after day and appears to be destructive of all things, *sleshma (kapha)* decreases day by day and *vayu (vata)* increases. Consequently, in this season, foods which taste salty, pungent, or sour, physical exercises, and exposure to sunlight, should be avoided. Foods which are sweet, light (easy to digest), fatty, cold, and liquids should be taken.

One should partake of corn flour mixed with very cold water and sugar after taking a bath in cold water. *Madya* (wine) should not be taken, or, if necessary, taken sparingly or diluted with water. Otherwise, it will cause emaciation, debility, a burning sensation, and delusion. Rice (boiled) white like *kunda* flower and *moon* should be eaten along with meat of desert animals. *Rasa* (meat juice) which is not very thick, *rasala* (curds churned with pepper powder and sugar), *raga* (syrup which is sweet, sour and salty), *khandava* (syrup which has many different kinds of tastes, prepared with many substances), and *paaka pancasara*, (syrup prepared with *draksa, mashuka, kharjura,* and *parusaka* fruits all in equal quantities, cooled and added with powder of *patra, tvak, ela* etc., kept inside a fresh mud pot, along with leaves of plantain and coconut trees, and made sour by fermentation), should be drunk in jugs (mugs) of mud and shells. Very cool water kept in a mud pot along with flowers of *patala* and *karpura* should also be used for drinking. *Sasanka kirana* (hollow, finger-like, fried pastry made of corn flour) should be eaten at night. Buffalo milk mixed with sugar and cooled by moonlight may be used for drinking.

The daytime should be spent in a forest having trees such as *sala or tala,* among others, which obstruct the hot rays of the sun, or in houses around which bunches of flowers and grapes are hanging from their vines. Sheets of cloth spreading sweet, scented water, are arranged (to fan the air). Bunches of tender leaves and fruits of *cuta* (mango) should hang all around. One should sleep on a soft bed prepared with petals of flowers of *kadali, kalhara, or munala,* among others. One should spend the day in places with fully blossomed flowers hanging, or remain inside the house cooled by water scented with *usira,* coming out from the well-shaped breasts, hands, and mouths of water fountain statues to get rid of the heat of the sun. At night, people should sleep on a terrace with plentiful moonlight.

Exhaustion (due to heat of the day) of a person of balanced mind will be relieved by anointing the body with paste of *chandana,* wearing garlands, avoidance of sexual activity, wearing very light and thin clothes, and by fanning with fans made of leaves of *tala* or large *padmini* (lilly) made wet with syringes sprinkling cool water softly. One should also use garlands of flowers of *karpura, mallika,* and pearls and beads of *harichandana* (white sandal paste), and enjoy children, the pleasant calls of the *sarika* (mynah bird) and *suka* (parrot), and beautiful women wearing bangles of lotus stalks, blossoms of lotuses in their hair, moving about nearby.

Varsa Ritu-Charya. In *varsa* (rainy season), the *agni* (digestive activity) though weak in people debilitated by the *adankala* (summer), undergoes further decreases and is vitiated by the *doshas*. They are aggravated by the effects of hanging, thick clouds full of water, the sudden blowing of cold wind and snow; ground water dirty from rain, the warmth of the earth, and the sourness and poor strength of digestive activity. The *doshas* start vitiating one another, causing many diseases. Hence, all general methods which mitigate the *doshas* and measures to enhance digestive activity should be adopted.

After undergoing purifying therapies (*vamana, virechana*) the person should also be administered *asthapana* (decoction enema therapy). One should use dry grains for food, meat juice processed with spices etc., meat of desert animals, soup, wine prepared from grapes, and fermented decoctions which are old or *mastu* (whey, thin water of curds processed with *souvarcala* and powder of *pancakole*). Rain water or boiled water from deep wells should be used for drinking. On days without sunlight, the food should be predominantly sour, salty, fatty, dry, mixed with honey, and easily digestible. People should go barefoot, travel only by vehicles, use perfumes, expose one's clothes to fragrant fumes, and dwell in the upper stories of the house, devoid of heat, cold and snow. River water, *udamantha* (a beverage prepared with flour of corn mixed with *ghee*), sleeping at daytime, exertion, and exposure to sun should be avoided.

Sarat Ritu Charya. In people who have become accustomed to the cold of *varsa* (rainy season), sudden exposure to the warm rays of the sun, causes the *pitta,* which has undergone increase in the body during *varsa* (rainy season) becomes greatly increased during *sarat* (autumn). In order to treat it, *tikta ghrita* (medicated *ghee* recipe described in the treatment of *kustha,* chapter 19 of *chikitsa sthana*), purgation therapy, and blood letting should be used.

When very hungry, the person should eat foods which are of bitter, sweet, astringent, and easily digestible, such as *sali* (rice), *mudga* ("green-gram"), *sita* (sugar) *dhatri* (*amalaka*), *patola, madhu* (honey), and meat of desert animals. The water which gets continuously heated by the hot rays of sun during day and gets cooled by the cool rays of the moon during night, has been detoxified by the rise of the star *Agastya*, and is pure, uncontaminated, and capable of mitigating the ruals (*doshas*) is known as *Hamsodaka*. It is neither *abhisyandi* (producing more secretions or moisture inside the minute channels so as to block them) nor dry (causing dryness by non-production of sufficient moistness in the channels). Such water is like *amarta* (nector) for drinking and other purposes.

Evenings should be spent on the terraces of houses which are painted white, anointing the body with the paste of *chandana, usira, and karpura,* wearing garlands of pearls and shinning dresses, and enjoying the moonlight.

Exposure to snow (mist), indulgence in alkaline substances, satiation from hearty meals, the use of *dadhi* (curds), *taila* (oil) *vasa* (muscle-fat), exposure to sunlight, strong liquors, and sleeping at daytime and the eartern breezes, should be avoided in this season. During *sita* (*hemanta and sisira* – winter and dewy season), and *varsa* (rainy season), the first three *rasas* (tastes such as sweet, sour and salt) should especially be used. The last three *rasas* (tastes such as bitter, pungent and astringent), should be used during *vasanta* (spring season), *svadu* (sweet) during *gharma* (summer); and *swadu, tikta and kasaya* (sweet, bitter and astringent) during *sarat* (autumn). Food and drink should be dry (moistureless and fatless) during *sarat* and *vasanta* (autumn and spring), cold during *gharma* (summer) and *ghananta* (end of rainy season), and hot in other seasons.

The habit of using all the (six) tastes every day is ideal for maintenance of health except during special seasons, when particular tastes suitable to the respective season should be used more often.

Ritusandhi – (Inter Seasonal Period). The seven days at the end and commencement of *ritu* (seasons) are known as *ritusandhi* (inter seasonal period). During that period, the regimen of the preceding season should be discontinued gradually and that of the succeeding season should be adopted gradually. Sudden discontinuance or sudden adoption gives rise to diseases by *asamyata* (non-habituation). The same have been discussed in detail by Srimad Vagbhata, son of Sri Viadyapati Simhagupta in the third *Sutrasthana* of Astanga Hridaya Samhita.

Diagnosis and Treatment in Ayurveda

Next, we shall discuss the concept of diagnosis and treatment in ayurveda. The ancient scholars used to diagnose a disease not depending upon "biochemical and radiological investigations", but with modest interrogation and the examination of *nadi*, i.e., examination of pulse. The science says that a physician should go to the house of the patient and observe, palpate, and question him. All of the five senses must be set to work at the time of examination (Su.1.10.4: AHR 1.1.21).

Much can be inferred by such an examination. According to Bhav 1.2.162f, the eyes should examined to know how the three *doshas* are affected. Similarly, a rough and cracked tongue shows the derangement of wind (*vayu*), and a red or blackish tongue derangement of the bile (*pitta*). A coated, moist, and white tongue shows derangement of the phlegm (*kapha*). The urine becomes whitish from *vayu*, red and blue from *pitta*. It turns only red by blood, or white and frothy by *kapha*.

The pulse examination (*nadi-pariksha*) has been fully described. The pulse-examination perhaps originated among the Arabians or Persians. On this subject, there exist special works under the title Nadipariksha, Nadiprakasa, and Nadivijnana. According to one of these works, the pulse of left side in women and that of right side in men should be examined, as a rule, only on the wrist. Yet, the pulses of the foot, neck, and nose are at times examined. The physician feels the pulse by pressing with the three middle fingers of his right hand. In *vayu*, the pulse beats either like a serpent or a leech, in *pitta* like a crow, quail, or a frog, in *kapha* like a swan, peacock, pigeon, or different kinds of cocks. The conditions are affected by the three *doshas,* and are incurable if the pulse is variably slow, weak, rapid, stopped, completely lost, or scarcely felt, continuously abandoning its natural pace and reappearing again. In diarrhoea, the pulse is cool and slow. In cholera, it is sometimes not detectable, and at other times palpable. In diseases of intestinal worms, the pulse is slow and weak, often irregular. In jaundice, it is alternatingly faint and then rapid as if "springing out". In hemorrhage, it is weak, stiff, and soft. In constipation, it shows varied movements, often feeble. In internal wounds of the chest, the pulse beats loudly, and rapidly; in a cough it is shaky.

Even at present, the *Kaviraja* in Bengal considers the pulse-examination as particularly important, and its capability to diagnose the nature of an ailment has been recognized by many physicians.

The definition of treatment in ayurveda, *upashaya*, is the widest imaginable by any system of medicine. A salubrious use of drugs (*aushadha*), diets (*anna*), and practices (*vihara*) are prescribed which are:

▶ contrary to the cause of the disease,
▶ contrary to the disease itself,
▶ contrary to both the cause and the disease,
▶ similar to the cause of the disease,
▶ similar to the disease, or
▶ similar to both the cause and the disease, constitutes treatment (*upshaya*).

The physical body, the mind, and the soul are three distinctive features of a human being. They are vitally connected and are one single entity. They are a total unit. A more pleasant state of well-being of the total unit results in a healthy life.

The maximum life span of an individual in this *Kali Yuga* (era) is stated to be hundred years. During this period, an individual should have a harmonious and coordinated pursuit of the three objectives of life:

▶ *Dharma* – the acquisition of religious merit,
▶ *Artha* – the acquisition of wealth and
▶ *Karma* – the satisfaction of the desires of love. Life from birth has three phases: *Balya* (childhood), *Yavvana* (adolescence), and *Vriddhavastha* (elderly age).

Vriddhapya

Old age may be considered as *Vriddhapya*. *Vridda* is *Vardhathi*, i.e., to grow, *Apya*, to reach. Attaining of highest stage of growth is termed as *Vruddhapya*. On average, it starts from ages 48 to 50. In this phase, the "tone" of all tissues gradually decreases, if not protected. How can we identify the commencement of *Vriddhapya*?

Physical Features. The physical features are:

▶ *ozokshaya* i.e., a gradual decrease of the "vital essence of the body" (loss of tone in muscles, looseness of joints, degenerative changes in the blood, loss of production of semen),
▶ *phalitakas* (wrinkling of the skin).

After *proudhavastha*, a woman who enters into a specific phase of life in which she experiences certain physical and psychological changes. It is termed *kshinarthawa avastha* and happens between 45 to 55 years of age. The internal and the external genitalia will gradually become atrophied and *mamsavridhi*, a slight deposition of fat at the *kati* (pelvis), *udara* (abdomen), and *vuru* (medial thighs) will occur. The woman gradually ceases her menstrual cycle, which is known as *nashtaarthava* (menopause).

Psychological Symptoms. 1) In later old age, an individual feels isolated. 2) Mentally, he is alert and his brain is capable of producing a spontaneous answer for a complex problem, but his mind may have difficulty with small tasks. 3) The individual develops strong emotions, including a sudden increase of temper and a gradual depression. There are frequently strong emotions because *vriddhapyavastha* is characterized by *yapanam* ("catabolism", or gradual loss of the *dhatus* of *deha* causing the body and mind to become weak).

What are the Changes in Age that Lead to Death?

- ▶ Sukra: heart diseases
- ▶ Mamsa: "New growth"
- ▶ Rakta: Brain disease
- ▶ Rasa: "congenia"

Causes of death:
- ▶ Hrudaya Vyadhis: diseases of heart
- ▶ Vriddhi Vyadhis (or Soadha and sopha syndrome): malignant neoplasms
- ▶ Prana Vaha Vata Vyadhis: cerebral vascular lesions
- ▶ Janmaja Vyadhis: diseases of early infancy
- ▶ Prameha complications: diabetes mellitus

The *vruddhapya* is classified as *akala vruddhapya* and *kala vruddhapya*. If the signs of aging start in one individual at an early age, it is termed as *akala vriddhapya*, (untimely and unacceptable), and can be caused by poor nutrition (*ahara vikriti*), an unprincipled life, improper or excessive physical activity, laziness, constant exhaustion of body and mind; constant anxiety or tension, or excessive indulgence in sexual activity (vihara vikriti).

The manifestations of aging, gradually starting from the fifteenth year, may be termed as *kala vruddhapya*. The clinical picture of aging (*Vruddhapya lakshanas*), is predominated by a vital force (*vata*) i.e., a dynamic force which controls the total higher functions and motor functions of human body, which includes the functions of CNS and PNS. The forces of *pitha*, a dynamic force, controls the "elementary system", gonadal, and reticuloendotherial system and *kapha* controls the total metabolism of the body. Weakness and tiredness at the end of the day due to *mamsa dhatu sosha*, i.e., muscular fatigue.

Characteristics of Aging

- ▶ Inability to keep up with routine mental and physical attitudes (*glani*)
- ▶ Decrease of memory mainly on specific information like names, dates etc., (*mano-glani*)

▶ Feeling of incapability (*sosha*)
▶ Irregular heart beating (*vataja hridaya*)
▶ Mild dysponea (*swasa*)
▶ Lightness of chest (*hridaya sunyata*),
▶ Complaints referring to the joints (*ama vata*)
▶ Decreasing concentration of hormones of the body and degenerative changes (*pitha vikritha lakshanas*)
▶ Ayurveda *Acharyas* says that the *sukra* may cease gradually after fifty years and results in *sukrakshaya lakshnas* ie., gradual decrease of production of semen and loss of libido.

If one fails to take care of oneself in this phase of life, "rapid aging syndrome" results, leading to mental degeneration, instability, paralysis, cardiac manifestations, and other manifestations which cause continuous sufferings. *Ayurveda Acharyas* (Acharya Charaka, the scholar of this science), says, in his works *Sutrasthana* and *Vimanasthana* says that *sukra* may cease after fifty years age, which indicates that the degenerative changes proceed gradually in all tissues which result in a gradual fall of both physical and mental vitality.

Can we Reverse these Degenerative Changes?

▶ As per modern medicine – the possibility is limited
▶ As per Ayurveda – the possibility unlimited

Adequate nutrients and food, limited intake of fat, regular consumption of green vegetables, fruits, and lean meat may create endogenous changes. Can we avoid aging? Physiologically, we cannot. However we can definitely avoid and reduce aging, and one can have a youthful life in our advanced age using *rasayana* therapy. *Rasa* means *dhatus* of the body and *ayana* means nourishment.

This unique treatment for aging syndrome rejuvenates the tissues – providing not only an internal nourishment of *rasa* (which is not merely a plasma) but the seven required vital tissues from *rasa to sukra*. If one applies a *nitya rasayana*, i.e., a simple self-applied *rasayana* therapy daily, and a *chikitsa rasayana*, periodically, an elderly person can maintain a state of complete physical, mental, and social well – being, not merely because of the absence of a disease.

Ayurveda advocates the state of *ojas*, a hidden force of human life. It is said that one's well-being depends upon the conditions of *ojas*. Stress, anxiety, and excessive exertion earlier in life may decrease the *ojas* pathologically. After sixty years of age, *ojas* gradually decreases physiologically. In recent times, it has been felt that a number of wasting syndrome are due to defective or deficient immunity of the human body, *ojakshaya*. The *ojas* is described as the human body's ability sustain the immunological system which maintain the integrity of vital functions of the body. It maintains life itself. If it is completely diminished, the entire vitality of life will be exhausted. All people do not possess the same degree of immunity. Thus, some people are prone to get diseases. Hence, every elderly person should try to regularly care for the condition of his *ojas* by avoiding exposure to disease. and, if frequently exposed, should to take steps to upregulate his *ojas*. *Ojovridhi* (enhancement of *ojas*) is indicated. One should monitor for any deviation from the normal condition of one's *agni* (a coordinated functional activity of all enzymes digestive and elementary tract). Many indigenous compounds are used in the enhancement of immunity, as described previously.

Disorders Common in the Elderly

The most common are *prameha* (diabetic) manifestations. Ayurveda (2000 B.C – 2001 A.D) is the first medical system in the world which diagnosed and managed diabetes mellitus (DM) under the name *madhu meha*. Charaka mentioned DM as hereditary. He has also underscored that a sedentary lifestyle, excessive consumption of sweets, and oily foods may lead to development of DM.

Deranged metabolism and obesity are known in Ayurveda as causes of DM and named it as *agni vaishamya*. Derangements in adipose tissue, muscle tissue and liver glucose are involved in the pathogenesis of DM. DM is characterized by polyuria and turbid urine. There is a two-step management of DM:

▶ *Sthula* or *parthyaraja* (non-insulin dependant DM) requires *vata-vardhana dravya* – e.g., *nimba* and *beejaka,*

▶ *Krisa* or *sahaja* (insulin-dependent DM) requires *vatha-hara dravya* e.g., *amalaki, gokshura.*

To tackle diabetes effectively, a comprehensive treatment is required. Conventional Western medical treatments provide temporary relief to diabetic patients but with short- and long-term complications like pancreatic beta-cell failure hypoglycemia, nephropathy, neuropathy, retinopathy, and cardiac disease which can result in increased mortality. Due to these clinical problems, throughout the world, the attention has been given herbal formulations, owing to their versatile role in DM without side-effects. These herbal medicines are undergoing intense research, and have been proven scientifically and clinically to have a potentially valuable role in treatment.

Herbs suitable for DM therapy are shown in Table 16.2.

The ingredients are also found to possess anti-oxidant, anti-hypertensive and hypocholesterolemic properties in addition to anti-diabetic properties.

With the following Do's and Do nots, one can have a suffering free life and control its clinical manifestations.

Table 16.2. Herbs suitable for DM therapy

Botanical Name	English Name	Hindi Name
Azadirachita Indica	Neem or Margosa	*Duk*
Boefhaavia diffusa	Spreading log weed	*Beshakapore Thikri*
Coccinea indica	Indian Shot	*Kanduriki*
Pterocarpus marsupium	Indian Kino	*Bijasar*
Tribulus terrestris	Small Caltrops	*Chota-gpkhru*
Emblica officinalis	Embilic Myrobalan	*Amla*
Terminalia	Beleric Myrobalan	*Bhaira*

Do's:

▶ Avoid anxiety which causes further complications.
▶ Have regular daily exercise, but moderate, forehead sweating should be an indication to stop the exercise.
▶ *Abhyangan*– every day massage of total body with *tilathaila* (ginger oil) for at least twenty minutes.
▶ *Abhyanga snana*, a total bath with hot water or *sirosnana* (head bath in a flowing water (i.e., a river) is ideal.
▶ Avoid stress.
▶ Avoid physical laziness in *vihara* (i.e., in physical movements).
▶ *Diva swapna* (daytime napping).
▶ Avoid root-foods.
▶ Take frequent baths.
▶ Avoid intake of sweets.
▶ Avoid large quantites of rice (foods containing many calories or carbohydrate.
▶ Avoid frequent sexual indulgence.
▶ Avoid waking at late hours.
▶ Strict control of diet.

The story of drugs in ayurveda goes back to the prehistoric days. The Indian sages invented drugs and their therapeutic uses long ago. *Rigveda*, the oldest document of Indian wisdom, contains material which shows the rational attitude towards the plant kingdom, and its exploitation for the benefit of the humanity. The *Atharvanaveda* has a more advanced outlook, and contains a large number of drugs used in many diseases. Atreya and his disciples, after a deep and concentrated effort, were able to make some generalizations about the rational explanations for drug actions, which form the basic concepts of *Dravyaguna*.

Frequently-tested, documented therapies for certain *vyadhis* i.e., disease:

Hridroga (Cardio Vascular Diseases).

▶ *Tila Panam*: warm drops of *tila tila* mixed with *kaanjikam* i.e, boiled rice and buttermilk, mixed with *sindhava lavana*;
▶ *Mrudhu swedana*: A moderate sweating process which is indicated as above.
▶ A powder of *harithakyadhi*: 250 mg with honey thrice a day maintains cardiac function.
▶ *Pushkara molladhi choornam*: 5 gms with honey mixed with *arjunaarista* maintains cardiac function.

The following ingredients have been found very helpful in the management of *Hridrogas*:

▶ *Punarnava* (Boerhaavia diffusa)
▶ *Guggulu* (Commiphora Mukul)
▶ *Amlaki* (Emblica officinalis)
▶ Arjuna (Teriminalia Arjuna)
▶ *Vibhitaki* (Terminalia Belerica)

▶ *Haritaki* (Terminalia Chebula)
▶ *Gokshura* (Tribulus Terrestris)
▶ *Draksha* (Vitas Vinifera)
▶ *Sunthi* (Zingiber Officinale)
▶ *Jatamansi* (Nordostachys jatamansi)

The following extracts of powders daily intake have also been found of value:
▶ *Karavellaka* (Momordica charantia Linn)
▶ *Badara* (Ziziphus mauritiana)
▶ *Bimbi* (Coccinia grandis Linn. Voigt)
▶ *Jivanthi* (Leptadenia reticulata)
▶ *Nimba* (Azadirachta indica A.juss)
▶ *Meshasringi* (Gymnema sylvestre (Retz) R.Br.ex Schult)

Vata and Joint Pains. Ayurveda texts have given an account of various joint disorders those affect individual more commonly after age 45. It has been believed that these are due to imbalance of *vatadosha*, one of the basic elements of the body, as well as metabolic activities taking place in the body. *Ama-vata* is the main causative factor for arthritis and other joint diseases. It happens due to improper functioning of *vata*, which is a result of improper digestion caused due to weakening of digestive power (*mandagni*). Ingestion of spicy, pungent, and heavy food, and lack of exercise are the root causes of these diseases, leading to impairment of digestive functions, resulting in formation of *ama*, the residual undigested food material in the digestive tract. This causes *vatadushti*, which in turn cause metabolic disorders, and spreads to other parts of the body, finally resulting in excruciating pain, swelling and stiffness of joints resembling arthritis. In some patients, *pitta* is also aggravated, which causes severe burning sensation around the joints. As the disease becomes chronic, it damages the joints and later also causes deformities.

Regulated gentle *taila abhyangam* with *thila thailam* (zinger oil) s one of the best therapies. Oil prepared like *dhanvanthari tailam, rasnadi, sahacharadhi, ksheerabala*, will help a lot.
▶ The decoction prepared of *rasna* 30 ml everyday maintains joint function.
▶ Garlic intake daily keeps the joints healthy.
▶ External application of warm castor oil followed with fomentation keeps the joints relaxed.

Useful herbs which help in management of *amavata*:
▶ *Salai Guggul* (Boswellia serrata);
▶ *Shuddha Guggulu* (Commiphora mukul)
▶ *Aswagandha* (Withania somnifera)
▶ *Chopchini* (Smilax china)
▶ *Gokshura* (Tribulus terrestris)
▶ *Guduchi* (Tinospora cordifolia)
▶ *Harida* (Curcuma longa)
▶ *Kulanjan* (Alpinia galanga)
▶ *Methi* (Trogonella foenum graeceum)

- ▶ *Nirgundi* (Vitex negundo)
- ▶ *Punarnava* (Boerhaevia diffusa)
- ▶ *Shuddha Shilajit* (Asphaltum)

Opthalmic. Susrutha says most eye diseases are curable with surgery only, but intake of *triphala gritham* and *anjanams* is very helpful (a preparation with *ghee* the meat of the coconut, and *sowveeranjanam*).

In addition, the following have been found to be of value:

- ▶ *Avarthaki* (Cassia auriculata Linn)
- ▶ *Thila thailam*
- ▶ *Haridra* (Curcuma longa Linn)
- ▶ *Wacha* (Acorus calamus Linn);

Constipation, Indigestion, Hyperacidity. Recommended medicines:

- ▶ *Kala namak* (Sodium chloride "impura")
- ▶ *Kutki* (Picrorrhiza Kurroa)
- ▶ *Nishoth* (Ipomoea Turpethum)
- ▶ *Bal harad* (Terminalia Chebula)
- ▶ *Sounth* (Zingibar Afficinate)
- ▶ *Sanay* (Cassia Lanceolata)
- ▶ *Isabgol* husk (Plantago Ispagula);
- ▶ *Shankh bhasma* (calcified conch shell) for increasing appetite

Skin Allergies.

- ▶ *Baybidang*(Embella Robusta)
- ▶ *Haldi* (Curcuma Longa)
- ▶ *Nishoth*
- ▶ *Chitraka* (Phumbago Zeylanica) – used in the treatment of hives

Epilepsy and Loss of Memory.

- ▶ *Brahmi* (Herpestis Monniera)
- ▶ *Malkangni* (Celastrus Paniculata)
- ▶ *Shankhpushpi* (EvolvulusAsinoides)

Respiratory Disorders.

- ▶ *Tulsi patti* (Ocimum sanctum)
- ▶ *Adusa* (Adhatoda Vaska)
- ▶ *Mulethi* (Glycyrrhiza Glabra);

Non Speficic Diarrhea and Dysentery.

- ▶ *Lodhra* (Symplocus Racemosa)
- ▶ *Aamgiri* (Mangifera Indica-kernel)
- ▶ Jayphal (Myristica Fragrans)
- ▶ *Belgiri* (Angle marmelos);
- ▶ *Falendra mingi* (Mangifera Indica)
- ▶ *Kutaj* (Holarrhena Antidysenterica)

Table 16.3. Symptomatic relief

Symptoms	Relased dosha	Active ingredients
Vasomotor symptoms, hot flashes, headache, palpitation, night sweats	Increased *vata* Increased *vata* and *pitta*	*Ashoka, Jeeraka, Mustaka, Chandanam, Jatamansi* and *Praval pishti*
Depression, insomnia, irritability, fatigue	Increased *vata*, functional debility of metabolic tissues	Ayurvedic anxiolytics and brain tonics i.e., *balya* and *madhya*, ingredients such as *aswagandha, jyotishmati* and *vacha*
Pruritus Vulvae	Increased *kapha*	Ingredients reducing itching (*kandughna*) such as *chandana* and *ashoka*
Vaginal discharge	Increased *vata*	*Raja-stambhak* ingredients reducing vaginal discharges such as *ashoka*
Arthralgia (painful joints)	Increased *vata*	*Vatashamak* ingredients reducing increased vata dosha such as *Rasna, Devadaru, Abhrakbhasma*

Table 16.4. Preventive management

Long term sequelae	Related dosha	Active ingredient
Osteoporosis	Increased *vata*	Ingredients reducing or retarding bone degeneration like *Asthiposhak* and *Balya*, drugs such as *Praval Pishti, godani shuddha* and *kukkutandwak bhasma*
Cardiovascular disorders	Increased *vata* and *pitta*	Cardiac tonics such as *hriddya*, incredients such as *arjun, guduchi* and *gokshura*

Feminine Disorders. Menstruation: In Ayurveda, menstruation (*raja-pravritti*) is the natural process or removal of excess *pitta dosha* in the form of menses (*raja*). *Raja-nivritti* is the state of gradual diminishing of *raja-pravritti* which ends as menopause. Ayurveda looks upon menopause as an imbalance of *pitta* and *vata doshas*. These two *doshas* accumulate, spread and localize in the vital metabolic tissues manifesting as symptoms and sequelae of menopause, such as reduced menses, osteoporosis, cardiac disease and emotional disturbance. Along with *ahaar* and *vihaar*, ayurveda promotes the management of menopause symptoms based on the following guidelines.

Symptomatic relief see Table 16.3.

For *preventive management* see also Table 16.4.

For sexual dysfunction: *Safed Musli* (chlorophytum arundinaceum), and the stimulants makardhwaj (also a diuretic) and *akarkara* (Anacylus pyrethrum) which are useful to treat both impotence and chronic gastrointestinal disorders.

For the safe treatment of common infections: *Tulsipatti, haldi, anwala* (Phyllanthus Emblica).

Breast Care. *Kasishandhy thaila* and *shriparni thaila* for the nourishment of breast tissue, which also makes the skin more sensitive and helps removes excess breast tissue. Extract of *manjuphal* and tannic acid makes organs firmer. Bach extract (Acorus Calamus): its volatile oil contains pinine and camphene which are bitter astringents and cause sweating on application so that the blood flow in the capillaries increase.

Premature Graying of the Hair. *Bhringraj* (Eclipta Alba), *chitrak mool* (Plumbago Zeylanica), *indrayan mool* (Citrullus Colocynthis) *chandanadhya thaila, yastimadyang thaila*, and *bhringraj thaila*, among others.

White Spots on the Skin. *Bavachi beej* (Psoralea Corylifolia), *elwa* (Aloe Indica); *pawad beej* (cassia Tora), *manjith, kushta*, and *rakshas thaila*.

Liver Disorders. *Sarfonka* (Galega purpuria), bhringaraj (Ellipta Eracta) for liver disorders and jaundice, *kutki* (Picrorrhiza kuroo) for "bilious fever", *kumari asava, arogya*, and *wardhini.*

Memory Enhancers. *Aswagandha* (withamia somnifera), *brahmi* (Herpestis monniera)

Rheumatic pains. *Indrayan beej* (citrullus colocynthis), kulinjan (Alpinia Galanga), *yougrajguggul, mahayogaraj guggul, mahapinda thaila, mahavishagarbha thaila* (for "sciatica" arthritis), *vat-har thaila*; and *guduchi thaila*. Massage oils prepared with the above are recommended for external use.

Depression. Ayurveda advocates as a preventative treatment a harmonious and coordinated pursuit of the three objectives of life (*dharma, artha* and *kama*) from childhood onwards. *Dharma* means the acquisition of religious merit, *artha* means acquisition of wealth and *kama* means the satisfaction of desires (these need not be only sexual but, rather, ambitions of higher states of mind and body). During *balyavastha* (childhood), one should be devote to education and acquisition of knowledge (*gnana*), which is necessary for future life. At this stage, one is termed *jnathi*. During *yuvvanastha* (youth), one should acquire wealth and satisfy passions, and during *vridhavastha* (old age) for one should acquire merit and release from one's "bondage" to the recurring cycle of birth and death.

Conclusion

I conclude this article on the great ancient Indian science called Ayurveda, which, like the four holy *Vedas*, offer knowledge with no beginning and no end. It is a subject as vast as an ocean, and my presentation here is similar to a drop of water in that vast ocean. Within stipulated limits, I have tried to present some unique features of the diagnosis, preventive approaches, clinical presentations, complications, and valuable natural compounds and herbs, which should be researched and developed for the chronic manifestations of aging, and associated diseases for the benefit of mankind. It is my earnest desire that this universal scientific medicine reaches its highest peaks in future, equaling the high levels obtained by other sciences through the contribution of intelligentsia and scholars.

References

1. Yoga Ratnakara
2. Charaka Samhitha
3. Susrutha Samhitha
4. Harita Samhitha
5. Kasyapa Samhitha
6. Madava Nidhana
7. Bhava Prakasa
8. Dravyaguna Vignanam (By P.V. Sharma)
9. Dravyaguna Vignanam (By Nisteshwar)
10. P.V.Tiwari
11. Indian Medicinal Plants (By Keertikar Basu)
12. Indian Materia Medica (By Nadakarni)
13. Shaw's Gynaecology
14. Savil's Medicine

17 Herbal Folk Medicine

E.P. Cherniack

A plethora of herbal extracts have been used in folk medicine [1]. Although few traditional medicines have been investigated, let alone in methodologically rigorous clinical trials in the elderly, some of its constituents have been found to have therapeutic properties in small trials. The results of these investigations may suggest potentially valuable medical uses.

Stinging Nettles

One of the best studied of these agents is extract of the stinging nettle plant (urtica dioica), which has several potential uses. One such use is as a diuretic. In a small investigation in rats, extracts of two different concentrations were shown to have diuretic and naturetic propertices [2].

Urtica extract has been used humans to treat disorders of the prostate. Benefits has been shown in a few studies in both mice [3, 4] and humans [5]. Urtica is commonly used as treatment for benign prostatic hypertrophy in Europe [6]. A multicenter double-blind controlled trial of more that four hundred subjects with benign prostatic hypertrophy (BPH) were treated with either a combination of urtica extract and saw palmetto or the conventional 5-alpha reductase inhibitor, finasteride [5]. Both groups had comparable increases in mean urinary flow and symptom scores. Improvements were greater for individuals with large prostates. Subjects treated with finasteride had more frequent adverse reactions than with the herbal compound. Since saw palmetto is known through several studies to have favorable effects on individuals with BPH, it is unclear if the urtica extract confers benefit to a degree beyond that which saw palmetto alone creates.

Urtica has been noted to have in vivo and in vitro antitumor activity as well. In one *in vitro* study, a 20% extract inhibited proliferation of prostatic tumor epithelial cells by thirty percent without a cytotoxic effect on the noncancerous stromal cells [7].

The utilization of urtica extract to treat joint pain has been described in a few small studies. In a placebo-controlled double-blinded crossover study, twenty-seven patients applied topical urtica extract on the base of their thumbs to treat osteoarthritis [8]. Significant improvements were observed in self-reported pain and disability scale scores. In another survey, a small number of self-selected urtica extract users were interviewed, and and it was noted more than ninety percent felt satisfied with relief of pain [9]. The incidence of side effects was negligible, a temporary rash being the most common [9].

A compound of many different herbs including urtica was used to treat diabetes in alloxan-induced non-obese diabetic mice [10]. Different concentrations of the compound reduced serum glucose by ten to twenty percent.

Two trials have examined the role of stinging nettles for allergic rhinitis [11, 12]. One, a double blind placebo controlled trial, was performed on its use at a school of naturopathy, showing improvement in patient symptom scores [11].

Stinging nettles have been used as folk medical treatment for hypertension in Morocco and for cancer in Turkey [13, 14]. No published reports of the efficacy of urtica for these indications have been forthcoming.

The safety of urtica has never been formally studied. There was one case report of a woman who had atropine poisoning from tea made from urtica [15].

Willow Bark

Compounds from willow bark have been used both in Native American and European folk medicine. As willow bark contains salicylates, many of the trials, albeit small, have been for pain control. The degree of inhibition of platelet aggregation induced by willow bark is less than that of acetylsalicylate [16]. There have been two small published clinical trials from Germany [17-19]. In one, a randomized, placebo controlled trial of almost eighty patients lasting two weeks, osteoarthritis pain scores were reduced by 14% [17, 18]. In a second, open, non-randomized investigation over 18 months, groups of approximately one to two hundred subjects each used different strengths of willow bark to treat low back pain1 [19]. More users of the higher strength received some benefit than those using the lower strengths. Borenstein, however, in a review of treatments for low back pain believed studies of willow bark show it gives a small amount of benefit [20]

Sassafras

Sassafras (sassafras albidum) is another plant that has been used in Native American and European folk medicine. Unfortunately, all of the published reports have described side effects of sassafras products such as diaphoresis and carcinogenicity [21-24].

Other Native American Medicines

Other Native American herbal extracts have been recently studied, and noted to medicinal effects. Goldenseal, in two in vitro studies, inhibited human cytochrome P450 [25] and relaxation of the guinea pig trachea [26]. Ledum groenlandicum has been shown to in one study to be an antimutagen. Juniper, which has *in vitro* antioxidant activities [27], is known to decrease the effect of oral anticoagulants [28]. Blood root (sanguinaria candensis) has been noted to have antimycobacterial effects [29]. Pine seed oil has been found to have antimicrobial and antiviral activity in mice [30]. The Carrier Indians of the Canadian northwest have compounds made of Picea glauca and pinus conorta which had *in vitro* antimicrobial activity, and extracts of alnus incana and sheperdia canadensis that were cytoxic to mouse cancer cells [31]. Extracts of the flowers and pods of tecoma sambucifolia, known among the Peruvian incas as "huarumo" have anti-inflammatory, antinociceptive and cytotoxic effects, when tested using *in vitro* assays, in human and hamster cells [32]. Uncaria tomentosa, also known in South American folk medicine as "una de gato", an herb used to treat infections, neoplasms, gastritis, and arthritis, has been made into extracts which have been found to inhibit the proliferation of a human breast cell cancer line [33]. Salmon berries (rubus spectabilitis), in one report, caused Stevens-Johnson syndrome [34].

European Folk Medicines

As mentioned previously, some of the herbs used in Native American folk medicines, such as willow bark and sassafras. As is the case with most folk medicines, these have been largely the subjects of small *in vitro* tests. Mixtures of mistletoe and other herbal products have been used as a cancer therapy in several European countries [35, 36]. Proven benefit has not been demonstrated, but anaphylactic reactions have been reported [35, 36].

African Folk Medicines

Over the past decade, there has been increasing interest in the plant species used in African folk medicines. Although most have not been subject to published trials in humans, many have *in vitro* medicinal properties that may make preparations derived from them ultimately the subject of human clinical trial.

The most frequent studied indication for these herbs has been the potential to prevent or treat infectious diseases. The plants which have been observed to have *in vitro* antibacterial properties include: bridella ferruginea [37], bridelia micrantha [38], alchormea cordifolia [38, 39], boerhavia diffusa [38], Pelargonium siodes [39], pelargonium reniforme [39], Aristolochia paucineveris Pomel [40], Dioscorea syvatica [41], dioscorea dregeana [41], cheilanthes viridis [41], veronia colorata [41], roureopsis obliquifoliolata [42] epinetrum villosum [42], cissus rubiginosa [42], solanum torvum fruit [43], bryophyllum pinnatum leaves [44], pterocarpus osun stems [4, 5], piliostigma thonningii stem bark [46], the stem bark of cleistropholis patens benth, also known in Nigerian folk medicine as the typhoid fever remedy "ogwu odenigbo" [47], erythrina caffra [48], erythrina humeana [48], erythrina lattisma [48], erythrina lysistemon [48], erythrina zeyheri [48], anacardium occidentale bark [49], calotropis procera [50], marulla bark and leaves [51], pentanisia prunelloides [52], mallotus oppositifolium [53], and cryptolepis sanguinolenta [54]. Masesa lanceolata has been observed to have antiviral properties [55]. Combretum molle stem bark, used in Ethiopian folk medicine, inhibited the growth of mycobacterium tuberculosis [56]. Harrisonia abyssinica roots [57], ximenia caffra roots [57], azadirachta indica stem bark [57], and zanha africana stem bark were fungistatic and fungicidal against Candida [57]. Spilanthes mauritiana roots and flowers [57] were fungistatic and fungicidal against Aspergillus. Ajuga remota also exhibited an antifungal effect [58]. Several plants were investigated and found to have antiparasitic activity: triclisia patens [59], and terminalia glaucescens [60], cryptolepis sanguinolenta root bark [61], cassia occcidentalis leaves [61], euphorbia hirta [61] garcinia kola stem bark and seeds [61], morinda lucida leata [61]. Phyllanthus niruri [61] had an antiplasmodial effect, vernonia colorata acted against toxoplasma [62] albizia gummifera [63], ehretia amoena [63], entada abyssinica [63], securingega virosa [63] and vernonia subuligera [63] had antitrypanisomal action, and asteracacae [64], ebenaceae [64], and meliaceae [64] were toxic to schistosomiasis.

Other tested indications for African folk medicine include neoplasms, arthritis, and gastrointestinal disorders. Twenty-two plant extracts from Zulu folk medicines inhibited a tumor cell line *in vitro* [65], Parkia biglobosa had some incomplete anti-inflammatory and analgesic effect on mice [66], and culcasia scandens leaves was antiinflammatory in rats [67]. A number of herbs have in vitro antiulcerative properties: taverniera abbysinica a. rich root extract [68], tetrapleura tetraptera schum et thonn. stem bark [68], guibourtia eheie leonard stem bark [68], diodia sarmentosa [69], cassia nigricans leaves [69], ficus exasperata leaves [69], synclisia scabrida [69], and voacanga africana [70]. Extracts of phyllantus amarus treated diarrhea in mice [71].

African folk medicines have been tested for several other indications. African mistletoe [72] and ocimum gratissimum [73] have hypoglycemic activity, and ajugarin Iand hibiscus [74] lower blood pressure [75]. Qat, an herbal psychogenic stimulant, can increase blood pressure [76]. Senecio latifoius has inhibited a human hepatocellular cell line [77]. Sclerocarya birrea hochst alters calcium cell signaling in rat muscle cells [78].

The use of traditional medicine in some regions of Africa is still quite popular. In one survey of almost three hundred patients using treatments for seizures in Nigeria, one of the most populous African nations, almost half used traditional folk medicine alone, one quarter used spiritual healing and folk medicine, and one-fifth used spiritual healing alone [79]. Relatives, friends, and neighbors had influenced 86% to use complementary and alternative medicine(CAM) other than spiritual healing. After hospitalization and conventional medical treatment, only about 15% continued to use CAM, but two-thirds of individuals who used spiritual healing persisted after starting conventional medication.

Toxicity from African folk medicine have been reported. In the early 1980s, slightly more than eighty percent of all poisoning cases reported in a South African hospital were the result of remedies prescribed by traditional healers [80]. There have been reports of herbal medicines contaminated with Salmonella bacteria [81]. Three plants, combretum erythrophyllum, gnidia kraussiana, and barlerii randii, were found to be mutagenic [81]. Inflammation and a burning sensation of the skin has been noted with dioscorea sylvatic [82] and urginea altissima [82], and poisoning has resulted from urginea sanguinea [83].

References

1. Turner N, Hebda R (1990) Contemporary use of bark for medicine by two Salishan native elders of southeast Vancouver Island, Canada. Journal of Ethnopharmacology 29(1): 59–72.
2. Tahri, Abdelhafid (2001) Acute diuretic, natriuretic, and hypotensive effects of a continous perfusion of aqueous extract of urtica dioica in the rat. Journal of Ethnopharmacology 73(1–2): 95–100.
3. Lichius J, Renneberg H, Blaschek W et al. (1999) The inhibiting effects of components of stinging nettles roots on experimentally induced prostatic hyperplasia in mice. Planta Medica 65(7): 666–668.
4. Lichius J, Muth C (1997) The inhibiting effects of urtica dioica root extracts on experimentally induced prostatic hyperplasia in the mouse. Planta Medica 63(4): 307–310.
5. Sokeland J (2000) Combined sabal and urtica extract compared with finasteride in men with benign prostatic hyperplasia: analysis of prostate volume and therapeutic outcome. British Journal of Urology International 86(4): 439–442.
6. Koch E (2001) Extracts from fruits of saw palmetto (Sabal serrulata) and roots of stinging nettle (Urtica dioica): viable alternatives in the medical treatment of benign prostatic hyperplasia and associated lower urinary tracts symptoms. Planta Medica 67(6): 489–500.
7. Hans-Helge M, Lenz C, Laubinger H et al. (2000) Antiproliferative effect of human prostate cancer cells by a stinging nettle root (urtica dioica) extract. Planta Medica 66(1): 44–47.
8. Randall C, Randall H, Dobbs F et al. (2000) Randomized controlled trial of stinging nettle for treatment of base-of-thumb pain. Journal of the Royal Society of Medicine 93(6): 305–309.
9. Randall C, Meethan K, Randall H et al. (1999) Nettle sting of urtica dioica for joint pain-an exploratory study of this complementary therapy. Complementary thearapies in medicine 7(3): 126–131.
10. Petlevski R, Hadzija M, Slijepcevic M (2001) Effect of 'antidiabetis' herbal preparation on serum glucose and fructosamine in NOD mice. Journal of Ethnopharmacology May;75(2–3):181–4
11. Mittman P(1990) Randomized, double-blind study of freeze-dried Urtica dioica in the treatment of allergic rhinitis. Planta Medica Feb; 56(1):44–7
12. Thornhill S, Kelly A (2000) Natural treatment of perennial allergic rhinitis. Alternative Medicine Reviews 5(5): 448–454
13. Ziyat A, Legssyer A, Mekhfi H, et al. (1997) Phytotherapy of hypertension and diabetes in oriental Morocco. Journal of Ethopharmacology 58(1): 45–54.
14. Samur M, Bozcuk H, Kara A, et al. (2001) Factors associated with utilization of nonproven cancer therapies in Turkey. A study of 135 patients form a single center. Supportive Care and Cancer 9(6): 452–458.
15. Scholz H, Kascha S, Zingerle H. (1980) Atropine poisoning from "health tea". Fortschritte der Medizin 98(39): 1525–1526.
16. Krivoy N, Pavlotzky E, Chrubasik S, et al. (2001) Effect of salis cortex on human platelet aggregation Planta Medica 67(3): 209–212.
17. Schmid B, Ludtke R, Selbmann H, et al.(2001) Efficacy and tolerability of a standardized willow bark extract in patients with osteoarthritis: randomized placebo-controlled double blind clinical trial. Phytotherapy Research 15(4): 344–350.
18. Schmid B, (2000) Effectiveness and tolerance of standardized willow bark extract in arthrosis patients. Randomized, placebo-controlled double blind study. Zeitschrift fur Rheumatologie 59(5): 314–320.
19. Chrubasik S, Kunzel O, Black A, (2001) Potential economic impact of using a proprietary willow bark extract in outpatient treatment of low back pain: an open non-randomized study. Phytomedicine 8(4): 241–251.
20. Borenstein D (2001) Epidemiology, etiology, diagnostic evaluation, and treatment of low back pain. Current Opinion in Rheumatology 13(2): 128–134.
21. Klepser T, Klepser M (1999) Unsafe and potentially safe herbal therapies. American Journal of Health Systems Pharmarcies. 56(2): 125–138.
22. Kapadia G, Chung E, Ghosh B et al. (1978) Carcinogenicity of some folk medicine herbs in rats. Journal of the National Cancer Institute. 60(3): 683–686.
23. Haines J (1991) Sassafras tea and diaphoresis. Postgraduate Medicine 90(4): 75–76.
24. Segelman A, Segelman F, Karliner J et al. (1976) Sassafras and herb tea. Potential health hazards. Journal of the American Medical Association 236(5): 477.
25. Budzinski J, Foster B, Vandenhoek S et al. (2000) An in vitro evaluation of human cytochrome P450 3A4 inhibition by selected commercial herbal extracts and tinctures. Phytomedicine 7(4): 273–282.
26. Abdel-Haq H, Cometa M, Palmery M et al. (2000) Relaxant effect of Hydrastis canadensis L. and its major alkaloids on guinea pig isolated trachea. Pharmacology and Toxicology 87(5): 218–222.

27. Idaomar M, El-Hamss R, Bakkali F et al. (2002) Genotoxicity and antigenotoxicity of some essential oils evaluated by wing spot test of Drosophilla melangaster. Mutation Research 513(1–2): 61–8.
28. Burits M, Asres K, Bucar F (2001) The antioxidant activity of the essential oils of Artemisia afra, Artemisia abyssinica, and Juniperus procera. Phytotherapy Research 15(2): 103–108.
29. Argento A, Tiraferri E, Marzaloni M (2000) Oral anticoagulants and medicinal plants. An emerging interaction. Annali Italiani di Medicina Interna 15(2): 139–143.
30. Newton S, Lau C, Gurcha S et al.(2002) The evaluation of forty-three plant species for in vitro antimycobacterial activities; isolation of active constituents from Psoralea corylifolia and Sanguinaria canadensis.Journal of Ethnopharmacology 79(1): 57–67.
31. Sakagami H, Yoshihara M, Fujimaki M et al. (1992) Effect of pine seed shell extract on microbial and viral infection. In Vivo 6(1): 13–16.
32. Ritch-Krc E, Turner N, Towers G (1996) Carrier herbal medicine: an evaluation of the antimicrobial and anticancer activity in some frequently used remedies. Journal of Ethnopharmacology 52(3): 151–156.
33. Alguacil L, de Mera A, Gomez J et al. (2000) Tecoma sambucifolia: anti-inflammatory and antinociceptive activities, and "in-vitro" toxicity of extracts of the "huarmo" of pervian incas. Journal of Ethnopharmacology 70(3): 227–233.
34. Riva L, Coradini D, DiFronzo G et al. (2001) The antiproliferative effects of Unicaria tomentosa extracts and fractions on the growth of breast cancer cell line. Anticancer Research 21(4A0: 2457–2461.
35. Steiner G, Arnold R, Roth R et al. (1991) Stevens-Johnson syndrome secondary to ingestion of salmon berries. Alaska Medicine 33(2): 57–59.
36. Irobi O, Moo0Young M, Anderson W et al. (1994) Antimicrobial activity of bark extracts of Bridellia ferruginea. Journal of Ethnopharmacology 43(3): 185–190.
37. Abo K, Ashidi J (1999) Antimicrobial screening of Bridelia micrantha, Alchormea codifolia and Boerhavia diffusa. African Journal of Medicine and Medical Sciences. 28(3–4): 167–169.
38. Ebi G. Antimicrobial activities of Alchornea cordifolia (2001) Fitoterapia 72(1): 69–72.
39. Kayser O, Kolodziej H (1997) Antibacterial actiivity of extracts and constituents of Pelargonium sidoides and Pelargonium reniforme. Planta Medica 63(6): 508–510.
40. Gadhi C, Weber M, Mory F et al. (1999) Antibacterial activity of Aristolochia paucinervis Pomel. Journal of Ethnopharmacology 67(1): 87–92.
41. Kelmanson J, Jager A, van Staden J (2000) Zulu medicinal plants with antibacterial activity. Journal of Ethnopharmacology 69(3): 241–246.
42. Otshudi A, Foriers A, Vercruysse A (2000) In vitro antimicrobial activity of six medicinal plants traditionally used for the treatment of dysentery and diarrhoea in Democratic Republic of Congo (DRC). Phytomedicine 7(2): 167–172.
43. Chah K, Muko K, Oboegvulem S (2000) Antimicrobial activity of methaolic extract of Solanum torvum fruit. Fitoterapia 71(2): 187–189.
44. Akinpelu D (2000) Antimicrobial activity of Bryophyllum pinnatum leaves. Fitoterapia 71(2): 193–194.
45. Ebi G, Ofoefule S (2000) Antimicrobial activity of Pterocarpus osun stems. Fitoterapia 71(4): 433–435.
46. Akinpelu D, Obuotor E (2000) Antibacterial activity of Piliostigma thonningii stem bark. Fitoterpia 71(4): 442–443.
47. Ebi G, Kamalu T (2001) Phytochemical and antimicrobial properties of constituents of "ogwu odenigbo", a popular Nigerian herbal medicine for typhoid fever. Phytotherapy Research 15(1): 73–75.
48. Pillay C, Jager A, Mulholland D et al. (2001) Cyclooxygenase inhibiting and anti-bacterial activities of South African Erythina species. Journal of Ethnopharmacology 74(3): 231–237.
49. Akinpelu D (2001) Antimicrobial activity of Anacardium occidentale bark. Fitoterapia 72(3): 286–287.
50. Larhsini M, Oumoulid L, Lazrek H et al. (2001) Antibacterial activity of some Moroccan medicinal plants. Phytotherapy Research 15(3): 250–252.
51. Eloff J (2001) Antibacterial activity of Marula Hochst. subsp. caffra bark and leaves. Journal of Ethnopharmacology 76(3): 305–308.
52. Yff B, Lindsey K, Taylor M et al. (2002) the pharmacological screening of Pentanisia prunelloides and the isolation of the antibacterial compound palmitic acid. Jounral of Ethnopharmacology 79(1): 101–107.
53. Ogundipe O, Moody J, Fakeye T et al.(2000) Antimicrobial activity of Mallotus oppositifolium extractives. African Journal of Medicine and Medical Sciences 29(3–4): 281–283.
54. Paulo A, Pimental M, Viegas S et al. (1994) Cryptolepis sanguinolenta activity against diarrhoeal bacteria. Journal of Ethnopharmacology 44(2): 73–77.
55. Apers S, Baronikova S, Sidambiwe J et al. (2001) Antiviral, hemolytic, and molluscicidal activities of triterpenoid saponins from Maesa lanceolata: establishment of structure-activity relationships. Planta Medica 67(6): 528–532.
56. Asres K, Bucar F, Edelsbrunner S et al.(2001) Investigations on antimycobacterial activity of some Ethiopian medicinal plants. Phytotherapy Research 15(4): 323–326.
57. Fabry W, Okemo P, Ansorg R (1996) Fungistatic and fungicidal activity of east African medicinal plants. Mycoses 39(1–2): 67–70.
58. Kariba R(2001) Antifungal activity of Ajuga remota. Fitoterapia 72(2): 177–178.
59. Marshall S, Russell P, Phillipson J et al. (2000) Antiplasmodial and antiamoebic activities of medicinal plants from Sierre Leone. Phytotherapy Research 14(5): 356–358.

60. Mustofa A, Valentin A, Benoit-Vical F et al. (2000) Antiplasmodial activity of plant extracts used in West African traditional medicine. Journal of Ethnopharmacology 73(1–2): 145–151.
61. Tona L, Ngimbi N, Tsakala M et al. (1999) Antimalarial activity of 20 crude extracts from nine African medicinal plants used in Kinshasa, Congo. Journal of Ethnopharmacology 68(1–3): 193–203.
62. Benoit-Vical F, Sanillana-Hayat M, Kone-Bamba D et al. (2000) Anti- Toxoplasma activity of vegetal extracts used in West African traditional medicine. Parasite 7(1): 3–7.
63. Freiburghaus F, Ogwal E, Nkunya M et al. (1996) In vitro antitrypanosomal activity of African plants used in traditional medicine in Uganda to treat sleeping sickness. Tropical Medicine and International Health. 1(6): 765–771.
64. Sparg S, van Staten J, Jagen A et al. (2000) Efficiency of traditionally used South African plants against schistosomiasis. Journal of Ethnopharmacology 73(1–2): 209–214.
65. Opoku A, Geheeb-Keller M, Lin J et al. (2000) Preliminar screening of some traditional Zulu medicinal plants for antineoplastic activities versus the HepG2 cell line. Phytotherapy Research 14(7): 534–537.
66. Kouadio F, Kanko C. Juge M et al. (2000) Analgesic and antiinflammatory activities of an extract from Parkia biglobosa used in traditional medicine in the Ivory Coast. Phytotherapy Research 14(8): 635–637.
67. Okoli C, Akah P (2000) A pilot evaluation of the anti-inflammatory activity of Culcasia scandens, a traditional antirheumatic agent. Journal of Alternative and Complemetary Medicine 6(5): 423–427.
68. Noamesi B, Mensah J, Bogale M (1994) Antiulcerative properties and acute toxicity profile of some African medicinal plant extracts. Journal of Ethnopharmacology 42(1): 13–18.
69. Akah P, Orisakwe O, Gamaniel K (1998) Evaluation of Nigerian traditional medicines: II. Effects of some Nigerian folk remedies on peptic ulcer. Journal of Ethnopharmacology 62(2): 123–127.
70. Tan P, Nyasse B (2000) Anti-ulcer coumpound from Voacanga africana with possible histamine H2 receptor blocking activity. Phytomedicine 7(6): 509–515.
71. Odentola A, Akojenu S (2000) Anti-diarrhoeal and gastro-intestinal potential of the aqueous extract of Phyllanthus amarus (Euphorbiaceae). African Journal of Medicine and Medical Sciences 29(2): 119–122.
72. Obatomi D, Bikomo E, Temple V (1994) Anti-diabetic properties of the African mistletoe in streptozocin-induced diabetic rats. Journal of Ethnopharmacology 43(1): 13–17.
73. Aguiyi J, Obi C, Gang S et al. (2000) Hypoglycaemic activity of Ocimum gratissimum in rats. Fitoterapia 71(4): 444–446.
74. Adegunloye B, Omoniyi J, Owolabi O et al.(1996) Mechanisms of the blood pressure lowering effect of the calyx extract of Hibiscus sabdariffa in rats. African Journal of Medicine and Medical Sciences. 25(3):235–238.
75. Odek-Ogunde M, Rajab M (1994) Antihypertensive effect of the clerodane diterpene ajugarin I on experimentally hypertensive rats. East African Medical Journal 71(9): 587–590.
76. Mion G, Oberti M, Ali A (1998) Hypertensive effects of qat. Medicine Tropicale. 58(3): 266–268.
77. Steenkamp V, Stewart M, van der Merwe S, (2001) The effect of Senecio latifolius a plant used as a South African traditional medicine, on a human hepatoma cell line. Journal of Ethnopharmacology 78(1):51–58
78. Belemtougri R, Constantin B, Cognard C et al. (2001) Effects of Sclerocarya birra hochst leaf extract on calcium signalling in cultured rat skeletal muscle cells. Journal of Ethnopharmacology 76(3); 247–252.
79. Danesi M, Adenji J (1994) Use of alternative medicine by patients with epilepsy: a survey of 265 epileptic patients in a developing country. Epilepsia 35(2): 344–351.
80. Venter C, Joubert P (1998) Aspects of poisoning with traditional medicines in southern Africa. Biomedical and Environmental Sciences 1(4): 388–391.
81. Sohni Y, Mutangadura-Mhlanga T, Kale P (1994) Bacterial mutagenicity of eight medicinal herbs from Zimbabwe. 322(2): 133–140.
82. Cogne A, Marston A, Mavi S et al. (2001) Study for two plants used in traditional medicine in Zimbabwe for skin problems and rheumatism: Dioscorea sylvatica and Urginea altissima. Journal of Ethnopharmacology 75(1): 51–53.
83. Fourkaridis G, Osuch E, Mathibe L et al. (1995) The ethnopharmacology and toxicity of Urginea sanguinea in the Pretoria area. Journal of Ethnopharmacology 49(2): 77–79.

18 Native American Elder Care

L. Mehl-Madrona

Introduction

As I wrote this essay, I found myself challenging biases and romantic prejudices in my search for what it was like in the past to be old in Native America. Being Native American, I found myself wanting our culture to be somehow better for the aged than that of our European invaders. We grow up with a variety of apocryphal stories about elders in pre-European times – about how we valued the elderly, even revered and respected them for their wisdom and teaching. My research for this essay revealed changing patterns of age relations even before the European invasion.

My own experiences of elders during my childhood colored how I started this essay. The older people I knew as children were a healthy lot. They walked extensively, even from village to village, refusing or unable to rely on automobiles to transport them. They ate a traditional diet. I remember "possum stew" and "squirrel stew," also called Brunswick stew. I remember the older women of our family picking greens for the evening meal from fields near our house. These included poke greens, mustard greens, collard greens, dandelion greens, and whatever else grew in the vicinity. We ate fresh berries. Both grandmother and great-grandmother canned extensively from our large garden, and the pressure cooker seemed to run constantly during late summer, leading to a large supply of canned squash, tomatoes, pumpkin, corn, okra, green beans, and many others that we ate all winter long. Our meat was mostly wild or locally raised, and therefore, free range. We ate corn bread as our staple carbohydrate, along with corn grits and corn on the cob.

The old people of my childhood had difficult access to medical doctors, and even less trust. They relied upon local healers, including my great-grandmother, to minister to their woes, mostly successfully, according to my childhood impressions.

Today's Native American elders are much different. Today diabetes runs over 50%. Heart disease is rampant. Diet consists of government surplus commodities, full of lard and sugar. White bread is the staple carbohydrate, along with soda pop and fried bread. Sugar consumption is massive, and meat quality is poor. Exercise is minimal, while smoking is prevalent. People's sense of dignity and meaning in life is compromised. Reservation life today tells us, unfortunately little about Native elders of yesterday.

Nevertheless, I have made an attempt to describe what is known, recorded, remembered, and discovered about our ancestors and their way of life, and have arrived at some startling (to me) conclusions – answers that I did not suspect before.

Age Roles: Script Negotiation

Every society tends to think about its elders in categorical ways, naturalizing and universalizing the concept, creating fixed images that prevent us from appreciating age as a variable social script, changing with the conditions of the moment.

From the Hollywood image of Eskimos sealing their aging members inside the igloo to die because he or she can no longer keep up with the tribe to the historical practice among the Lakota people for the oldest woman to have absolute veto power over the war council, we construct a series of perceptions of age in Native America. These perceptions become inappropriately fixed.

The process by which societies conceive age and translate this concept into social roles is a fundamental dynamic of history and social life, much as Bruhns and Stothert (1999) have described for gender.

The men and women who participate in social life use age to assign roles and status, open and close opportunities, empower and constrain. The negotiation of age relations can be viewed as script writing by the various involved generations. The parties seek to gain advantage or minimize disadvantage as they invent technologies, alter economies, change social relations, develop different politics, and generate ideology. These creative activities are what humans do as they solve the problems of organization and survival. All societies create cultural scripts that bind people and their activities together in ways that work to solve the basic problems of subsistence, mental and physical survival, and personal satisfaction.

What remains hard for each culture to appreciate is the extent to which roles maintained for the elderly are just that, and not biologically requisite activities.

What is different about elders in ancient America when compared to elders in modern America?

▶ Without a written language, among hunter/gatherers, the memory of elders was vital for interpreting events and for constructing survival strategies, since the elderly had the longest memory for events and how the people had previously, successfully responded to changing conditions of the environment, and to other challenges.

▶ Intuitive or shamanic societies value experience and the wisdom thereby accruing more than written-language based societies that value texts.

▶ Elders had more exercise, sense of purpose and dignity, and extended family relations in the past.

Necessary roles for elders included:
▶ Historian
▶ Repository for stories and ceremonies.
▶ Interpreter of natural events.
▶ Extended childcare and home care provider
▶ Family laborer.

Modern U.S. society differs from traditional Native American society in that it
▶ is more driven by products and the need to consume them,

▶ values those members of society who consume the most (have the most disposable income),

▶ constrains access to income (and status) by age (aging is associated with physical restrictions and social restrictions, e.g., mandatory retirement, limited social security income),

▶ equates "successful" aging with the maximum accumulation of wealth, thereby mitigating against traditional values of individual sacrifice for the group and the valuing of cooperation over competition,

▶ needs a mobile work force which breaks up extended families and leaves elders alone,

▶ emphasizes youth, since youth are more easily manipulated to consume than are the elderly. Ego drives that sense of needing "toys," and mating-related concerns sells beauty products, clothing, etc.,

▶ devalues elders in relation to their decreasing desire for accumulating more "stuff", a natural consequence of healthy aging as we become comfortable with what we have, valuing relationships over things,

▶ values youth as a source for necessary warriors to protect the boundaries and economic interests of the modern state (a bargaining force in international relations, business, and competition).

The evidence indicates less stratification of age (and gender) roles in pre-agricultural societies than in our current society.

Culture and the Elderly

One immediately available, modern representative of ancient hunter-gatherer societies, are the Inglalik people of Alaska, who represent a material culture in which the elderly were integral, honored members. This culture seems to be representative of hunter-gatherer societies, even of thousands of years ago. The Inglalik, also called Deg Hit'an, an Athabascan group, strongly engender and promote cooperation and mutual dependence among men and women, young and old. The primary foods and sources of material for artifacts are wild species. Manufacturing involves hand labor and individual skills applied to locally available raw material. This material culture carries nonmaterial ideological elements. Artifacts are not just aids to material living, but also means to achieve social cooperation and interdependence (Osgood 1940). "Differentiation of tasks and artifacts associated with these tasks was accompanied by a model of integration. This model represents how most hunter-gatherer societies of North and South America probably lived."

Hunter-gatherer societies have less differentiation of age and sex roles from emerging agricultural societies. Among hunter-gatherer, age-related restrictions eventually limit a man's ability to hunt, propelling him into other activities, but women's roles remain relatively constant despite age. Less scripting of roles is observed with people contributing to the common survival and community life as they are able.

With some notable exceptions such as the Hopi, pre-European Native communities were mobile. Small settlements or villages of up to a few hundred people formed and disbanded as the seasons and food availability changed. During spring, which was the berry-picking, root-digging, and fish-spawning season, many kinship networks would gather and form a dense settlement for a brief period of time. Later in the fall, the same people would gather into smaller bands and hunt throughout a wide geographical area. Even tribes involved in agriculture were fairly mobile. After the crops were planted in the spring and after the first or second weeding, groups moved to other planting and gathering sites. In general, women were responsible for planting and caring for the fields and for gathering wild nuts, berries, and other plants. Late summer and fall would bring the groups back together to harvest corn and other crops, and to gather nuts and other wild plants (Jackson 1994).

Elders had to be mobile to participate in this life, since dogs were the largest domesticated animals. Skeletal remains suggest general healthiness and mobility, despite some degenerative conditions encountered.

Respect for the Aged and the Dead

Ancient Native American solutions to the problems of living are relevant to all of us today. They are examples of ways of being that move us and satisfy our curiosity. The study of ancient America has the potential to instruct us about the patterns that characterize everyone's ancestors on all continents (Bruhns and Stothert 1999, p. 277).

The bones of the dead had special meaning for ancient perople. The archaic Las Vegas people of coastal Ecuador are a well-studied example (Ubelaker 1980, nd). For example, a single individual found buried under the threshold of an early Las Vegas shelter was a woman, well over age 45. Archaeological evidence has suggested that she was accorded an important role as lineage head and authority, which would accrue to the oldest members of a group.

Veneration of ancestors improves the status of the elderly, evidenced by the Zapotec and Mixtec religions, who believed that the ancestors propitiated the forces of nature (Marcus 1983; Marcus and Flannery 1996).

Health in Native America

Health is crucial to aging. Successful aging includes good health, and good health promotes longevity. Traditional Native American cultures perceive health as a state of balance of spirit, mind, and body. Illness is the result of disharmony or imbalance in spirit, mind, body, and environment. Illness requires treatment at the many levels, including personal, family, community, and spirit. Traditional medicine has included herbalists, shamans, purification ceremonies, healing rituals, emotional therapies, manipulative medicine, teas, herbs, and special foods (Jackson 1994).

Aztec curing, for example, consisted of medicines or mechanical manipulations, along with incantations, prayers, and rituals. Women healers were prominent at the time of Conquest, but their roles were reduced by Christian pressure, which defined traditional medicine systems as witchcraft (Ortiz de Montellano 1990). Nevertheless, Aztec healers were more advanced than their European conquerors in the treatment of injuries, broken bones, pregnancy, and childbirth. Much of this knowledge was lost due to the Christian healers. The belief in owls as supernatural helpers, for example, was virtually completely suppressed.

Native American surgeons repaired lacerations with bone needles and human hair. They set bones in plasters made of downy feathers, gum, resin, and rubber. They lanced boils, removed tumors, amputated legs, made artificial legs, removed teeth, castrated men and animals, sucked out venom to treat snake bites, and used tourniquets and cauterization. They concocted emetics, purgatives, febrifuges, skin ointments, deodorants, toothpaste, and breath fresheners. They gave enemas with rubber hoses. The bulb syringe made of rubber was invented in the Amazon. North Americans used animal bladders for the same purpose of irrigating wounds and suctioning mucous.

Most Native people took daily baths in rivers, lakes, streams, ponds, or elaborate medicinal baths. Sweathouses and steam rooms abounded in North America, called *timescalli* by the Aztec, who built beehive shaped structures of stone and brick. Stones were heated outside and brought into the structure where the patient rested inside. Herbs were burned for smoke or added to steam. Body massage was aided by leaves and ointments. Every village had one or more *timescale*, used to treat everything from fever and boils to insect allergies, snakebites, exhaustion, and aching muscles.

Hot springs were used as sacred *huaca* by Quechua speakers and others for ceremonial and medicine bathing.

Sweathouses or sweat lodges were ubiquitous, from California to Delaware, from the Arctic to the tip of Chile. Both Californians and Delaware peoples built semi-subterranean earthen structures entered by a tunnel. The Alaskans built similar baths covered by logs. The Creek people used hides and mats. People of the southeastern United States slept all night in sweat houses in the winter months, and then jumped into cold creeks, ponds, or rivers in the morning. Plains people covered their lodges with branches and leaves, and later blankets. Some tribes included elaborate ceremonies as part of the sweat bath (Lakota, Cree), while others simply sat together in fellowship (Couer d'Alene, Spokane).

Interestingly, Europeans of that time (Spaniards, English, French) thought that frequent bathing was harmful and debilitating, leading to terrible diseases. Colonial officials outlawed bathing as harmful to the Native peoples whom they had conquered. Bathing decreased disease, and may have accounted for some of the general freedom from epidemic diseases among Native peoples before European conquest. The destruction of sweat houses and the forbidding of bathing contributed to the rapid spread of Old World epidemics in the New World.

Food and Health in Native America

Indigenous life-styles (hunter-gatherer) throughout the world naturally decrease the incidence of free radical diseases (which increase with aging, increasing morbidity and mortality, and decreasing longevity; Harman 2001). Inherent in the indigenous lifestyle is food restriction, a lack of ionizing radiation, and a high proportion of antioxidant consumption, while minimizing grain and diary intake. Diets consumed by North and South American Natives had high levels of antioxidants.

Following discovery by Columbus of the Americas, Native American spices, condiments, and foods had a very strong impact on the European diet. Prior to the introduction of American tomatoes and sweet peppers, the Italians endured a dreadfully dull diet. Cooks had few choices of sauces to ladle onto their pasta. Affluent diners had meats and gravies flavored with black pepper. The less affluent had cheeses and cream sauces; the poor had a few herbs and vegetables. Spaghetti with carrot sauce or lasagna made with beets lacked the sparkle of their contemporary counterparts.

With the arrival of the first foods from America, Italian cuisine exploded with new ideas, and the tables of rich and poor alike groaned under the weight of many marvelous new dishes. Yellow, orange, green, and red tomatoes from cherry to almost melon size and in round and oblong shapes found their way into the Italian kitchen to be pickled, sliced, chopped, diced, dried, pureed, and made into hundreds of sauces, The Italians added a diverse set of American sweet peppers, varying in more sizes and shapes than the tomatoes and named bell, banana, and cherry peppers because their shapes reminded the cooks of something already familiar to them, With virtually no other ingredients, the Italians had the perfect sauce for spaghetti, ravioli, lasagna, and a host of other noodle dishes, as well as for meats.

Italians liked at least one of the American squashes. They adopted a long, thin, green one, calling it zucchini, the diminutive of the Italian zucca, or "gourd." They added American beans to their diet, including the green bean and the kidney bean. These beans and peppers along with broth and some noodles became the standard ingredients in minestrone, the unofficial national soup of Italy (Weatherford 1988).

Casein (the main protein of milk) exposure was uncommon in the North American diet. Current studies have shown decreased life expectancy when casein is the only source of protein, theoretically due to its high levels of easily oxidized amino acids (Harman 1978). Replacing casein with soybean protein increased life expectancy by 13 years. Indeed, controversy continues over whether Native Americans are genetically able to process dairy. Clearly, pre-European elders did not eat dairy, perhaps contributing to health and longevity.

Periods of caloric restriction were also inherent in the hunter-gatherer life style of North America. Decreases in caloric intake are associated with proportionate decreases in oxygen utilization, decreasing mitochondrial superoxide radical formation, and ATP production (Harman 2001). The former decreases the aging rate (Harman 1994, 1993, 1995), thereby increasing life span. The latter decreases energy input, resulting in adapted metabolic changes in an effort to sustain body maintenance and function (Harman 2001). The interaction of these adaptations with the sudden appearance of the modern European diet, explains much of the sudden collapse in health found among colonized and assimilated Native populations.

Inevitably the nutrient in shortest supply was fat, since wild game were lean. The major sources of fat were nuts, sunflower seeds, and, for some tribes, cotton seeds (Jackson 1994).

Cooking methods included boiling, roasting, steaming, and baking, but not frying, since fat was scarce. Boiling was the preferred method for cooking most foods. Meat, fish, corn, wild rice, and other foods were boiled in clay pots, birch bark pots, or any container that would hold water. Both stone-boiling (putting heated stones into a container of liquid) and boiling by directly heating a container of liquid were used. Some foods, such as clams, were steamed in a pit lined with hot rocks and wetted with plant materials. Root vegetables, such as wild turnips, were roasted over hot coals or baked in hot ashes. Meat and fowl were barbecued by handing pieces on sticks near a fire. Foods were preserved for later use by drying.

Despite times of caloric restriction, the writings of immigrants to North America tell of abundant food supplies. Early explorers encountered numerous wild plants, roots, berries, nuts, and lichens. When de Soto's expedition landed in Florida in 1539, the Spaniards found the area "... cultivated with fields of Indian Corn, beans, pumpkins and other vegetables, sufficient for the supply of a large army" (Spellman 1948).

The early Spanish explorers who reached the Southwest in the 1550's witnessed extensive farming of the staple crops of corns, beans, and squash. In 1601, while visiting the Wichita communities in what is now south central Kansas, don Juan de Onate found the villages surrounded by fields of corn, beans, squash, sunflowers, tobacco (Carlson 1992). The Wichita People also gathered seeds, berries, roots, greens, pinon nuts, and acorns in season and hunted deer and small animals such as rabbits and prairie dogs.

Sharing food was basic to traditional Indian cultures. The 18th century naturalist, W. Bartram (Bartram 1955) conveyed the strong communal focus of the post-harvest activities among the Choctaws, Creeks, Chickasaws, and Cherokees:

"There is a large crib or granary, erected in the plantation...and to this each family carries and deposits a certain quantity, according to his ability or inclination, or none at all if he chooses. [This produces] a public treasury, supplied by a few and voluntary contributions, and to which every citizen has the right of free and equal access, when his own private stores are consumed; to serve as a surplus to fly to for succour; to assist neighboring towns, whose crops may have failed; accommodating strangers, or travelers, afford provisions or supplies, when they go forth on hostile expeditions; and for all other exigencies of the state ..."

One mid-day meal was the usual practice among Native peoples. Morgan (1891) described the home life of Native people of the late 1880's as follows:

"The meal was prepared and served usually before the noon-day hour – 10–11:00. After its division at the kettle, it was served warm to each person in earthen or wooden bowls. They had neither table or chairs, nor plates, nor any room in the nature of a kitchen or a dining room, but ate, each by himself, sitting or standing or where most convenient for the person. Food which remained, was reserved for any member of the household when hungry. Toward evening the women cooked hominy, and put aside to be used cold for lunch in the morning or evening or for the entertainment of visitors. They had neither formal breakfasts or suppers. Each person when hungry ate whatever food the house contained. They were moderate eaters." This is a fair picture of Indian life in general in America when discovered.

What were the traditional foods of North America? As mentioned, still most popular among the world's cuisines is the pepper – from mild to spicy. Tomatoes are a close second. Prior to Columbus, the only known pepper to Europeans was the black powder made by grinding the dried berry fruit of the plant *Piper nigrum*. If the outer shell of the plant was removed before grinding, the powder was white. Native Americans used a completely unrelated plant, *Capsicum frutescens*, its fruits ranging from dark greens through bright oranges, purples, and yellows (Weatherford 1988). Hot peppers (including cayenne) were an important part of the diet along with potatoes, sweet potatoes, yams, and many fruits – American passion fruit, avocado, Squashes, including zucchini, were important along with green beans, kidney, and other beans. Corn and beans were staples, along with venison, poultry, and other game. Maple sugar and syrup provided sweetening. Seafood was plentiful along the coast, replaced by fresh water fish, inland. Clams were cooked by the Massachusetts Natives in earthen ovens with seaweed. The Narragansetts boiled together whole corn kernels with lima beans in a mixture called succotash. Cranberries accompanied wild turkey. Corn meal was fried into thick cakes much like Mexican tortillas, called pone by the Algonquins, or Shawnee-cake by Europeans settlers. Spoonfuls of cornmeal were cooked in pots of hot bear fat, later called hush puppies. Jerusalem artichokes were cultivated in the south, along with tapioca from the cassava plant and native American pecans. Southeastern natives, such as the Taino of what is now called Puerto Rico, basted meats and fish with special sauces and cooked them over outdoor fires.

The traditional North American diet did not include wheat or breads (except from nuts or corn – after about 1100 A.D.) and only minimal dairy. Means were wild and free-range.

The Indian red bean was used by the Choctaw in what is now called Louisiana, along with gumbo file, a sassafras flavoring, made from the leaves of the Sassafras tree, mixed with shrimp, crayfish, and other fish. Catfish stew involved potatoes and tomatoes, alongside this unusual American fish with a skin instead of scales. Squirrel stew was popular in what is now called Virginia and North Carolina, the meat being combined with corn, tomatoes, and beans. Jerky and dried meat sticks were common. A popcorn nut mixture dipped in maple syrup formed a snack that was the precursor of "Cracker Jacks." Chocolate and vanilla were used commonly. "Trail mix" was commonly eaten – a mixture of nuts, seeds (sunflower, pumpkin, and others) and dried fruits. Dried meat was sometimes added.

Native fruits included pineapples and papayas, persimmons, papaws (*Asimina triloba*), and the maypop fruit (*Passiflora incarnata*).

Less known to Europeans are the chayote, a vine (*Sachium edule*) vegetable resembling yellow-green squash, representing a family of various shapes, sizes, colors and textures. The Aztecs called in chayotili, while the Mayans called it pataste. Central American Natives ate virtually the entire plant – root, leaves, fruit, and seeds. Pokeweed was an important green.

The Muskogee and Creeks used 11 varieties of hickory nut, several of black walnut (from the tree *Juglans nigra*). Acorns were the staple of California Native diet, along with pine nuts. Forty-seven types of berries have been found, further subdivided into 20 varieties of blueberries, 12 varieties of gooseberries, choke cherries (*Prunus serotina*), wild currants (*Ribes inebrians*) 4 varieties of elderberry (*Sambucus melano-*

carpa, S. mexicana, S. neomexicana, and *S. coerulea*), wild grapes (*Vitis arizonica* and *V. californica*), ground cherries (*Purpalis pubescens* and *P. fendleri*), hockberries (*Celtis pallida, C. reticula, C. douglasa*), manzanita (*Arctostaphylos pringlii* (*A. pringens, A. patuli*), and squaw berry (*Rhus trilobata*).

Health, Hunter-Gatherers, and the Transition to Agriculture

While estimates place the average life expectancy at birth in ancient Rome to about 30 years with a maximum life expectancy of 122 years, the descriptions by early explorers of North American suggest healthier aging for this continent (Ames et al. 1993; Kaltreider 2000). My review of the literature has suggested that the introduction of agriculture introduces warfare, degrades the status of women and the aged, and decreases health.

Beginning about 10,000 years ago in the post-glacial period, foragers began to harvest some wild plants and animals more intensively than others, and to engage in experiments designed to encourage the growth of their favorite species. This period of development, called the Formative Age in the New World (Neolithic in the Old World), was associated with increased cultivation, animal husbandry, and the crafts of pottery and weaving. Permanent settlements eventually developed, along with larger trading networks, and complex societies. Population density increased with the creation of communities, associated with diarrheal and other infectious diseases with their various vectors and parasites. Tapeworms and pinworms increased leading to debilitation, poor absorption of food, malnutrition, anemia, and death.

This transition to agriculture was not necessarily healthy or desirable. For example, 9,000 to 2,000 years ago, Chinchorro foragers of the desert coast of northern Chile and southern Peru were studied by Sonia Guillen and Marvin Allison, who found them to be generally healthier than later agricultural people of the same area. Their skeletal remains showed that women and men had a good life expectancy for that time period. Some lived well over fifty years. Guillen's study of the Chinchorro cemeteries found little evidence of pathology in their skeletons (the normal pattern for foragers living in small groups and eating well).

Women were affected by spinal arthritis, found in one-third of all their skeletons. One-fifth of women suffered from compression fractures in their spines due to osteoporosis, perhaps aggravated by multiple pregnancies. Forty percent suffered from severe leg infections that actually damaged their bones.

Among 51 Chinchorro skeletons from around 2000 B.C., 86.4% of adults had Harris lines, indicating some periods of starvation (4.8 per person) and/or nutritional stress. Eighty-six percent of children had these lines (6.1 per individual).

Thoughts about elders were definitely influenced by their belief in the importance of the dead as continuing participants in community life. Women and men, living and dead, participated in important social activities (Guillen 1992; Allison 1984; Rivera 1995). Excavations indicate a general respect for the elder, with much less differentiation between the living elderly and the deceased than encountered in today's modern culture. Deceased family members were expected at ceremonies and meals, and were buried in the family compound, presumably because they continued to participate in family life.

An analysis of 200 skeletons of the La Paloma site on the desert coast of Peru (7,000 to 4500 years ago) showed that ancient people were healthy by pre-ceramic standards, though they did suffer from tuberculosis, cancer, and frequently broken foot bones, osteoarthritis of the spine, and back problems (Quilter 1989). As these people moved toward agriculture, the elderly became less numerous and less healthy. Longevity fell.

Worldwide, women who contribute to subsistence agriculture by cultivating plants, introduce solid foods to infants earlier than hunter/gatherers. Grinding cultivated seeds and boiling them in water in ceramic vessels permits early weaning. Giving an infant gruel for lunch allows a woman greater mobility and relieves the stress of producing milk. But this practice also shortens the birth interval and spurs population growth, resulting in increased elderly mortality and decreased longevity (Crown and Wills 1995). The average life span, for example, at Grasshopper Pueblo, from 1275 to 1400 AD, in Arizona, was 38 years (Ezzo 1993), dramatically lower than what had been found for earlier hunter-gatherer peoples. Increasing agriculture led to decreasing life expectancy. Among the early Formative Valdivia people of coastal Ecuador (ca. 3000–1500 BC), comparative early adoption of horticulture led to a life expectancy at age 15 that was the lowest of all studied Ecuadorian populations – that of 38.7 years for men and 32.3 years for women. Increased mortality was related to increased infection, trauma, and interpersonal violence. Warfare and domestic violence dramatically increases with the acceptance of the agricultural lifestyle and its concomitant demands. Increased dental hypoplasia, caries, and abscesses were also noted in skeletal reamins (Ubelecker 1980, nd). This pattern of health and disease mirrors the patterns seen with increased sedentary life styles, increased population densities, changing diet toward grains, and increased warfare, all of which are associated.

Changes in activities, scheduling, sex roles, and age roles, all evolved concomitantly with changes in food-producing technology and the development of crafts, also called "human domestication." Agriculture promoted "survival of the fittest," and decreased the status of elders. Gathering populations were more respectful of the contributions provided by the elderly whose memories included where to search for food and how to survive (Cohen and Armeledge 1984; Cohen, et al. 1993).

Early classic Mexico showed similar changes and relationships at Teotihuacan, long in ruins when the Aztecs entered the Valley of Mexico. This city covered 29 square miles of densely packed buildings. Its citizens lived in apartment compounds. Adult women were malnourished and carried a high parasite load (Thomsen 1969; Spence 1974). Old people participated in spinning and weaving of textiles, among the most labor intensive and time consuming tasks performed in the home. By the late years of the city, investigators at the site, Tlajinga 33, found virtually everyone living in compounds, with 30–40% infant mortality, and 50% of family members dead by age 15. Deaths were highest at ages 3 to 5, related to weaning stress. Half of the inhabitants of Tlajinga were dead by age 40. Most of the remainder died within the next 15 years. Women's work was shared by the handful of elderly women available. The city collapsed by the 7th Century AD.

Anemia was frequently seen in the bones, manifesting as porotic hyperostosis and cribra orbitalia, related to nutritional stress. It was common among maize dependent populations. These signs are also seen among people with diets low in animal products.

Native American Herbal Pharmacology

No review of Native American aging and elder care is complete without a discussion of the medical practices that kept people healthy. Herbs were part of this medical practice.

Native herbal pharmacology was well-developed when Europeans arrived in the Americas. From the Amazon came the cure for malaria – the Peruvian bark, which contained quinine, previously used for many ailments, including cramps, chills, and heart rhythm disorders (Taylor 1965, p. 78). This plant was called quina-quina, by its cultivators, the Quechua-speaking Incas, living from 3000 to 9000 feet. Paradoxically, Sir Ronald Ross received a Nobel Prize for discovering how malaria was transmitted, but the Quechua received no credit for curing it.

Amazon natives used ipecac, a Quechua term for *Cephalaelis ipecacuanha* or *acuminata*, for expelling poisons and toxins and for ritual purifications. Ipecac became a cure for amebic dysentery. The Amazonians also used curare, a member of the genus *Chondodendron*, to treat lockjaw.

High-altitude Quechua speaking Incas used chilca (*Baccharis pentlandii*), a shrub of high, cold altitudes (1,000 to 3,000 meters), to treat inflammation, rheumatism, and bone and joint injuries. Coastal Incas used Pacific kelp, *Macrocystis*, to cure and prevent goiter.

Pine bark and needles were used to prevent and to cure scurvy, coming to European attention in 1535, when Jacque Cartier (1491–1557) became stuck in the ice with his three ships at the Huron city of Hochelaga (now Montreal). While the Europeans thought scurvy to be an infectious disease, the Hurons knew it was a nutritional malady, and treated it with their pine concoction called *annedda*. It contained a massive dose of vitamin C, anti-oxidants, bioflavinoids, and pycnogenol. Lind (1716–1794) received credit for curing scurvy after reading Cartier's account and bringing it to the attention of the British Navy.

Northern California and Oregonian Indians used Rhamnus purshiana, a shrub, to cure constipaiton. Called cascara sagrada, by the Spanish, for sacred bark, the herb is still in widespread use.

Northeastern Americans used *Spigelia mainlandia*, a vermifuge pinkroot, to treat intestinal worms. North American dogwood (genus *Cornus*) was administered to reduce fevers. Bloodroot (*Sanguinaria Canadensis,* or *puccoon*) was used as an emetic, along with lobelia. Wild geranium (*Heuchera americana*) was used as an astringent (also called alumroot). Boneset (*Eupatorium petrolatum*) was used as a stimulant (Driver 1969).

The bark of the poplar tree or the willow tree was used for headaches and other aches and pains. This bark is now known to contain salicin, a relative of salicylate, and a powerful anti-inflammatory agent. Witchhazel bark and leaves (*Hamamelis virginiana*) were used as an astringent, and as a balm to soothe strained or tired muscles. Dried flowers of plants in the genus *Arnica*, were applied to sprains and bruises to relieve pain and swelling. Petroleum jelly was widely used, called "Indian petrolatum," by early European settlers.

Native Americans and Substance Use

Substance abuse affects aging and longevity. Current Native American communities suffer greatly from tobacco and alcohol abuse, while drug abuse abounds among the youth. Potential substances of abuse abounded in the New World, actual abuse was rare. Woodland Natives of North America smoked dried tobacco in pipes, but only for ceremonial purposes and did not inhale. Mexican Natives and Southwestern US Natives rolled tobacco into cornhusk cigarettes and cigars for ceremonial use. The cigar was the ceremonial object for Caribbean Natives and those of the Southeastern United States. Northern Pacific Coasts peoples chewed tobacco with lime. Aztecs ate tobacco leaves. Creek Natives mixed tobacco with *Ilex cassine* leaves and other herbs to make the "Black Drink" used it rituals. Cherokee laws were particularly harsh on public intoxication as were those of the Aztecs. The practice almost never occurred.

Why did Europeans bring to the world the abuse of these many substances – from the coca leaves of the Andes to American tobacco? Today's Natives would argue that the Europeans lacked a spiritual context for these powerful medicines, and therefore imbued them with evil energies. Be that as it may, substance abuse affects aging, decreasing longevity and quality of life.

Other examples of spiritual and highly controlled use of potentially substances of abuse include the use of *Lophophora williamsii* in Mexico and peyote or mescal cacti in Texas as spiritual hallucinogens. The Native American Church currently uses peyote in its ceremonies, just as ancient Aztec priests did. The milder cactus, Dona Ana, or *Coryphantha macromeris*, Aztec *pipintzintli* (the leaves of *Saloia divinorum*), ololiuqui (seeds of *Rivea corymbsa* vine), and mescal beans of the Texas mountain laurel (*Sophora secundiflora*) were also used as spiritual hallucinogens. The Mayans and the Aztecs used *Psilocybe mexicana* and *Psilocybe cubensis* in ceremonies. The Aztecs also used *Paneolus campanulatus, or teonanacatl,* which translates as "food of the Gods," in ceremonies. Canadian plains peoples used a drink from the root of the marsh plant *Acorus clamus*, also called *cakanies*. Jimsonweed was used in the same way in North America. It was a hallucinogen from the genus *Datura*, and was named for its use in Jamestown, Virginia.

Native peoples in the Americas made wines and beers, but never with more than 3 to 4 percent alcohol. Ancient Mexicans fermented *Agave* and *Dasyliron* plants to make *pulque*, a vitamin-rich, fermented beverage. The Tahono O'odham and the Papago peoples of southern Arizona and northern Mexico made cactus wine and beer from mesquite, screwberries, maize, and even corn stalks. Atlantic Coast peoples made persimmon wine, popular with the European colonists. North America boasted over 40 different types of alcoholic drinks at the time of Columbus' landing, all made from fruits and plants, including palm, plum, pineapple, mamey, and sarsaparilla wines (Driver, p. 110). Mayan mead was called *balche* and came from the fermented honey of a stingless bee.

Plants like Oregon grape root and pine bark were widely used and are now known to contain pycnogenol – a unique mixture of phenols and polyphenols, broadly divided into monomers such as catechin, epicatechin, and taxifolin, and condensed flavinoids, such as procyanidin B1, B3, B7. Pycnogenol also contains phenolic acids, such as caffeic, ferulic, and para-hydroxybenzoic acid as minor constituents (Packer et al. 1999). Pycnogenol prolongs the lifetime of the ascorbyl radical (Cossins et al. 1998) and protects endogenous vitamin E (Virgili et al. 1998) and glutathione (Rim-bach, et al. 1999) in human endothelial cells from oxidative stress. It modulates nitric oxide metabolism in stimulated macrophages by inhibiting both NOS mRNA expression and its activity (Virgili, et al., 1998). This means that it provides powerful anti-oxidant protection, thereby reducing the severity of or preventing the onset of chronic degenerative diseases. Antioxidants are known to delay the onset or to reduce the severity of diabetes, independent of other risk factors. Antioxidants like pycnogenol reduce the severity of slow the development of arteriosclerotic cardiovascular disease and are effective protectors against cancer promoters and mutagens.

Scientific Confirmation. Studies are appearing on many different Native American herbs and herbal formulations. One of the most studied ancient remedy is St. John's Wort (*Hypericum perforatum*), which has received publicity as therapy for depression. The first report on St. John's Wort to appear in the scientific literature described 6 women with depression, aged 55–65, who were treated in an open trial with active hypericine complex, a derivative of St. John's Wort. A significant increase in the urinary output of 3-methoxy-4-hydroxyphenylglucol, a metabolite of norepinephrine and dopamine which is considered indicative of antidepressant action, followed. Together with an additional 9 cases, after 4 weeks of treatment, the SGAC (Clinical Assessment Geriatric Scale) and DSI (Depression Status Inventory) scores showed a significant improvement in anxiety, dysphoric mood, loss of interest index, anorexia, hypersomnia, insomnia, obstipation and feelings of worthlessness ($p<0.01$ to $p<0.05$; Arnheim Forsch 1984).

The next major landmark was a meta-analysis of 25 controlled studies of the antidepressant action of Hypericum (St. John's wort) on 1,600 patients. Doses ranged from 300–900 mg/d of Hypericum extract for 2–6 weeks. Most studies were double-blind, comparing Hypericum with placebo or conventional antidepressant drugs. The most common instrument used to assess depression was the Hamilton Depression Scale. For mild-to-moderate depression, Hypericum was equivalent to imipramine and maprotiline. Severe depression was much less prone to respond. 2.5% of patients complained of side effects.(Journal of Geriatric Psychiatry and Neurology 1994).

In a third meta-analysis of 23 randomized studies of Hypericum for mild to moderately severe depression encompassing 1,757 patients, the probability that St. John's Wort would be better than placebo was 2.7 (95% CI 1.78–4.01). Single botanical remedies were as effective as common antidepressant pharmaceuticals (OR 1.1, 95% CI.93–1.31); combinations were more effective (OR 1.52, 95% CI 0.78–2.94). There were 4% dropouts for side effects in the Hypericum groups v. 7.7% in drug groups (OR 0.6, 95% CI 0.27–1.38) and side effects were reported in 20% and 53% respectively (OR 0.39, 95% CI 0.23–0.68; BMJ, 1996).

Mind-Body Therapies in Native America

Mind-body therapies, including meditation, guided imagery, visualization, and what is now hypnosis were especially common in North America. An Arikara word translates as "putting them to sleep so that they dream like they're asleep, but they're really awake." Modern people call this hypnosis.

Contrary to Hollywood's stereotypes, the actual practice of Native American healing was counseling intensive, with long discussions of the patient's emotional and family life, problems within the community, and behavior. Healers work with spirits who advise them about the patient and help the healer to make behavioral prescriptions for how the patient must change lifestyle, relationships, and behavior. Broken taboos must be repaired. In *Coyote Medicine* (Mehl-Madrona 1997), I wrote about a community ceremony in which the spirits reveal that an incest taboo has been broken. The involved uncle confesses and begs for forgiveness. The community witnesses the healer drive the evil out of the uncle's body, and then agrees to his penance, which consists of a series of selfless acts for the community which will restore balance and therefore relieve an illness in the niece. This did in fact happen, and was in interesting example of the community dealing with a serious problem in a healing manner without involvement of police or legal authority and in such a way that the perpetrator's position in the community was restored along with the honor and health of the victim.

Studies are continuing to reveal the efficacy of psychological therapies, so much the mainstay of Native American healing.

Exercise in Native America

Physical activity was common among the elderly prior to European conquest. Since dogs were difficult to ride, walking was the chief means of transportation. Elders expected to walk and did. Physical fitness was important. Obesity was rare (Jackson 1994).

Evidence continues to accumulate to support the role of physical activity in maintaining wellness through old age. Life-long physical activity is important. Less active elders have more degenerative disease, decreased longevity, increased pain, and more arthritis complaints than more active elders.

Spiritual Therapies in Native America

Spiritual therapies, including ceremonies, were among, and continue to be, the most powerful examples of Native American healing. Many studies support the importance of religious commitment to longevity and health. Other studies are beginning to appear on the effect of prayer on health. Byrd (1994), for example, studied 393 patients in the coronary care unit of the San Francisco General Hospital of the University of California at San Francisco Medical Center. All received standard medical care but were randomized to two groups. The group who received distant prayer (even though they weren't knowledgeable that were receiving such prayer, fared better than those who did not prayer.

Manipulative and Energy Therapies in Native America

Manipulative therapies were the hallmark of Native American medicine. Unfortunately, many of these therapies have disappeared, though a few devoted practitioners try to maintain them. Cherokee, for example, practiced an intricate form of manual therapy that still rivals the best of European osteopathy. Cherokee healing also including energy medicine with oils, crystals, and hands-on and hands-above the body techniques. Scientific evidence does exist to support the utility of manipulative and energy therapies.

Agriculture and Health

The study of the skeletal pathologies consistently show that the switch from hunter gatherer to agriculture resulted in worsening health and increasing morbidity and mortality (Dickel et al. 1984). The Central Valley California Archaic people provide well-researched evidence for this trend. Acute stress decreased with these changes, presumably due to a reduction in seasonal inadequacies of nutrition. Archaic people may have created a new system (agriculture) in response to the problem of seasonal inadequacies, not perceiving the delayed negative health consequences of agricultural life. They achieved resource stabilization, but at the cost of increased infant and maternal death, and overall worsened mortality due to increased population density and disease.

Studies of the ancient peoples of the Ohio Valley show many healthy adults over age 30 (Cassidy, 1987). Easy mobility with only seasonal occupation of villages may have contributed to this relative longevity, related to its prevention of poor hygiene and its consequences. Between 400 to 500 AD, warfare appeared in the Ohio Valley related to competition for scarce resources (Seeman, 1979). Still, feasting with the dead was considered important, and the aged and the dead were respected. Warfare, however, decreased the value of the old. Young, strong warriors increased in value, at the expense of their elders.

Around 500 AD, endemic syphilis appeared to affect both sexes, indicating a 50% prevalence, related to both long-distance travel and trade.

Despite the Victorian era belief that ladies should not sweat, most human societies assigned grueling labor to both sexes. By the time of first European contact, all agriculture was done by women. Men hunted, made war, and traded.

Maize began to become important around 800 AD. After 1100 AD, maize was the staff of life for Indians all over the East. It was the basis for the development of complex chiefdoms along the Mississippi and the Ohio River Valleys (Cook, 1984).

Increasing agricultural and the cultivation of corn was associated with more arthritis of the left arm and the spine among skeletons analyzed from the post-1100 AD time frame.

Corn decreased childhood health related to:

▶ Less healthy environment of villages.
▶ Possible negative health consequences of grains.
▶ Immunoreactivity to grains.

The disease load increased, along with crowding, competition, and war. By 1200 AD, 25,000 people or more, lived in the city of Cahokia, on the Mississippi River, suffering under crowded and unsanitary conditions, all of which fostered disease. These included no clean drinking water and no controlled sewage removal. Urban concentration was responsible for a dramatic increase in the prevalence of tuberculosis in North America. Dental disease increased with agriculture related to the presence of a sticky carbohydrate staple (Buikstra 1984; Buikstra et al. 1986).

Food production, compared to gathering, more effectively expanded through technological innovation and increased labor investment. Consequently, people worked much harder, as evidenced in their skeletons. Complex communities resulted along with payment of tributes and taxation. The status of women and of the aged decreased as a result of corn and agriculture. Women became subordinate to men in the Eastern U.S. by the time of first European contact. Women were overworked and poorly nourished. Mortality increased, and the aged were less valued, due to their limited ability to produce crops or wage war. Life expectancy decreased. By first contact, for example, the average life span for women was 15 years and for men, 17 years, at the Averbach site in Tennessee.

Eighteenth and nineteenth century Plains Indians' rank and status came from participation in aggressive activities. The Plains people had been river bottom farmers and food hunters, which quickly changed when horses appeared. War had been common, but horses and rifles resulted in an escalation of earlier patterns. Tribal ideology came to be associated with male military, political, and religious roles, which gained ascendancy late in prehistory, with relative de-emphasis of metaphors involving creation, nurturance, motherhood, fertility, and sex (Medicine 1983).

Oriental Medicine: Similarities to Native American Practice

It is helpful to compare systems of indigenous medicine, and Chinese medicine has perhaps become the best known in North America – even better known than the continent's own indigenous healing systems. Traditional Chinese medicine practitioners work within the grand hypotheses of yin-yang and the Five Elements, believed to control all natural phenomena, including human life (Chang and Chi 1999). What is similar with North American beliefs is the importance of balance among all the elements. North American principles emphasize seven principles, symbolized by the sphere, including the four directions (North, East, South, West), the Center, the Sky, and the Earth. Medicine wheels illustrate these concepts in two dimensional shapes, similar to Chinese drawings to represent the interaction of the five elements. Sky and Earth, male and female, resemble with close correspondence the Chinese concept of yang and yin. Energy is stressed in Native medicine, as it is in Chinese medicine. Even the Lakota name for the highest spiritual Being, Taku skan skan, translates literally as "that which moves what moves." The concept refers to what makes movement, which is energy.

Chinese medicine selects herbs to maintain a balance between yin and yang in the interaction of the Five Elements (five organ systems: the heart, kidney, liver, lung, and spleen systems) of human physiology. Native medicine selects herbs to restore balance within the seven directions of the body. When pathogenic factors of either external (bad chi) or internal factors (the seven emotions) alter the human body, yin and yang are said to be out of balance. In Native America, when illness occurs, imbalance or disharmony are diagnosed. When illness results from too much yang, a doctor prescribes an herb with yin properties or vice versa (Liu and Mau 1980). Similar principles exist in Native American medicine with herbs being selected for their personality and the effects of their personality upon the patient.

Related to aging, in Chinese Medicine, the kidney system and the chi circulation work less effectively in most elderly people. Chi is best translated as the vital energy necessary to maintain body health. Chi is believed to be derived from a combination of Heaven chi (air needed for respiration) and earth chi (nutritional sources from food). Chi circulates through meridian paths throughout the body to supply vital energy (Xie 1999). When the circulation of chi is impeded due to aging or a shortage of chi results from illness, various ailments, and reduced body functions manifest. Tonic type formulas are often given to the elderly to elevate the state of chi to a sufficient rate of circulation.

Place, Health, Modern Corporatization, and Aging

Despite migratory patterns, the concept of place was important to Native peoples, who had extensive traditions about how to interact with the land upon which they roamed. Migration, of course, was limited by the absence of any mode of transportation except feet and small boats.

Unlike the Native American concept of the individual as subservient to place and existing within the environment in a complex web of inter-relationships, the nineteenth century liberal ideal of the good society situated the individual at the center of the social world. This individual was neither old nor young, but was poised to take control of his world with an iron grip (Jonsson 2000). A healthy environment was seen as a result of an organic equilibrium between individuals pursuing their own interests. Concern for the larger community emerged only when it was in the interests of the individual to be altruistic. Self first; community later, was the motto and the culture of the conquerors of the Americas.

Native American culture stands in stark contrast to this society of the individual with its community focus in which the young and the old are both important, with those of middle age intent on providing service to them. The modern idea of society, however, is very different from the community of individuals which constitutes a tribe (Rabinow 1989). This society is vague, abstract, and determines the details of the individual's everyday life (Jonsson 2000). Individuals struggle against their fates determined by society.

Corporatization is the opposite of tribal life. The rigidity of corporatization is stifling, suppressing the wildness of individual creativity, and ultimately annihilating humanity. Today's modern corporation is the antithesis of Native American life, and, of course, cannot include the elderly, except as stockholders. Corporate life requires an abrogation of the sense of the power of place, for good corporate employees move readily to anywhere that the company needs them. It breaks the web of relationships of person to other people, animals, plants, and even the stones of a natural environment. Modern corporate life captures the individual, dispossessing her of everything personal, putting to psychological death the person, by an immense social machinery. This includes the loss of place and the loss of the ability to grow old in one place. Modern life equates aging with Florida, for example, and not with a stable place of birth, adulthood, and death.

Corporatization is also antithetical to the well-being of elders. Tribal life with its close knit relationships provides a crucible for healthy aging that corporate cultures (notably the United States) do not provide. Inadequate social programs cannot compete with life-long tribal participation for creating the sense of meaning and purpose so crucial to mental, physical, and spiritual health.

Native American life was more akin to post-modernism than to the philosophies of its European conquerors. Post-modern life is characterized by frequent deviations from linear paths. Post-modernism recognizes that chaos is necessary to maintain adaptability. Post-modernism explodes corporatization, restoring the disorder needed for human survival. Modernism operates from rules and algorithms, containing instructions for every possible encounter. Post-modernism recognizes that novel encounters continually emerge to defy the rules. Success and survival come from creative adaptability, not from following the rules. In the writing of Musil (MWQ, p. 505), the military character, General Stumm von Bordwehr, expresses this phenomenon differently, when he says, "Somehow or another, order, once it reaches a certain stage, calls for bloodshed." The creativity of the human psyche erupts volcanically when sufficiently bridled.

Within corporative society, the rules for elder behavior are constrained and limiting. These include mandatory retirement and exclusion of the elderly from active participation in the lives of their children and grand-children, so essential to Native America. Creative adaptability was essential to hunter-gatherer survival, and the living memory of the elders served as a repository of possible and historical responses. Rigidity of rules increases with the capacity to write them down. Agriculture, warfare, and modern corporatization have been the downfall of healthy aging, from a Native perspective.

Consider this poetic rejection of modern corporatization (Musil, p. 162): "Within the frozen, petrified body of the city, he felt his heart beating in its innermost depths. There was something in him that had never wanted to remain anywhere, had groped its way along the walls of the world, thinking: 'There are still millions of other walls; it was this slowly cooling absurd drop 'I' that refused to give up its fire, its tiny glowing core.' When that pilot light is extinguished, the soul has died."

This passage captures the alienation of modern corporative life that was not present in Native America. Continuous, active participation by the elderly in the survival and operations of the tribe provided a radically different life experience from the alienating retirement and exclusion of the elderly from corporate life. Paradoxically, unlike Native society, where the elderly were essential providers of childcare, corporative society also excludes the elderly from the lives of children. The less the family is included in modern corporati-zation, such as is seen for recent immigrants where all generations live together, the less this occurs. Nevertheless, the American ideal marches toward an exclusion and separation of generations that is anathema to Native American culture.

I wonder about those of us who cannot corporatize. Besides "unruly Natives," the ranks of those who cannot assimilate into corporate culture include artists, maverick doctors, alternative healers, shamans, alcoholics, drug addicts, geniuses, and criminals – just those whose repository of radical responses provide a range of behaviors to save society when conditions change. Such deviants were more readily accepted into tribal life, perhaps related to conscious or unconscious awareness of the need to have a great range of adaptability, manifesting as a wide response set. Corporatization is death to the soul. It excludes wild, unpredictable, uncontrollable practices such as shamanic healing and ceremony. Characterized by the empty, repetitive motions of the assembly line, corporate culture applies rigid standard to individuals, forcing compliance.

In post-modernism, inner and outer reflect each other. The macrocosm and the microcosm are mirrors. The shape of a small section of a beach mirrors the shape of the California coastline.

The sense of personal belonging is lest with corporate culture. Personal belonging means that the land owns you, not that you own the land. It means that you and the land are inseparable. It means that the person and his or her family cannot be considered as divisible and separable. It means that membership in the tribe is for life. Place and position cannot be lost except by the most extreme behavior with punishment by banishment, a fate considered worse than death, since the dead continued to participate in tribal life.

Today's Situation

Elder care is dismal in North America today. Diabetes and other degenerative diseases are rampant. Nutrition is poor. Health has suffered.

Diets in Native America are not currently conducive to healthy aging. They are high in refined carbohydrates, fat, and sodium, and low in meats, eggs, cheese, milk, vegetables, and fruits (Kumanyika and Hellitzed 1985). Many dishes are combinations of meat and starch, and many foods are fried.

A study of food intake patterns of members of the Standing Rock Reservation in the Dakotas in 1970 showed a high consumption of coffee, bologna, potato chips, and carbonated beverages. Frying and boiling were the most common methods of food preparation. Traditional foods were reserved for special occasions (Bass and Wakefield 1974).

A dietary survey of 420 Hopi women and children conducted in 1974–1975 revealed that the contemporary Hopi diet consisted primarily of meat, mutton, eggs, potatoes, some canned vegetables, fruits and fruit juices, lard and other fats, coffee, tea, milk, and several commercial pastries and sweets (Kuhlein 1981). Only one-fourth of those studied had eaten a traditional food during the 24 hours prior to the study.

Similar dietary intakes were found for Navajo women in 1979–1980, with infrequent use of traditional Navajo foods. Coffee, tortillas or fry bread, potatoes, eggs, and sugar were the foods most commonly consumed, followed by sweetened drink mixes or soft drinks, store-bought bread, mutton, beef, milk, butter or margarine, bacon, luncheon meat, chicken, and tea (Wolfe and Sanjur 1988).

In Contrast to the Hopi and the Navajo, 98.6% of Eastern Cherokee households questioned in a food practice survey conducted in 1982 stated that the obtained food from traditional sources such as hunting, fishing, and gathering wild foods. The most frequently consumed Native foods were corn, squash, beans, trout, pumpkin, and wild greens. Non-native foods frequently consumed included coffee, milk, eggs, wheat bread, soft drinks, potatoes, bacon, fruits, and fruit juices (Terry and Bass 1984).

Like the Eastern Cherokee, Taos Pueblo residents continue to eat a variety of traditional foods (Aspenland and Pelican 1992). Four varieties of corn are cultivated – sweet corn and yellow, blue, and white corn – and are used in a variety of dishes. Pumpkins, wild greens, wild plums and chokecherries, pinto beans, and other traditional foods are widely consumed.

Nevertheless, for the country as a whole, Native American elders are eating poorly and are partaking of a diet conducive to diabetes, heart disease, and other degenerative disorders.

References

1. Allison MJ. 1984. Paleopathology in Peruvian and Chilean Populations. In Paleopathology at the Origin of Agriculture, ed. MN Cohen and GJ Armelagos, 515–530, Orlando: Academic Press.
2. Ames BN, Shigenaga MK, Hagen TM. 1993. Oxidants, antioxidants, and the degenerative diseases of aging. Proc Natl Acad Sci USA 90: 7915–7922.

3. Anderson MM. Kafka's Clothes: Ornament and Aestheticism in the Habsburg frin de siecle. New York: Oxford University Press, 1992, pp. 98–122.

4. Arzheim Forsch Sep 1985; 35(9): 1459–65.

5. Artzheim Forsch 1984; 34(8): 918–20.

6. Aspenland S, Pelican S. Traditional food practices of contemporary Taos Pueblo. Nutrition Today 1992; 27: 6–12.

7. Bass MA, Wakefield LM. Nutrient patterns and food patterns of Indians on Standing Rock Reservation. J American Dietetics Assoc. 1974; 64: 36–41.

8. BMJ Aug 31 1996: 313(7052): 253–58.

9. Buikstra JE. 1984. The Lower Illinois River Region. A prehistoric context for the study of ancient diet and health, In Paleopathology at the Origins of Agriculture, ed., Mark N. Cohen and George R. Armelagos, 307–45, Orlando: Academic Press.

10. Buikstra JE, Koningsberg LW, Bullington J. 1986. Fertility and the Development of Agriculture in the Prehistoric Midwest. American Antiquity 51(3): 528–46.

11. Bridges PS. 1989. Changes in Activities with the Shift to Agriculture in the Southeastern United States. Current Anthropology 30: 385–94.

12. Bridges PS. 1991. Skeletal Evidence of Changes in Subsistence Activities between the Archaic and Mississippian Time Periods in Northwestern Alabama. In What Mean These Bones? Studies in Southeastern Bioarchaeology, ed. Mary Lucas Powel, Patricia S. Bridges, and Ana Maria Wagner Mires, 89–101. Tuscaloosa: University of Alabama Press.

13. Bruhns Stothert. Women in Native America. 1999.

14. Byrd RB. Positive therapeutic benefit of intercessory prayer in a coronary unit population. South Med J 1988; 81: 826–829.

15. Carlson PH. Indian agriculture, changing subsistence patterns, and the environment on the Southern Great Plains. Agricultural History 1992; 68: 52–60.

16. Cassidy C. 1987. Monod Skeletal Evidence for Prehistoric Subsistence Adaptation in the Central Ohio Valley. In Paleopathology at the Origins of Agriculture, ed., Mark N. Cohen and George R. Armelagos, 307–45, Orlando: Academic Press.

17. Chang I-M, Anti-aging and health-promoting constituents derived from traditional Oriental herbal remedies. Information retrieval using the TradiMed 2000 DB. In Park SC, Hwang ES, Kim H-S, Park W-Y. Healthy Aging for Functional Longevity: moledular and cellular interactions in senescence. Ann NY Acad Sci 2001; 928: 281–286.

18. Chang IM, Chi JG. 1999. Harmonization of traditional Oriental (Chinese) medicine and modern medicine: a step forward with TradiMed Database 2000. In Cha K-Y (ed.) Traditional and Allopathic Medicine in the 21st Century. Pochun Cha University. Seoul, Korea, 151–160.

19. Cohen MN, Armelagos GJ., 1984, Editors Summation. In Paleopathology at the Origins of Agriculture, ed., Mark N Cohen and George R Armelagos, 393–424 Orlando: Academic Press.

20. Cohen MN, Bennett S. 1993. Skeletal Evidence for Sex Roles and Gender Hierarchies in Prehistory. In Sex and Gender Hierarchies, ed., Barbara Diane Miller, 273–96. Cambridge and New York: Cambridge University Press.

21. Cook DC. 1984. Subsistence and Health in the Lower Illinois Valley: Osteological Evidence. In Paleopathology at the Origins of Agriculture, ed., Mark N Cohen and George R Armelagos, 235–69. Orlando: Academic Press.

22. Crown PL, Wills WH. 1995. The Origins of Southwestern Ceramic Containers: Women's Time Allocation and Economic Intensification. J Anthropol. Res 51:173–86.

23. Dickel DN, Schulz PD, McHenry HM. 1984. Central California: Prehistoric Subsistence and Health. In Paleopathology at the Origins of Agriculture, ed. Mark N. Cohen and George R. Armelagos, 439–62. Orlando: Academic Press.

24. Driver HE. Indians of North America, 2nd edition. Chicago: University of Chicago Press, 1969, pp. 557–58.

25. Ezzo JA. 1993. Human Adaptation at Grasshopper Pueblo, Arizona: Social and Ecological Perspectives. Intl Mongraphs in Prehistory, Archaeological Series 4. Ann Arbor.

26. Guillen SE. 1992. The Chinchorro Culture: Mummues and Crania in the Reconstruction of pre-ceramic coastal adaptation in the South Central Andes. Ann Arbor: University Microfilms.

27. Harman D. Free radical theory of aging: nutritional implications. Age 1978; 1:145–152.

28. Harman D. Free radical involvement in aging: pathophysiology and therapeutic implications. Drugs and Aging 1993; 3: 60–80.

29. Harman D. Free radical theory of aging: role of free radicals in the origination and evolution of life, aging, and disease processes. In Free Radicals, Aging, and Degenerative Diseases. Johnson Jr JE, Walford R, Harman D, Miquel J, eds. New York: Alan R. Liss, pp. 3–49, 1995.

30. Harman D. Aging: prospects for further increases in the functional life span. Age 1994; 17: 119–146.

31. Harman D. Aging: Overview. In Park SC, Hwang ES, Kim H-S, Park W-Y. Healthy Aging for Functional Longevity: Molecular and cellular interactions in senescence. Ann NY Acad Sci 2001; 928: 1–21.

32. Jonnson S. Robert Musil and The History of Modern Identity: Subject without Nation. Durham: Duke University Press, 2000, p. 64.

33. Jackson MY. Diet, culture, and diabetes. In Joe J, Young R. (ed.) Native American Diabetes. New York: New Babylon Press, 1994.

34. Kuhnlein HV. Dietary mineral ecology of the Hopi. J Ethnobiology 1981; 1: 84–94.

35. Kumanyika S, Hellitzed D. Nutritional status and dietary patterns of racial minorities in the United States. Background paper for the U.S. DHHS Task Force on Black and Minority Health, 1985, p. 27.

36. Liu F, Mau LY. Chinese Medical Terminology. 1980 Hong Kong: Commerical Press.

37. Marcus J. 1983. Rethinking the Zapotec Urn. In The Cloud People, ed. Kent V. Flannery and Joyce Marcus, 144–48. Orlando: Academic Press.

38. Marcus J, Flannery KV. 1996. Zapotec Civilization: How Urban Society Evolved in Mexico's Oaxaca Valley. London: Thames and Hudson.

39. Medicine B. 1983. Warrior Women: Sex Role Alternatives for Plains Indian Women, In The Hidden Half: Studies of Plains Indian Women, ed. Patricia C. Albers and Beatrice Medicine, 267–80. Lanham, Maryland: University Press of America.

40. Mehl-Madrona L. Coyote Medicine: Lessons for Healing from Native America. New York: Scribner, 1997.

41. Morgan LH. Houses and house life of American aborigines. In: Contributions to North American Ethnology, Rocky Mountain Region, Vol. 4. Washington, D.C.: Government Printing Office, 1891.

42. Musil R. The Man without Qualities. Translated by Sophie Wilkins and Burton Pike. New York: Knopf, 1995, p. 392.

43. Ortiz de Montellano B. 1990. Aztec Medicine, Health, and Nutrition. New Brunswick: Rutgers University Press.

44. Osgood C. 1940. Ingalik Material Culture. Yale University Publications in Anthropology, No. 22, New Haven.

45. Packer L, Rimbach G, Virgili F. Antioxidant activity and biological properties of a procyanidin-rich extract from pine (Pinus maritime) bark, pycnogenol. Free Radical Biol. Med 1999; 27: 704–724.

46. Quilter J. 1989. Life and Death at La Paloma. Iowa City: University of Iowa Press.

47. Rabinow P. French Modern: Norms and Forms of the Social Environment. Cambridge, MA: MIT Press, 1989, 12 ff.

48. Rimbach G, Virgini F, Park YC, Packer L. Effect of procyanidins from Pinus maritime on glutathione levels in endothelial cells challenged by 3-morpholinosyndonime or activated macrophages. Redox Rep 1999; 4: 171–177.

49. Rivera MA. 1995. The Pre-ceramic Chinchorro Mummy Complex of Northern Chile: Context, Style, and Purpose. In Tombs for the Living: Andean Mortuary Practices, ed., TD Dillehay, 43–78. Washington, DC: Dumbarton Oaks.

50. Seeman MF. 1979. Feasting with the Dead: Ohio Hopewell Charnel House: Ritual as a Context for Redistribution in Hopewell Architecture. In Hopewell Archaeology: The Chillicothe Conference, ed., David S. Brose and Niomi Greber, 39–46. Kent: Kent State University Press.

51. Spellman CW. The agriculture of the early north Florida Indians. Florida Anthropology 1: 37 and 41–42.

52. Spence MW. 1974. Residential Practices and the distribution of skeletal traits in Teotihuacan, Mexico. Man 9: 262–73.

53. Taylor N. Plant Drugs That Changed the World. New York: Dodd Mead, 1965.

56. Terry RD, Bass MA. Food practices of families in an Eastern Cherokee township. Ecology and Food Nutrition 1984; 14: 63–70.

57. Thomsen M. (1969). Living Poor: A Peace Corps Chronicle. Seattle: University of Washington Press.

58. Ubelaker DH (No date). Health Issues in the Early Formative of Ecuador: Skeletal Biology of Real Alto. In The Formative of Ecuador, ed., Richard Burger and Scott Raymond. Washington, DC: Dumbarton Oaks.

59. Ubelaker DH (1980). Human Skeletal Remains from Site OGSE-80, a Pre-ceramic Site on the Santa Elena Peninsula, coastal Ecuador. J Washington Acad Sci 70(1): 3–24.

60. Virgili F, Kim D, Parker L. Procyanidins extracted from pine bark protect alpha tocopherol in ECV 304 endothelial cells challenged by activated RAW 264.7 macrophages: role of nitric oxide and peroxynitrate. FEBS Lett 1998; 431: 315–318.

61. Virgili F. Kobuchi H, Packer L. Procyanidins extracted from Pinus maritime (Pycnogenol): scavengers of free radical species and modulators of nitrogen monoxide metabolism in activated murine RAW 264.7 macrophages. Free Radical Biol Med 1998; 24: 1120–29.

62. Weatherford J. Indian Givers: How the Indians of the Americas transformed the world. New York: Fawcett Columbine, 1988.

63. Wolfe WS, Sanjur D. Contemporary diet and body weight of Navajo women receiving food assistance: An ethnographic and nutritional investigation. J Amer Dietetics Assoc 1988; 88: 822–827.

64. Xie Z. Selected terms in traditional Chinese medicine and their interpretation (IX). Chinese J Integrated Trad. Western Med 1999; 5: 300–302.

19 Looking After Our Elders: Healthcare and Well-being of the Elderly from the Perspective of Gwich'in and Other First Nations of Canada

R. Welsh, N.J. Turner

Introduction

We had fun with our elders ... We loved them and in caring for them we also had a lot of joy in doing this (Ruth Welsh)[1].

The Gwich'in are an Athapaskan-speaking First Nation of Canada's Yukon and Northwest Territories, with their traditional lands extending into eastern Alaska. For countless generations, from time immemorial, they have lived on the land, relying on fishing in the Mackenzie River and in the numerous other rivers and lakes that traverse their territory, as well as hunting caribou, moose, beaver, muskrat, and geese, and gathering a variety of plants for food, materials and medicine (Andre and Fehr 2001). In many ways, their's is a hard existence, with long, dark, cold winters and short, but intense summers. Nevertheless, the Gwich'in have been, by their own assessment, a happy and healthy people. They delight in the company of family and friends, and appreciate stories, jokes and games, as well as teachings that help them to survive in the harsh environment.

The Gwich'in, like other First Nations, cherish older people for their knowledge, experience, and wisdom. In Gwich'in communities, all people take responsibility in caring for their elders. Health and well-being is seen holistically. It is dependent on diet, on physical activity, and on spiritual, emotional and mental fitness as well as on physical condition. According to Gwich'in accepted wisdom, an active elder who goes for walks, socializes with friends and family, and who knits or sews or practices some other creative activity, generally has a positive outlook on life and will not often become sick or ailing.

Increasingly, however, Gwich'in concepts of health and disease are converging with those of conventional Western society. One of the big concerns for the Gwich'in today is that since most of the people moved and settled into permanent towns in the mid-1900's, they have adopted the food and lifestyle of mainstream society, and this is proving to be detrimental to their overall health, including the health of elderly people.

In this chapter, we discuss the various ways in which elders are cared for by members of their community, with supplemental relevant information from some other First Nations of Canada.

---

[1] The quotations from Alestine Andre and Ruth Welsh come from a conversation recorded on Saturday, March 24, 2001 in Victoria, B.C. Both women are Gwich'in; Alestine lives in Tsiigehtchik, Northwest Territories, and Ruth lives in Tagish, near Whitehorse, Yukon.

As Gwich'in people, our well-being is taught to us from a very early age, so that good health will stay with us for the rest of our lives. For us, prevention is stressed, first and foremost, rather than having to depend on medication. In many cases, we are taught, we can avoid use of medicines if we look after our diet and keep active in our lives. This was the number one lesson in our upbringing. Happy thoughts and humour are also an important part of our well-being. We are always taught to remember the good things, rather than dwelling on things that did not turn out so well. When we prepare medicines for a member of our community, the extra medicine is given to our elders. We spend time with our elders and try to include them in all our community activities and events (Alestine Andre).

Gwich'in children were taught to think about their elders and to give them priority at all times. Alestine remembers from her childhood:

"...When we came back from the residential school ... The plane landed, ...we no sooner got in the door when my mother told us..., 'Go and see so-and-so, your grandmothers. Go and see them, go and see all of them.' So there'd be a little pack of us. My brother and my two sisters and myself, the four of us would go across to their houses or to their tent or wherever and we'd go in there and just visited with them. ... And then later on, we might do some work for them, like see if they had enough water, or see if they had enough wood ..."

The Gwich'in have always been a caring people; thoughtfulness for others' needs was a value instilled in a child by her parents:

"I remember growing up and my mother telling me to always look after people that were orphans - *Chiitee* ["orphan"] and those that [were] older, *anjoo* ["older people"], like the real older people... She always said, "visit them or help them when they needed help.": If we're talking about taking care of our elders, we took care of everybody ..." (Alestine Andre).

This caring attitude was a general one for First Nations across the country. Dr. Mary Thomas, elder of the Secwepemc (Shuswap – Interior Salish) Nation of south central British Columbia, recalled from the time when she was growing up, in the 1920s, "... Our communities were very, very strong. Everybody helped each other." Families and neighbors would gather together to help each other with gardening, ploughing or other big chores, and everyone looked out for elderly people in the community (lecture, University of Victoria, February 2001).

Food and Nutrition

Good nutrition is seen by Gwich'in and other First Nations people as essential to good health. In general, the traditional diet of northern peoples was well balanced and healthy, including a wide diversity of foods consumed over the course of the year, although there might be lean times, especially in the early spring (Johnson 1997; Kuhnlein and Turner 1991; Nuxalk Food and Nutrition Program 1984).

An illustration of the close relationship between traditional diet, health and longevity recognized by indigenous people, is in a description of a 112-year-old Aniishenabe elder from Ontario. He had remained in good health in his first 107 years, and attributed his longevity to diet, saying he never touched store-bought food until he was in his 50s (Vancouver Sun, July 3, 1982). Gwich'in and others also attributed long life to 'bush people' being very active, and therefore being very fit, strong and healthy.

Obviously, because providing elders with nutritious food is crucial to their care, it has been a virtually universal practice among First Nations to ensure that the best foods are prepared and provided for elders. At communal dinners and feasts, it is usually the elders who are served first, before anyone else. This is a reflection of the respect for elderly people, which is a part of all traditional teachings. Alestine Andre recalled, for example, "... At our camp out in the bush, we also took special care of my grandmother, ... when we went for berries, one of us would lead her, out of the boat and help her up the hill. And she was in her eighties. She was still young ... then half way we'd stop or we'd stop along the way and we had water, so we'd give her water ... So we're always around her."

Even today, Gwich'in elders and others in need are routinely provided with game and other wild food. Generally, the families know what type of food the elders like, and they provide them with one serving dish at a time, already cooked. "We know the type and part of fish, caribou, moose, muskrat, rabbit, ptarmigan, grouse, meat or fish broth, or western food like chicken, bannock, hamburger or soups that our elders favor" (Alestine Andre). Depending on the food, elders enjoy country foods that are either boiled or roasted. The elders who are not able to get out and therefore not very active, prefer medium portions, whereas those who lead an active outdoor life eat three hearty meals a day. The older an elder gets, the less food they want, as their appetite seems to wane. Too much solid food for someone who is not active will cause constipation and a sick feeling. Then, medicine is need to relieve the constipation, and sometimes another medication to counteract the first.

One practice to alleviate such problems is to chop solid foods finely in a blender. In traditional culture, too, meat and fish are boiled and the broth, sometimes lightly salted, is drunk instead of eating solid flesh. Broth is always given to those who are bedridden or who cannot walk[2]. Many Gwich'in seniors and elders use drink broth daily to help keep them strong and healthy. Another healthy traditional food that people commonly use is wild berries. "We have many berries that we use fresh, dried, frozen, canned as fruit or made into jams. Juice is also made from the berries, which we use instead of buying juice from the store. This is the reason, I am sure, that we stay healthy and active and are able to take care of ourselves well into our 80s and 90s and are still very much enjoying our lives" (Ruth Welsh).

Stomach and digestive tract ailments and obesity are two recognized problems directly related by Gwich'in to diet; both of these can be treated by eating specific foods to cleanse the stomach, or by reducing or refraining from other foods, such as those high in fat. In any case, Alestine notes, "We are always cautioned not to overeat favored foods otherwise we will end up with a tummy ache. For example, we are told not to overeat berries, loche fish liver, bear root plant (*Hedysarum alpinum*)[3], black duck,

---

[2] It is also given to very young children to help wean them off the breast or bottle, giving them a good start to a healthy diet (Ruth Welsh).

[3] Note that there is another species, "wild sweetpea" (*H. boreale; syn. H. mackenzii*), which is said to be quite toxic and has caused poisoning to those who mistake it for the edible type (Kuhnlein and Turner 1991).

animal bone marrow, and duck grease. More recently, we are starting to associate poor diet with processed foods or foods brought from the community stores, versus the more traditional country food. The awareness of nutrition, health, physical activity, and food is starting to emerge".

Elders in other indigenous communities are similarly cared for nutritionally. Mary Thomas recalled that in her household and others in her Secwepemc culture, there was always a pot of bones simmering on the stove. When anyone came into the house, her mother would say, "Pour out some broth for grandma, [or for grandpa]." Mary Thomas said, "It's the food that they ate that made them healthy. They didn't ever fry food. They boiled, barbecued, or baked it in the oven (pit-cooked it). Now, we fry everything. ...We were never sick when we were kids. It guess it's when the diet changed, that's when people started getting sick." (pers. comm. to NT, January 1996).

Aboriginal children of all Nations were instructed always to be generous with whatever they obtained, especially to elders. When a boy caught his first salmon or procured his first deer, he would give it away to an uncle or grandparent (Arvid Charlie, pers. comm. to NT, December 1999). Likewise, a girl who had made her first basket, would be taught to fill it with berries and then give it away to an older relative (Mabel Joe, pers. comm. to NT, 1995).

These teachings, of providing food for elderly people, whether at feasts or out in the bush, or in their homes, were deeply engrained. Chief Adam Dick of the Kwakwa̲ka̲'wakw Nation of the Northwest Coast recalled that any time his people went hunting for seal or deer, or fishing for salmon, they were sure to provide for those who could not go out for it themselves: "The first of everything always went to the old people... They let them have their winter supply before we'd go out for the rest of the village." (pers. comm. to NT, 2001).

In general, the elders know and trust that whatever favorite food is prepared for them is good for their health. Gwich'in and other elders are always thankful for what food is brought to them, and especially enjoy the traditional food. This appreciation for traditional foods as opposed to imported market foods is diminishing and this trend poses serious concerns for the nutritional health of future generations of elders (Kuhnlein 1989a, 1989b).

Shelter and Living Requirements

As well as ensuring that elderly people were provided with nutritious food, it has been important for the Gwich'in and other First Nations to provide adequate shelter and accommodation for elders. There are no beliefs among the Gwich'in, as in the *fengshui* Chinese tradition of house orientation, that housing *per se* influences health. The structure of the family unit determined the house style and size in the old days, before the mid-20th Century. The Gwich'in lived on the land year round in small and extended family units and they all lived in one room. Originally, they lived in large caribou skin tents, or large "moss houses" (subterranean houses), and more recently in canvas tents and one-room log cabins. The family unit was together, and this was an important factor in the emotional and mental health of elders, because they were included as part of all the daily activities.

Over the last 50 years or so, as people have moved into permanent communities, circumstances have changed. The modern houses have walls and separate rooms, and the lifestyle in town has caused a separation between and among family members, even when they are all still living under one roof. Elders can feel more isolated; they may no longer have such close contact with children and other family members.

Elders living on their own were also cared for. Ruth Welsh recalled the help and comfort they used to provide as children for the home of one old woman, Mrs. Drymeat:

"When they were in tents, … she had boughs on the floor. And we'd go out every second week or so, a bunch of us … Some of them were grown up, some of us were small and we'd just tagged along. [We] pitched right in and we'd get fresh boughs for her … [or] the next time we would just add [boughs] on top … You'd do this a couple of times and then you take it all out and start all over again. It was always nice and fresh in there. It smelled so-o Christmasy in there! …. [with] those little wood stoves, camp stoves … It was nice and toasty warm."

The care of the Gwich'in elders was overseen by community leaders like Alestine's father, Hyacinthe Andre, when he was a chief at Tsiigehtchic. For example, one year at Christmas time, some of the elders decided to stay in town instead of going out in the bush after Christmas; they wanted to stay in their tents. Alestine's father assigned each of the young people to get a load of wood for each of the older people who were staying in town. The elders helped themselves, too, as much as they could. They enjoyed going out. "They wanted to get out and get that exercise and fresh air and just clear their mind." (Ruth Welsh). They would pack dried willow twigs and other wood home whenever they were out. One old woman, Alestine recalls, used to go across the Arctic Red every day to get one or two pieces of driftwood from a big wood pile there, having her one-dog sled to help her bring it home.

Adam Dick recollected, similarly, how the young Kwakwaka'wakw people would be organized to check on the elders and their needs:

"My grandfather, he'd call these young people in and tell them to check on that house, check on this house, and see what they need. If they need wood, go get 'em. … And water, too. 'Cause we were getting water from the river. They used to have pails and they packed them up, firewood, anything… The old Kwaxsistala [Adam's grandfather] used to make sure that the elder people got their supplies first, especially in this time of year. You'd see wood stacked up in front of the old peoples' houses. … They don't have to ask for it." (pers. comm. to NT, 2001)

Not only food, shelter, firewood and water, but the other needs of the elders were routinely looked after. For example, the Gwich'in elders' clothing was made "by our women, by the women of the community, to make sure they stayed warm" (Ruth Welsh).

Self Sufficiency, Self Esteem and Respect

The elders of Aboriginal communities, as with elders everywhere, like to keep themselves occupied, and to feel that they are useful, contributing members of the family. This feeling of worth, and the respect that Aboriginal people have for their elders' knowledge and wisdom, is critical to elders' health and well-being.

Many Gwich'in elders, even those of very advanced in years, took pride in their sewing, tanning hides, carving, or helping to process food. All they needed was some assistance with certain aspects of this work. Ruth Welsh recalls as a child and young adult helping thread needles for the elderly women who still made their own moccasins, their own mukluks [hide boots] and their own hand-sewn dresses from fabric they bought at the local store. "...They enjoyed doing those things, it gave them a lot of independence ... The only problem was they couldn't see well enough to thread a needle, so we would thread quite a few and long thread on it so that they wouldn't have to thread them all." (Ruth Welsh).

Children were taught to be polite to elders at all times. Alestine noted that when they visited the elders as children, "...it was a time, too, when we just clustered around the doorway and we didn't run all over the house." Ruth added, "No. That was not allowed in those days." Alestine recalled that when their grandmother came to their house for their Sunday prayers, "... we see her little head bobbing along the window, ...We knew she was coming, so we just ran around and we made a place for her, a little mat. We'd have a special mattress for her to sit [on] ..." Ruth noted that the first thing they did as children returning to Fort McPherson on the boat from school would be to go as a whole group and visit all the older people in the community. "I think silently they [our parents] were teaching us through example, how to respect and to care for our elders." After awhile, Ruth recalled, the young people would automatically go to look after the elders, getting their wood, water, ice or snow or whatever they needed. "There came a point and time where no one had to tell us. We did it." They didn't expect any payment. "You didn't even think of being paid for something like that. And we'd sit down with them and they'd tell us stories and that was better than any money in the world." Sometimes though, the elders would give the children who helped them a small gift like an orange, or a cup of tea, water or some bannock.

Elders were included in every community event, dance or feast; they were never left out. Older people were brought along to the fish camp, or on any other trips they wanted to come on. The elders would have their own tent and the children could learn from watching them and listening to them.

The skills that elders had were always appreciated by younger people. Even the knack of positioning a piece of food in an outside fireplace to make the fire burn better was something that developed with experience; Alestine was always amazed at her grandmother's abilities to maintain a perfect fire. Ruth Welsh noted:

"They were excellent guides as far as teaching us how to make things – how to cut fish, how to make the smokehouse, and get the bark of the trees for the roof and around the house. Sometimes we'd use willows, all around [the house], because you needed that air circulating. They stressed how important that was. And every story that they told us over the years, whether it was an old, old story or whatever, there was always a moral to those stories, ...and now it's finally teaching us how to do things and how to live. I always couldn't wait for the end, because I want to figure out what the moral was. It was right there, you couldn't miss it!"

Intervals out in the bush, and feasts, potlatches and other community events, were important times for elders to be able to talk, to recollect their experiences and to teach others the knowledge that had been passed on to them by a previous generation of elders. After every feast, Alestine recalled, an elder always spoke to them. "The whole community, everybody in that center or hall sat and listened. It didn't matter whether it was a man or a woman elder.... The eldest [person] spoke, spoke to all of us. And we sat there and we listened." In societies where knowledge is traditionally communicated orally, these teachings from older to younger generations are particularly significant.

In a similar vein, Chief Earl Maquinna George, a Nuu-Chah-Nulth hereditary chief of Ahousaht on the West Coast of Vancouver, talked about learning from the elders speaking at feasts from the time of his childhood, in the 1930s:

"There was another old man called *Tushka*. He had a cane, and after the dinner was... eaten, he got up and banged the cane on the floor, and he was the start of what was going on. He announced what the feast was for, who it was for, and the reason why the feast went on. He started, with the historical stories of where our people came from. And this was *Tushka*. He must have been one of the leading historians of our culture. He knew about the songs, and the dance that go with each family. There were various types of feasts that went on a lot. The people were proud of the many things that were said through the long talks by *Tushka* ..." (pers. comm. to NT, 1999).

Earl George explained that even the smallest children were made to sit still and listen when the elders spoke like that. It was both in respect for the elders, but also to ensure that the knowledge they held would be passed on and absorbed by the youngest generation.

Medicine and Healing Needs

Many contemporary Aboriginal people remember having gathered and prepared medicines for their elders, when they were young; it was routine to do this. Both Alestine Andre and Ruth Welsh recalled bringing medicine, as well as food and other supplies, to their elders. (Alestine still does this for elders in her community.) The elders would ask for certain medicines, and the younger people would go out and gather them, and often would prepare the medicine to order, or dry medicinal plants for the elders to use during the wintertime. Medicinal herbs were prepared in different strengths, depending on the nature or seriousness of the ailment. For example, spruce cone tea is made as an infusion for the common cold, whereas spruce pitch tea, which is much stronger, is prepared and administered to an elder suffering from influenza. It is also used for stomach ulcers, and upset stomach, and "too much bile", according to Ruth. Usually about a one week's supply of any type of medicine – whether for tea, salve or poultice – was prepared at a time, and only the quantity of medicine needed for one series of treatments was collected, prepared and provided to the elder.

To provide care for elders and others, the Gwich'in might employ several health practices at once, including visiting a sick elder, ensuring that they are warm and comfortable, that they have enough fuel, water and food, and, finally, bringing whatever herbal medicines might be good for their illness. Alestine, in preparing and delivering a traditional plant medicine treatment, would recommend that both the patient *and* their resident caretaker (wife, husband, etc.) take the medicine, since a medicinal tea, while alleviating the illness of the sick person, will also help maintain the health of the caretaker. If the ailing person or couple is elderly, Alestine will prepare and deliver the medicinal teas to their home and, if necessary, will bring more again after three or four days when she knows the first batch has been completely used[4].

The Gwich'in and other indigenous people who use traditional herbal medicine believe in its healing powers. Some individuals will make traditional plant medicines (e.g. Labador or muskeg tea – *Ledum groenlandicum*) and drink them routinely as a general tonic for good health, while other individuals will take the medicinal teas, salves, poultices only when they feel sick or when they need to treat a cut or infection. Those who take these treatments are very happy with them, and deeply appreciative of the ones who gather and prepare the medicines for them.

Some traditional medicine preparations are common knowledge amongst most older and middle-aged Gwich'in. Everyone knows, for instance, that the spruce cone tea is good for colds and is a good tonic to help maintain general good health. There are numerous people, both women and men, who collect and prepare such medicinal teas to treat themselves as required, or who drink a daily portion of medicinal tea to stay healthy. However, there are a few individuals in each of the four Gwich'in communities, who are widely recognized as having an extended and specialized knowledge of traditional medicine, including salves, poultices and stronger medicines. For serious ailments, the elders and other people in the community will seek these specialists out and request their help specifically.

In other Aboriginal communities, too, younger people help and support the elders in preparing and administering their medicines. For example, Nlaka'pamux elder Mabel Joe recalled as a young wife helping her elderly, crippled mother-in-law to treat her arthritis in the sweat lodge. At her mother-in-law's request, she gathered four large bundles of stinging nettles. Her mother-in-law sat inside the sweat lodge and took each bundle from Mabel in turn, hitting her arthritic joints with the stinging leaves and repeating the process four times. By the time she had finished this treatment, her arthritis had improved so much that she was able to discard her cane and walk normally (Turner et al. 1990). Mary Thomas also remembers her mother treating elders in their Shuswap community at Neskonlith (Salmon Arm), making them medicinal tea or poultices, or whatever else they needed (pers comm. to NT 2001).

---

[4] For younger ailing people, Alestine will prepare the medicine and deliver it to their home, and in this case will provide written instructions on how to collect, prepare the traditional plant medicine tea so they can prepare the treatment themselves in the future. She will often suggest that individuals make and drink the teas even when they are not sick.

Adam Dick talked about how the younger Kwakwaka'wakw people were instructed by his grandfather as headman of the village to harvest and then dry the medicines for their elders to use: "They go..., in the season when it comes, like the spring, through the summer, [they get]...like the *ixwm'i* [devil's club – *Oplopanax horridum*] – you can dry it.... Like the *m'umt'eni* [grand fir – *Abies grandis*], you can take it, put it in pails or sacks. They can be dried, to be used in the winter months. You soak them, and drink it.... (pers. comm. to NT, 2001).

The types of medicines taken by elderly people were similar to those taken generally. However, some tonics and other medicines were specifically recognized for keeping older people fit and healthy. For example, one Kwakwaka'wakw elder from Fort Rupert used to drink a tonic tea of grand fir bark every day. He was about 75 years old at the time he was interviewed (1969), but he looked about 50, and his youngest child was about 10 years old (Turner and Bell 1973).

Elderly people tend to suffer more from chronic diseases such as rheumatism and arthritis, and other ailments such as cataracts of the eyes, that were treated with specific traditional medicines such as devil's club or solutions of different kinds of tree bark (Turner 1982; Turner and Hebda 1990).

No known scientific trials have been done to date that confirm the efficacy of Gwich'in medicines specifically, although most people in the past have relied on them and have believed them to be effective. Other indigenous peoples of northern Canada and other regions of North America have similar health practices, and many of them use the same types of medicinal plants in comparable preparations, and some of these have been demonstrated to show antibiotic activity (Turner et al. 1990; McCutcheon et al. 1992, 1994; Ritch-Krc et al. 1996a, b; Johnson 1997; Bannister 2000; Moerman 1998; Marles et al. 2000). Clinical studies of some related herbal medicines, particularly those used in Germany and elsewhere in Europe and in traditional Chinese herbal medicine (Blumenthal 2000), demonstrate efficacy for many of them. In general, however, indigenous herbal specialists caution against applying their particular traditional medicines more widely. They believe that "the traditional health practices of Native North American peoples using traditional plant medicine treatments belong to the Aboriginal groups for their use. All groups have a common unwritten rule that we will only take and use the traditional plant that we need to take care of a particular ailment." (Alestine Andre).

Changes

Today, health care for Gwich'in and other Aboriginal elders is different from that of the past. A choice of "western" or "traditional" medicine is available to most people. Western medicine includes both what the physicians at the health clinics prescribe for illness, and the medicines one can buy off the drugstore shelves. Traditional medicine, on the other hand, is the medicine that has been used locally for thousands of years, gathered and prepared by family members or local herbal specialists.

There are definite advantages with the ready availability of western pharmaceutical drugs, and with modern surgery, and other medical advancements. Traditional medicine, however, is considered more dependable, especially for minor ailments and "first aid", and is "free" to those who know where to find it and how to use it. Many elders use both western and traditional medicine, although some use only traditional medicine. Even today some people, especially the older elders, prefer the healing power of spruce pitch salve and tea, and spruce cone tea, to that of prescription drugs.

People still retain a holistic view of health and well-being: "The most important way for us to stay well and active as we grow older is to be as active as we can daily by walking, gardening, sewing, cooking our meals, using foods that we can grow ourselves or by buying foods that we know are grown organically. We should try to get as much of our vitamins, minerals, proteins and everything else that our body needs for our daily well being from our food intake" (Ruth Welsh).

As mentioned earlier, the well-being of elders is partly due to their feelings of self esteem, of being valued by their families and communities. Alestine Andre and Ruth Welsh regard the times of their own childhood and the elders they knew then with great affection. Ruth recalled a tiny old woman named *Vigiighe'* who stayed in town at Fort McPherson in a tent year round. The young people helped her put up her tent, got her firewood and ice for her, and check on her fire. " She was a happy, happy little lady.... we'd sit there and listen to her stories." Sometimes she wanted to go down to the store, and about six teenagers would go with her. "We had so much fun with her. We went and got a toboggan and one person was on the back with her; she was sitting down in the toboggan. The rest of us were her dogs, just like dogs in a harness! ... Only it was only a rope that we were holding. And we'd run. And she'd be so excited, she'd be giggling." They would stop in from of the Hudson's Bay store, go in with her, and pack home her groceries. "We had fun with our elders. We weren't vicious in any way, you know. We loved them, and in caring for them we also had a lot of joy in doing this."

As an elder now herself, Ruth is anxious about her future. She worries that elders are not as well looked after as they used to be. "It's scary even for me now. I almost panic sometimes thinking you know. I don't have any children. I'm by myself now. I wonder what's going to happen if I live that long. Will I be cooped up in some old folks' home by myself and not have anyone come and see me? It's frightening." Alestine, who is younger than Ruth, and already has her father living with her, reassures her: "I'll take you in. You can live with us!"

Despite medicare and perhaps better access to health clinics and social services, the attitudes of younger Gwich'in people have changed, their priorities have changed, and the elders sometimes do not receive such kind attention and respect in the community that they used to get. Peoples' diets are also changing (Berkes and Farkas 1998), and, for indigenous elders everywhere, this represents a serious health problem. Incidence of heart disease, diabetes, obesity and other indicators of high risk are increasing (Hopkinson et al. 1995; Stephenson et al. 1995).

Many of the changes to traditional systems of care for the elderly in indigenous societies started to occur with the imposition of the residential school system. For Secwpemc elder Mary Thomas, for example, her close relationship with her grandmother was virtually severed when she was taken away to the residential school in Kamloops.

... I was about six and a half years old when I was taken away from my grandmother. ... We practically lived with Grandma. Oh, it was so good! She was so kind to
us, yet she was firm. Just out of the blue, they took us away from there and put us in the
residential school. And there were nights I cried myself to sleep. I was lonely. I missed
my grandmother. ... The way I grew up... we were always asking questions: "Grandma,
what is this? Grandma, what are you doing? Grandma, why do you want it?" ... We were
allowed to talk as much as we could. In the residential school, we were not allowed to
speak. ... I didn't know English. How can I communicate if I don't know the language?
... And when I got caught speaking [Shuswap language], I got strapped, five strokes on
each hand... It drew blood on the wrist.

... My grandmother ... taught us pride ... in our people. There [at residential school]
we were taught totally the opposite. We were told that this type of teaching – the
teaching of my grandmother – was the work of the devil and that we were to throw it
away. We were not allowed to even hum an Indian song... We were totally cut off from
studies that we learned from our grandparents (Lecture, University of Victoria, February 2001).

The trauma Mary felt at being taken away from her grandmother, and at having all
of her grandmother's teachings devalued, must have had as much of an impact on her
grandmother as it did on her. The residential schools began a process of disruption, of
enforced turning away from traditional values and teachings, which has occurred to a
greater or lesser extent in Aboriginal communities everywhere.

Chief Adam Dick reflected on the situation in his own community, in which people
have forgotten many of the traditional ways:

And it's gradually changing and changing and changing ... It changes, you know, in
a community like Kingcome ... They don't listen to their elders ... they think they know
it all. But they don't do [traditional activities] anymore. ... I know for sure that they
don't even know about the *ts'ats'ayim* [eelgrass – *Zostera marina*, one of the traditional
foods from the ocean] anymore. They don't know how to handle fish anymore. They
don't pick berries anymore. They don't dry berries any more like they used to do.
And I said to ... one of the boys, "What's the matter with them people?" "Adam, they're
getting lazy. They just go to the store and buy them." They don't ... even know how to
bake bread anymore, he was telling me, some of the people ... I guess all the villages are
the same ... They depend on the way things are now today, you know, the superstores
and all that ...

When asked about caring for the elders, and making sure that they got enough
good food, firewood and other necessities, Adam replied:

"They don't do that anymore. ... As I said before, things are changing. Even, at Alert
Bay, I heard that somebody was supposed to go fishing. And some of the people
go down there, to see if they could get some. "No, no. We've just got enough for our
family ... Can't give you any." ... they don't help each other any more ... (pers. comm. to
NT, 2001)

As an elder today, like Ruth Welsh, Adam worries about the future. Kim Recalma
Clutesi explained that today's elders, who, when they were young, took such good
care of their own elders have an expectation that they would be looked after when
they grew older. This makes the changing attitudes of younger people even harder to
accept.

Thus, although specific treatments for physical ailments of Gwich'in and other elders are available, the other aspects of health, seen to be equally important for their overall well-being – good nutrition, strong social support, feelings of being a valued and respected member of the family and community – are not as positively reinforced as in earlier times.

Over the recent decades as Gwich'in people have started living permanently in towns, families have become separated. Instead of being altogether in one room, telling stories and in conversation, the family now occupies different spaces; the parents or grandparents are sitting in the living room watching television, while the children or grandchildren are in their own rooms playing Nintendo or other video games. As well, many young people, adults and even close relatives, will often ask for payment for doing chores for their parents or elders like chopping and hauling wood, shoveling snow in their yard, or getting ice. Most of the young people do not seem to be interested in learning traditional ways like sewing, making sleds, canoes, and log homes, or traveling on the land.

Gwich'in communities suffer from elder abuse when children and grandchildren bother their parents and grandparents for money when their pension cheques arrive in the mail each month. Drug, alcohol and gambling addictions are realities in many indigenous communities, and this makes it a challenge for Gwich'in and others to work with and revive traditional languages and cultures. Elders are also affected, and some are caught up in this cycle.[5]

In fact, often a person who does not consume alcohol, does not do drugs or gamble, and tries to be positive in their approach to life is seen as "abnormal." It takes tremendous energy to work in these communities where negativity, complaining, mistrust, and strained relationships within and among families are common. Nevertheless, a few elders and younger people who emulate them are still healthy – in the broadest sense of the word – and continue to talk to the ones who express or demonstrate an interest in the Gwich'in way.

Throughout North America there are many initiatives among First Nations communities to support and recognize elders, drawing on traditional practices but within a contemporary context. For example, S'ul'hween Quw'utsun' (the Elders Program) of the Cowichan Nation on Vancouver Island, was started in 1993 to enhance the health and well-being of elders through providing them with meals of traditional food (e.g. salmon and clams), opportunities for social interaction and decision-making, and sharing teachings with younger people.

There are four components of a person's health, and the elders promote an holistic approach to the health and well-being of all. The Elders Program reflects these for components. The spiritual goals are to support the free expression of spirituality and to facilitate the feeling of support by the elders for the community in matters of spiritual experience, growth, and traditional values. Emotionally, the goal is to encourage participation in community life by providing a place for socializing and the development of friendship, and by providing caregiver support. Also important is the pride

---

[5] Ruth Welsh notes, "Taking alcohol while on medication does a lot of harm. We know that one can counteract the other and be fatal at times. A drink now and then is fine but don't over do it. At least, not to the point of making you have a headache or sick to your stomach."

and feeling of ownership and self worth that the elder people enjoy from making central program decisions ... discussed and made by the group as a whole (Modeste et al. 1995).

This program exemplifies a recent trend towards developing new mechanisms to enable communities to care for their elders in ways that reflect continuity of cultural values even in the face of monumental social, demographic and economic change. There is a widespread recognition that changing times have left gaps in the traditional modes of ensuring elders' well-being. Seniors' centers, elders' circles and weekly elders' meetings, where older people can come together and enjoy social exchange in a culturally comfortable way, are facilitated in almost every Aboriginal community across Canada. In British Columbia, an Elders' Gathering is hosted annually in different communities throughout the province, and younger community members help with the travel and accommodation arrangements for their elders. Canadian Aboriginal elders have been hosted internationally as well, by indigenous communities and organizations in the United States, United Kingdom, New Zealand and elsewhere.

Hence, the special, honored place traditionally occupied by elders in Gwich'in and other First Nations communities has been retained and in some cases strengthened even in the face of change. The positive effects of traditional practices on their overall health and enjoyment of life are undeniable, and, in understanding these traditional approaches to health, many lessons can be learned by Society as whole in the care and support of elderly people. The final words go to Ruth Welsh who, as a Gwich'in elder, expresses at once a traditional approach to elders' healthcare and a recommendation for the future[6]:

"Many older people still go out and pick the berries, fish and hunt with their families and have a great time doing these things with them. It gives them time to teach the younger ones about taking care of themselves and each other and also teaching them how to survive off the land. Happiness for these people is being with family – grandchildren. Happiness is teaching.

Our mental attitude has much to do with our well-being. Look around you. Many people cannot see, period. Enjoy each new day, watch the dawn, the sunrise, the clouds, the rain, the snow falling, the ice forming or melting. Each has a story to tell. Listen to the birds in flight or singing or talking. We must try to understand them. Are they singing because they are happy? Is it a distress call? There could be a change in the weather. Who knows? Maybe we don't but we can try. It is a good mental exercise.

Take care of your body. It is the only one that we get! We cannot change the way that we were build, therefore let us be good to our selves. Treat yourselves as you would your best friend. You would, I'm sure, give your best friend nothing but the best. Do likewise for yourself. Don't put into your body anything that would harm you. We all know that cigarettes and alcohol used to excess harms us in many ways, such as asthma, emphysema, cancer, liver and kidney problems and heart disease to name a few. Do we really need these things?

[6] Acknowledgements: We would like to say "*mahsi' choo*", thank you very much to many people for helping us with this project, and in particular: Arvid Charlie, Chief Adam Dick (Kwaxsistala) and (7OqwiloGwa), Chief Earl Maquinna George, Mabel Joe, Agnes Mitchell, Dr. Daisy Sewid-Smith, Martina Slaven; Hyacinthe Andre; and Dr. Mary Thomas. We are also indebted to Dr. Paul Cherniack, for initiating this project and providing helpful guidance. We also acknowledge financial support for this research from Global Forest Science to Alestine Andre (GF-18–2001–156).

Think happy thoughts. If you have raised your family, think of all the good times that you had with them. Don't dwell on the bad times or the hard times. Those things are in the past. You gave it your best so be proud of that. We cannot change what was in the past but we can change a lot of things now and try to make the best of things to come."

References

1. Andre, A. and Fehr A. 2001. Gwich'in Ethnobotany. Plants used by the Gwich'in for food, Medicine, Shelter and Tools. Gwich'in Social and Cultural Institute, Tsiigehtchic, NT and Aurora Research Institute, Inuvik, NT.
2. Bannister, K.. 2000. Chemistry Rooted in Cultural Knowledge: Unearthing the Links between Antimicrobial Properties and Traditional Knowledge in Food and Medicinal Plant Resources of the Secwepemc (Shuswap) First Nation. Doctoral Dissertation, Department of Botany, The University of British Columbia, Vancouver, B.C.
3. Berkes, F. and Farkas C.S. 1998. Eastern James Bay Cree Indians: Changing patterns of wild food use and nutrition. Ecology of Food and Nutrition 7(3): 155–172, 1978
4. Blumenthal, M. 2000. Herbal Medicine. Expanded Commission E Monographs. American Botanical Council, Austin, TX.
5. Hopkinson, J., P.H. Stephenson, and N.J. Turner. 1995. Changing Traditional Diety and Nutrition in Aboriginal Peoples of Coastal British Columbia. Pp. 129–166, in: Stephenson et al. (Editors). 1995. A Persistent Spirit: Towards Understanding Aboriginal Health in British Columbia. Canadian Western Geographic Series, Vol. 31, Department of Geography, University of Victoria, BC.
6. Johnson, L.M. 1997. Health, Wholeness, and the Land: Gitksan Traditional Plant Use and Healing. PhD Dissertation, Department of Anthropology, Edmonton, Alberta.
7. Kuhnlein, H.V. 1989a. Change in use of traditional foods by the Nuxalk Native people of British Columbia. In: Pelto G.H. and Vargas, L.A. Perspectives in Dietary Change. International Nutrition Foundation, Cambridge, UK.
8. Kuhnlein, H.V. 1989b. Factors influencing use of traditional foods among the Nuxalk People. Journal of the Canadian Dietetic Association 50: 102–108.
9. Kuhnlein, H.V. and Nancy J. Turner. 1991. Traditional Plant Foods of Canadian Indigenous Peoples. Nutrition, Botany and Use. Volume 8. In: Food and Nutrition in History and Anthropology, edited by Solomon Katz. Gordon & Breach Science Publishers, Philadelphia, Pennsylvania.
10. Marles, R., C. Clavelle, L. Monteleone, N. Tays, and D. Burns. 2000. Aboriginal Plant Use in Canada's Northwest Boreal Forest. UBC Press, Vancouver and Toronto.
11. Modeste, D., D. Elliott, C. Gendron et al. 1995. S'huli'utl Quw'utsun/The Spirit of Cowichan: A Journey Through the Tsewultun Health Centre/ Huy'tseep qu no Siiye'yu kwun's 'i m'i ewu'u Tuna Tsewultun. Pp. 331–256, in: Stephenson et al. (Editors). 1995. A Persistent Spirit: Towards Understanding Aboriginal Health in British Columbia. Canadian Western Geographic Series, Volume 31, Department of Geography, University of Victoria, BC.
12. McCutcheon, A.R., S.M. Ellis, R.E.W. Hancock and G.H.N. Towers. 1992. Antibiotic Screening of Medicinal Plants of British Columbian Native Peoples. Journal of Ethnopharmacology 37: 213–223.
13. McCutcheon, A.R., S.M. Ellis, R.E.W. Hancock and G.H.N. Towers. 1994. Antifungal Screening of Medicinal Plants of British Columbian Native Peoples. Journal of Ethnopharmacology 44: 157–169.
14. Moerman, D.E. 1998. Native American Ethnobotany. Timber Press, Portland, OR.
15. Nuxalk Food and Nutrition Program. 1984. Nuxalk Food and Nutrition Handbook, Nuxalk Nation Council, Bella Coola, BC.
16. Ritch-Krc, E.M., S. Thomas, N.J. Turner & G.H.N. Towers. 1996a. Carrier herbal medicine: traditional and contemporary plant use. Journal of Ethnopharmacology 52: 85–96.
17. Ritch-Krc, E.M., Turner & G.H.N. Towers. 1996b. Carrier herbal medicine: an evaluation of the antimicrobial and anticancer activity in some frequently used remedies. Journal of Ethnopharmacology 52: 151–156.
18. Stephenson, P., S.J. Elliott, L.T. Foster, and J. Harris (Editors). 1995. A Persistent Spirit: Towards Understanding Aboriginal Health in British Columbia. Canadian Western Geographic Series, Volume 31, Department of Geography, University of Victoria, BC.
19. Turner, N.J. 1982. Traditional use of devil's-club (Oplopanax horridus; Araliaceae) by Native Peoples in western North America. Journal of Ethnobiology 2(1): 17–38.
20. Turner, N.J. and M.A.M. Bell. 1973. The ethnobotany of the southern Kwakiutl Indians of British Columbia. Economic Botany 27(3): 257–310.
21. Turner, N.J. and R.J. Hebda. 1990. Contemporary use of bark for medicine by two Salishan Native elders of southeast Vancouver Island. Journal of Ethnopharmacology 229 (1990): 59–72.
22. Turner, N.J., L.C. Thompson, M.T. Thompson and A.Z. York. 1990. Thompson Ethnobotany. Knowledge and Usage of Plants by the Thompson Indians of British Columbia. Royal British Columbia Museum, Memoir No. 3, Victoria, British Columbia.

20 Complementary and Alternative Medicine Use Among Latinos

D. Salas-Lopez, A. Natale-Pereira

Present day Latin American culture has been shaped by its Indian, African, and Spanish origins. Health beliefs and knowledge about disease stem from the com-bination of Spanish traditions introduced by the colonizers, the health practices of indigenous groups and African slaves, and learned biomedical knowledge. As such, the use of complementary and alternative medicines in the form of herbs, massage, prayer, and magic is prevalent and represents an important element of the health practices of Latinos, particularly the elderly, that can not be underestimated [1, 9–12].

The Latino culture takes a holistic view of health and illness. The mental and physical well being of the individual seems to be inseparable. Latinos comprise a heterogeneous group of people that use an explanatory model of illness generally associated with social, psychological, and physical domains. These beliefs are reinforced within the family, and family members play a major role as resource of informal health information. Traditional or folk healing among Latinos, as is the case of non-Western cultures is common practice and is transferred through generations [9, 11, 12].

As a diverse group, not all Latinos hold the same beliefs or engage in similar health behaviors. Some practices may be ubiquitous among some groups but minimally used among others. Even within subgroups, there are cultural and heritage differences in the use of alternative medicines. Nevertheless, most Spanish speaking countries share similar practices in the use of traditional herbal medicines regardless of their differences in culture.

For the most part, Latinos believe in disease as a disturbance of the balance between physical and social well being. Folk diseases such as mal de ojo (evil eye, or dangerous imbalances in social relationships), empacho (upset stomach, or stress during or after eating) and ataques de nervios (nerve attacks, or expression of strong emotions) are some of the most consistent examples shared among the different subgroups [1].

For example, Central Americans believe that illness may be the result of an imbalance between the environment and an individual, extremes of emotions, and outside forces. Mexican Americans also view ill health as an imbalance between the individual and the environment, with variables such as emotions and spiritual factors. On the other hand, Puerto Ricans view illness as a lack of personal attention to health, punishment for sins, or evil [1, 10, 11].

Folk illnesses, which are perceived to arise from a variety of causes, often require the services of a folk healer. There are a number of different types of folk healers within the system that varies by subgroup. Examples include curanderos, sobadores, santeros, herbalists, or spiritualists. These traditional healers prescribe specific teas, ointments, and compresses to cure illness. They may also be consulted to carry out spiritual rituals to prevent or cure disease. The use and acceptance of folk healers varies among the different Latino subgroups [1, 10, 11].

Curanderismo as a system has evolved from spiritualist, homeopathic, Aztec, Spanish, and other Western foundations. Curanderos use rituals, prayers, pledges, or herbal bathes for cleansing and healing. Other healers such as the sobadora use massage therapy to manipulate bones and joints. A bruja, brujo, and hechicero practice magic rituals. The yerbalista prescribes herbal remedies that may be used topically or ingested in a variety of ways [1].

The use of complementary and alternative treatments is underestimated in Latino populations. The extensive use of such therapies is driven, in large part, by the belief that these treatments come from nature, have fewer side effects, are less expensive, and easy to purchase in local botánicas and bodegas. In addition, there is anecdotal evidence for their effectiveness that comes from heritage and family tradition. Most of these treatments exist in tablet form, teas, or ground substances and are purchased on the advice of traditional healers. This chapter will focus on herbal therapies commonly used by many Latino subgroups [1].

The following is a list of commonly used herbal treatments for a variety of ailments and illnesses in this population. While this list is not exhaustive, it represents those treatments used most often by Latinos. It is not recommended that they be used without the advice of a physician since many of these have active ingredients that may have interactions with other prescribed medications and treatments [2–6].

Uña de Gato (Cat's Claw)

Cat's claw grows in the rain forests of the Andes Mountains in South America, particularly Peru. It may take more than two decades to mature. It grows thorns resembling the claws of a cat (hence its name). It is popular in South American folk medicine. In order to protect this highly valued herb, the Peruvian government restricts harvesting of the root. Only the inner bark is harvested, leaving the root untouched and able to regenerate for many years to come. The root bark is used as medicine by many to treat inflammation, rheumatism, gastric ulcers, tumors, dysentery, and as birth control. Although cat's claw has become very popular in North America and is used for AIDS and HIV, little scientific evidence supports the use of cat's claw for these conditions. A cat's claw tea is prepared from 1 gram of root by adding water and boiling for ten to fifteen minutes. After cooling and straining, one cup is drunk three times per day. No serious adverse effects have been reported. Cat's claw may be contraindicated in diseases such as multiple sclerosis and tuberculosis [2, 4, 5].

Menta (Mint)

Mint grows in many parts of the world. The two varieties most used by Latinos are menta negra, which has violaceous leaves and has a high oil content, and menta blanca, which has pure green leaves and a milder taste. Mint has been used to treat indigestion, colic, gingivitis, irritable colon, and tension headaches. It is primarily used as a tea although it is also used topically as an oil for pain and minor cuts. The tea is prepared by boiling 1 cup of water with 5 grams of dry menta leaves for five to ten minutes. After cooling and straining, three to four cups daily relieves indigestion and stomach ailments. Mint is also available in tablet form, which is taken three times a day for irritable colon. A combination of mint and eucalyptus in an oil base is used topically for headaches. Although no serious adverse side effects have been reported, large quantities may cause gastrointestinal distress and dermatitis [2, 4, 5].

Rabo de Gato (Cat's tail)

Cat's tail is a tall plant with lemon colored flowers. It grows at high altitudes in Mediterranean countries such as Spain. Cat's tail is used for dyspepsia, gastritis, and minor skin infections. It is commonly used by farmers and country veterinarians for minor skin abrasions in animals. It is believed to have active ingredients that are anti-inflammatory. A tea is prepared with thirty to forty grams of the flower. This tea is cooled and strained and can be used topically with compresses. No serious side effects have been reported.

Rompepiedras (Stone busters)

This is a common plant in Cuba, Philippines, Nigeria, Guam, and Central India. It grows up to sixty centimeters and all of the plant parts are used therapeutically, including its yellow leaf. It is used by Ayurveda and increasingly by Latinos, for the treatment of hepatitis, gonorrhea, diabetes, edema, and skin irritation. It is thought to contain antiviral ingredients that act on liver cells. It is used most commonly for hepatitis B infections and in one study was found to reduce hepatitis B antigen in 59% of chronic carriers. It is available in granules, which are taken in quantities of 900–2,700 mg per day for three months. There are no known side effects.

Cola de Caballo (Horse Tail)

This plant grows in the northern hemisphere and in Europe. It is a wine colored, cone shaped plant that grows in the summer and fall and resembles the asparagus species. It is used for a variety of ailments including, in-grown toe nails, edema, osteoarthritis, osteoporosis, and rheumatoid arthritis. Horsetail has also been used for kidney stones, cystitis, bleeding ulcers, and tuberculosis. It is thought to contain many naturally occurring elements including silica, potassium, aluminum, and manganese. This is felt to be responsible for it's varied use. Horsetail is prepared as a tea by adding one to four grams in boiling water. Two to six cups three times a day is the usual dose. There are no known side effects.

Diente de Leon (Lion's teeth)

This plant is found worldwide. Reaching heights of up to thirty centimeters, this plant produces yellow flowers year round. The leaves and flowers are used for alcohol withdrawal symptoms, constipation, edema, and indigestion. Lion's teeth, is rich in vitamins A, B, C, and D and minerals such as iron, silica, manganese, zinc, potassium and magnesium. It is felt to have diuretic properties although its mechanism of action is not understood. Three to five grams of dry root yield five to ten milliliters of Lion's teeth extract. This extract is used three times a day. Side effects are more common in patients with gall bladder disease and peptic ulcer disease thought to be due to over stimulation of bile acids.

Rusco (Butcher's Broom)

Butcher's broom is a spiny plant that grows in the Mediterranean region and Northern Europe. It's roots and young leaves are used for arteriosclerosis, venous insufficiency, hemorrhoids, and varicose vein. The plant is also used as a broom by butcher's (hence it's name). It is thought that the active ingredients decrease vascular permeability. Studies on its extract have shown improvement in patients with chronic venous insufficiency when used in combination with Vitamin C. Butcher's broom extract is used in 50–100 mg per day. There are no known side effects [7].

Gordolobo (Mullein)

Mullein is a biannual white plant that grows wild in the Spanish mountains. Its leaves are harvested in the spring, it's flowers in July and September, and it's roots in March and October. It is used as a treatment of respiratory infections, chronic obstructive pulmonary disease, cough, and ear infections. It is also used as a topical preparation for skin burns and infections. It is ingested as a tea by boiling one cup of water with five to ten grams of leaves or dry flowers. The tea is taken three to four times a day. It can be used in combination with other herbs for cough. Mullein extract is used by some as an oil preparation for ear infections. There are no known side effects.

Yuca (Yucca)

This plant grows in the dry regions, particularly the Southeastern United States. Its stem and root are used for osteoarthritis and rheumatoid arthritis [8]. Native Americans have used yucca bathes for skin disorders, including alopecia and dandruff. Yucca is available in tablet form and is used twice a day. Higher doses are used for rheumatoid arthritis. Alternatively, six to seven grams of yucca leaves can be boiled with one cup of water. This can be ingested three to five times a day. Side effects known to occur with higher doses include weakness and leg cramps. Additionally, hemolytic reactions have been reported.

Verdolaga (Pursley)

An annual herb, this plant has thick stems with long round leaves. Pursley grows in dry sandy regions close to water bodies in many areas in Europe. It is also found in the continental United States. Pursley is used for constipation, cystitis, conjunctivitis, and blepharitis. Farmers who grow the leaves have also used it in salads. It is thought to contain Vitamin C, laxative properties, and anti-inflammatory characteristics. It can also be used topically for conjunctivitis and blepharitis. The plant is soaked in one liter of water. Two to four cups of the mixture are used daily.

Trebol de Agua (Buckbean)

This is an aquatic plant that grows up to 30 centimeters in length. Its long leaves have white and pink flowers. Buckbean is found in lagoons and around other water bodies in Europe and some parts of North America. It has been used for chronic gastritis, loss of appetite, and menstrual cramps. Buckbean tea is taken prior to every meal as a tea. Known side effects include vomiting and diarrhea.

Helecho macho (Male fern)

This plant has lancet like leaves that are divided in oblong segments united at the base. It grows in forest in Europe and North and South America. It is used mainly for intestinal parasites. Although it is not specific for any particular parasite, it has been used primarily for ancylostoma duodenale. Its active ingredients are felt to paralyze the musculature of the parasite resulting in detachment from the intestinal lining. When male fern is combined with laxatives the parasite is expulsed. Male fern root is prepared by dissolving three to five grams in water. This is done twice a day followed by a laxative at night. Side effects include nausea, vomiting, and diarrhea. It is also contraindicated in anemia, cardiac disorders, and gastric ulcers.

Avena (Oatmeal plant)

This plant grows worldwide and is one of the most commonly used herbs. The wild form of the oatmeal plant is harvested, using only the green leafy portion and the fruit of the plant. It is used for high triglycerides, eczema, high cholesterol, insomnia, skin irritations, and nicotine withdrawal. The seed or fruit of the plant is thought to be rich in iron, manganese, and zinc. Oatmeal plant is used as a food supplement or as a tea. Oatmeal tea is prepared by boiling 30 grams in one cup of water. After cooling and straining, it is ingested twice a day. It is also used topically as a bathe for many skin disorders. There are no known side effects. It is contraindicated in patients with gluten sensitivity.

Cilantro (Coriander)

This is an annual plant that can grow up to 90 cm tall with white or pink flowers. It is found in many Mediterranean countries, the Orient, North and South America. Coriander is used as a condiment, in salads, and for medicinal purposes. Its uses include indigestion, intestinal gas, loss of appetite, and halitosis. Approximately, 25 to 30 grams of coriander seeds are dissolved in one liter of water. One cup of this mixture is ingested after each meal. Narcotic-like side effects have been reported.

Hierba centella (Cowslip)

Cowslip is a plant that grows in rain forests and coastal regions of Europe and the Americas. It's kidney shaped leaves and yellow flowers can reach heights up to 40 cm and a diameter of 4 cm. It is used for rheumatoid arthritis and other inflammatory illnesses. Cowslip leaves are ground and used topically over the affected joints two to three times daily for ten to fifteen minutes. Side effects include skin irritation.

Migranela

The leaves of migranela are ubiquitous in Europe and North America. It has been used for headaches, fever, arthritis, and menstrual cramps. It is thought to increase serotonin levels and inhibit platelet aggregation. Pulverized migranela can be purchased in tablet form and taken daily for headaches and other ailments. Side effects include nervousness and gastrointestinal distress.

Amapola

The amapola plant is an annual herb that grows up to 80 cm tall. Its beautiful flower is the part that contains medicinal properties. Amapola has been used for insomnia, anxiety, and cough. Its active ingredients include papaverine that is thought to be useful in anxiety. It can be used as a tea by boiling flower petals in water and drinking one to two cups per day. There are no known side effects.

References

1. Molina, CW, Aguirre-Molina, M. "Latino Health in the US: A Growing Challenge", 1994 American Public Health Association.
2. Aquino R, De Feo V, De Simone F, et al. Plant metabolites, new compounds and the anti-inflammatory activity of Uncaira tormentosa. J Nat Prod. 1991; 54:453–59.
3. Foster S. Herbs for Your Health. Loveland, CO: Interweave Press, 1996, 72–73.
4. Bradley, PR, Ed British Herbal Compendium, vol.1. Bournemouth, Dorset UK: British Herbal Medicine Association, 1992, 174–76.
5. Tyler VE. Herbs of Choice: The Therapeutic Use of Phytomedicinals. Binhamton, NY: Pharmaceutical Products Press, 1994, 56–57.
6. Castleman M. The Healing Herbs. Emmaus, PA: Rodale Press, 1991, 219–21.
7. Rudofski G, Diehm C, et al. Chronic venous insufficiency; Treatment with ruscus extract. MMW 1990; 132–205–10.
8. Bingham R, Bellew BA. Bellew JG. Yucca plant saponin in the management of arthritis. J Appl 1 1975; 27:45–50.
9. Boyle, J.S. (1996). Central Americans. In J.G. Lipson, S.L. Dibble, & P.A. Minarik (Eds.), Culture and nursing care: A pocket guide. San Francisco: UCSF Nursing Press.
10. De Paula, T., Lagana, K., & Gonzales-Ramirez, L. (1996), Mexican Americans. In J.G. Lipson, S.L., Dibble, & P. A. Minarik (Eds.), Culture in nursing care: A pocket guide. San Francisco: UCSF Nursing Press.
11. Juarabe, T. (1996) Puerto Ricans. In J.G. Lipson S.L. Dibble, & P.A. Minarik (Eds.), Culture and nursing care: A pocket guide. San Francisco: UCSF Nursing Press.
12. Spector, R.E. (1991), Cultural diversity in health and illness (3rd ed.). Norwalk, CT: Appleton & Lange.

21 Diet and Lifestyle Modification for the Elderly

E.P. Cherniack

In this chapter, the potential role of many different types of alternative medical therapies and their implications for the elderly will be discussed. The phrase "diet and lifestyle modification" is a poor attempt to summarize the concepts behind all these treatments, they include, in addition to the use of the use of diet and red wine to improve health, techniques of mental self-control ("mind/body" therapies) and use of touch and thought by others to improve a patient's health (massage and "energy healing techniques).

Diet

Other than the Ornish diet, which will be discussed extensively in the next chapter. A lot of other popular diets might potentially used by the elderly. One of the oldest diet, and one which has been supported by some experimental evidence is the Pritikin diet.

Developed several decades ago, the Pritikin diet relies on protein and especially fat restriction as cornerstones of the regimen. Users consume mostly vegetables and whole grains, increase fiber intake and try to reduce fat intake to less than ten percent. While it is not simple to follow, several studies have purported to have shown benefit several decades ago. Virtually all of the studies, however, have been performed by Dr. Pritikin or colleagues who are proponents of the diet.

One study examining the health effects specifically in the elderly was conducted by Weber et al., who examined seventy persons at least 70 years old (mean age close to 79) who followed a diet and daily exercise and resided for a month at center for participants in a Pritikin program [1]. This small trial was uncontrolled and unblinded. During their stay, they were reported to have lost an average of 2.2 lbs., reduced mean serum cholesterol from 222 to 179, and decreased triglycerides from 156 to 141. In addition, their exercise capacity increased.

Several other smaller studies were also conducted using the diet. Although not specifically conducted in the elderly, they noted reductions in cholesterol and fecal bile acids, and increased ventricular function [2–5]. A double-blind trial compared lipid reductions in subjects with peripheral vascular disease over one year between a diet similar to the Pritikin diet (low-fat, high fiber and complex carbohydrate) and an American Heart Association Hyperlipidemia diet (low-fat and cholesterol, high-fiber) [6]. There was significant improvement in walking distances in the users of both the less complicated American Heart Association diet and more complicated high-complex carbohydrate diet after one year, with no significant changes in lipid profile.

Theoretically, users might receive some of the possible benefits of those observing the Ornish diet, namely protection against atherosclerotic disease. Nevertheless, it also possible that dieters might receive minimally sufficient quantities of fat from the diet with such an extreme fat restriction to sustain adequate health. Long-term studies of the diet's safety, have not been done in the general population nor the elderly, and is not clear how readily older persons might adhere to such a diet.

The Atkins diet is another popular diet that is relatively simple to follow. Relying on decreasing caloric intake through carbohydrate restriction, followers can eat any foods they want other than carbohydrate-rich foods. The diet has been used for more than twenty-five years. Published studies on the outcome of the Atkins diet have yet to be performed, but the unpublished results of several trials comparing the Atkins diet to others have been present at scientific meetings. Some of the trials, supported by diet proponents, noted that adherents did lose weight, but they but differed on total and low-density lipoprotein (LDL) cholesterol [7, 8]. In theory, elderly users of this diet might to vulnerable to suffer manifestations of atherosclerotic disease, although no long-term studies have been performed on the elderly. In addition, there is concern that the degree of ketosis that might ensue from the degree of carbohydrate restriction might be harmful [9, 10].

Another carbohydrate restriction diet is the Zone diet. Unlike the Atkins diet, the degree of carbohydrate restriction and protein intake is dependent on the activity level of the person, with active persons being allowed more protein and carbohydrates. Thus, it is a more complex diet for users to follow. In addition, the assumption that active individuals require a higher protein input has been challenged, and it might be true that the elderly need a greater intake of protein than implied by their level of activity alone 11]. The use of the Zone diet has not been studied in trials published in peer-reviewed scientific journals.

The Sugar Busters diet relies on reduction of intake of sugar, processed or natural to create caloric reduction. Based on the benefits conferred to diabetics who follow a sugar-restricted diet, it is unclear whether similar benefits are conferred on nondiabetic participants in the program. Again the diet has never been tested in published investigations, nor in the elderly.

There are some individuals who attempt to adhere to an American Diabetic Association calorie restriction diet in effort to lose weight. However, no data is available on the effects of the use of such a diet by nondiabetic individuals.

Anderson et al. considered the potential benefits and risks of a number of popular diets. He predicted that higher fat diets would place individuals at a higher risk for atherosclerotic disease from increased cholesterol levels, low-carbohydrate diets would decrease risk for disease, but the greatest benefit would be provided by low-fat, high-carbohydrate, and high-fiber diets [12].

Red Wine

Population studies have observed that there is an association between alcohol intake and numerous diseases included atherosclerotic illnesses, cancer, hypertension, macular degeneration, osteoporosis, peptic ulcer disease, nephrolithiasis and cholelithiasis [13, 14]. The relationship or relative risk of illness and consumption has been characterized as a J- or U-shaped curve, implying that moderate consumers of alcohol are at lowest risk [13, 15, 16]. These have been studies of large populations that have included but have not been exclusive to the elderly.

Red wine has been reported in vitro to have several health benefits, such as inhibiting platelet aggregation and preventing LDL oxidation [17, 18]. The benefits may be derived from chemical compounds known as flavonoids, which have antioxidant properties, reservatrol, caffeic or protocatechiuic acid [18–24]. Reservatrol has been noted to have anti-tumor activity, and stimulates cytokines, natural killer, and T cell function [25, 26]. Resveratrol has also been shown to inhibit the growth of pathogenic bacteria and fungi on the skin [27]. Several investigations indicate that these benefits might also be conferred by grape juice without the alcohol [28, 29].

In vivo benefits have also been observed. Red wine has been reported to improve conductance in coronary arteries [30] and to have cardioprotective effects in animal models [31–33]. These include limitation of infarct size [32] and inhibition of endothelin-1 which promotes atherosclerosis [33]. Red wine was reported to increase serum antioxidant concentrations in elderly women [34], and many of the illnesses that red wine or the compounds found within might impact upon, are major causes of illness in the aged [35].

Mind/Body Therapies

The term "mind/body" therapies refer to use of one's own thought to promote health. It comprises a variety of techniques including meditation, yoga, biofeedback, hypnosis, guided imagery, and relaxation therapy.

There have been few randomized controlled trials of many of the therapies, but a number of investigations have been conducted on the use of these methods to treat disorders commonly encountered by older persons.

Biofeedback

Biofeedback refers to a process by which an individual attempts to self-regulate functions normally controlled involuntarily by the autonomic nervous system. Typically the involuntarily processes are measured by a device that gives a signal, perhaps by beeping or pulsing, to the person. The user then attempts to alter the signal through an exercise. Biofeedback has been extensively studied and reported to treat numerous disorders such as fecal and urinary incontinence, headaches, hypertension, and strokes.

There are several possible uses for biofeedback that may be important for the elderly. The treatment of fecal incontinence is probably the most extensively studied that has particular implications for the elderly, and biofeedback has also been used to treat urinary incontinence, pain, and hypertension. The use of biofeedback to treat constipation has yielded mixed results [36, 37].

Fecal incontinence has been noted to occur in just over two percent of the community-dwelling patient population and forty-five percent of nursing home residents [38]. Although there are a plethora of trials, most of them have been small and uncontrolled [39–45]. Nevertheless, those that have been conducted appear to show benefit in three-quarters of all subjects, though there has been cure in only one-half [38, 46]. Patients who undergo biofeedback have improve their thresholds for perception of the urge to defecate [46].

Biofeedback was utilized in several trials including two randomized trials to treat urinary incontinence. The incidence of incontinence was reduced by eighty-percent, which was significantly more effective than medication [47–49].

Several small investigations have examined the role of biofeedback for several other possible uses, such as the rehabilitation stroke victims, treatment dysphagia, of healing foot ulcers, and treatment of pain [50–54].

Some other small studies indicated a promising role for biofeedback in the treatment of hypertension [55–58], but a meta-analysis of studied noted that the effect was small [59].

Yoga

Yoga is a group of systems of philosophy and physical discipline which is several thousands of years old. As applied to improve health, it generally consists of the use of a regimen of body postures and breathing exercises. In a small investigation, the use of yoga decreased the heart rate and altered the baroreflex sensitivity of healthy elderly persons [62].

However, when one-hundred elderly were randomized to receive either aerobic exercise or yoga, the aerobic exercise received benefits in oxygen consumption, anaerobic threshold, diastolic blood pressure, and improved cholesterol after four months that was not conferred on the group that performed yoga [60]. Yoga was also used as a control intervention in studies in the elderly of a behavioral therapy for chronic tinnitus and exercise to improve glucose tolerance [61].

Attempts have been made to use yoga to treat hypertension, cardiovascular disease, epilepsy, and asthma among other illnesses, in investigations done mostly in India [60, 63]. Studies, mostly involving small numbers of subjects have been conducted on the use of yoga to treat hypertension [63, 64]. In studies that included elderly subjects, yoga exercises improved some symptoms of carpal tunnel syndrome and osteoarthritis of the hands [66, 67].

A Cochrane database review of the use of yoga to treat seizures found one trial that met the appropriate review criteria with only a small number of subjects [68].

Meditation

Meditation has been defined as the "self-regulation of attention" [69]. Subjects who practice meditation characteristically focus their attention on a single subject (for example, the sensations in one's leg), and techniques are used to return attention to focus if the mind becomes distracted. Meditation can be classified as concentration meditation, in which there is a single object of attention, or mindfulness meditation, in which the objects of meditation are changed.

Two forms of concentration meditation that have been the subject of investigation are Transcendental Meditation (TM), and "relaxation response". TM, a popular form of meditation and probably most extensively studied, albeit by TM proponents, is based on concepts of traditional Indian philosophy and will be discussed more completely in another chapter.

Relaxation response describes meditation that was created in the 1970s in which practitioners try to achieve the "relaxation response", which is a reduction in sympathetic nervous system arousal [69]. The relaxation response has been used to treat pain and anxiety, but has been seldom studied in the elderly. At least one small, uncontrolled study showed that this method, combined with more conventional techniques, decreased symptoms of chronic pain in almost sixty percent of all subjects [69, 70].

Mindfulness meditation has also been utilized to treat chronic pain, depression, and anxiety [69]. Several small studies, mostly self-controlled and in younger patients, have shown some benefit [71].

Hypnosis

Hypnosis describes a therapy in which a therapist induces certain perceptions, thoughts, or behaviors in a subject through relaxation, imagery, or by altering the focus of his concentration [69]. There is often a multi-step process including instructions for relaxation, followed by directing one's concentration, suggestion of a behavior, and a posthypnotic phase in which the suggestion is reinforced. Hypnosis has been used to treat pain, hypertension, insomnia, and obesity among other medical conditioned.

There is a paucity of studies using hypnosis for the elderly as a distinct subject population, and most of the investigations have involved only small numbers of subjects. Conditions common to the elderly for which hypnosis has been studied include post-operative and cancer pain [77, 78]. In one single-blinded investigation, in which self-hypnosis was compared to standard care (attention training that was also part of the hypnotic therapy). Both groups had improvement, with the self-hypnosis group receiving the greatest pain relief [79]. Two meta-analyzes of the use of hypnosis to achieve weight loss also showed some efficacy, with an average weight loss of between two and seven pounds [80].

Guided Imagery

In guided imagery, which is similar to hypnosis, a therapist suggests images for the subject to picture to improve his emotional state. It has been used to relieve pain in terminally ill patients and help rehabilitate stroke victims [82]. One randomized study of 130 patients observed that patients having colorectal surgery who listened to guided imagery tapes needed fifty percent less narcotic medication perioperatively to relieve pain [69]. Guided imagery has also been used in numerous studies to provide pain relief for terminally ill patients. Many of the trials of guided imagery however, employ guided imagery in conjunction with other methods, and so it is difficult to discriminate between guided imagery and the effects of other techniques. Nevertheless, one meta-analysis rated guided imagery as higher in efficacy than other cognitive techniques [69, 83].

Massage

Massage therapy refers to the rubbing of the hands by a practitioner on a patient's body for healing purposes. There are many different types of massage therapies: reflexology (stroking of the subject's body to alter "energy" generated by a given point on a subject's body), Swedish massage, which uses oil rubbed onto a patient's body on a table, and the Trager method, in which limbs are held to the side or above the body, and then rocked or held [84]. Franke et al [85] compared Swedish massage to acupuncture and standard exercise in the treatment of low back pain, but only acupuncture proved better than control. Massage therapy was found to be the most common form of alternative medicine used by patients with osteoarthritis, but few formal trials have been conducted on its use [84]. Foot reflexology decreased pain and anxiety in an uncontrolled trial in oncology patients [86].

Distant Healing

Distant healing is a term describing methods of treatment of disease in which the practitioner does not make physical contact with the patient. It includes Therapeutic Touch, energy healing, prayer, and other forms of spiritual healing. A review of these therapies noted that most of the trials that have been conducted thus far showed some benefit, but methodologic problems precluded definitive determination of benefit [87]. A meta-analysis of therapeutic touch did not show any advantage [88].

Some forms of distant healing are know as "energy healing". This describes systems of therapy in which a patient's body is presumed to generate "energy fields" and practitioners attempt to treat disorders by manipulating these "energy fields". Such systems include reiki, qi gong, and polarity therapy. While a complete discussion of the theories behind these systems is beyond the scope of this chapter, there have been few formal clinical trials of the effects of these treatments. Lee et al. randomized forty elderly subjects with chronic pain in an unblinded study to receive "qi therapy" or standard pain reduction, and found significantly decreased pain in the qi-treated group [89].

Aromatherapy

Fragrances have been investigated in the treatment of a number of disorders that might be beneficial for the elderly, such as the relief of chronic pain [90] and relief of anxiety in terminally ill individuals [91]. A review of investigations conducted thus far did not find enough evidence to support its use for relief of anxiety [94]. In one randomized double-blinded trial, it was also successful as a treatment for alopecia areata [92]. In one case study, aromatherapy and massage was used to treat behavioral disturbance in demented patients with mixed results [93]. There have been reports of allergic reactions to aromatherapy [95, 96].

References

1. Weber F, Barnard R, Roy D (1983) Effects of a high-complex-carbohydrate, low-fat diet and daily exercise on individual 70 years of age or older.
2. Rosenthal M, Barnard R, Rose D et al. (1985) Effects of a high-complex- carbohydrate, low-fat, low-cholesterol diet on levels of serum lipids and estradiol. American Journal of Medicine 78(1): 23–7.
3. Mattar J, Salas C, Bernstein D et al. (1990) Hemodynamic changes after an intensive short-term exercise and nutrition program in hypertensive and obese patients with and without coronary artery disease Arquivos BrasileirosCardiologia 54(5): 307–312.
4. Barnard R, Massey M, Cherny S, O'Brien L et al. (1983) Long-term use of a high-complex carbohydrate, high-fiber low-fat diet and exercise in the treatment of NIDDM patients. Diabetes Care 6(3): 268–273.
5. Reddy B, Engle A, Simi B, et al. (1988) Effect of a low-fat, high-carbohydrate, high-fiber diet on fecal bile acids and neutral sterols. Preventive Medicine 17(4): 432–439.
6. Hutchinson K, Oberle K, Crockford P, Grace M et al. (1983) Effects of dietary manipulation on vascular status of patients with peripheral vascular disease. Journal of the American Medical Association 249(24): 3326–3330.
7. Yancy W, Bakst W, Bryson K et al. (2002) Effects of a very-low-carbohydrate diet program compared with a low-fat, low-cholesterol reduced-calorie diet. February 23–27. Abstract of the North American Association for the Study of Obesity, Abstract 100541, San Diego CA.
8. Clifton P, Noakes M, Parker B (2002) The effect of a high protein weight loss diet in overweight subjects with type 2 diabetes. February 23–27. Abstract of the North American Association for the Study of Obesity, Abstract 100543, San Diego CA.
9. Hirschel B (1977) Dr Atkins' dietetic revolution: a critique. Schweizerische Medizinische Wochenschrift 17(29): 1017–1025.
10. Forster H (1978) Is the Atkins diet safe in respect to health? Fortschritte der Medizin 96(34): 1697–1702.
11. Lemon P (2000) Beyond the zone: protein need of active individuals. (2000) Journal of the American College of Nutrition 19(5 suppl): 513s-521S.
12. Anderson J, Konz E, Jenkins D (2000) Health advantages and disadvantages of weight-reducing diets: a computer analysis and critical review. Journal of the American College of Nutrition 19(5): 578–590.
13. de Lorimer A (2000) Alcohol, wine, and health. The American Journal of Surgery 180(5): 357–361.
14. St. Leger A, Cochrane A, Moore F (1979) Factors associated with cardiac mortality in the developed countries with particular reference to the consumption of wine. Lancet 1: 1017–1020.
15. Rimm E, Klatsky A, Grobee D et al. (1996) Review of moderate alcohol consumption and reduced risk of coronary heart disease: is the effect due to beer, wine, or spirits? British Medical Journal 312: 731–736.
16. Gaziano J. Gaziano T, Glynn R et al. (2000) Light-to-moderate alcohol consumption and mortality in the physicians' health study enrollment cohort. Journal of the American College of Cardiology 35(1): 96–105.

17. Wang Z, Huang Y, Zou J et al. (2002) Effects of red wine and wine polyphenol resveratrol on platelet aggregation in vivo and in vitro. International Journal of Molecular Medicine 9(1): 77–79.
18. Nigdikar S, Williams N, Griffin B et al. (1998) Consumption of red wine polyphnols reduces the susceptibility of low-density lipoproteins to oxidation in vivo. American Journal of Clinical Nutrition 68(2): 258–265.
19. Nijveldt R, van Nood E, van Hoorn D et al. (2001) Flavonoids: a review of probable mechanisms of action and potential applications. American Journal of Clinical Nutrition 74(4):418–425.
20. Abu-Amsha R, Croft K, Puddey I et al. (1996) Phenolic content of various beverages determines the extent of inhibition of human serum and low-density lipoprotein oxidation in vitro: identification and mechanisms of actions of some cinnamic acid derivatives from red wine. Clinical Science 91: 449–458.
21. Frankel E, Kanner J, German J et al. (1993) 341: 454–457. Inhibition of oxidation of human low density lipoprotein by phenol substances in red wine. Lancet 314: 454–457.
22. Meyer A, Yi O, Pearson D et al. (1997) Inhibition of human low-density lipoprotein oxidation in relation to composition of phenolic antioxidants in grapes (Vitis vinifera) Journal of Agricultural and Food Chemistry 45: 1638–1643.
23. Caccetta R, Croft K, Beilin L et al. (2000) Ingestion of red wine significantly increases plasma phenolic acid concentrations but does not acutely affect ex vivo lipoprotein oxidizability. American Journal of Clinical Nutrition 71(1): 67–74.
24. Natella F, Ghiselli A, Guidi A (2001) Red wine mitigates the postprandial increase of LDL susceptibility to oxidation. Free Radical Biology and Medicine 30(9): 1036–1044.
25. Potter G, Patterson L, Wanogho E (2002) The cancer preventative agent resveratrol is converted to the anticancer agent piceatannol by the cytochrome P450 enzyme CYP1B1 British Journal of Cancer 86(5): 774–778
26. Falchetti R, Fuggetta M, Lanzilli G et al. (2001) Effects of resveratrol on human immune cell function. Life Sciences 70(1): 81–96.
27. Chan N (2002) Antimicrobial effect of resveratrol on dermatophytes and bacterial pathogens of the skin. Biochemical Pharmacology 63(2): 9–104.
28. Freedman J, Parker C, Perlman J et al. (2001) Select flavonoids and whole juice from puple grapes inhibit platelet function and enhance nitric oxide release. Circulation 103(23):2792.
29. Miyagi Y, Miwa K, Inoue H (1997) Inhibition of human low-density lipoprotein oxidation by flavonoids in red wine and grape juice. American Journal of Cardiology 80(12):1627–31
30. Rendig S, Symons J, Longhurst J (2001) Amsterdam EA Effects of red wine, alcohol, and quercetin on coronary resistance and conductance arteries. J Cardiovascular Pharmacology 38(2):219–27
31. Bernatova I, Pechanova O, Babal P et al. (2002) Wine polyphenols improve cardiovascular remodeling and vascular function in NO-deficient hypertension. American Journal of Physiology: Heart and Circulatory Physiology 282(3): H942-H948.
32. Hale S, Kloner R (2002) Effects of resveratrol, a flavinoid found in red wine, on infarct size in an experimental model of ischemia/reperfusion. Journal of Studies on Alcohol 62(6): 730–735.
33. Corder R, Douthwaite J, Lees D et al. (2001) Endothelin-1 synthesis reduced by red wine. Nature 414(6866): 863–864.
34. Cao G, Russell R, Lischner N (1998) Serum antioxidant capacity is increased by consumption of strawberries, spinach, red wine or vitamin C in elderly women. Journal of Nutrition 128(12):2383–90
35. Ceriello A, Bortlotti N, Motz E et al. (2001) Red wine protects diabetic from meal-induced oxidative stress and thrombosis activiation: a pleasant approach to the prevention of cardiovascular disease in diabetes. European Journal of Clinical Investigation 31(4):322–328.
36. Heyman S, Wexner S, Vickers D et al. (1999) Prospective, randomized trial comparing four biofeedback techniques for patients with constipation. Diseases of the Colon and Rectum 42(11): 1388–1398.
37. Rieger N, Wattchow D, Sarre R et al. (1997) Prospective study of biofeedback fo treatment of constipation. Diseases of the Colon and Rectum 40(10): 1143–1148. Diseases of the Colon and Rectum
38. Whitehead W, Wald A, Norton N (2001) Treatment options for fecal incontinence. Diseasese of the Colon and Rectum 44(1):131–142.
39. Ryn A, Morren G, Hallbrook O et al. (2000) Long-term results of electromyographic biofeedback training for fecal incontinence. Diseases of the Colon and Rectum 43(9): 1262–1266.
40. Glia A, Gylin M, Akerlund J et al. (1998) Biofeedback training in patients with fecal incontinence. Diseases of the Colon and Rectum 41(3): 359–364.
41. Mimura T, Roy A, Storrie J et al. (2000) Treatment of impaired defecation associated with rectocele by behavioral retraining (biofeedback). Diseases of the Colon and Rectum 43(): 1267–1272.
42. Rieger N, Wattchow D, Sarre R et al. (1997) Prospective trial of pelvic floor retraining in patients with fecal incontinence. Diseases of the Colon and Rectum 40(7): 821–826.
43. Patankar S, Ferrara A, Larach S et al. Electromyographic assessment of biofeedback training for fecal incontinence and chronic constipation. Diseases of the Colon and Rectum 40(8): 907–911.
44. Patankar S, Ferrara A, Levy J et al. (1997) Biofeedback in colorectal practice: a multicenter, statewide three-year experience. Diseases of the Colon and Rectum 40(7): 827–831.
45. Ko C, Tong J, Lehman R, et al. (1997) Biofeedback is effective therapy for fecal incontinence and constipation. Archives of Surgery 132(8): 829–833.
46. Chiaroni G, Bassotti G, Stegagnini S et al. (2002) Sensory retraining is key to biofeedback therapy for formed stool fecal incontinence. American Journal of Gastroenterology 97(1): 109–117.

47. Burgio K, Locher J, Goode P et al. (1998) Behavioral vs. drug treatment for urge incontinence in older women: a randomized controlled trial 280(23): 1995–2000.
48. McDowell B, Engberg S, Sereika S et al. (1999) Effectiveness of behavioral therapy to treat incontinence in homebound older adults. Journal of the American Geriatrics Society. 47(3): 309–318.
49. Burgio K, Locher J, Goode P (2000) Combined behavioral and drug therapy for urge incontinence in older women. Journal of the American Geriatrics Society 48(4): 370–374.
50. Geiger R, Allen J, O'Keefe J et al. (2001) Balance and mobility following stroke: effects of physical therapy interventions with and without biofeedback/forceplate training. Physical Therapy 81(4): 995–1005.
51. Edwards C, Sudhakar S, Scales M et al. (2000) Electromyographic (EMG) biofeedback in the comprehensive treatment of central pain and ataxic tremor following thalamic stroke. Applied Psychophysiology and Biofeedback 2594): 229–240.
52. Reddy M, Simcox D, Gupta V et al. (2000) Biofeedback therapy using accelerometry for treating dysphagic patients with poor laryngeal elevation: case studies. Journal of Rehabilitation Research and Development 37(3): 361–372.
53. Rice B, Kalker A, Schindler J et al. (2001) Effect of biofeedback-assisted relaxation training on foot ulcer healing. Journal of the American Podiatric Medical Association 91(3): 132–141.
54. Hasenbring M, Ulrich H, Hartmann M et al. (1999) The efficacy of a risk factor-based cognitive behavioral intervention and electromyographic biofeedback in patients with acute sciatic pain. An attempt to prevent chronicity. Spine 24(23): 2525–2535.
55. Henderson R, Hart M, Lal S et al. (1998) The effect of home training with direct blood pressure biofeedback of hypertensive: a placebo-controlled study. Journal of Hypertension 16(6): 771–778.
56. Hunyor S, Henderson R, Lal S et al. (1997) Placebo-controlled biofeedback blood pressure effect in hypertensive humans. Hypertension 29(6): 1225–1231.
57. Nakao M, Nomura S, Shimosawa T et al. (1997) Clinical effects of blood pressure biofeedback treatment on hypertension by auto-shaping. Psychosomatic Medicine 59(3): 331–338.
58. Nakao M, Nomura S, Shimosawa T et al. (1999) Blood pressure biofeedback treatment, organ damage and sympathetic activity in mild hypertension. Psychotherapy and Psychosomatics 68(6): 341–347.
59. Eisenbeg D, Delbanco T, Berkey S et al. (1993) Cognitive behavioral techniques for hypertension: are they effective? Annals of Internal Medicine 118: 964–972.
60. Blumenthal J, Emery C, Madden D et al. (1989) Cardiovascular and behavioral effects of aerobic exercise training in healthy older men and women. Journal of Gerontology 44(5): M147-M157
61. DiPietro L (1998)Moderate-intensity aerobic training improves glucose tolerance in aging independent of abdominal adiposity. Journal of the American Geriatrics Society. 46(7):875–9.
62. Bowman A, Clayton R, Murray A et al. (1998) Effects aerobic exercise training and yoga the baroreflex in healthy elderly persons. Journal of the American Medical Association 280(18): 1601–1603.
63. Patel C (1975)12-month follow-up of yoga and biofeedback in the management of hypertension Lancet 1(7898): 62–64
64. Patel C (1975) Randomised controlled trial of yoga and bio-feedback in management of hypertension. Lancet 2(7925):93–95.
65. Garfinkel M, Singhal A, Katz W et al. (1998) Yoga-based intervention for carpal tunnel syndrome: a randomized trial. Journal of the American Medical Association. Nov 11;280(18):1601–1603.
66. Garfinkel M, Schumacher H, Husain A, (1994) Evaluation of a yoga based regimen for treatment of osteoarthritis of the hands. Journal of Rheumatology (12):2341–2343
67. Garfinkel M, Schumacher H, (2000) Yoga. Rheumatologic Disease Clinics of North America. 26(1):125–132.
68. Ramaratnam S, Sridharan K (2000) Yoga for epilepsy. Cochrane Database Systems Review 2000;(3):CD001524
69. Barrows K, Jacobs B (2002) Mind-body medicine: an introduction and review of the literature. Medical Clinics of North America 86(1): 11–31.
70. Jacobs G, Benson H, Friedman R (1996) Perceived benefits in a behavioral-medicine insomnia program: a clinical report. American Journal of Medicine 100: 212–216.
71. Kabat ref 48, 49 in barrows, miller, speca,teasdale
72. Kabat-Zinn J, Lipworth L, Burney R et al. (1987) Four-year follow-up of a meditation-based program for the self-regulation of chronic pain. Clinical Journal of Pain 2: 159–13.
73. Kabat-Zinn J, Massion A, Kristelle J et al. (1992) Effectiveness of a meditation-based stress reduction program in the treatment of anxiety disorders. American Journal of Psychiatry. 149L 936–943.
74. Miller J, Fletcher K Kabat-Zinn J (1995) Three-year follow-up and clinical implications of a mindfulness meditation-based stress reduction intervention in the treatment of anxiety disorders General Hospital Psychiatry 17: 192–200.
75. Speca M, Carlson L, Goodney E et al. (2000) A randomized, wait-list controlled clinical trial: the effect o a mindfulness meditation-base stress reduction program on mood and symptoms of stress in cancer outpatients. Psychosomatic Medicine 62: 613–620.
76. Teasdale J, Williams J, Soulsby J et al. (2000) Prevention of relapse/recurrence i major depression of mindfullness-based cognitive therapy. Journal of Consulting and Clinical Psychology 68: 615–623.
77. Montgomery GH, Weltz CR, Seltz M, Brief presurgery hypnosis reduces distress and pain in excisional breast biopsy patients. Int J Clin Exp Hypn. 2002 Jan;50(1):17–32.
78. Lynch D Jr., (1999) Empowering the patient: hypnosis in the management of cancer, surgical disease and chronic pain. American Journal of Clinical Hypnosis. 42(2):122–30

79. Lang D, Benotsch E, Fick L et al. (2000) Adjunctive non-pharmacological analgesia for invasive medical procedures: a randomized trial. Lancet 355: 1486–1490.

80. Allison D, Faith M. (1996) Hypnosis an adjunct to cognitive-behavioral psychotherapy for obeisity: A meta-analytic reappraisal. Journal of Consulting and Clinical Psychology 62: 513–516.

81. Tusek D, Church J, Fazio V, (1997) Guided imagery as a coping strategy for perioperative patients AORN Journal Oct; 66(4): 644–9 82.

82. Page S, Levine P, Sisto S, Johnston M (2001) A randomized efficacy and feasibility study of imagery in acute stroke Clinical Rehabilitation 15(3):233–240

83. Fernandez E, Turk D (1989) The utility of cognitive coping strategies for altering pain perception: a meta-analysis. Pain 38: 123–135.

84. Field T (2002) Massage therapy. Medical Clinics of North America 86(1): 163–171.

85. Franke A, Gebauer S, Franke K et al. (2000) Acupuncture massage vs. Swedish massage and individual exercise vs. group exercise in low back pain sufferers–a randomized controlled clinical trial in a 2×2 factorial design Forschende Komplementarmedizin und Klassiche Naturheilkunde 7(6):286–293

86. Stephenson N, Weinrich S, Tavakoli A (2000) The effects of foot reflexology on anxiety and pain in patients with breast and lung cancer. Oncology Nursing Forum 27(1): 67–72

87. Astin J, Harkness E, Ernst E (2000) The efficacy of "distant healing": a systematic review of randomized trials. Annals of Internal Medicine 132(11): 903–910.

88. Winstead-Fry P, Kijek J (1999) An integrative review and meta-analysis of therapeutic touch research. Alternative Therapies in Health and Medicine 5(6): 58–67.

89. Lee M, Yang K, Huh H et al. (2001) Qi therapy as an intervention to reduce chronic pain and to enhance mood in elderly subjects: a pilot study. American Journal of Chinese Medicine 29(2): 237–245.

90. Buckle J (1999) Use of aromatherapy as a contemporary treatment for chronic pain. Alternative Therapies in Health and Medicine 5(5): 42–51

91. Wilkinson S, Aldridge J, Salmon I et al. (1999) An evaluation of aromatherapy massage in palliative care. Palliative Medicine 13(5): 409–417.

92. Hay I, Jamieson M, Ormerod A (1998) Randomized trial of aromatherapy. Successful treatment for alopecia areata. Archives of Dermatology 134(11): 1349–1352.

93. Brooker D, Snape M, Johnson E et al. (1997) Single case evaluation of the effects of aromatherapy and massage on disturbed behaviour in severe dementia. British Journal of Clinical Psychology 36(Pt 2): 287–296.

94. Cooke B, Ernst E (2000) Aromatherapy: a systematic review. British Journal of General Practice 50(455): 493–496.

95. Katsarou A, Armenaka M, Kalogeromitros D et al. (1999) Contact reactions to fragrances. Annals of Allergy, Asthma, and Immunology 82(5): 449–455.

96. Schaller M, Korting H (1995) Allergic airborne contact dermatitis from essential oils used in aromatherapy. Clinical and Experimental Dermatology 20(2): 143–145.

22 The Benefits of Lifestyle Modification for Older People

A.L. Silberman

Introduction

Where should we focus our efforts to improve our health care system? This is no longer the million-dollar question. In today's health care environment, it is the multi-billion-dollar question.

For obvious reasons, the focus should be where the payback is greatest – and the greatest payback in terms of health and quality of life is in lifestyle modification. Despite the impressive technological advances of traditional Western medicine, we still fail to adequately promote the basic, common-sense choice of lifestyle modification as a treatment option, even though the scientific arguments for clinical and cost effectiveness are clear.

Lifestyle modification means improving nutrition, physical activity levels, psychological well-being, stress management skills and safety practices, decreasing tobacco usage, and adopting other behavioral practices that positively affect health. There is a direct relationship between lifestyle modification, reduced health risk and reduced health cost. Given the overwhelmingly poor state of our nation's lifestyle practices, and our economic and humanitarian responsibilities, the need to devote serious attention to lifestyle modification is undeniable.

While maintaining a healthier lifestyle is important for everyone, it is especially critical for older people. A 1996 U.S. Surgeon General's report on physical activity and health stated that people of all ages could improve their quality of life through moderate physical activity [1]. Particularly in older people, significant health problems can set off a downward health spiral – they become less active, causing their health to deteriorate, which in turn leads to isolation that can result in a reduced quality of life and increased risk factors for disease, disability and death. It is a sad truth that much of this decline is preventable by adopting and adhering to healthier lifestyle practices.

For example, excessive weight often affects older Americans. A recent report by the American Academy of Family Physicians (AAFP) estimates the average weight of an American who is 5'4" and more than 50 years old at 160 pounds, while the optimum range is 111 to 146 pounds [2]. In contrast, older European adults weigh an average of 145 pounds. The reason? To cite just one factor, elderly Europeans are more active than Americans. Instead of relying on cars, for instance, Europeans cycle or walk more frequently as a means of transportation. So we know that many healthy seniors can maintain their optimum weight with healthy nutrition and moderate exercise.

One promising trend is the growing proactivity of older consumers, who are more receptive than ever to the benefits of healthy living. Patients are looking for less invasive solutions than traditional Western therapies offer. The medical community should recognize this trend, and deliver the message that smart health choices are critical to health outcomes.

Often, just the opposite occurs – physicians do not discuss lifestyle modification with older patients because they mistakenly assume that the elderly are resistant to change. It is incumbent upon the clinical community to confront and dispel the misconception that once a person reaches a certain age, it is too late to benefit from lifestyle modification.

We must communicate the critical fact that older people can control risk factors, reduce pain and avoid adverse events by improving their lifestyle practices. Many seniors desperately want to maintain their independence, are highly motivated, and are willing to invest the time required to improve their health practices – they want to stack the deck in their favor in every possible way, especially if it means preserving their independence.

It is our responsibility to inspire confidence, not take it away. It is our duty to counsel older patients about the truth, not just what we believe will be easiest for them. People of every age deserve accurate scientific information, including a complete range of therapeutic options, so they can make intelligent choices about the risks, benefits, costs and side effects of all possible therapies, including lifestyle change. If prevention of pain, risk and unnecessary expense is an objective of the treatment plan, then lifestyle modification and conventional medicine are complementary and inseparable.

More than two decades ago, Dean Ornish, M.D. and his colleagues at the Preventive Medicine Research Institute (PMRI) demonstrated that intensive lifestyle modification can slow, stop, or reverse the progression of coronary artery disease. Dr. Ornish's premise is straightforward – since coronary artery disease develops over time and from a variety of factors, these underlying factors must be addressed to successfully treat the disease. The Dr. Dean Ornish Program for Reversing Heart Disease simultaneously addresses the prominent behaviors that contribute to heart disease – high-fat diets, lack of exercise, unmanaged stress and lack of social support.

The success of the Ornish Program in helping individuals stop or reverse the effects of some forms of heart disease provides an important demonstration of the power of lifestyle change and its role in successfully managing and improving the health of older people.

Prevention is Intervention

Preventive medicine is logical, efficient and the least expensive treatment available. Lifestyle modification is fundamental to primary, secondary and tertiary prevention, at any age. Consider the ways preventive measures may be utilized as part of a comprehensive treatment plan:

▶ Primary Prevention (preventing or delaying the onset of disease) – Primary prevention reduces the risk of disease and injury. For example, weight management can prevent or delay the onset of Type II diabetes, and wearing seat belts can prevent accidental injury.

▶ Secondary Prevention (detecting and treating disease early) – Lifestyle modification is important for the prevention of atherosclerotic disease morbidity and mortality. For example, detecting and treating high blood pressure can prevent stroke.

► Tertiary Prevention (managing or reversing the progression of disease) – Lifestyle modification can be a valuable, complementary treatment option. For example, the Ornish Program can slow, stop or reverse cardiovascular disease through lifestyle modification of diet, physical activity, stress and psychosocial status.

While incremental modification of lifestyle practices leads to modest improvements, major changes often lead to impressive clinical results. Older adults can benefit immensely from a comprehensive treatment plan that includes lifestyle modification interventions that address nutrition, physical activity, stress management, psycho-social support, smoking cessation and safety.

A Health Insurance Company Pays for Prevention

Increasingly, insurance providers are recognizing the health and economic benefits of preventive therapies, including lifestyle modification. This recognition has been slow in coming, but the movement toward reimbursement for lifestyle modification continues to gather momentum.

Historically, prevention received "lip service", but few resources. However, in 1997 Highmark Blue Cross Blue Shield in Pittsburgh, Pennsylvania, made medical payer history when it began to provide the Ornish Program free-of-charge to members with any Highmark health insurance product.

The decision to offer the Program as part of its comprehensive health promotion and disease prevention delivery system was firmly rooted in Highmark's mission. Knowing that heart disease is the leading killer of men and women in the United States, and knowing that lifestyle behavior is a significant underlying cause, Highmark decided it was the clinically, socially and fiscally responsible thing to do.

The Science – A Program That Works

Highmark selected the Ornish Program because it had been scientifically proven to reverse heart disease. Dr. Ornish and his colleagues at the non-profit Preventive Medicine Research Institute (PMRI) conducted a series of scientific studies and randomized clinical trials demonstrating, for the first time, that the progression of coronary artery disease can be reversed through comprehensive changes in patients' lifestyles.

To prove the power of this inexpensive, low-tech alternative, researchers used high-tech medical technologies such as computer-analyzed quantitative coronary arteriography and cardiac PET scans to track the progress of Ornish Program participants. Within 12 months of making lifestyle changes, patients reported a 91 percent average reduction in the frequency of angina. Most of the patients became pain-free, including those who had been unable to work or engage in routine daily activities due to severe chest pain. Within a month of beginning the program, blood flow to the heart increased. Within a year, even severely blocked coronary arteries began to improve in 82 percent of participants in the PMRI study [3].

As reported in the December 1998 issue of the *Journal of the American Medical Association*, most of the study participants were able to maintain comprehensive lifestyle changes for five years [4]. On average, participants demonstrated even greater reversal of heart disease after five years than after one year. In contrast, the patients in the comparison group, who made only moderate lifestyle changes, worsened after one year and their coronary arteries became more severely clogged after five years. Also, the incidence rate of cardiac events – including heart attacks, strokes, bypass surgery and angioplasty – was 2.5 times lower after 5 years in the group that made comprehensive lifestyle changes.

These impressive outcomes have particular significance for older Americans. Dr. Ornish's research demonstrated that older people who commit to positive lifestyle changes do just as well as younger people – in fact, the oldest patient in the study, who is now 88, showed the greatest amount of reversal of symptoms. Dr. Ornish demonstrated that age is not a factor because the primary determinant of improvement in coronary artery disease was neither age nor the severity of disease, but adherence to the preventive lifestyle – the more extensive their lifestyle changes, the more they improved. This finding offers new hope and new choices for older patients, since the risks of bypass surgery and angioplasty increase with age.

The increasing risk that comes with age is confirmed by a number of studies:

▶ Mortality for bypass surgery is 5.5 percent for the elderly vs. 1.0 percent in younger patients during the first five post-operative days [5].

▶ Hospital stays, complications and mortality increase in direct correlation to age following bypass surgery [6].

▶ A 10-year follow-up study of 21,516 patients aged 50–79 concluded that, "Age was the most important correlate of death after PTCA, with a 65 percent increase in risk of death for each 10 year increase in age. Age has an independent effect on early and late survival after PTCA (percutaneous transluminal angioplasty)" [7].

▶ Post-PTCA patients over age 65 (compared to under age 65), are more likely to require emergency CABG (5.4 percent vs. 2.8 percent) or elective CABG (3.9 percent vs. 1.6 percent). In-hospital death rates were higher in the elderly (3.9 percent vs. 1.6 percent). Two-year mortality was also higher in the elderly (8.8 percent vs. 2.9 percent). These rates remained significant when adjusted for risk factors and co-morbidities [8].

▶ Elderly patients, post-PTCA with stent, have higher mortality (2.2 percent vs. 1.2 percent), procedural MIs (2.9 percent vs. 1.7 percent), and emergency CABGs (3.7 percent vs. 1.4 percent) [9].

These increased risks are due to the greater prevalence of co-morbidities in the elderly such as:

▶ Lower ejection fraction.
▶ Higher left ventricular and diastolic pressure.
▶ History of previous myocardial infarction.
▶ Increased renal dysfunction.
▶ Chronic obstructive pulmonary disease.

▶ Greater incidence of hypertension.

▶ Greater incidence of diabetes.

Bypass surgery (CABG) and angioplasty (PTCA) can alleviate angina, but neither can prevent future recurrence of plaque formation. The Ornish Program can and does reduce the reformation of arterial plaque. Program results demonstrate that the positive benefits of lifestyle modification can enable patients to avoid invasive treatments, providing a powerful opportunity to stop or reverse the debilitating effects of heart disease, as they regain control of their health – and their lives.

The Ornish Program

Based on solid scientific evidence, Highmark Blue Cross Blue Shield made the Ornish Program available to members with documented coronary artery disease and to those with a combination of risk factors.

The Program's objectives are to improve blood flow to the heart, reduce cholesterol and other risk factors, improve exercise capacity, avoid adverse cardiac events, and avoid the need for initial or repeat invasive procedures.

The Ornish Program is based on four equally important lifestyle components – moderate exercise, stress management, group support and a low-fat plant-based diet. By committing to major changes in their lifestyles, patients can achieve significant results. In the short term, participants experience symptom relief, such as less-frequent and less-severe angina, and improved risk factors. Over the long term, they are better protected from the progression of heart disease and may experience reversal of their condition.

Through education and hands-on instruction, the Program format is effective in facilitating lifestyle changes. It is conducted in a supportive atmosphere and provided by a professional team that includes a physician, exercise physiologist, registered dietitian, nurse case manager, certified stress management specialist and behavioral health clinician.

High levels of adherence to the Program often surprise clinicians, but the rewards for patients are usually immediate and pronounced. Instead of hoping for potential benefits in the future, they experience noticeable benefits in the first few weeks of the Program, reinforcing their reasons for adopting a new lifestyle and their commitment to maintaining it for the long-term.

Significant, sustained reductions in angina within weeks and the ability to work, walk or enjoy sexual activity without pain or fear are powerful motivators. For most patients who adopt and maintain the lifestyle changes, the reductions in frequency of angina are comparable to those achieved by revas-cularization. It is easy to understand their dedication when you consider that many participants are facing the prospect of cardiac surgery or death.

The Ornish Program Components

The Ornish Program addresses the underlying causes of heart disease by teaching patients to adopt comprehensive lifestyle changes in four inter-related areas: moderate exercise, stress management, group support and nutrition.

Moderate Exercise

Regular physical activity reduces the risk of death from coronary artery disease. People of all ages experience beneficial physiologic adaptations to physical activity. As part of the Program, an exercise prescription based on individual fitness is developed and monitored for each participant. This moderate aerobic exercise regimen provides participants with a number of health benefits including:

▶ Increased heart efficiency.
▶ Increased ability of muscles to use oxygen efficiently.
▶ Decreased oxygen requirements of the heart.
▶ Decreased resting blood pressure.
▶ Increased ability to exercise at higher workloads for longer periods of time before experiencing fatigue, shortness of breath or chest pain.
▶ Decreased triglyceride levels and increased HDL cholesterol levels, which make it more difficult for fats to collect inside artery walls.
▶ Decreased blood sugar.
▶ Decreased ability of blood to clot and stick to vessel walls.
▶ Increased mobility, making it easier to perform daily activities.
▶ Decreased body fat.
▶ Increased metabolism.

Strength training is an important element of the exercise component. After age 20, people who do not exercise begin to lose muscle mass. The most significant loss comes after age 60 and contributes to frailty – as we age, we need our muscles even more. Research studies conducted by Maria Fiatarone, M.D. and colleagues at the Center for Aging at Tufts University demonstrated that people in their 80s and 90s can achieve strength gains of at least 100 percent with just a few months of resistance training [10].

Strength training works on the "overload principle," which makes the muscles work harder by increasing resistance to movement or increasing the frequency and duration of activity. In the past, strength training was used primarily by athletes to improve performance or for physical rehabilitation after an injury. This type of training was once considered unsafe for populations such as the elderly or people with cardiovascular disease. However, recent studies demonstrate that, when appropriately prescribed and supervised, strength training is safe and effective for both populations.

Strength training provides a number of important benefits including:

▶ Increased functional capacity.
▶ Increased lean tissue.
▶ Increased bone density.
▶ Improved balance and stability.

- ► Improved ability to perform work and leisure activities.
- ► Improved metabolism.
- ► Increased strength.

The Ornish Program guidelines for exercise include three to five hours of moderate aerobic exercise and two to three sessions of strength training per week.

Stress Management

Stress is an automatic reaction to change or demand. Usually, it is this reaction that is harmful, not the situation itself. When prolonged and unmanaged, stress causes powerful chemicals like adrenaline and cortisol to be released by the adrenal glands, with multiple negative effects including:

- ► Increased heart rate.
- ► Increased blood pressure.
- ► Spasms of blood vessels.
- ► Disturbances in heart rhythm.
- ► Increased stomach acid.
- ► Decreased blood flow.
- ► Increased muscle tension.
- ► Increased blood clotting and viscosity.
- ► Short, shallow breathing.
- ► Abnormalities in the immune system.

These effects are adaptive in the short term and help a person prepare for danger. When stress is chronic, these physical reactions can cause disease. For a person with heart disease, reactions to stress may lead to angina, shortness of breath, palpitations or sudden blockages of coronary arteries. Other stress-related conditions include insomnia, sexual dysfunction, increased muscle tension, ulcers, chronic headaches, high blood pressure, neck aches and backaches. In addition, psychological reactions to stress may include anxiety, depression (especially when stress is chronic), anger, hostility, irritability and decreased concentration and memory.

Numerous studies demonstrate that emotional responses to stress increase risk for coronary artery disease. A study published in the American Heart Association Journal, *Circulation*, found that the risk of heart attack increased by 2.3 times in the two hours following an anger episode [11]. In an analysis of more than 45 studies, hostility has emerged as one of the most important personality variables in coronary artery disease [12].

Stress also may lead to maladaptive coping behaviors such as overeating, isolation, inactivity, sleep disorders and substance abuse or addiction, which create additional risk.

The Ornish Program equips patients with adaptive tools that help them remain calm, despite stressful challenges through the daily practice of:

- ► Yoga postures.
- ► Meditation.

▶ Deep breathing.
▶ Progressive relaxation.
▶ Guided imagery/visualization.

These stress-management techniques provide a number of positive benefits including:
▶ Decreased blood pressure.
▶ Decreased heart rate.
▶ Decreased respiratory rate.
▶ Increased mind/body awareness.
▶ Improved concentration.
▶ The ability to discover inner sources of tranquility, peace of mind and well being.

Group Support

A number of studies demonstrate that patients who lack social support are at higher risk for premature mortality, independent of other risk factors, and support the hypothesis that social interaction reduces the incidence or severity of cardiovascular disease. For example, Kawachi and colleagues studied middle-aged health professionals for four years and found that men who were not married, had few friends or relatives, and were not members of community groups were at increased risk for cardiovascular death, independent of conventional risk factors [12]. In another study, Nancy Frasure-Smith and her colleagues found that social support reduces the risk of death from depression in elderly cardiac patients [14].

In Dr. Ornish's book, *Love & Survival – 8 Pathways to Intimacy and Health*, numerous research studies are cited that correlate isolation and lack of social support with increased rates of illness and death. Conversely, love and intimacy are among the most powerful healing factors. He concludes, "I am not aware of any other factor in medicine – not diet, not smoking, not exercise, not stress, not genetics, not drugs, not surgery – that has a greater impact on our quality of life, incidence of illness, and premature death from all causes" [15].

The Ornish Program reflects this conviction by utilizing group support to address patients' psychosocial needs. Patients meet twice a week for one hour in group support sessions led by a behavioral health clinician. The purpose is to let down their defenses, talk about their feelings and listen to the feelings of others. The sessions emphasize interactive skill-building, including:
▶ Learning to identify and pay attention to feelings.
▶ Developing comfort in expressing feelings.
▶ Developing the ability to listen with empathy and compassion to the feelings of others.
▶ Improving coping abilities.

The sessions teach patients to listen in ways that enable others to feel that they have been heard. When we feel heard, we feel regarded and connected, an important part of the healing process, because it reduces the feelings of isolation that first lead to stress and illness.

The group sessions create an atmosphere of support and respect in which members feel comfortable expressing their feelings. As individuals gain the courage to share their feelings with the group, others feel safer in opening their hearts as well. The resulting connection and intimacy enrich patients' lives and are essential to the healing process. Participating in group support helps them develop meaningful relationships and learn to generalize this social intimacy and expression to other aspects of their lives.

Nutrition

The risks imposed by high-fat, animal protein-based diets are widely known. Ornish Program patients may enjoy a variety of low-fat foods in abundance including:

▶ Whole Grains – breads, cereals, brown rice, pasta, bulgur, kasha, barley and other whole grains.
▶ Vegetables – vegetables and vegetable juices.
▶ Fruits – fruits and fruit juices.
▶ Legumes – dried peas, dried beans, meat substitutes made from legumes.
▶ Non-Fat Milk Products[1] – non-fat milk, yogurt, cottage cheese, cheese, sour cream, cream cheese.
▶ Egg Whites – egg whites added to foods, egg white omelets, eggbeaters.
▶ Non-Fat Sweets[1] – cookies, cakes, pies, frozen yogurt, candy.
▶ Alcohol[2] – beer, wine, liquor

The Ornish Reversal diet is a plant-based, whole foods eating plan with no more than 10 percent of calories from fat and no added cholesterol, which is present only in foods of animal origin (that also are usually high in saturated fats). In contrast, a plant-based diet is high in fiber and rich in antioxidants such as vitamins A, C, E and beta-carotene.

In a study conducted by R.B. Singh and colleagues, 406 patients who had myocardial infarctions or unstable angina were randomized to either a conventional, low-fat diet or a plant-based, low-fat diet. After one year, patients assigned to a plant-based, low-fat diet experienced fewer cardiac events (50 plant-based, low-fat diet patients vs. 82 conventional, low-fat diet patients) and lower mortality (21 plant-based, low-fat diet patients vs. 38 conventional, low-fat diet patients) [16].

Plant-based nutrition is also linked to lower rates of breast, prostate and ovarian cancers. Scientists studying nutrition believe that the thousands of protective and beneficial properties that whole foods contain – fiber, isoflavones, carotenoids, bioflavinodes and lycopene – contribute to good health and protect from disease. Vegetarian diets also correlate with reduced incidence rates of osteoporosis, Type II diabetes and obesity.

---

[1] Amount restricted.
[2] Allowed, but not encouraged; amount restricted.

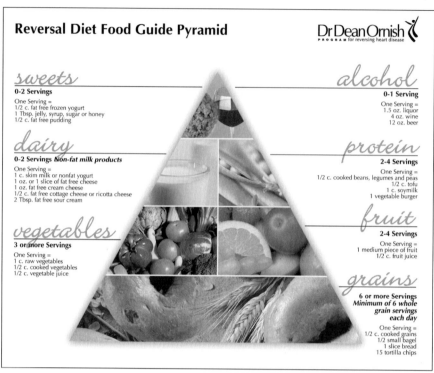

Figure 22.1. Reversal Diet Food Guide Pyramid

In addition, plant versions of estrogen, called phytoestrogens, found in soy products such as tofu, are believed to be protective because they contain antioxidants that prevent cholesterol oxidation and reduce the likelihood of it depositing in the arteries (Fig. 22.1).

While nutrition is an important aspect of the Ornish Program, it is just one component of an integrated treatment. Dr. Ornish's research shows that the best outcomes are achieved when patients adhere to all four treatment modalities.

An Integrated Approach

The Ornish Program is a synergistic approach incorporating exercise, stress management, group support and a low-fat, vegetarian diet. While each component offers powerful benefits in its own right, combining and coordinating them enhances the benefits of each and gives patients the power to transform, adopt and maintain new lifestyle practices. Adherence in one area promotes adherence in the others. For example, exercise releases the tension that causes overeating, stress management releases hostility to improve group support sessions, and so on.

Daily Schedule

Patients participate two days a week, four hours per day, for 12 weeks. To facilitate close relationships among patients and the provider team, groups are limited to approximately 15 people. While the program is conducted at various times throughout the day and evening to accommodate patients' needs, a typical schedule is:

▶ Hour 1: Exercise
▶ Hour 2: Stress management
▶ Hour 3: Lunch/lecture
▶ Hour 4: Group support

Risk Stratification

Baseline data on each patient is collected prior to program entry. At 12 weeks, a second set of stress tests, lipid panels, and psychosocial information is completed to gauge each patient's progress. (See the indicators presented in Table 22.1.) Based on the re-

Table 22.1. Highmark Dean Ornish Program: 12 week outcomes for the first 13 cohorts (n=326), December 7, 2001

	Number of Participants[a]	Average Score at Baseline	Average Score at 12 Weeks	Average Change	Percent Change [%]	P Value[b]
Experienced Angina in Past 30 Days	338	79 People	40 People	N/A	-49.4	p<.0001
Total Cholesterol [mg/dl]	365	192.2	170.3	-21.9	-11.4	p<.0001
HDL Cholesterol [mg/dl]	362	44.3	39.9	-4.4	-9.9	p<.0001
LDL Cholesterol [mg/dl]	342	111.7	95.31	-16.4	-14.7	p<.0001
Triglycerides [mg/dl]	364	187.7	177.7	-10	-5.3	p<.05
Oxygen Capacity [METS]	341	9.69	11.8	+2.2	+22.9	p<.0001
Weight [lbs.]	377	197.6	187.4	-10.2	-5.2	p<.0001
Body Composition [% body fat]	357	31	28.5	-2.5	-8.1	p<.0001
Systolic Blood Pressure [mmHg]	349	132.9	123.2	-9.7	-7.3	p<.0001
Diastolic Blood Pressure [mmHg]	349	80.5	73.4	-7.1	-8.8	p<.0001
Minutes Exercise/week	349	111	222.7	+111.7	+100.6	p<.0001
Minutes Stress Management/week	325	49.6	318.7	+269.1	+542.5	p<.0001
Depression Scale [CES-D]	362	11.8	6.1	-5.7	-48.3	p<.0001
Hostility Scale (Cook-Medley)	362	8.4	6.8	-1.6	-19.0	p<.0001
Perceived Stress Scale	360	14.8	9.6	-5.2	-35.1	p<.0001

[a] Participants missing either baseline or 12 week data were not included in the analysis. [b] Angina analysis is McNemar's test for paired samples. All remaining analyses are 2-tailed paired t-tests.

sults and program compliance, patients are risk-stratified according to established protocols and case managed for the remainder of the year. For example, a patient requiring additional stress management support will continue to attend that program component beyond the original 12-week timeframe.

Close case management and participation in a self-directed community/support group helps patients remain committed to the program and to one another. Biometric data, psychosocial surveys and improvements in risk factors are communicated to the patient's physician, who maintains control of medication and other clinical issues throughout the course of the Program. Open communication with patients' physicians helps ensure that they understand the complementary value of the Program.

Retreat Model

Patients who lack access to or are unable to participate in the one-year program can participate in an alternative five-day retreat. While not yet scientifically proven to reverse heart disease, the retreat is designed to expose participants to lifestyle modification and its short-term benefits, which ideally will lead to full Program participation and/or integration of permanent lifestyle changes.

The Payback

The benefits for Ornish Program participants is usually significant, both in terms of physical improvements and improvements in psychosocial measurements. The following outcomes, which were achieved in 12 weeks by Highmark Blue Cross Blue Shield participants in Pittsburgh and Windber, Pennsylvania, demonstrate significant reductions in blood pressure, cholesterol, weight, body fat and measurements of stress, hostility and depression.

Ornish Program Site List

- ▶ Alegent Health, Omaha, NE
- ▶ Allegheny General Hospital, Pittsburgh PA
- ▶ Camden Clark Memorial
- ▶ Charleston Area Medical Center, Charleston, WV
- ▶ City Hospital, Martinsburg, WV
- ▶ DuBois Regional Medical Center, DuBois, PA
- ▶ Good Samaritan Health System, Kearney, NE
- ▶ Hamot Hospital, Erie, PA
- ▶ Jameson Hospital, New Castle, PA
- ▶ Lehigh Valley Hospital, Allentown, PA
- ▶ Monongahela Valley Hospital, Monongahela, PA
- ▶ Ohio Valley Medical Center, Wheeling, WV
- ▶ Pinnacle Health System, Harrisburg, PA

▶ Princeton Community Hospital, Princeton, WV
▶ St. Joseph's Hospitals, Parkersburg, WV
▶ St. Mary's Hospital, Huntington, WV
▶ SwedishAmerican Health System, Rockford, IL
▶ United Hospital Center, Clarksburg, WV
▶ West Virginia University Hospitals, Morgantown, WV
▶ Westmoreland Regional Health System, Greensburg, PA
▶ Wheeling Hospital, Wheeling, WV

National Rate of Cardiovascular Procedures and Adverse Events/Cost

Cardiovascular diseases rank as America's leading cause of death and the major cause of disability and health care expenditures in the United States.

Often, invasive procedures are finger-in-the-dike efforts. According to a study published in the *New England Journal of Medicine*, 63 percent of patients receiving PTCA have repeat procedures within three years and 13 percent of those having bypass surgery need a second procedure within three years [17]. Another study published in the *Journal of the American College of Cardiology* demonstrated that restenosis occurs in 30 to 50 percent of angioplastied lesions within six months of initial treatment [18]. When this occurs, then these procedures are often repeated, at additional expense and at greater risk.

In contrast, the Ornish Program has enabled participants to delay or avoid invasive procedures altogether by directly addressing the underlying causes of heart disease through lifestyle modification to mitigate these risks.

Prevention Yields Significant Cost Savings

In terms of living better, the payback for lifestyle modification – freedom from pain and the ability to regain control of one's life and health – is incalculable. In terms of cost avoidance, the payback can be quantified and presents a compelling business case for lifestyle modification. The investment in lifestyle modification is minimal – it costs very little to eat a healthful diet, walk and manage stress. The only side effects are beneficial. There is a truism that also applies to lifestyle improvement education: If you think education is expensive, try ignorance.

Several studies confirm the Ornish Program's financial payback:

Multicenter Lifestyle Heart Trial Demonstration Project (Mutual of Omaha Study) [19]. In a study published in the *American Journal of Cardiology*, 333 patients presenting for revascularization (CABG or PTCA) were reviewed. A total of 194 entered the Ornish Program, while 139 in the control group underwent revascularization (66 PTCA, 73 CABG).

In addition to initial revascularization, the control group required 34 additional procedures in the following three years (23 PTCA and 11 CABG), a total of 173 procedures (89 PTCA and 84 CABG) in the three-year trial period at an estimated cost of $ 6.6 million ($ 47,647 per patient). This number reflects only the cost of the procedures and no other medical expenses, such as emergency department visits or medication, etc.

The Ornish Program group underwent a total of 57 procedures (31 PTCA and 26 CABG) during the three-year study period at a total cost of $ 3.5 million (or $ 18,119 per patient). Overall costs for the Ornish Program group of patients were 47 percent lower at $ 3.1 million ($ 29,000 per patient) over a three-year period.

David Eddy, M.D., Ph.D. Review of Literature [20]. In his report, *Assessment of Intensive Lifestyle Changes for the Treatment of Coronary Artery Disease*, Dr. Eddy completed a meta-analysis of existing literature on the Dean Ornish Program. He concluded that, "... the program is at least cost-neutral, and is probably cost saving, is robust under a wide range of assumptions and sensitivity analyses. While it is never possible to know the exact financial effects of a treatment, all the available evidence suggests that the comprehensive lifestyle program is highly likely to be cost saving, and extremely unlikely to be cost increasing."

Highmark Blue Cross Blue Shield Data. In an analysis of the impact of the Ornish Program on Highmark members, Highmark's actuarial staff used data from the Mutual of Omaha study to project actual cost savings at Highmark. They concluded that the Ornish program is likely to save $ 16,186 per capita over a three-year period for patients who are ill enough to require intervention (PTCA or CABG).

In another study, Highmark reviewed 110 patients for whom complete claims data were available for one year prior to entering the program and one year after entering the program.

Participants were required to have documented evidence of heart disease with a history of PTCA or CABG. Claim costs for study participants, which averaged $546 per member per month (PMPM) for the year prior to entering the program, dropped to $273 PMPM for the year after they entered the Ornish Program.

An additional Highmark study reviewed office visits and hospital admissions for 88 patients in managed care programs (with similar benefit structures) for which complete claims data were available for a two-year period (one year prior to entry into the Ornish Program and one year post-entry, Table 22.2).

Table 22.2.

	Prior Year	Year After Entry	% Change
ED Visits (chest pain/angina)	150	121	-19.3
ED Visits (all causes)	451	201	-55.4
Admissions (chest pain/angina)	123	13	-89.4
Admissions (all causes)	505	80	-84.1

In addition to the results listed here, at least one patient waiting for a heart transplant due to ischemic cardiomyopathy improved enough to be removed from the heart transplant list. Avoiding a heart transplant saves more than $300,000 per patient – plus a lifetime of anti-rejection medication and, it saves the patient from the significant risk of physical and emotional trauma resulting from transplant surgery.

Federal Participation – The Medicare Lifestyle Modification Program Demonstration

Administrators of government health programs recognize the importance of a measurable return on health care expenditures.

The Centers for Medicare and Medicaid Services (CMS), formerly the Healthcare Financing Administration (HCFA), conducted its own internal peer review of the Ornish Program and agreed to move forward with a demonstration project to confirm the Program's clinical and cost effectiveness in the Medicare population. The Medicare Lifestyle Modification Program demonstration was implemented by CMS to confirm that this comprehensive lifestyle program may be a cost effective alternative to customary medical treatments. The demonstration will study up to 1,800 Medicare beneficiaries who satisfy clinical admission criteria.

Better Health and Lower Costs at any Age

Simply put, lifestyle modification works.

Lifestyle modification contributes to better health at any age, without risk and with relatively little expense for the health and economic benefits achieved. While many people in crisis or with severe or unstable heart disease benefit immediately from cardiac surgery, billions of dollars could be saved if even a small percentage of these patients were able to avoid invasive procedures by making lifestyle changes instead. It is both clinically and fiscally irresponsible to deprive people of information about the health benefits of lifestyle modification.

The health and economic advantages of lifestyle modification programs are undeniable. Self-help often makes more clinical sense than institutional help, and this option has been proven in a statistically significant, replicable and scientific context. Both Highmark Blue Cross Blue Shield and Mountain State Blue Cross Blue Shield proactively identify and offer their members a treatment option that is clinically proven to reverse heart disease. Recognizing the clinical and economic benefits, Medicare is also conducting a demonstration program. Throughout the national health insurance community, more payers are reimbursing for the Ornish Program as a starting point for improving health status, decreasing utilization, achieving market differentiation and setting a new standard for services that reach beyond traditional approaches.

However, these early successes have only scratched the surface, meeting but a fraction of the population's need for effective alternative treatments that work. The United States' health care system excels at the high tech fix – treating acute disease and trauma – but lags behind much of the developed world in addressing the underlying causes of disease, many of which are lifestyle-based. Our system of passively paying for illness and disease and reimbursing physicians for treating only sick patients creates a conflict between revenue goals and optimal health outcomes.

The reality of today's health care environment calls for a new delivery model that includes incorporation of and reimbursement for proven lifestyle modification interventions. Research-based evidence on the benefits of lifestyle modification is not materializing fast enough in medical practice or in third-party payer support. The gap between principle and practice is wide, and it is taking too long for our healthcare system to commit to the obvious. Lifestyle Advantage was formed to accelerate the process – its mission is based on these facts, and on the recognition that the incorporation of lifestyle modification as a critical element of comprehensive health care cannot be accomplished soon enough.

Common sense and good business dictate that our national health care delivery system utilize lifestyle modification – because it is effective, because it makes economic sense, and most important of all, because it positively affects the health and well being of those whom we are sworn to serve.[3]

References

1. U.S. Department of Health and Human Services (1996) Physical Activity and Health: A Report of the Surgeon General. U.S. Department of Health and Human Services, Centers for Disease Control & Prevention, National Center for Chronic Disease Prevention & Health Promotion, Atlanta, Chapter 4 p. 2–3.
2. O'Toole CH (2001) Eating to win, a nutritional game plan is important for good health – particularly after the age of 50. Pittsburgh Magazine, September 2001: 96–101.
3. Ornish DM, Brown SE, Scherwitz LW, et al (1990) Can lifestyle changes reverse coronary atherosclerosis? The lifestyle heart trial. The Lancet 336: 129–133.
4. Ornish DM, Scherwitz L, Billings J, et al (1998) Can intensive lifestyle changes reverse coronary heart disease? Five-year follow-up of the lifestyle heart trial. Journal of the American Medical Association 280: 2001–2007.
5. Paone G, et al (1998) Does age limit the effectiveness of clinical pathways after coronary artery bypass graft surgery? Circulation 98(19 suppl): 1141–5.
6. Peigh P, et al (1994) Effect of advancing age on cost and outcome of coronary artery bypass grafting. Annals of Thoracic Surgery 58(5): 1362–7.
7. Taddei CF, et al (1999) Influence of age on outcome after percutaneous transluminal coronary angioplasty. American Journal of Cardiology 84(3): 245–51.
8. Kelsley S, et al (1990) Results of percutaneous transluminal coronary angioplasty in patients greater than or equal to 65 years of age. American Journal of Cardiology 66(15): 1033–8.
9. DeGregario J, et al (1998) Coronary artery stenting in the elderly: short-term outcome and long-term angiographic and clinical follow-up. Journal of the American College of Cardiology 32(3): 577–83.
10. Nelson ME, Fiatarone MA, Morganti CM, Trice I, Greenberg RA, Evans WJ (1994) Effects of high intensity strength training on multiple risk factors for osteoporotic fractures. A randomized controlled trial. Journal of the American Medical Association 272: 1909–14.

[3] Acknowledgements: I want to extend my appreciation to the following individuals for their contributions to the Ornish Program, Lifestyle Advantage and the content of this chapter: Dean Ornish, M.D., Aaron Walton, George Grode, Daniel Lebish, Bryce Williams, Lee Lipsenthal, M.D., Mark Fuller, MD, Ken Melani, MD, Sue Boyle, Robert Crytzer, Terri Merritt-Worden, Melanie Elliott-Eller, Brent O'Connell, M.D., Brad Pifalo, M.D., Dave Lambert, Marlene Janco, Glenn Perelson and James Billings, Ph.D.
Please call Lifestyle Advantage at 1–800–879–2217 to arrange a site visit, obtain a schedule of retreats or for program materials, at no charge.

11. Rozanski A, Blumenthal JA, Kaplan J (1999) Impact of psychological factors on the pathogenesis of cardiovascular disease and implications for therapy. Circulation 99: 2192–2217.

12. Ornish DM (1998) Love & Survival: The Scientific Basis for the Healing Power of Intimacy. HarperCollins, New York: Harper Collins, p. 58–59.

13. Kawachi I, Colditz GA, Ascherio A, Rimm EB, Givannucci E, Stampfer MJ, Willett WC (1996) A prospective study of social networks in relation to total mortality and cardiovascular disease in men in the USA. Journal of Epidemiology and Community Health 50(3): 245–51.

14. Frasure-Smith N (1989) Long-term follow-up of the Ischemic Heart Disease Life Stress Montoring Program. Psychosomatic Medicine 51(5): 485–513.

15. Ornish DM (1998) Love & Survival: The Scientific Basis for the Healing Power of Intimacy. HarperCollins, New York: Harper Collins, p. 2–3.

16. Singh RB, et al (1992) An Indian experiment with nutritional modulation in acute myocardial infarction. American Journal of Cardiology 69: 879.

17. King SB, Lembo NJ, Weintraub WS, Kosinski AS, Barnhart HX, Kuntner MH, Alazraki NP, Guyton RA, Zhao XQ (1994) A randomized trial comparing coronary angioplasty with coronary bypass surgery. Emory angioplasty versus surgery trial. New England Journal of Medicine 331: 1044–1050.

18. Hirshfeld JW, Schwartz JS, Jugo R, Macdonald RG, Goldberg S, Savage MP, Bass TA, Vetrovec G, Cowley M, Taussig AS, Whitworth HB, Margolis JR, Hill JA, Pepine CJ (1991) Restenosis after coronary angioplasty: A multivariate statistical model to relate lesion and procedure variables to restenosis. Journal of the American College of Cardiology 18: 647–656.

19. Ornish DM (1998) Avoiding revascularization with lifestyle changes: The multicenter lifestyle demonstration project. American Journal of Cardiology 82: 72T-76T.

20. Eddy, DM (2000) Assessment of intensive lifestyle changes for the treatment of coronary heart disease.

C Common Medical Problems of the Elderly and CAM

23 Treatments for Arthritis: Conventional Drugs versus Complementary Alternative Medicines

Yuan Lin

Introduction

Arthritis comes in many forms. Two of the most common ones are osteoarthritis and rheumatoid arthritis. *Osteoarthritis (OA)*, which afflicts 16 million Americans, is a degenerative disease of the joints that eventually causes morbidity and disability especially in the elderly. The incidence of the disease increases with age and can be accelerated by joint injuries. Osteoarthritis may begin at a young age but by the age of 70, a large part of the population has some form of the disease [1]. *Rheumatoid arthritis (RA),* affecting over 2 million Americans, is an autoimmune disease of unknown origin. RA is a chronic systemic inflammatory disease marked by painful swelling of the joints. It is a potentially crippling and debilitating illness that can occur at any age but the incidence increases with age and affects females over males in a 2.5/1 ratio [2].

The etiology of these two types of arthritis is different. Both are usually characterized by inflamed, painful and swollen joints with RA mostly in the peripheral joints and OA frequently in the hand, hip and knee joints. Once the disease is diagnosed, the conventional drug treatments, mainly for the relief of pain, are similar. Non-steroidal anti-inflammatory drugs (NSAIDs), either by prescription or over-the-counter, are the most frequently used for symptomatic relief of arthritis but have major adverse effects and might even worsen the disease progression. Many patients thus turn to complementary alternative medicines (CAM) for effective and safer treatment. A number of such "unconventional" treatments have received much attention and gained popularity among arthritis patients; among them are the use of glucosamine and chondroitin, acupuncture and herbal medicine. In recent years, a large number of placebo-controlled clinical trials have been carried out to demonstrate the utility and safety of these CAM treatments. These studies will be the focus of this chapter.

The Etiology of OA and RA

OA used to be considered as a simple "wear and tear" of joints due to aging and cartilage degeneration. OA is now regarded as a result of both mechanical and biological events that destabilize the normal coupling of degradation and synthesis of articular cartilage chondrocytes and extracellular matrix and subchondral bone [3]. Cartilage matrix, mainly composed of type II collagen and proteoglycan, is constantly in a process of synthesis and degradation. Such a process is in balance in healthy individuals. Failure to maintain such balance, increased degradation or reduced synthesis, is considered to be the cause of the disease [1].

Age is considered as the strongest determinant of OA. Women are at a higher risk of developing OA than men particularly after menopause. Obesity and sport injuries are also risk factors for hip and knee OA. Most common clinical symptoms include joint pain, morning stiffness, bone enlargement and limitation of range of motion. Pain in the joint area is what brings the patients to the doctor. The clinical diagnosis is usually confirmed by finding typical radiographic changes of OA including marginal osterophytes, asymmetrical joint-space narrowing, subchondral bone sclerosis, subchondral cyst formation and in severe cases, deformity of bone ends [1].

RA is an autoimmune disorder of unknown etiology [2, 4]. It affects 1% of the adult population, and is the most destructive to synovial joints. Unlike OA, it involves primary tissue inflammation rather than joint degeneration. RA is a chronic, progressive, systemic, inflammatory disease of connective tissue characterized by spontaneous remissions and flare-ups. If left untreated, it can result in progressive joint destruction, deformity, disability and premature death. Clinical features of RA include morning stiffness, swelling of joints and wrist, fatigue, depression, the presence of rheumatoid nodules and an increased level of serum rheumatoid factor. The clinical course of the disorder is extremely variable among RA patients. Clinical diagnosis depends on radiographic evidence of change and more sensitive magnetic resonance imaging. Unfortunately there seems to be a poor correlation between clinical assessment and disease progression and thus a correct diagnosis may be difficult in the earlier stages. The American College of Rheumatology recommends early consultation with a rheumatologist and periodic assessment of disease activity and course of treatment program [5].

Conventional Drug Treatments for OA and RA

To date, there is no known cure for both types of arthritis and no means of preventing the onset of these diseases. Optimal management requires early diagnosis and timely introduction of agents that reduce the probability of irreversible joint damage [5].

Current treatment of OA is mostly directed to control symptoms such as pain and limitation of function because there are no disease-modifying OA drugs available. The most common management of OA is the "pyramid approach", with layers of the pyramid added one to another in a stepwise fashion [1]. Treatment should be individualized based on the severity and progression of the disease. The layered management begins with patient education, physical and occupational therapy, weight reduction and exercise. Non-steroidal anti-inflammatory drugs (NSAIDs) in low dose can be added to a regime of paracetamol and a topical capsaicin cream; intra-articular corticosteroid injection can be given to patients already on paracetamol and NSAIDs. The NSAIDs used are mainly for the control of pain and are often associated with side effects such as gastropathy [6]. An earlier study also indicated some bone destruction due to the use of NSAID [7]. There is no clear evidence to suggest superiority of one NSAID over another. A meta-analysis by Henry et al. [8] found that piroxicam, ketoprofen, tolmetin and azapropazone were associated with greater risk of serious gastrointestinal complications, such as perforation, ulcers and bleeding than other NSAIDS, especially low–

dose ibuprofen. The general principle is to use the minimum effective dose; avoid using more than one NSAIDs simultaneously and stop using the drug if no pain is felt. A number of cyclooxygenase-2 (COX-2) inhibitors have come to the market recently. These inhibitors exert anti-inflammatory effects by blocking the COX-2 enzyme but not the COX-1 enzyme which is needed to protect the stomach lining. Thus, they might provide a safer drug for patients with OA and will improve management of symptoms (see next section). The safety of long term use of COX-2 inhibitors and their superiority over the older NSAIDs remains to be seen.

The underlying causes leading to the onset of OA and RA are different. Until recently, the management of both types of arthritis was similar – the same pyramid management scheme involving the initial conservative management with a low dose of pain relief medications for several years. Recently, there has been a paradigm shift in the treatment of RA [2]. In addition to a more aggressive treatment using NSAIDs in the early stage of disease progression, a number of disease-modifying antirheumatic drugs (DMARD) are used, sometimes in combination. Also studies suggest that early aggressive treatment may alter the disease course [9] and most rheumatologists who care for RA patients favor aggressive treatment early in the course of the disease.

It is not known which is the best initial DMARD for patients with RA. Hydroxychloroquine or Sulfasalazine is often the initial choice for patients with mild disease. Methotrexate is selected for patients with severe disease and has the most predictable benefits. However, it can cause myelosuppression and in rare cases hepatotoxicity and pulmonary toxicity thus there is a need for laboratory monitoring. The early results of combination use of DMARDs yield conflicting results [10]. Other studies showed the slowing of joint erosions with combination therapy suggesting that concurrent use of several DMARD agents is a valid form of disease management [11]. A number of COX-2 specific NSAIDs have been approved by FDA recently for use in RA. A recent report [12] demonstrated that treatment with rofecoxib (a COX-2 inhibitor) was associated with significantly fewer upper GI incidents than one of the NSAID drug, naproxen. However, in the same study, it also showed that the COX-2 drug has a higher risk of myocardial infarction. Recently, a new biological response modifier– anti-tumor necrosis factor (TNF)-alpha has generated enthusiasm due to its potential as a totally new class of drugs for RA [13]. TNF-alpha has a variety of pro-inflammatory activities and plays a central role in RA. Anti-TNF-alpha works by blocking the natural TNF receptor from attracting inflammatory cytokines to the affected joints thus provides therapeutic intervention. However, this excitement is tempered by the potential for long-term side effects and toxicity.

Complementary and Alternative Treatments for Arthritis

In most cases, conventional chemical drugs are effective in controlling pain and inflammation but they have side effects, some of which could be severe. The search for safer and effective alternative treatments is needed. A survey by Eisenberg et al. [14] concluded that alternative medicine use and expenditures increased substantially between 1990 and 1997, attributable primarily to an increase in the proportion of the population seeking alternative therapies. CAM treatment for arthritis was found to be the fourth most common application after back problems, allergies and fatigue. Three forms of non-conventional treatments: Glucosamine and chondroitin sulfate, acupuncture and herbal medicines are the most commonly used CAM treatments for arthritis in the US. The analysis in the following sections on these three CAM for arthritis is based on clinical studies that were performed using modern clinical trial protocols in patients with either OA or RA. Other forms of CAM treatments for arthritis, such as physical manipulation, exercise and change of diet and life style have also been shown to be helpful in patients with arthritic conditions.

Glusoamine and Chondroitin Sulfate

Glusosamine, the amino sugar derivative of glucose, is a normal constituent of glycosaminoglycans in cartilage matrix and synovial fluids. Chondroitin sulfate, a polysaccharide, predominates in the ground substance of cartilage, bone and blood vessels and other connective tissues. It consists of repeating disaccharide units in specific linkage, each composed of a glucuronic acid residue linked to a sulfated N-acetylgalactosamine residue. The idea that these compounds may act as disease modifiers for OA originated from the notion that consumption of cartilage derivatives could provide substrates for cartilage repair. However, there is doubt about the absorption of these substances and their underlying mechanism of action raising skepticism among many health professionals [15].

The commercial forms of these compounds are produced by extraction from shellfish shell (glucosamine) and cow cartilage (chondroitin) and have been used to treat OA in Europe for over a decade and is gaining substantial popularity in the US. They are sold in Europe as drugs and in the US as dietary supplements for a number of years. A large number of clinical trials to evaluate the clinical effectiveness of these substances for the treatment of OA has been carried out. Recently, McAlindon and his colleagues [16] performed a meta-analysis combined with systematic quality assessment of clinical trials (from 1966–1999) of these preparations for OA. At least 37 clinical trials were performed during this period of time, but only 15 trials met their criteria (double blind, randomized, placebo-controlled for 4 or more weeks) and were included in the analysis. The author used the global pain score or the Lequesne index in the index joint as the primary outcome measure and considered the trial positive if improvement in the treatment group was equal to or greater than 25% compared with the placebo group, and was significant ($p>$ or $=0.05$). The trials demonstrated that glucosamine and chondroitin preparations for OA collectively demonstrate moderate to large treatment effects on symptoms compared with placebo, (39.5%, SD 21.9 for glucosamine, 40.2%, SD 6.4 for chondroitin sulfate). The authors also concluded that the assessments of methodological aspects of these studies suggested that the actual efficacy of these products is likely to be more modest. Furthermore, the efficacy was smaller when measured after only 4 weeks of treatment, suggesting that full therapeutic benefit may take longer than one month. Nevertheless, even modest efficacy could have clinical utility, given the safety of these preparations.

In another analysis, Towheed and Anastassiades [17] reviewed nine randomized, controlled trials of glucosamine in the treatment of OA. In 7 of the trials, in which they compared gluosamine with placebo, glucosamine was always superior. In two trials comparing glucosamine to ibuprofen, glucosamine was superior in one and equivalent in the other. Methodologic problems, including lack of standardized case definition of OA and lack of standardized outcome assessment led the authors to conclude that further studies are needed.

The amounts generally administered are glucosamine, 1500 mg, and chondroitin sulfate, 1200 mg daily. Although glucosamine has been described as effective when used alone, it is probably reasonable to use the combination pending further studies. Deal and Moskowitz [18] raised the issue that these agents are not FDA-evaluated or recommended for the treatment of OA. They are available as health food supplements and the number of studies of toxicity, particularly with respect to long-term evaluation, is limited.

One of the most encouraging result came from a study of long-term effects of using glucosamine for OA in a 3 year randomized, placebo-controlled clinical trial [19]. Two hundred and twelve patients with knee OA were randomly assigned to either 1500 mg glucosamine-sulfate once daily or placebo for 3 years. One hundred and six patients on placebo had a progressive joint-space narrowing of −0.31 mm (−0.48 to −0.13 mm). There was no significant joint-space loss in those on glucosamine sulfate: −0.06 mm (−0.22 to 0.09 mm). As assessed by WOMAC scores, symptoms worsened slightly in the placebo group and improved in patients taking glucosamine. The trial indicated that long-term administration of this compound can prevent joint structure change in patients with OA of the knee with a significant improvement in symptoms.

A number of studies suggested that chemical drugs worked faster than either glucosamine of chondroitin; but they also found that several months after treatment ended, the analgesic effect of the supplement remained stronger. None of the studies so far has found any serious side effects from either supplements. One of the animal studies suggested that glucosamine may worsen insulin resistance, a major cause of diabetes. Chondroitin can cause bleeding in people who have a bleeding disorder or take a blood thinning drug.

To date, there is no evidence for the effectiveness of these agents for the RA patients since cartilage damage plays a lesser role in the etiology of the disease.

Acupuncture

Acupuncture has been a key element of health care in China for at least 2000 years. The general theory of acupuncture is based on the premise that there are patterns of energy flow (Qi) through the body and the critical balance of the energy flow is essential for health. Acupuncturists believe that illness results from imbalance of bodily energy that can be corrected by insertion of thin needles through the skin to open hidden channels or meridians in the body and thus restore health. Acupuncture has grown enormously popular in the US in recent years. In 1993, the Food and Drug Administration estimated that over 1 million Americans were spending $500 million a year on the practice. Acupuncture has gradually entered the medical mainstream in the US and many states have accredited licensure programs and some insurance companies in many states already pay for the treatment particularly if it is prescribed by physicians.

Acupuncture is becoming a common technique within the physiotherapy profession as a treatment modality for pain management [20]. In November of 1997, a panel convened by the Office of Alternative Medicine, at the National Institutes of Health concluded that there is clear evidence to indicate that acupuncture therapy is useful in easing nausea associated with cancer chemotherapy and some forms of pain. Acupuncture has been used in both OA and RA patients for many years either alone or as an adjunct to conventional drug treatment. However, there are some inherent problems in clinical trials with acupuncture [21]. Trials of acupuncture can only be single blinded since the clinician giving the acupuncture is aware of which is the true treatment and which is the control. In addition, there is difficulty with the control procedure. Frequently, a "sham" or "mock" acupuncture is used in which the needles are placed at nearby non-classical points, as a placebo. However, in a number of trials, the sham control appeared to have an analgesic effect not too different from the real procedure [22]. Even with these drawbacks in mind, a number of clinical studies were made to test the effectiveness of acupuncture in the treatment of arthritis.

A limited number of clinical trials in RA patients, gave conflicting results as to the effectiveness of acupuncture. A randomized control study by Davis and his colleagues [23] enrolled 64 patients and used a single point (Li3) needle insertion, 4 minutes each time for 5 treatments. The outcome measures included the inflammatory markers (erythrocyte sedimentation rate and C-reactive protein), pain, swollen joint count and general health questionnaires. The results demonstrated that there is no significant difference between the treatment and control groups. The negative results were challenged by Tukmachi [24] in a letter to the editor. He cited flaws in test design including the selection of the Li3 point, the short duration and limited number of treatments, all of which do not conform to the theory and practice of acupuncture for the treatment of pain. In another study by a Swedish group [25], they observed improvements in RA patients treated either with deep electrical acupuncture or superficial needle insertion. Fifty eight patients with RA were assigned to either treatment and received 10 treatments during 5 weeks. Both treatments showed significant improvements in sickness impact, pain, general well-being, upper and lower limb impairment, grip strength and joint tenderness. Even though the use of acupuncture in the treatment of RA is one of the treatments of choice in China, the difficulties in modern clinical trial design and the limited number of studies available render the utility of acupuncture in treating RA inconclusive and point to the need for more randomized controlled trials.

There is however, moderately strong evidence that acupuncture is beneficial in treating OA patients [26]. Two recent clinical studies using acupuncture on patients with OA of the hip showed significant improvement after treatment. Thirty two patients were randomly allocated to either 6 sessions of acupuncture lasting up to 25 minutes (A) or given advice and exercise (B) over a 6 week period [27]. Patients were assessed for pain and functional ability. There was a significant improvement in group A as indicated by the decrease in WOMAC pain score immediately after treatment and this was maintained at the 8 week follow-up. There was no significant change in group

B. In another study [28], 67 patients were separated in 2 groups: group 1 had traditional needle placement and manipulation while with group 2, needles were placed away from classic positions and not manipulated. In both groups needles were placed with the L2 to L5 dermatomes. For all parameters (pain, functional impairment, activity in daily life) there was a significant improvement versus baseline in both groups, 2 weeks and 2 months after treatment but there is no sig-nificant difference between the two treatment groups. In another study, Singh and colleagues [29] recruited 73 patients with symptomatic OA of the knee to determine whether demographic, medical history, or arthritis assessment data may influence outcome and rate of decay after being treated with acupuncture twice weekly for 8 weeks. Using two different scoring systems, patients in the treatment group show improvement at 4, 8 and 12 weeks. Scores were stable regardless of the baseline severity of the OA. The group with the least disability and pain rebounded to original levels to a greater degree than did those who initially were more disabled. They concluded that acupuncture for patients with OA of the knee may work best when used early in the treatment plan, with a methodical decrease in frequency in treatment once the acute treatment period is completed to avoid a rebound effect. Demographic and medical history data were not mediating variables.

Herbal Medicines

Herbal medicine has been used both in Eastern and Western civilizations for maintaining health for thousands of years. In China, the practice of traditional Chinese herbal medicine is based on the comprehensive collection of ancient medical books and records. Books over 1000 years old still are in existence and are still used as a guide to treat diseases [30]. Herbal medicines have become popular in the US due to the general belief that they are safer than chemical drugs. According to a survey by Eisenberg et al. [14], herbal medicine is one of the most commonly used CAM therapies and the use of CAM therapy for rheumatic diseases is highly prevalent and increasing. Their popularity have prompted many clinical studies and publications in most mainstream journals. [31, 32].

In a recent comprehensive review by Long et al. [33], 12 randomized controlled trials and two systematic reviews fulfilled the inclusion criteria of the authors. Studies were limited to randomized controlled trials with OA patients. They found promising evidence for the effective use of some herbal preparations in the treatment of OA. In addition, evidence suggested that some herbal preparations can reduce the consumption of NSAIDs. The reviewed herbal medicines appear relatively safe.

In these trials the following herbs were reported to be able to relieve pain in OA patients.

For oral use

▶ *Articulin-F* (an Ayurvedic herbal-mineral formulation): Forty two OA patients were assigned to treatment group (2 capsules of Articulin F) or control group (2 capsules of placebo) for 3 months. Treatment group showed significant improvement in pain severity and disability score [34].

▶ *Extract of avocado/soybean unsaponifiables* (ASU): ASU is made of unsaponifiable fractions of avocado oil and soya bean oil. One hundred sixty four OA patients (either hip or knee) were randonly assigned to one 300 mg ASU a day or a placebo capsule. After 6 months, the ASU group showed a significantly improved pain score and functional disability score. In another study, ASU also significantly reduced NSAID consumption and delayed resumption of NSAID after stoppage in regular NSAID users [35, 36].

▶ *Devil's claw:* Devil's claw is a medicinal plant native to Africa. Its pain reducing activity was attributed to a group of compounds, iridoid glycosides. There were two double-blind control trials on OA patients, one with 400 mg of Devil's claw extract (containing 1.5% iridoid glycosides) for 3 weeks; one with 335 mg of Devil's claw extract (containing 3% iridoid glycosides) for 2 months. In both trials, results revealed a significant drop in pain intensity and increase in mobility [37, 38].

▶ *Willow bark extract:* Willow bark contains salicin, the precursor of salicylic acid more commonly known as aspirin. Seventy eight inpatients with OA of hip or knee were either treated with willow bark extract (containing 240 mg salicin) or with placebo for 2 weeks. A significant but moderate analgesic effect was confirmed by the physician and by the patients [39].

▶ *Ginger extract:* Comparing two groups either with 170 mg ginger extract or placebo, there were no significant differences in pain relief [40].

For topical applications

▶ *Capsiacin cream* (0.025%): Capsiacin is derived from hot chilli peppers. It is the most popular topical cream for the treatment of pain. A meta-analysis of 3 placebo controlled, double-blind clinical trials [41–43] favored capsacin cream for improvements in pain and articular tenderness, although only one of these trials reached a statistically significant level.

▶ *Stinging nettle leaf:* In a small trial with 27 OA patients, the application of stinging nettle leaf on the painful areas for one week showed pain and disability scores significantly lower as compared to placebo [44].

There are no undesirable side effect associated with taking these herbal products with the exception of a few patients who, after taking Articulin-F, experienced nausea, dermatitis and abdominal pain.

RA is an autoimmune disease characterized by synovial inflammation. Herbs used to treat RA are mostly immunosuppressive agents. A number of animal models and clinical studies have been performed with traditional Chinese herbal medicines (TCM) as immunosuppressive agents for the treatment of lupus erythematosus, rheumatoid arthritis, atopic eczema and organ transplantation [45].

Tripterygium wilfordii Hook F (TWHF) is the most commonly prescribed TCM in China for the treatment of RA. One placebo-controlled double blind trial has clearly demonstrated efficacy [46]. The immunosuppressive activity has been attributed to components such as triptolide, tripdiolide, triptonide and triptophenolide [47]. In a double blind controlled study with 70 RA patients, the treatment group was given a TWHF extract for 12 weeks and compared to either baseline or placebo treated group.

Of the TWHF group, 82–93% noted improvement in different clinical criteria or laboratory tests indicative of inflammation. Another Chinese herb, *Sinomenium acutum*, and its active component, sinomenine have been used extensively in China. Using animal models Liu and his colleagues [48] demonstrated that sinomenine was able to significantly improve the arthritic score, hind paw swelling and erythrocyte sedimentation rate. In author's lab, the use of whole herb extract was able to reduce pain and swollen joints as well as improving serum factors in a small group of patients with RA [49]. This study was an outcome study and neither the care- giver or the patients were blinded. Further clinical studies are needed to demonstrate the effectiveness of this preparation. In another study, a Japanese-Chinese herbal mixture (Keishi-sushi-to) was used for RA. Oral administration of this mixture to a rat model resulted in a reduction in the severity of the arthritis especially if it was administered at least 7 days prior to the induction of arthritis [50].

The adverse reactions that derived from the use of these herbs were not well documented, Zhang and Ni [51] reported a few cases of nephrotoxicity from ingestion of *T. wilfordii* and labels on isolated sinomenine indicated the possibility of its causing allergic dermatitis.

Most of the studies confirm the notion that herbal medicines when used properly are generally safe. However, there are few available data bases on adverse reactions. Prior to solid clinical data becoming available, some key points must be observed in patients contemplating taking herbal preparations [52]:

▶ "Natural" does not necessarily mean safe.
▶ Interactions between herbal medicine and single chemical drugs do occur.
▶ Lack of standardization, quality control and regulation may result in variability in herbal content, contamination during manufacture and potential mis-identification of plant species.
▶ Patients must heed the recommended dosage and length of treatment.

Thus all patients should be encouraged to discuss their use of herbal therapies and other dietary supplements with their doctors and report any adverse reactions associated with the use of these therapies.

The efficacy and safety of herbal medicines requires well designed and executed clinical trials. It is however important to recognize that clinical trials which use products that are not standardized make comparisons difficult. Variability in herbal preparations are likely to be the single major contributing factor to conflicting results.

Conclusion

Arthritis is a major cause of pain and disability in the elderly. Drug intervention includes non-opioid analgesics such as paracetamol, NSAIDS, topic analgesics, intra-articular steroid injections. Such treatments offer quick relief for pain, but may prove ineffective in some patients and NSAIDs often have serious adverse effects. Alternative and complementary medicine have thus become popular among arthritis patients.

Table 23.1. Comparison of modern chemical drug treatment and complementary alternative medicine (CAM)

	Chemical drug treatment	**CAM**
Human body	Cells and tissues	Holistic function
Objective	Treatment of disease and/or symptoms	Restoring homeostasis
Action	Fast; acute diseases	Gradual, chronic diseases
Patient	Considered as a group	Individualized therapy

Conceptually, we are faced with two fundamentally different philosophies of medicine, the conventional single chemical drug and CAM (Table 23.1). In practice, these lead to very different views of medical treatment.

However, both types of treatments share a common view that health is associated with homeostasis or functional balance. Critical disturbances at target tissues or organs can often be speedily dealt with by the powerful technologies and single chemical entities of western medicine. Such forceful intervention though successful in treating acute symptoms can lead to further loss of homeostasis with resulting side effects often at sites far removed from the original disease. On the other hand, CAM emphasis on maintaining and restoring balance may be more appropriate to disease prevention and the handling of chronic conditions without an unacceptably high level of collateral damage. An open-minded philosophy would not force a choice of one over the other, but examine how the advantages of one can complement the strengths of the other.

Physicians and patients are beginning to accept an integrated approach of treatment for arthritis. Results from many studies discussed in this chapter are encouraging. Disease modifying drugs and new drugs with fewer side effects are emerging. On the CAM treatment side, positive results were demonstrated in the use of glucosamine and chondrotin, acupuncture and selected herbal medicines. Unfortunately, most of the CAM treatment modalities are not well characterized by well-designed clinical trials and are not yet approved by FDA for the treatment of arthritis. This review is intended to select clinical studies that have been carried out mostly with placebo control and when possible double blinded to critically evaluate the effectiveness and safety of the treatments for OA and RA. The disease progression varies greatly among OA and RA patients and one needs to weigh all factors before choosing the most effective and safe program for the management of the disease.

As pointed out by Fontanarosa and Lundberg [53] "There is no alternative medicine. There is only scientifically proven, evidenced-based medicine supported by solid data or unproven medicine, for which scientific evidence is lacking". A significant body of work on CAM over the past 25 years has shown that modern scientific and clinical can be used to validate those practices that are safe and effective. Further stringent CAM clinical trials offer the hope of novel treatments for arthritis patients.

References

1. Creamer P, Hochberg MC (1997) Osteoarthritis. Lancet 350: 503–509
2. Lee DM, Weinblatt ME (2001) Rheumatoid arthritis. Lancet 358: 903–911
3. Kuetner K, Goldberg VM (1995) Osteoarthritic disorders. Rosemont: Academy of Orthopaedic Surgeons.
4. Wallace DJ, Metzger AL, Ashman RF (1995) Rheumatic diseases. In Lawlor G, Fischer TJ, Alderman DC (eds) Manual of Allergy and Immunology 3rd ed. Little, Brown & Company, Boston/NY, p303–352
5. Arthritis and Rheumatism (1996) Guideline for RA management, ACR clinical guideline Committee Vol 39, p713–722
6. Zeudler H (1991) Epidemiology and NSAID induced gastropathy. J Rheumatol 28:2–5
7. Newman NM, Ling RS (1985) Acetabular bone destruction related to NSAIDs. Lancet 2:11–14
8. Henry D, Lim LL, Garcia-Rodriquez LA, et al. (1996) Variability in risk of gastrointestinal complications with individual NSAIDs: results of a collaborative meta-analysis. BMJ 312:1563–1566
9. Van de Heide A, Jacobs JW, Bijlsma JW, et al. (1996) The effectiveness of early treatment with «second line» anti-rheumatic drugs: a randomized, controlled Trial. Ann Interm Med 124:1308–1315
10. Wilkens RF, Urowitz MB,/stablein DM, et al. (1992) Comparison of azathioprine, methotrexate and the combination of both in the treatment of rheumatoid arthritis: a controlled clinical trial. Arthritis Rheum 35: 849–856
11. Lipsky PE, van der Heijde DM, St. Clair EW, et al. (2000) Infximab and methotrexate in the treatment of rheumatoid arthritis. New Engl J Med 343: 1594–1602
12. Bombardier C, Laine L, Reicin A, et al. (2000) Comparison of upper gastrointestinal toxicity of rofecoxib and naproxen in patients with rheumatoid arthritis. N Engl J Med 343:1520–1528
13. Moreland LW, Baumgartner, SW, Schiff MH, et al.(1997) Treatment of RA with a recombinant human tumor necrosis factor receptor (p-75)-Fc fusion protein. N Engl J Med 337:141–147
14. Eisenberg DM, Davis RB Ettner S, et al (1998) Trends in alternative use in the United States, 1990–1997. JAMA 280:1569–1575
15. Constantz RB (1998) Hyaluronan, glucosamine and chondroitin sulfate: roles for therapy in arthritis? In Kelley WN et al. (eds) Textbook of Rheumatology. Philadelphia, WB Sanders.
16. McAlindon TE LaValley MP Gulin JP Felson DT (2000) Glucosamine and chondrotin for treatment of OA: a systematic quality assessment and meta-analysis. JAMA 283:1469–1475
17. Towheed TE and Anastassiades TP (2000) Glucosamine and chondroitin for treating symptoms of OA JAMA283:1483–1484
18. Deal CL, Moskowiz RW (1999) Nutraceuticals as therapeutic agents in OA. The role of glucosamine, chondroitin sulfate and collagen hydorlysate. Rheum Dis Clin North Am 25:379–395.
19. Reginster JY, Deroisy R, Rovati LC, et al. (2001) Long-term effects of glucosamine sulfate in OA progression: a randomized, placebo controlled clinical trial. Lancet 357: 251–256
20. Lee TL (2000) Acupuncture and Chronic pain management. Ann Acad Med Singapore 29:17–21
21. Lewith GT, Vincent C (1996) On the evaluation of clinical effects of acupuncture: A problem reassessed and a framework for future research. J Altern Complement Med 2:79–90
22. Lewith GT, Machin D (1983) On the evaluation of clinical effects of acupuncture. Pain 16: 111–127
23. David J, Townsend, DJ, Sathanathan, R, et al. (1999) The effect of acupuncture on patients with rheumatoid arthritis: a random placebo-controlled cross-over study. Rheumatology 38: 864–869
24. Takmachi E (2000) Acupuncture and RA. Rheumatotoloty 39:1153–1154.
25. Mayer M, Nisell R, Stenstrom CH, et al. (2001) Sensory stimulaion with acupuncture in rheumatoid arthritis: a randomized, controlled study. The Web-Journal of Acupuncture
26. Berman BM, Swyers JP, Ezzo J (2000) The evidence for acupuncture as a treatment for rheumatologic conditions. Rheum Dis Clin North Am 26:103–115
27. Haslam R (2001) A comparison of acupuncture with advice and exercise on the symptomatic treatment of osterarthritis of the hip- a randomized controlled trial. Acupunct Med 19:19–26.
28. Fink MG, Wipperman, B and Gehrke A (2001) Non-specific effects of traditional Chinee acupuncture in osteoarthritis of the hip. Complement Ther Med 9:82–89
29. Singh BB, Berman BM, Hadhazy V et al. (2001) Clinical decision in the use of acupuncture an an adjunctive therapy for osteoarthritis of the knee. Altern Ther Health Med 7: 58–65
30. Hui YZ (2000) Approaching traditional Chinese medicine: Inheritance and exploration. In Drug Discovery and Traditional Chinese Medicine, Lin Y (ed) Kluwer Acad Publishers, Boston/Dordrechet/London, p1–12
31. JAMA, November 11 issue, 1998
32. Yuan R, Lin Y (2000) Traditional Chinese medicine: an approach to scientific proof and clinical validation. Pharmacology and Therapeutics 86:191–198
33. Long L, Soeken K, Ernst E (2001) Herbal medicines for treatment of OA: a systematic review. 40:779–793
34. Kulkarni RR, Patki PS, Jog VP et al (1991) Treatment of OA with herbal medicine. J Ethanopharmacol 33:91–95
35. Maheu E, Masieres B, Valat JP et al (1998) Symptomatic efficacy of ASU in the treatment of OA of the knee and hip. Arthritis Rheum 41:81–91.
36. Blotman F, Maheu E, Wulwik A et al (1997) Efficacy and safety of ASU in the treatment of OA of the knee and hip. Rev Rhum Engl Ed 64: 825–834
37. Guyader M (1984) Les plantes antirhumatismales. Univertite Pierre et Marie Curie, Ph.D. Thesis
38. Lecomte A, Costa JP (1992) Harpagophytum dans l'arthrose. 37°2 Le Magazine 15:27–30

39. Schmid B, Tschirdewahn B, Kotter I et al (1998) Analgesic effect of willow bark extract in OA. Focus Alternative Complementary Ther 3:86
40. Biddal H, Rosetzky A, Schlichting P et al (2000) A randomized, placebo-controlled, cross-over study of ginger extracts and ibuprofen in OA. Osteoarthritis Cartilage 8:9–12
41. Deal CL, Schnitzer TJ, Listein E et al (1991) Treatment of arthritis with topical capsaisin: a double blind trial. Clin Ther 13:383–393
42. McCarthy GM, Mccarty DL (1992) Effect of topical capsaisin in the therapy of painful OA of the hands. J Rheumatol 19:604–607
43. Altman RD, Aven A, Holmburg CE et al (1994) Capsaisin cream 0.025% as monotherapy for OA: A double blind study. Semin Arthritis Rhum 23(Suppl.):25–33
44. Randall C, Randall H, Dobbs F et al. (2000) Randomized controlled trial of nettle sting for treatment of base-of-thumb pain. J R Soc Med 93: 305–309
45. Ramgolam V, Ang SG, Lai YH et al. Traditional Chinese medicines as immunosuppressive agents. Ann Acad Med Singapore 29:11–16
46. Lipsky PE, Tao XL (1997) A potential treatment for RA: Thunder god vine. Semin Arthritis Rheum 26: 713–723
47. Tao XL, Cai JJ, Lipsky PE (1995) The identity of immunosuppressive components in the ethyl acetate extract and chloroform methanol extract of T. wilfordia Hook F. J Phar Exp Ther 272:1305–1312
48. Liu L, Buchner E, Beitze E et al. (1996a) Amelioration of rate experimental arthritides by treatment with the alkaloid sinomenine Int J Immunopharmacol 18:529–543
49. Yuan, R. Marco Polo Technologies: a model for a modern TCM company. In Drug Discovery and Traditional Chinese Medicine, Lin Y (ed) Kluwer Acad Publishers, Boston/Dordrechet/London, p191–200
50. Wakabayashi K, Inoue M, Ogihara Y (1997) The effect of keishi-bushi-to on collagen-induced arthritis. Biol Pharm Bull 20:376–380
51. Zhang JZ, Ni RZ (1985) Four cases of nephrotoxicity by *Tripterygium wilfordii*. Chin J Dermatol 18:231–232
52. Cirigliano M, Sun A (1998) Advising patients about herbal treatments. JAMA 280:1565–1566
53. Fontanarosa PB, Lundberg GD (1998) Alternative medicine meets science. JAMA, 280:1618–1619

24 Alternative and Complementary Treatments in Respiratory Diseases in the Elderly

N.S. Cherniack

Introduction

As with diseases affecting other systems of the body, the aim of alternative and complementary treatments of respiratory diseases is prevention, relief of symptoms, and improving function. While treatments in orthodox medicine are formulated specifically for each disease etiology, treatment in alternative medicine is designed specifically for each individual with little consideration of differences in the types of pathogens involved. Thus bacterial diseases are handled quite differently from viral diseases in conventional medicine, but diseases caused by a specific bacteria are treated pretty much the same in different patients; on the other hand alternative medicine therapeutic approaches would be customized for each patient but might not be different for viral versus bacteria respiratory infections in the same patient. These differences in the overall holistic philosophy and individualized approach underlying alternative versus conventional medicine create problems in designing studies on effectiveness. In addition the possibility of placebo effects and the choice of the proper placebo for some alternative medicine techniques like acupuncture complicates the assessment of treatment efficacy.

All these impede the gathering of valid data testing the value of alternative treatments. So that in general there is insufficient data that meet orthodox medicine criteria to decide whether a particular alternative medicine approach is effective; and this creates the real possibility that truly effective treatments may be overlooked. Despite the paucity of reliable efficacy data the use of alternative techniques is increasingly popular both among younger and older individuals.

Reasons for use of alternative treatments by elderly include the cost of conventional treatments and medication, lack of treatment in orthodox medicine, and the perception that conventional medicine is too impersonal. A large fraction of the elderly use alternative techniques to prevent rather than to treat illness [1, 2].

Types of Respiratory Disease

Diseases of the respiratory system are prevalent in the older population and alternative and complementary methods have been likely used to treat all the known respiratory diseases. However published reports of these treatments have mainly dealt with four types of respiratory disease and the review will focus on these.

Respiratory infections where the treatments aim at preventing colds and other upper and lower respiratory tract infections, and the relief of symptoms such as coughing and chest congestion.

Asthma used to be considered a disease of young people arising in childhood and persisting in some into adulthood. But it is now recognized that asthma can appear for the first time in late middle age. Asthma is a disease characterized by reversible airway obstruction caused by increased reactivity of the smooth muscle to a variety of stimuli, which produces wheezing, coughing and shortness of breath. It is thought to be a chronic inflammatory condition and now is treated conventionally by agents, which exert an anti-inflammatory effect. Edema of the airway epithelium and constriction of the airway smooth muscle as well as hypersecretion of mucus characterize an asthmatic episode many of which have an allergic basis. But other triggers of asthma include respiratory infections, cigarette smoke, chemical dusts and vapors, animal dander, heavy exercise, and exposure to cold air. Anxiety and psychological stress are well known provocateurs of asthma. For example some asthmatic patients allergic to cat dander will develop an attack when shown a picture of a cat. Asthma is quite common in adults. It has been estimated that almost 25% of people over 65 wheeze, but there are many other causes of wheezing besides asthma. In older people asthma may be confused with COPD or heart disease but all three can occur together. While many effective medications have been developed in recent years to prevent and to relieve bronchospasm, alternative treatments are still frequently used perhaps because of treatment costs or fear of the imagined and real hazards of using "unnatural substances".

Chronic obstructive lung diseases such as bronchitis and emphysema. Although these have a genetic component powerful environmental factors like smoking exist [3]. Despite intensive study and a good understanding of the causes of the disease, there is no cure or an accepted way of slowing disease progress, or even of relieving major symptoms such as dyspnea. It is the fifth leading cause of death and affects about six percent of the U.S. Population and is common in the elderly. About half of affected individuals die within ten years. It is slowly progressive causing hypoxia, often hypercapnia, and dyspnea, weakness, and weight loss. The diseases are characterized by largely irreversible air way obstruction with glandular hyperplasia and increased secretion of mucus in the airways (bronchitis) and/or loss of lung elasticity (emphysema) which increases the tendency of the airways to collapse during expiration and produces air trapping, an expanded lung, and a shortening of the muscle fibers of the diaphragm, external intercostals, and other inspiratory muscles. Diaphragmatic shortening and foot-ward displacement by the over-inflated lung decreases the force of diaphragm contraction and heightens tendencies for diaphragm fatigue all of which promote and intensify dyspnea. Conventional treatment, which is often ineffective, includes bronchodilators, like beta-2 agonists, acetylcholine antagonists, agents such as aminophylline, anti-inflammatory agents like steroids given by inhalation or systemically, antibiotics, oxygen, and rehabillative procedures such as exercise conditioning and respiratory muscle training. Opiates have been used with quite limited success in the treatment of dyspnea in COPD because ventilatory depression is a common adverse side effect increasing the severity of hypoxia and hypercapnia [4–7]. Lung volume reduction surgery or transplantation is sometimes considered and performed in patients with severe COPD, but often has a poor outcome in patients over 75 [8].

Lung cancers also occur mainly in the elderly and can be divided into small and non-small cell carcinomas. Small cell cancers metastasize rapidly through the blood and are treated by chemotherapy but life expectancy remains low despite treatment, about a year after diagnosis. Localized non-small cell tumors can be surgically removed but more widespread tumors require radiation and chemotherapy. Although treatment has been substantially improved in recent years five-year survivals remain quite low. While conventional treatments are generally type specific and aim at arresting or eradicating the tumor, alternative treatments are mainly used to control symptoms such as dyspnea, pain, weakness, nausea and vomiting.

As shown below, a wide variety of alternative method techniques have been used to manage respiratory disease. While asthma and respiratory infections are quite effectively treated by orthodox medicine, chronic obstructive lung disease and cancer are not. The widespread use of alternative medicine by asthmatics is somewhat surprising.

Types of Alternative Treatments of Respiratory Diseases

▶ Botanicals (Chinese, Ayurvedic, e.g. Ma huang [ephedrine], Magnolia, minor blue dragon, ginko, ginseng, pirorrhiza, ahhota vasca, forskolin, scutellaria, onion)
▶ Nutritional (vitamins, magnesium, zinc, acetylcysteine, omega-3 fatty acids)
▶ Acupuncture
▶ Homeopathic (e.g. oscillococcinum)
▶ Breathing maneuvers

Not only are lung diseases more common in the elderly, but aging also compromises lung function and the ability of the respiratory system to respond to stress. Perhaps some, in an attempt to retard the effects of aging, have used alternative techniques. Thus far, there have been no studies of whether any of these alternative medicine modalities in fact slow the decreases in lung function that are outlined in the next section.

Effects of Aging on Respiratory Function

Aging causes a progressive deterioration in almost all aspects of lung function [9]. But in the non-smoker, there is sufficient reserve so that respiratory symptoms do not occur. The elasticity of the lung decreases and elastic recoil increases mainly because of a decrease in lung surface area; while the chest wall becomes stiffer so that greater muscle force is required to expand the lungs. At about 55 to 60 years of age, respiratory muscle strength and endurance also lessen but perhaps at a slower rate in individuals who regularly exercise. As a consequence, there is a decline in vital capacity and the rate at which air can be maximally expired from the lung in one second (FEV1). In non-smoking normals, FEV1 declines at a rate of about 30 ml. per year but this is greatly accelerated in smokers. The loss of lung elasticity also allows small peripheral airways to collapse at low lung volumes interfering with gas exchange and the distribution of inspired air in the lungs. Diffusion capacity, the ability to transfer oxygen and carbon dioxide across the alveolar membranes into the blood, decreases gradually after about age 40. As a result of these changes, the partial pressure of oxygen in the lung decreases according to the equation $PaO_2 = 109 - (0.43 \times age)$, but carbon dioxide tension in the arterial blood remains relatively constant. Pulmonary arterial pressures and vascular resistance also rise with age. The ventilatory response to both hyper-capnia and to hypoxia also tends to fall with age. It is of interest that the ability of the elderly to recognize impediments to breathing is also diminished perhaps delaying their contacting medical help. While maximum exercise capacity is diminished in the elderly, a decrease in muscle mass and in circulatory function rather than respiratory performance is responsible. A decrease in the rate of mucociliary transport and loss of the cough reflex decreases ability to defend against infection and exposures to oxidants and other pollutant in the air over the years further damages the lung. All these changes reduce the ability of the geriatric patient to adjust and compensate when lung infections and chronic lung diseases occur.

Treatment of Respiratory Infections by Alternative Method Techniques

Alternative medicine has been used in two ways with respect to respiratory infections to prevent infection and to alleviate symptoms such as congestion or cough [10–14].

Vitamins, zinc, etc. are used to prevent infections. High doses of Vitamin C sometimes more than 500 mg are taken by the elderly to prevent colds and other respiratory illness, but there has been no well designed study indicating that Vitamin C is of value. However, it may reduce the duration of cold symptoms [15].

Supplemental zinc in doses of 23 mg of the ionized form has been reported to reduce the duration and severity of cold symptoms in older adults but not children. It has been recommended that zinc lozenges may be helpful during colds in community-dwelling older patients [16]. However, the evidence is not convincing that zinc either reduces the severity or adverse effects of colds. Patients taking the lozenges were more likely to complain of mouth irritation, unpleasant taste, feeling sick, and diarrhea.

Despite the lack of convincing data, botanicals of various types have been used mainly to treat the cough, sneezing, fever, and chest congestion occurring with respiratory infections [17]. A variety of herbal tea mixtures have been used to treat colds symptomatically.

Echinacea has been used in patients who have frequent colds. In a study of 108 such patients for two months, no difference was found in the frequency of colds between Echinacea and placebo treated patients. Other herbals used to prevent and treat colds include garlic, golden seal, ginseng, hyssop, licorice, and elderberry.

Allium septa and onion are used to treat coughs and chest colds in Latin America. A number of onion extracts, like thiosulfinates and cepaenes, have been shown to have anti-inflammatory and anti-asthmatic actions.

Aloe is used for many medical conditions including asthma, cold and coughs. Interpretation of efficacy studies of botanicals in respiratory infections and in other respiratory diseases are made more complex because of difficulties in precisely defining the purity and actual dose of the agents used, since there are few if any standards of quality for herbal or other botanical products Also, botanicals often contain one or more chemicals that can be extracted and account for therapeutic effects. The quantity of specific chemicals in a given botanical may vary considerably depending in on such factors as rainfall, intensity of exposure to the sun, and the chemical composition of the soil in which the plants were grown [18].

Oscillococcinum a homeopathic patented, commercially available medicine has been advocated for the prevention and treatment of asthma. Based on the homeopathic principle that like should cure like, the medicine is made from wild duck heart and liver, a well-known reservoir of influenza virus. A recent Cochrane review found that there was no evidence that oscillococcinum prevents influenza, but it did seem to reduce the length of the illness slightly by about one-quarter day [19].

Steam inhalations with eucalyptus, wintergreen, or peppermint, a kind of aromatherapy, have been used for many years to relieve chest congestion.

Alternative Treatments of Asthma

Fourty-one percent of respondent asthmatic patients use complementary and alternative medicine techniques according to a survey carried out in Great Britain. The three most prevalent techniques were herbalism, homeopathy, and breathing maneuver. Similar findings were obtained in a study performed in the U.S. [2, 20–24].

A diverse group of herbs and other botanicals have used to treat asthma and allergic symptoms in different parts of the world. At times, various botanicals are used in combination. Extracts of some of these herbs have been shown in animal studies or in vitro to have anti-inflammatory, anti-allergic, or smooth muscle relaxing effects and the active substance in the herb has been identified. See Table 24.1 for some examples. Many act as diaphoretics, suppress coughing, or are used as tonics. (Qi) There have been only a handful of controlled studies in humans. When they have been compared to traditional bronchodilators in the treatment of asthma, the botanicals have been less effective An excellent and comprehensive review of these agents by Bielory and Lupoli can be consulted for detailed information on studies that have been performed [25]. In addition alternative treatments are used to reduce symptoms produced by rhinitis [24–32].

Ma huang is used for asthma and hay fever and may be combined with other herbs like apricot, gypsum, and licorice. It contains ephedrine an alpha and beta agonist and is a well-established bronchodilator. Ephedrine has many side effects, which can be quite hazardous. These include vasoconstriction, hypertension, and tachycardia. It can also cause mydriasis and insomnia. Synthetic ephedrine is available Minor blue dragon is a mixture, which includes ma huang, and asarum, which has an analgesic and anti-bacterial action and in addition licorice and ginger, which have some, cough suppressant effect [25].

Table 24.1. Active ingredients found in some herbals used to improve respiratory system health

Herbal	Active Ingredient	Biological Effect
Ma huang	L-ephedrine	Alpha and beta receptor agonist
Licorice	Terpenoids	Stimulates cortisol activity, inhibits11beta dehydroxyehydrogenase
Ginkgo bilboa	Ginkgolides	Platelet activating factor antagonist
Onions	Cepaenes, thiosulfinates	Anti-anaphylactic activity may suppress LB4 and TX4 synthesis
Malabar Nut	Vascine	Anti-histamine activity
Coleus forskoli	Forskolin	Increases cyclic AMP
Salboku-to	Magnol	Inhibits 11beta dehydoxysteroid dehydrogenase
Tylophora	Tylophorine	Inhibits passive cutaneous anaphylaxis
Picrorrhiza kurroa	Androsin	Inhibits bronchocostriction induced by latelet activating factor

Herbs commonly used for a number of different reasons have also been tried by asthmatics. Ginko bilboa is claimed in traditional Chinese Medicine to have an anti-tubercular and anti-bacterial effect and to help expel phlegm and prevent wheezing. Ginkolides extracted from the leaves of ginko biloba antagonize platelet-activating factor but in one study seemed to have no effect on exercise induced asthma.

Ginseng has been used in asthmatics to adjust qi and improve adaptation to stress, including that caused by labored breathing Licorice is used as an expectorant. Excess ingestion may prolong the action of cortisol and even produce Cushing-like signs. It contains triterpenes, which may have an anti inflammatory effect because of their similarities in structure to corticoids [24, 25].

Other more unfamiliar herbs used in Chinese, Japanese, Indian, and Latin American folk medicine have been tried in asthma and used to treat allergies [24, 25]. Scutellaria is used in traditional Chinese Medicine for allergies, upper respiratory infections, and inflammations. Some animal experiments suggest it inhibits the PCA reaction. Picrorrhiza kurroa is used in India to relieve asthmatic symptoms. However, a double-blind study found no improvement in lung function or reduction in clinical attacks with its use. Alkaloids made from adhatoda vasica, the malabar nut, have been shown to have a weak antihistaminic action in guinea pigs and to produce respiratory stimulation in dogs. The malabar nut is used to treat bronchitis and asthma in Ayurvedic medicine.

Tylophora asthnatica and tylophora indicum are ayurvedic medicines, which have been used in diseases in which there is sputum accumulation. The leaves of the tylophora plant are chewed or an alcoholic extract of the leaves are made. Side effects include sore mouth, loss of taste and vomiting. Although some studies of humans have reported good results with tylophora, a double-blind investigation found no benefits.

Forskolin a derivative of the plant coleus forskholi, which is used as an expectorant antitussive, and febrifuge in India, has been reported to increase airway conductance but the effect is more transient than that of fenoterol.

Saiboku-To, a combination of two herbal preparations sho-saiko-to and hange-kaboku-to contains 10 different herbs. Although it can cause pneumonitis, animal experiments suggest that it has multiple effects that might be beneficial in asthmatics. It suppresses histamine release and Type I reactions as well as having an inhibitory effect on PAF and leukotriene production It has been studied in clinical trials in Japan in steroid dependent asthma and reported to have useful actions.

Solanum xanthocarpum, Kantari, is used in Ayurvedic Medicine as an expectorant, anttussive and bronchodilator. Bector and Puri studied 60 patients with chronic lung disease and concluded that there was slight to significant improvement in cough and other clinical symptoms [30].

On the other hand, herbals can have adverse effects in asthmatics and occasionally are a cause of occupational asthma in those employed in the food industry [32, 33]. Garlic dust for example has been reported to be a cause of occupational asthma.

Older patients frequently take dietary supplements including multivitamins. Nutritional non-herbal supplements such as omega-3 fatty acids have been used in asthmatics [34, 35]. These are essential long-chain fatty acids which are not synthesized by humans but come from fatty fish, wild game, and plants. Omega-3 fatty acids compete with omega-6 fatty acids and impede the formation of prostaglandins, leukotrienes, and thromboxane. They also have anti-inflammatory and anti-thrombotic effects and alter cytokine production. Omega-3 fatty acids have been shown to reduce triglyceride levels, and decrease the incidence of ventricular arrhythmias. They can lower blood pressure. There haven't been enough clinical trials to decide whether omega-3 fatty acids will be useful in asthma, but an anti-inflammatory effect has been demonstrated in rheumatoid arthritis. High daily doses can cause nausea and vomiting, and blood glucose elevations. However, in a small study in 14 asthmatic patients, those who took perilla seed oil, which contains n-3 fatty acids for 4 weeks had significant increases in vital capacity and forced vital capacity(one second) but not those who took corn oil which contains n-6 fatty acids.

It is encouraging that there are increasing reports from studies that aim at elucidating the cellular effects of herbals and their constituents. The active ingredients of some of the herbs have been identified and their biological effects assessed

Acupuncture has had mixed effects in the treatment of asthma [36–42]. Frequently, improvement in symptoms has been reported, but few studies have observed any change in lung function [43–50]. There is a substantial problem in determining the proper use of placebos with acupuncture that tends to cloud findings [51–54]. Nonetheless, acupuncture was considered to be possibly effective in asthma by an NIH consensus panel, but a Cochrane review concluded that there was not enough evidence to reach a firm conclusion [54].

The successful treatment of asthma using a homeopathic approach has been reported and homeopathy is frequently used by asthmatic patients in Great Britain [2, 19]. Homeopathy involves the use in a very diluted form of substances which cause symptoms when undiluted. A Cochrane review of 3 placebo controlled trials of homeopathic treatment of 154 patients found that in two to the three trials the homeopathic patients fared better, in one because symptom severity was less, and in the other there was a greater improvement in lung function [19].

Breathing exercises have been said to be helpful in the treatment of asthma, but the term has been used in many different ways in both Eastern and Western medicine making it difficult to decide whether they are really useful [55–60]. Lehrer and co-workers are exploring the usefulness of biofeedback techniques in the treatment of asthma [57, 58]. They have evidence supporting the hypothesis that biofeedback to increase respiratory sinus arrhythmia decreases respiratory impedance in asthmatic patients. Peak flow variability was decreased in asthmatics that practiced daily Qigong-Yangsheng a traditional Chinese medicine technique that combines movements, mental exercise and breathing techniques. Buteyko therapy teaches deliberate under-breathing as a technique for preventing asthma. Hyperventilation with consequent lowering of arterial PCO_2 has a constrictive effect on airways. In Buteyko, all astmatic attacks are believed to result from hyperventilation, which in turn causes decreased cortisol levels. There is no evidence that supports this relationship or demonstrates a beneficial effect of Buteyko. Yoga has been tried as a technique to prevent asthma attacks. Yoga reduced sympathetic reactivity in a study in nine asthmatics but had no effect on pulmonary function.

A number of alternative medicine techniques like massage and hypnosis have been tried in children but not in the elderly and appear to provide some relief although more studies are needed.

Alternative Treatments of Chronic Obstructive Lung Disease

Many of the herbal preparations used in asthma are also used by patients with COPD since the two diseases have many symptoms in common. For example, Solanum xanthocarpum, Kantari, is used in Ayurvedic Medicine as an expectorant, anti-tussive and bronchodilator. Bector and Puri studied 60 patients with chronic lung disease and concluded that there was slight to significant improvement in cough and other clinical symptoms [30].

In COPD, unlike asthma, symptoms are persistent. Dyspnea in asthma is episodic and reversible, but not in COPD. Dyspnea, or shortness of breath, is defined as the perception of increased difficulty breathing or an unpleasant awareness of breathing. Sometimes in patients whose blood is poorly saturated with oxygen, inhalation of oxygen-enriched mixtures attenuates the dyspnea. A rigorous trial of exercise training sometimes combined with exercises to specifically improve the strength and endur-ance of the respiratory muscles relieves dyspnea, but requires a commitment that many patients are unwilling or unable to make [61–67]. Dyspnea occurs in many patients with COPD. Dyspnea seems to occur when the force generated by the res-piratory muscles is too great or inappropriately too large, relative to the increase of the tidal volume demanded by the activity or exercise [68–71]. Such an imbalance between the magnitude of inspiratory effort and the resultant inspiratory volume often occurs when pulmonary disease causes a structural alteration in either the lung parenchyma or the airways. It is clear that humans can estimate accurately their tidal volume, and the force and tension of the respiratory muscles. Studies in which muscles have been temporarily paralyzed show that the magnitude of nervous discharge to the paralyzed muscle can also be sensed. While earlier studies suggest that increased respiratory work (i.e. pressure times volume) produces dyspnea, more recent studies indicate that the most important factor is the pressure produced by respiratory muscle contractions per breath expressed as a percent of the maximal pressure a subject can generate. Inspiratory pressure is also more dyspnogenic than changes in either the respiratory rate or the inspiratory duty cycle, that is, the ratio of inspiratory time/total time of the respiratory cycle. This idea that dyspnea is a function of pressure developed by the inspiratory muscles considered as a percent of maximal pressure – may explain dyspnea in patients with neuromuscular disorders. It has been shown that CO_2 itself is dyspnogenic and probably hypoxia as well. These effects of oxygen and CO_2 tension are independent of their effects on respiratory muscle contraction and, most likely, are mediated by increases in the nervous discharge to the muscles It has been suggested that actual levels of ventilation may be selected so as to minimize the sense of dyspnea (or effort) used in breathing yet prevent excessive increase in CO_2. This principle would affect both the ventilation level and its pattern and would vary with the mechanical properties of the lung and chest wall. For example, ventilation may be adjusted to minimize both excessive ventilation and CO_2 elevation. In addition, the respiratory pattern at any given level of ventilation, that is the selection of a tidal volume and respiratory rate, may serve to minimize the force exerted with each breath while at the same time assuring an adequate tidal volume to avoid or minimize hypoventilation and CO_2 retention. In addition, ventilation is substantially affected by both behavioral factors such as alertness, which increases ventilation, and emotional factors such as anxiety, which may increase breathing frequency by shortening expiratory time.

Acupuncture (or acupressure) is sometimes effective in relieving the dyspnea associated with chronic airway obstruction [49, 72–74]. A review of 16 studies by Jobst, half of which were randomized clinical trials, suggested that traditional Chinese acupuncture could relieve dyspnea in over half of patients with chronic disabling breathlessness who received treatment [49]. Acupuncture also facilitated the reduction of the use of pharmacological agents for dyspnea in some patients.

Difficulties in study design may explain the mixed results in previous studies [49, 51, 55, 66]. In most studies, the real acupuncture points used in treatments of dyspnea were the same in all patients; in only two studies reviewed by Jobst were the points individualized as recommended in traditional acupuncture practice. Thus, in some studies, the treatment may not have been given optimally. Some of the studies quoted by Jobst used as a control stimulation of genuine acupuncture points thought not to be important for relief of dyspnea [49]. In other studies, needling supposedly ineffectual points relatively distant from genuine points produced sham acupuncture. However, the points used in both these types of sham acupuncture have been thought by some to have an effect on the lung or dyspnea so that they were not good controls.

If the acupuncture and sham acupuncture results are combined, acupuncture was more effective than the regimen in which neither was used. Another problem in acupuncture studies is deciding on treatment points for needling. Additionally, studies of acupuncture effectiveness have tended to use the same set of points in all patients tested, while in practice the points to needled by therapist trained in traditional Chinese medicine varies among individuals even those being treated for the same disease.

Alternative Treatments of Pulmonary Carcinoma

There are 165,000 new cases of lung cancer each year in the United States, of which more than 50,000 are inoperable. Although striking therapeutic advances have been made both in the treatment of small and non-small cell lung cancer, only about 13% of all patients with lung cancer survive more than 5 years. In addition elderly patients are less likely to tolerate some commonly used chemotherapy combinations.

Alternative treatments of cancer with a number of different plant and animal products have been tried. For example, Jin Fu Kang, a herbal mixture in oral liquid form, was reported to produce 8 partial remissions and one complete remission in 96 patients with non-small cell lung cancer tested. Garlic extracts have been found to have an apoptotic effect on non-small lung cancer cells in vitro. Extracts of shark cartilage are purported to have anti-angiogenic effects, which could be useful in treating lung and other cancers [76–78]. In addition there are a number of alternative treatment methods which involve special diets, nutritional supplements, and sometimes vaccines.

More often, alternative treatments have been tried to ameliorate some of the major symptoms of cancers. The most frequent symptom in a study of 129 geriatric patients with lung cancer were fatigue (82%), cough (67%) dyspnea (61%), pain (59%) and weakness (55%) [79]. Physical functioning in lung cancer patients is negatively correlated with age. Older patients have more comorbid conditions. Loss of weight after diagnosis of lung cancer is associated with increased symptom distress.

Except for the least advanced forms of lung cancer (without metastases and nodal spread) not beyond the bronchopulmonary nodes), conventional treatment requires chemotherapy and radiation therapy, sometimes in conjunction with surgery. These therapies themselves can at least temporarily worsen symptoms.

Dyspnea occurs in 75% to 85% of patients with lung cancer. To a lesser degree, patients with cancer of other organs report dyspnea as well [3, 4]. 70% of cancer patients report some degree of breathlessness in their last six week of life. Direct or indirect tumor effects can cause dyspnea, or it can be treatment related. Dyspnea is more prominent in patients with pulmonary cancer who have involvement of the mediastinal nodes rather than involvement of the airways or alveoli.

While a measure of lung volume (vital capacity) correlates weakly with the degree of dyspnea reported by patients with cancer, lung involvement as observed on either chest x-ray or clinical examination is a better predictor of dyspnea than is the measured lung function in such patients. Furthermore, anxiety is independently correlated with dyspnea in patients with all cancers. Loss of muscle mass and decreased strength in patients with lung cancer can exacerbate dyspnea. There is at present no good treatment for dyspnea, even though it can become severely disabling.

Acupuncture has been used in several studies to relieve pain in patients with lung disease not caused by cancer, and in a much smaller number of studies in lung cancer patients with mixed success [49, 51]. Relief of pain in cancer patients may become a serious problem because of fears of harming the patient arising from the side effects of too much analgesia or of causing addiction. In addition to standard acupuncture, auricular acupuncture has been used for the relief of cancer pain. However, none of these have been adequately controlled. Acupuncture also is reported to be helpful in reducing nausea and vomiting after cancer chemotherapy.

As a treatment modality, acupuncture has the following advantages:

▶ it has few side effects;
▶ it can be used even in weakened patients; and
▶ it has shown to be effective in cancer (though not lung cancer) in reducing pain and nausea, both common symptoms of lung cancer or its treatment, chemo or radiation therapy.

Pain itself can limit respiratory excursions and produce dyspnea while nausea interferes with proper nutrition.

Acupuncture studies have often lacked appropriate controls. The need for appropriate control groups is critical, for the efficacy of a placebo has been well demonstrated in the treatment of dyspnea in cancer patients [75].

Cigarette smoking is the major risk factor for lung cancer. Acupuncture has been tried in smoking abstinence programs. In one study of 85 patients, 71% stopped smoking.

Other alternative methods have been used to improve well-being in seriously ill cancer patients. In a controlled study, transcutaneous electrical stimulation of nerves resulted in a significant decrease in the sense of patient's fatigue and with also some lessening of pain. Relaxation therapies have also been reported to bring about pain relief, as has self-hypnosis.

Green tea has been advocated as a cancer preventive in humans. Epigallocatechin gallate, a polyphenol, the main constitutient of tannin in green tea, has anti-tumor activity. Beta-carotene supplementation in a large study among US physicians found no efficacy in reducing over all cancer risk.

Summary

Respiratory diseases are quite common in the elderly and are a frequent cause of disability and death. In addition, some respiratory diseases cannot at the present time be adequately treated. It is not surprising then the elderly have tried alternative methods of dealing with respiratory illness. Some of these treatments are risky and to the extent they delay consultation with a physician, all are dangerous. The efficacy of alternative methods is uncertain. Differences in approach to the patient and the divergence in the approach to treating disease may make it quite difficult to adequately assess alternative treatment methods in patients, But with some modalities like acupuncture, results are promising but as yet inconclusive. At another level progress has been made in assessing the biologic actions of a number of herbals and nutritional supplements. Slow but steady progress is being made in incorporating useful alternative techniques in orthodox medicine.

References

1. Kaptchuk, TJ, Eisenberg DM, The persuasive appeal of alternative medicine. Ann. Int Medicine 129: 1061–1065, 1998
2. Blanc PD, Kuschner WG, Katz PP, Smith S, Yelin EH The use of herbal products, coffee or black tea, and over-the-counter medications as self-treatments among adults with asthma. J Allergy Clin Immunol.100: 789–91, 1997
3. Celli B. Pathophysiology of chronic obstructive pulmonary disease. In Cherniack NS, Altose MD, and Homma I (eds.): Rehabilitation of the Patient with Respiratory Disease New York, McGraw-Hill, 1999: pp. 105–113
4. Marin JM, Montes de Oca M, Rassulo J et al. Ventilatory drive at rest and perception of exertional dyspnea in severe COPD. Chest 115: 1293, 1999.
5. Schwartzstein RM, and Manning HL. Mechanisms of Dyspnea. In Cherniack NS, Altose MD, and Homma (eds.): Rehabilitation of the Patient with Respiratory Disease New York, McGraw-Hill, 1999; pp. 191–203.
6. Gift AG, Plaut M, Jacox A. Psychological and physiological aspects of dyspnea in chronic obstructive lung disease. Heart Lung 15: 595, 1986
7. Bellman MJ, Botnic WC, Shin JW. Inhaled bronchodilators reduced dynamic hyperinflation during exercise in patients with chronic obstructive pulmonary disease. Am J Respir Crit Care Med 153: 967, 1996.
8. Martinez FJ, Montes de Oca M, Whyte RI et al. Lung-volume reduction improves dyspnea, dynamic hyper-inflation, and respiratory muscle function. Am J Respir Crit Care Med 155: 1984, 1990
9. Crapo,roCampbell EJ Aging of the respiratory system in Fishman's Pulmonary Diseases and Disorders 3rd Edition Chapter 19, 251–264 1998 McGraw-Hill, NY
10. Hunt C, Cratravarty NK, Anron G, Habibzadeh N, Sharan CT. The clinical effect of vitamin C supplementation in elderly hospitalized patients with acute respiratory infections. Int J Vitamin. Nutr. Res. 64: 212–9, 1994
11. Menzel DB Antioxidant vitamins and prevention of lung disease. Ann. NY Acad of Sci. #: 141–155, 1992
12. Massad A, Sherif B et al. Zinc gluconate lozenges for treating the common cold Ann Int Med. 125: 281–289, 1996
13. Crone C, Gabriel G, Wise TN. Non-herbal nutritional supplements – the next wave. Psychosomatics 42: 285–299, 2001
14. Brinker F The rational treatment of cough with botanical medicines. Phytotherapy 3; 101–111, 1994
15. Douglas RM, Chalker EB, Treacy B. Vitamin C for preventing and treating the common cold. The Cochrane Library Issue 1, 2001
16. Marshall I. Zinc for the common cold. The Cochrane LIBRARY, issue 1, 2001
17. Brinker, F Rational treatment of coughs with botanical medicines Brit. J. of Phytotherapy 3: 101–111, 1994
18. Murch SJ, KrishnaRaj S, Saxena PK. Phytopharmaceuticals: Mass-production, standardization, and conservation. Scientific Review of Alt Med 4: 39–43, 2000
19. Vickers AJ, Smith C. Homeopathic oscillococcinum for preventing and treating influenza and influenza like syndromes. The Cochrane Library Issue 1, 2001
20. Rowane WA, Rowane MP. An osteopathic approach to asthma. J Am Osteopath Assoc 1999;99: 259–64
21. Linde K, Jobst KA. Homeopathy for chronic asthma. The Cochrane Library, Issue 1, 2001
22. Ernst E. Breathing techniques-adjunctive treatment modalities for asthma? A systematic review. Eur. Respir J 2000; 15: 969–72
23. Ernst E. Complementary therapies for asthma: what patients use. J Asthma 1998: 35: 667–71
24. Huntley, A, Ernst E. Herbal medicines for asthma: a systematic review. Thorax 55: 925–929, 2000
25. Bielory L, Lupoli K. Herbal interventions in asthma and allergy Journal of Asthma 36; 1–65, 1999
26. Lewith GT, Watkins AD. Unconventional therapies in asthma(review) Allergy 51: 761–769,1996
27. But P, Chang C. Chinese herbal medicine in the treatment of asthma and allergies(review) Clin. Rev. Allergy Immunol. 14: 253–269, 1996
28. Huang KC. The pharmacology of Chinese herbs CRC Press, Boca Raton, Florida 1993 pp 310
29. Davies, A, Lewith G, Goddard J, Howarth P. The effect of acupuncture on non allergic rhinitis; a controlled pilot study. Alternative Therapies in Health and Medicine 4: 70–74, 1998
30. Bector NP, Puri AS. Solanum xanthocarpum (Kantakari) in chronic bronchitis, bronchial asthma, and non-specific unproductive cough. J Assoc Physicians India 19: 741–744, 1971
31. Gupta S., George P, Gupta V et al. Tylophora indica in bronchial asthma-double blind study. Indian J Med Res 69: 981–989, 1979
32. Hudd P. Adverse reactions to herbal treatments. J R Soc Med. 1999, 92: 547
33. Tamoki J, Kondo M, Tagaya E, Takemura K, Konno K. Zizyphi fructus, a constituent of antiasthmatic herbal medicine, stimulates airway epithelial ciliary motility through nitric acid generation. Exp Lung Res 22:255–66, 1996
34. Crone C, Gabriel G, Wise TN. Non-herbal nutritional supplements – the next wave. Psychosomatics 42: 285–99, 2001
35. Okamoto M, Mitsunobu F, Ashida K, Mifune T, Hosaki Y, Tsugeno H, Harada S, Tanizaki Y. Effects of dietary supplementation with n-3 fatty acids compared to n-6 fatty acids on bronchial asthma. Intern Med 39: 107–111, 2000
36. Chow, Shao J, Ding Y. Clinical observation on 111 of asthma treated by acupuncture and moxibusion. J Tradit Chin Med 5: 23, 1985
37. Lemiere C, Cartier, A, Lehrer SB, Malo JL. Occupational asthma caused by aromatic herbs. Allergy 51: 647–9, 1996
38. Yu DC, Lee SP. Effect of acupuncture on bronchial asthma. Clin Sci Mol Med 51; 503, 1976
39. Tandon MK, Soh PFT, Wood AT. Acupuncture for bronchial asthma? A double-blind crossover study. Med J Aust 154: 409, 1991.
40. OKW, SO SY, Lam WK et al. Effect of acupuncture on exercise-induced asthma. Lung 161: 321, 1983
41. Dias PLR, Subramaniam S, Lionel NDW. Effects acupuncture in bronchial asthma. J R Soc Med 1982; 75: 245–8
42. Christensen PA, Lauren LC, Taudorf SC et al. Acupuncture and bronchial asthma. Allergy 39: 379,1984

43. Berger D, Nolte D. Acupuncture in bronchial asthma: body plethysmography measurements of acute broncho-spasmolytic effects. Alt Med East West 5: 265, 1977.

44. Tahskin DP, Bresler DE, Kroening RJ et al. Comparison of real and simulated acupuncture and isoproterenol in methacholine-induced asthma. Ann Allergy 39: 379, 1977.

45. Hu J. Clinical observation on 25 cases of hormone dependent bronchial asthma treated by acupuncture. J Tradit Chin Med 1998; 18(1): 27–30.

46. Tandon MK and Soh PFT. Comparison of real and placebo and placebo acupuncture in histamine induced asthma; a double-blind crossover study. Chest 1989; 96: 102–5

47. Kleijnen J, Ter Riet G, Knipschild P. Acupuncture and asthma: review of controlled trials. Thorax 1991; 46: 799–802

48. Zwolfer W, Keznickl-Hillebrand W, Spacek A et al. Am J Chin Med 1993; 21(2): 113–7

49. Jobst KA, Chen JH, McPherson K et al. Controlled trial of acupuncture for disabling breathlessness. Lancet 2: 416, 1986

50. Sliwinski J. Matusiewicz R. The effect of acupuncture on the clinical state of patients suffering from chronic spastic bronchitis and undergoing long term treatment with corticosteroids. Acupuncture Eletrother Res 9: 9, 1984

51. Jobst KA. A critical analysis of acupuncture in pulmonary disease: efficacy and safety of the acupuncture needle. J Alt Comp Med 1(1): 57, 1995

52. Fung KP, Chow OKW, So SY. Attenuation of exercise-induced asthma by acupuncture. Lancet 2: 1419, 1986

53. Tashkin DP,Bresler DE et al. Comparison of real and simulated acupuncture and isoproterenol in the methacholine-induced asthma. Ann. Allergy 1997, 76: 855–863

54. Linde K, Jobst K, Panton J. Acupuncture for chronic asthma. The Cochrane database of systemic reviews 2000 (2) CD000008

55. Bhole MV. The treatment of asthma by yoga methods. Spectrum: the journal of the British Wheel of Yoga. Autumn 1999 9912–14

55a. Vincent C, Lewith G. Placebo controls for acupuncture studies. J Roy Soc Med 1995; 88: 199–202

56. Mass R, Richter R,Dahme B. Biofeedback-induced voluntary reduction of respiratory resistance in severe bronchial asthma. Behav. Res Ther 43: 815–19, 1996

57. Lehrer P, Carr RE, Smetankine A, Vaschillo E, Peper E, Porges S, Edelberg R, Hamer R, Hochron S. Respiratory sinus arrhythmia versus neck/trapeziuz EMG and incentive inspirometry biofeedback for asthma: a pilot study. Appl Psychphysiol Biofeedback 1997: 2295–109

58. Lehrer PM, Hochron SM, Mayne TM, Isenberg S, Lasoski AM, Carlson V, Gilchrist J, Porges S. Relationship between changes in EMG and respiratory sinus arrhythmia in a study of relaxation therapy for asthma. Appl Psychophysiol. Biofeedback 1997, 63: 183–91

59. Bowler S, Green A, Mitchell C. Buteyko breathing and asthma; a controlled trial. Medical J. of Australia. 169, 575–578, 1998

60. Blanc PD, Trupin L, Earnest G, Katz PP, Yelin EH and Eisner MD. Alternative therapies among adults with a reported diagnosis of asthma or rhinosinusitis. Chest: 120; 1461–1467, 2001

61. Weiner P, Magadle R, Berar-Yanay N et al. The cumulative effect of long-acting bronchodilators, exercise and inspiratory muscle training on the perception of dyspnea in patients with advanced COPD. Chest 118: 672, 2000.

62. Bourjeily G, Rochester CL. Exercise training in chronic obstructive pulmonary disease. Clin Chest Med 21(4): 763, 2000.

63. ACCP/AACVPR Pulmonary Rehabilitation Guidelines Panel. Pulmonary rehabilitation: joint ACCP/AACVPR evidence-based guidelines. Chest 112: 1363, 1997.

64. Carter R, Nicotra B, Clark L et al. Exercise reconditioning in the rehabilitation of patients with chronic obstructive pulmonary disease. Am Phys Med Rehab. 69: 118, 1988

65. O'Donnell DE, Webb KA, McGuire MA. Older patients with COPD: benefits of exercise training Geriatrics 48: 59, 1993.

66. Lacasse Y, Wong E, Guyatt GH et al. Meta-analysis of respiratory rehabilitation in chronic obstructive pulmonary disease. Lancet 348: 115, 1996.

67. Leblanc P, Bowie DM, Summers E, Jones NL, Killian KJ. Breathlessness in exercise in patients with cardiorespiratory disorders AM Rev Dis. 133: 21–25, 1986

68. Gandevia SC. Neural mechanisms underlying the sensation of breathlessness: kinesthetic parallels between respiratory and limb muscles. Aust NZ J Med 1988; 18: 83–91

69. Chonan T, Mulholland MB, Altose MD, Cherniack NS. Effects of change in level and pattern of breathing on the sensation of dyspnea. J Appl Physiol 1990; 69: 1290–1295.

70a. Kurtz ME, Kurtz JC, Stommel M, Given CW, Given BA. Symptomatology and loss of physical functioning among geriatric patients with lung cancer. J Pain Symptom Management 2000; 19:249–256.

70. Bradley TD, Chartrand DA, Fitting JW, Killian KJ, Grassino A. The relation of inspiratory effort sensation to fatiguing patterns of the diaphragm. Am Rev Respir Dis 1986; 134: 1119–1124.

71. Lavietes MH, Sanchez CW, Tiersky LA, Cherniack NS, Natelson BH. Psychological profile and ventilatory response to inspiratory resistive loading. Am J Respir Crit Care Med 2000; 161: 737–744

72. Bruera E, Schmitz B, Pither J, Neumann CM, Hanson J. The frequency and correlates of dyspnea in patients with advanced lung cancer. J Pain Symptom Management 2000; 19: 357–362.

73. Yamashita H, Tsukayama H, Hiroshi BA, Tanno Y, Nishijo K. Adverse events related to acupuncture. J Amer Med Assoc 1998; 280: 1563–1564.

74. Ernst E, White AR. Prospective studies of the safety of acupuncture: a systematic review. Am J Med 2001; 110: 481–485.
75. Kleinhenz J, Streitberger K, Windeler J, Gubbacher A, Mavridis G, Martin E. Randomised Clinical trial comparing the effects of acupuncture and a newly designed placebo needle in rotator cuff tendonitis. Pain 1999; 81: 235–241.
76. Pan CX, Morrison RS, Ness J, Fugh-Berman A, Leipzig RM. Complementary and alternative medicine in the management of pain, dyspnea, and nausea and vomiting near the end of life. J Pain Symptom Management 2000; 20: 374–387.
77. Wu W, Bandilla E, Ciccone DS, Yang J, Cheng S-Cs, Carner N, Wu Y, Shen R. Effects of Qigong on late-stage complex regional pain syndrome. Alternative Therapies 1999;5:45–54
78. Cooley ME. Symptoms in adults with lung cancer. J Pain Symptom Management 2000; 19: 137–153.

25 The Use of Complementary and Alternative Therapies in Older Women

F. Milan, K. Montgomery

Introduction

Menopause is a natural, inevitable process in most women. Physiologically, there is decreasing development of ovarian follicles, which causes a significant drop in production of estradiol and other hormones. Ultimately, there is cessation of menses. During the years surrounding the final menses, a majority of women experience some symptoms related to the declining hormone levels such as hot flashes, vaginal dryness, irregular menses, and mood swings or irritability. In the years following menopause other health problems arise due to the long-term consequences of decreased hormone production. Bone loss occurs at a rapid rate perimenopausally, then continues at a slower rate throughout the rest of a woman's life. With the average age of menopause being 50 years, most women will have over thirty years to lose bone. Estrogen replacement therapy has been used successfully to prevent and treat osteoporosis [1, 2].

After menopause, there is also an increased risk of coronary heart disease. Estrogen appears to have an effect on the coronary vasculature beyond its established beneficial effect on lipids [3]. There is evidence that estrogen may act on coronary vessels via several rapid effects including the bioavailability of endothelial-derived nitric oxide, promoting vasodilation and inhibiting fibrinolysis. These effects may result in long-term decreases in atherogenesis [4].

Estrogen replacement is extremely effective at reducing the severity and frequency of hot flashes [5]. It has been suggested that estrogen replacement therapy may decrease the risk of colon cancer [6], cognitive decline and dementia [7], and diminish symptoms of arthritis [8] and urogenital atrophy [9].

Estrogen replacement therapy, however, has some significant risks and side effects associated with it. There appears to be an increased risk of breast cancer, endometrial cancer, venous thrombosis, and cholelithiasis. In women with an intact uterus, there can be vaginal bleeding. Other side effects of estrogen include breast tenderness, bloating and possibly weight gain. The optimal duration of therapy is unclear. The maximal benefit for the bones and heart appears with continued, long-term use, while the risk of breast cancer increases with the length of therapy.

There are many possible reasons for women to choose alternative therapies for the treatment of symptoms and consequences of menopause and aging. After weighing the risk/benefit ratio for estrogen replacement therapy, many women do not begin the medication. We know that up to a third of women never fill their prescription for hormone replacement and 20% of those who do discontinue the medication within the first year 10). Side effects, especially irregular vaginal bleeding, also cause many women to discontinue estrogen. Other women feel that menopause is a natural process and resist "medicalization" of a normal phase of their lives. Many women feel that the use of natural hormones may be safer, have less side effects, and be equally effective as estrogen in treating symptoms of menopause [11]. There has been a great deal of negative public sentiment around the treatment of horses in the marketing of esterified equine estrogens. Advertising for herbs, vitamins and soy products marketed for older women can be found on TV, radio and in magazines. These dietary supplements are readily found at most conventional pharmacies (see Table 25.6).

This chapter discusses some of the complementary and alternative therapies commonly used by older women and the evidence to support or reject their use. The topics covered include: herbal therapies, phytoestrogens and soy products, "natural" progesterone and estrogen products, vitamins, minerals, exercise, relaxation therapy and acupuncture.

Herbal Medicine

Introduction

Herbs can be defined in several different ways. In the botanical nomenclature, herbs are non-woody seed producing plants that die back at the end of the growing season. In the culinary arts, herbs are vegetable products used to add flavor or aroma to food. Herbal medicine (also called botanical medicine, phytomedicine) is the use of plant materials (medicinal herbs, medicinal botanicals, etc.) to treat disease states or to improve health. There is physical evidence that the use of herbal medicine dates back to Neanderthal man [12]. All cultures have long folk medicine histories that include the use of plants. One quarter of our modern pharmaceuticals are derived from plant materials and the use of many of those originated from the herbal lore of native peoples [12]. Herbal medicines are considered by many to be dilute drugs with multiple active chemicals in any given plant. The active component(s) are actually not known for most herbal remedies and therapeutic effects are often known to differ within different parts of the same plant (i.e. stem, root, leaf, and berry).

According to several surveys on use of complementary and alternative therapies in the U.S., herbal medicines are used by 12–20% of the general population and the majority of that use is without the input of either a conventional or alternative health care provider [13–16]. However, in 1994, Congress passed the Dietary and Supplements Health and Education Act of 1994 (DSHEA) which severely restricted the FDA's authority over these products. Under this legislation, no standardization of manufacturing or premarket safety evaluation of herbs is required. Several studies on the inconsistent quality of herbal products and reports of herb-drug interactions have heightened concerns about the safety of the use of these products as medicines [17]. However, the amount of quality research on herbal medicines has paralleled its use by the public. There is a rapidly growing literature suggesting efficacy of a number of herbal products in treating a variety of health problems. In this section we will describe some of the individual herbal products used by older women and some of the combination herbal products marketed for the treatment of medical problems and symptoms common in this age group.

Black Cohosh (Cimicifuga racemosa)

Black cohosh is a member of the buttercup family and perhaps the single most popular herb used for menopausal symptoms. It is native to the forests of eastern North America and has been used as a medicinal herb for hundreds of years. There are references to black cohosh in early 18th century medical writings documenting how physicians of the time learned of the herb's medicinal properties from the Native Americans of eastern North America [18].

Chemical studies of the herb date back as far as 1827. Use of black cohosh as a phytotherapy for "femal problems" became popular in Europe in the 1930s and in the 1940s the first clinical experiments were done to evaluate its estrogen-like effects. Remifemin, an alcoholic extract of black cohosh root, was developed in Germany in the 1950s [18] and remains the most commonly used black cohosh preparation. This has made the literature on black cohosh quite unique in the world of herbal medicine. There are studies dating back 50 years and almost all done using the same standardized extract.

Since the 1950s there has been a debate as to whether black cohosh has a hormonal effect as it's mechanism of action. The data in this area remains mixed. All the studies on black cohosh to date have been done in Europe, mostly in Germany. One randomized study demonstrated that black cohosh suppressed LH secretion in a group of 110 post-menopausal women who received Remifemin for 2 months [19]. Another double-blind randomized clinical trial looked at the effects of 2 different doses (40 mg vs. 127 mg) of Remifemin in 152 women with menopausal symptoms. Neither group had any changes in their LH, FSH, SHBG, prolactin or estradiol levels or their vaginal cytology [20].

For years, many authors had insisted that black cohosh contained isoflavones (genistein and formononetin). More definitive research done recently seems to refute that claim [21].

Most of the clinical trials assessing black cohosh's effectiveness in treating menopausal symptoms have been uncontrolled and unblinded. At least one double-blind randomized controlled trial has been done in Germany. 80 women were given either 625 mg of CEE, 8 mg of Remifemin or placebo for 12 weeks. The black cohosh and estrogen groups showed significant and comparable improvement in the Kupperman menopausal index, the Hamilton Anxiety Scale and vaginal epithilium proliferation. The black cohosh group did not experience significant side effects [22].

Occasional and mild gastric discomfort has been reported with black cohosh. After the many years of studies on the herb and more than 60 years of clinical use in Europe, there is probably good reason to consider black cohosh well tolerated. However, there is still no good long-term data to confirm that it is safe in patients with a history of breast cancer. However, there is in-vitro data showing that black cohosh did not stimulate the proliferation of ER positive breast cancer cells and also augmented the anti-proliferative effect of Tamoxifen [18].

While more double-blind randomized controlled trials are needed to firmly establish the efficacy and safety of black cohosh, the data to date seems to indicate that it may be a reasonable alternative to estrogen replacement therapy for patients with menopausal symptoms.

Dong Quai (Angelica sinensis)

Dong Quai is a popular traditional Chinese medicine used frequently in Chinese herbal formulations for gynecologic disorders, menopausal symptoms and often recommended as a general "female tonic". In traditional Chinese medicine teachings, Dong Quai is not felt to have "estrogenic" properties. The daily dose of Dong Quai is usually 4–15 g of the root in oral formulations. Like other Chinese medicines, it is used in combination with several other herbs (with as many as 4 or more) to achieve synergy and balance with the different components.

There are several chemical components of Dong Quai that may account for its pharmacological activity. Ferulic acid has been found to have inhibitory effects on contractions of the rat uterus [23]. Dong Quai also contains coumarins which can act as vasodilators and antispasmodics. These coumarins also make Don Quai dangerous for people on warfarin. It has been shown to increase the INR of animals treated with warfarin [24].

There is very limited data regarding the clinical efficacy of Don Quai. A double-blind randomized-controlled trial [25] done in treated 71 post-menopausal women (45–69 years of age) with either 4.5 gm of Dong Quai root daily taken divided into three doses or placebo for 24 weeks. The groups were monitored with transvaginal ultrasounds to measure endometrial thickness, vaginal smears for cytologic examination, a diary of menopausal symptoms and evaluation by a clinician with completion of a Kupperman index [26]. At 6, 12 and 24 weeks there was no significant difference between the treatment and placebo groups for any outcome. This study has been criticized for using Don Quai alone and measuring estrogen-related variables. In traditional Chinese medicine, it is usually used in combination with other herbs and is it's mechanism of action is not felt to be due to estrogenic properties. The bottom line is that there is insufficient evidence to either prove or disprove the effectiveness and safety of Don Quai.

Evening Primrose Oil (Oenothera biennis)

Evening primrose oil is obtained from the seed of the plant *oenothera biennis* and contains gamma-linolinic acid (GLA) and dihomo-gamma-linoleic acid (DGLA). GLA and DGLA are both precursors of prostaglandins E1 and E2. Administration of GLA and DGLA affect prostaglandin production in a way that increases the non-inflammatory to inflammatory ratio of prostaglandins [27]. Evening primrose oil, therefore, is also thought to be useful in a variety of inflammatory and prostaglandin mediated conditions like arthritis, dysmenorrhea, mastalgia and PMS. Anecdotally evening primrose oil is thought to be helpful for menopausal hot flashes.

The very limited evidence for evening primrose oil's usefulness for hot flashes, however, is negative. There was a double-blind, randomized controlled study done in the UK which treated half of 56 women with hot flashes with 500 mg of evening primrose oil and 10 mg of Vitamin E twice a day and the other half with placebo for 6 months. The placebo group actually showed a greater but not significant improvement in hot flashes than the treatment group [28].

Evening primrose oil is generally very well tolerated. Large doses can cause loose stools and abdominal cramping. It is definitely contraindicated in pregnancy and there have been some reports of seizures in patients with schizophrenia concomitantly taking anti-psychotic medication [27].

Valerian (Valeriana officinalis)

There is a historical record of Valerian's use dating back to Hippocrates and Galen. Valerian is currently used as an anxiolytic and a sleep aide. There are a great variety of valerian preparations made from the root including, extracts standardized to anywhere from 0.15% to 1% valerenic acid, full strength root tinctures and pure root. A tea can be made by steeping 2–3 grams of dried root in 150 ml of boiling water. Many commercial products marketed for stress, sleep, and "for women" contain valerian in combination with Ginseng, Kava Kava, Evening Primrose and Passion Flower. The dose ranges greatly based on preparation. 400–900 mg of valerian root extract can be taken 1–2 hours before bedtime.

There are many constituents thought to be responsible for the sedating and anxiolytic properties of valerian. Valerenic acid and other sesquiterpenes are the best studied. There is some evidence that these compounds inhibit the catabolism of GABA and may also bind loosely to benzodiazepene receptors [29]. Most of the studies evaluating valerian's effect on sleep in normals and those with insomnia have been small, done in Germany and have used differently prepared valerian root extracts. There have been, however, at least 2 randomized, blinded, crossover studies that used polysomnography to evaluate the effect of valerian on sleep architecture. They found that after several doses of valerian, patients with insomnia had improved sleep latency [30] and quality with an increase in REM sleep compared to the placebo study period [31]. There is insufficient data to comment on valerian's effectiveness in treating anxiety.

Clinical studies done on over 12,000 patients for as long as 14 days have reported few significant adverse effects of valerian. There may be some sedation or morning drowsiness at higher doses [29]. However, extended use has been associated with a withdrawal syndrome similar to that seem with benzodiazepenes [32]. There is a theoretical danger of mixing Valerian with other sedating substances with common mechanisms of action such as: alcohol, benzodiazepenes and barbiturates.

Kava (also known as Kava Kava [Piper methysticum])

Kava has a long folk tradition of use for sedation and anxiety. It has been used throughout the Polynesian Islands for ceremonial rituals for thousands of years. It is used similar to the way alcohol is used in Western societies. It's use for anxiety and stress has been increasing and it is a very common ingredient in the compound herbal preparations marketed for this purpose and "for women's problems". Most kava root extracts are standardized to between 30–70% kava-lactone content. It can also be taken as a tea made from 2–4 grams of dried root and 150 ml of boiling water. In the Polynesian Islands a drink is prepared by masticating the roots and mixing the resulting liquid with water. For kava root extract products standardized to 70% kava lactones, the recommended dose is 100 mg three times a day. A cup of tea three times a day can be used with the tea made by adding boiling water to 2–4 grams of root.

The active ingredients in kava are called kava lactones or pyrones. Their mode of action is unknown. They are not thought to effect benzodiazepene or GABA receptors. There are several small European trials done to assess the efficacy of Kava in the symptomatic treatment of anxiety. One systematic review and meta-analysis [33] reported that all 7 double-blind randomized controlled studies meeting their strict methodological criteria found kava to be superior to placebo in treating anxiety. Pooled data from three of the studies found significant improvement in HAM-A (Hamilton Anxiety Rating Scale for Anxiety) scores with kava.

While short-term use is felt to be safe, long-term use has been associated with "kawaism" or kava addiction and Kava dermopathy (a pellagra-like syndrome unresponsive to therapy with niacin) in the Polynesian Islands. Kava can cause drowsiness and impaired motor reflexes but is not felt to impair cognitive function like benzodiazepenes [34]. There has been a report of coma resulting from the combined intake of kava and alprazolam [35]. There is also a theoretical danger of mixing kava with other sedating substances such as: alcohol and barbiturates.

Ginseng (Panax ginseng, Panax quinquefolius)

There are several different types of Ginseng that are used for medicinal purposes. *Panax ginseng* is grown or cultivated in China and is known as Chinese or Asian ginseng. There are less commonly used forms of ginseng from Korea and Japan. *Panax quinquefolius* is American ginseng and grows wild in the hills of the Southeastern U.S. Wild American ginseng is so widely sought after that it is classified as an endangered species. American ginseng is now being commercially cultivated. *Eleutherococcus sentcosus* commonly known as Siberian ginseng, is not a true ginseng.

Asian Ginseng is typically used as a powder of root extract. American ginseng is used as the pure root. Because of the decreasing availability of ginseng, especially American ginseng, products are often adulterated with other herbs and sometimes do not contain any detectable ginseng at all. In addition, ginseng products are rarely standardized. Studies done by Consumer Reports [36, 37] on ginseng products revealed variations of ginseng contents from 5% to 140% of the labeled amounts. Ginseng is now being added to some food products (i.e. fruit juice, bottled water, breakfast cereal) as a "neutraceutical".

The cost of ginseng can be high especially for true American ginseng ($ 30–50 per month) while Asian ginseng or Korean Ginseng is often less expensive ($ 10–40 per month). For American ginseng the recommended dose is 0.25–0.5 grams of root two times daily. For Asian Ginseng, the recommended dose is 0.6 to 3.0 grams of powdered root extract 1–3 times a day.

For thousands of years, Ginseng has been used throughout Asia for medicinal purposes. It has been used throughout the world as an "adaptogen" or a substance that can help the body to adapt to the stress it encounters in its environment. In other words "it's good for what ails you". It is also used to increase energy, decrease glycemia and as an aphrodisiac. It is often marketed to older people as a way to "feel young" and to older women as a treatment for menopausal symptoms.

The active ingredients in ginseng are known as either ginsenosides or panaxans of which there are many subtypes. Ginsenoside Rb-1 is thought to be responsible for the hypoglycemic effect of ginseng by decreasing islet cell insulin concentration [38]. The mode of actions of the other ginsenosides is unknown.

A review of 16 studies on Ginseng for multiple indications (i.e. physical performance, psychomotor performance, cognitive function) found "no compelling evidence for any of these indications" [39]. There was a recent double-blind randomized placebo-controlled study done in Canada which found that American Ginseng significantly decreased the glycemic response when taken 40 min before a glucose challenge in normals or when taken either 40 min before or at the time of a glucose challenge in diabetics [40]. There are no studies documenting its effects on menopausal symptoms or other problems of aging.

Little is known about the safety of long-term ginseng use. There are few consistently reported or validated adverse effects despite previous concerns about estrogenic effects. There have been case reports of post-menopausal vaginal bleeding in women taking ginseng [41].

Drug interactions are a concern with ginseng. Ginseng has been reported to lower the INR in patients on coumadin [42]. There is a theoretical risk of causing hypoglycemia in diabetics by augmenting their hypoglycemia therapies.

Cranberry (vaccinium macrocarpan)

In the 1920s it was reported that eating large amounts of cranberries produced a more acidic urine. It was then postulated that eating cranberries or drinking their juice would hinder bacterial growth and be useful in the prevention and treatment for urinary tract infections [43]. When cranberry juice cocktail was introduced to the market it became a very popular home remedy for UTIs. It was then discovered that the mechanism by which cranberry worked in urinary tract infections was not based on its effect on urinary pH. The two active components of cranberry are fructose and proanthocanidins. They both work by inhibiting the fimbrial adhesion activity of E. coli, which prevents it from sticking to the epithelium of the urinary tract [44].

The evidence supporting cranberry's ability to prevent UTIs is convincing. A double-blind randomized controlled trial done several years ago showed that older women who drank 300 ml a day of cranberry juice cocktail for 6 months had significantly reduced bacteriuria and pyuria than the placebo group [45]. A more recent trial done in Finland randomized 150 women with a history of UTIs to drink 50 ml of cranberry-lingonberry juice concentrate or lactobacillus GG drink or control for 6 months. The group who drank the juice had a 20% reduction in absolute risk for recurrent UTI over the lactobacillus and control groups with recurrence rates of 16% vs. 39% vs. 36%, respectively [46]. Cranberry has not, however, been proven to be effective in the treatment of UTIs.

Cranberry is now available as whole fruit (with a variety of sweet coatings to make it more palatable), whole fruit juice and capsules or tablets of concentrated cranberry. Recommended doses for prevention are 3 oz of juice a day, 1.5 oz of whole cranberries, 6 capsules of dried cranberry concentrate. The dose for treatment of a UTI is less clear with the recommendation being about 4–10x the quantity for prevention. While drinking cranberry juice is generally accepted as safe and well tolerated, some concerns have been raised over the concentrated cranberry products. In an uncontrolled trial, 5 healthy volunteers consumed cranberry tablets "administered according to the manufacturer's recommended dosage" for 7 days. All of the volunteers experienced a significant increase in urinary oxalate levels (average by 43%) as measured in a 24-hour urine sample. None of them had any clinical evidence of a urinary stone [47]. This is a small and uncontrolled study, however, this finding probably warrants further research.

Phytoestrogens

Introduction and History

Phytoestrogens are a group of naturally occurring plant derived non-steroidal compounds which bind to estrogen receptors. There are 3 main classes of phytoestrogens: isoflavones, coumestans and lignans. While there is some overlap, isoflavones are found in legumes and beans (highest concentrations in soybeans). Lignans are found mostly in flaxseed with some found in other cereals, fruits and vegetables. Coumestans are found in clover and sprouts (alfalfa and soybean sprouts). Isoflavones have the most potent estrogenic activity and have therefore received the most attention by the medical community [49].

The first report of a bioassay revealing estrogens in plant extracts was in 1926. In the 1940s phytoestrogens had an enormous biological impact on the sheep industry of Australia. An outbreak of infertility in sheep grazing on subterranean clover devastated the industry and came to known as "Clover Disease" [49]. Since that time a large body of literature exploring the effects of phytoestrogens on animals and humans has developed.

Active Ingredients and Mechanism of Action

Isoflavones have emerged as the most interesting class of phytoestrogens as they have the most potent estrogenic activity as well as an extensive range of biological actions. Isoflavones have a common diphenolic structure that resembles the structure of the potent synthetic estrogen diethylstilbesterol [50], physiologic estrogen 17 beta estradiol and synthetic antiestrogen tamoxifen [51]. The major isoflavones, genistein, glycetein and daidzein occur in plants as inactive glycosides. They are also derived from precursors biochanin A and formononetin. The estrogenically active lignans are enterodiol and enterolactone and are derived from the compounds secoisolariciresinol and matairesinol found in plants.

In humans, lignans and isoflavones must undergo complex enzymatic metabolic conversions in the gastrointestinal tract in order to become compounds with estrogenic activity [49]. For example, in some individuals, daidzein, is converted to equol, a potent isoflavone metabolite [52]. Clover sprouts also contain the isoflavone formonetin which is metabolized in the GI tract to daidzein. [52]. The extent of those metabolic reactions can vary among individuals from 5–70% of the precursors becoming metabolized into active compounds [50]. The variability is affected by gut microflora, diet and concomitant intake of medications especially antibiotics [52]. Absorption of isoflavones are decreased by both H2 Blockers and proton-pump inhibitors [50]. A diet rich in carbohydrate results in more extensive biotransformation of isoflavones by increasing intestinal fermentation [48].

Phytoestrogens have demonstrated numerous biochemical properties. The level and direction of their estrogenicity depend on the target tissue, the receptor status of the tissue and the level of endogenous estrogen. Phytoestrogens, including isoflavones are essentially weak estrogens. They bind selectively and with high affinity to ER beta receptors [53]. In pre-menopausal women who have high circulating levels of endogenous estrogen, phytoestrogens have an anti-estrogenic effect when they bind to estrogen receptors. In post-menopausal women they are binding to otherwise empty receptors and have an estrogenic effect [48]. Isoflavones also stimulate SHBG synthesis in the liver like estrogen [48]. Isoflavones have also been found to inhibit tyrosine kinase, which may account for their nonestrogenic effects on bone [54]. Other proposed mechanisms of action of isoflavones include: antioxidant effects on lipoproteins and DNA, effects on glucose transport, cell proliferation and cell differentiation [51].

Food Sources of Phytoestrogens

To best understand the phytoestrogen interventions being used in the literature as well to advise patients with regard to diet, it is useful to discuss the food sources of soy, soy protein and isoflavones. Soybeans and food products made from soybeans have the highest concentration of isoflavones but there is enormous variation depending on where the soybean is grown and how it is prepared (Tables 25.1 and 25.2). Isoflavones are more bioavailable from fermented soy products (i.e. tempeh) than other soy products or other fruits and vegetables [55]. Lentils, peanuts, chickpeas alfalfa and barley all have isoflavones but at a concentration of 0.01% to 0.1% of that found in soybeans (Table 25.3).

The Epidemiology of Soy

Soy products are a staple in the diet of East Asian countries. East Asian diets typically include 20–150 mg a day of isoflavones whereas Western diets include only 2–5 mg a day [52]. In these populations with soy-enriched diets, epidemiological studies reveal lower incidences of diseases that have been linked with female hormones such as: breast and ovarian cancers, osteoporosis and coronary heart disease [56]. Asian women also report fewer and less severe menopausal symptoms than Western women.

Table 25.1. Food Sources of Soy Protein and Isoflavones. (From: Phytoestrogens for the Prevention and Treatment of Osteroporosis (1999) Alternative Medicine Alert, 12Vol. 2, No.12, p.139; published by American Health Consultants 1 (800) 688–2421; reproduced with permission)

Soy Food	Serving Size	Protein g/100 g	Genistein g/100 g	Daidzein g/100 g	Total Isoflavone1 mg/serving
Mature soybeans (uncooked)	1/2 cup	37.0	73.76	46.64	175.6
Roasted soybeans	1/2 cup	35.2	65.88	52.04	167.0
Soy flour	1/2 cup	37.8	96.83	71.19	43.8
Textured soy protein	1/2 cup	18.0	78.90	59.62	27.8
Green soybeans (uncooked)	1/2 cup	16.6	72.51	67.79	70.1
Soy milk	1 cup	4.4	6.06	4.45	20.0
Tempeh (uncooked)	4 oz	1 7.0	24.85	17.59	60.5
Tofu (uncooked)	4 oz	15.8	13.60	9.02	38.3
Soy isolate (dry)	1 oz	92.0	59.62	33.59	56.5
Soy concentrate (dry)	1 oz	63.6	5.33	6.83	12.4
Soy cheese	1 oz	7.0	20.08	11.24	31.3

ᵃThe above isoflavone content is a mean estimate. It varies widely among soybean varieties and manufacturers.

Table 25.2. Isoflavone contents of soybeans

Soybean Type	Mg Isoflavones in 1/2 cup serving
Japanese dry	222 mg
U.S. dry	93–188 mg
U.S. fresh	23 mg
U.S boiled	18 mg
U.S. frozen	77 mg

Table 25.3. Isoflavone Content of Selected Foods (From: Vincent A, Fitzpatrick LA. (2000) Soy Isoflavones: Are they Useful in Menopause? Mayo Clin Proc;75:1174–1184; reproduced with permission)

Food	Daidzein(µg/100 g dry weight)	Genistein(µg/100 g dry weight)
Barley	14	7.7
Clover seed	178	323
Peanut	58	64
Soybean	10,500–85,000	26,800–120,500
Chickpea	11–192	69–214
Lentil	3–10	7–19
Alfalfa	62	5
Broccoli	6	8
Cauliflower	5	9

While there are obviously a number of other explanations for this difference, women in Western countries have approximately an 80% incidence of hot flashes, Asian women living in China have an incidence of only 20% [51]. The Study of Women's Health Across the Nation (SWAN) surveyed 12,479 women ages 40–55 years and found that Japanese American and Chinese American women were 40% less likely to experience hot flashes [57].

Clinical Evidence

Introduction

The literature on the clinical effects of a soy-enriched diet and isoflavone supplements is large and growing (Table 25.4). It is currently one of the best researched areas in complementary and alternative medicine. DBRCTs have been done evaluating the effect of soy on menopausal symptoms, cardiovascular disease and lipids, and breast cancer. Interpreting the literature is difficult because many trials evaluating phytoestrogens fail to clarify the type and concentration of soy or isoflavone intervention used. Others use the terms phytoestrogens, soy, soy protein, isoflavones interchangeably. While isoflavones are phytoestrogens, the reverse is not always true. The term soy refers to use of the whole soybean whereas soy protein refers to protein extracted from the soybean. Soy products and soy protein contain isoflavones in varying amounts. There are also isoflavone extracts which contain just individual compound(s), most commonly genistein and/or daidzein. There are standardized isoflavone extracts being evaluated that are made from red clover which is also a source of the phytoestrogen group coumestans.

Efficacy of Soy and Isoflavones for Menopausal Symptoms

Conventional estrogen replacement therapy has been shown to decrease hot flashes by about 70% [48]. It has been clearly documented that in studies done on hot flashes, placebo alone reduces hot flashes by 15–50% [48]. This renders uncontrolled studies on treatment for hot flashes fairly useless and makes it a challenge for investigators to find a significant effect over placebo. There have been several placebo-controlled

Table 25.4. Phytoestrogen dosing

	Hot Flushes	Osteoporosis	Cholesterol
Diet (soyprotein)	40–60 gm/d	20–30 gm/d	40–50 gm/d
Isoflavone supplements	75 mg/d	40 mg/d	40 mg/d
Ipriflavone	200 mg TID	200 mg TID	?

trials evaluating the effectiveness of soy supplementation with foods or extracts for treating symptoms of menopause (Table 25.5). Most studies have used some outcome measure to assess effect on vasomotor symptoms and many have looked at vaginal symptoms and/or cytology. A few have included either transvaginal ultrasound or endometrial biopsy to look for estrogenic effects on the endometrium. The studies have been fairly small and have ranged in length from 6–24 weeks. The studies using supplements or extracts have been double-blind and randomized, the control groups receiving a placebo to match the intervention (tablets, capsules or flour). The trial that evaluated the use of whole soy foods [63] was randomized but unblinded.

The majority of the trials using soy products or isoflavones from soy have shown a significant reduction in vasomotor symptoms for the women in the control groups (by 40–45%) over the treatment groups (25–30%). The studies of isoflavones from red clover have not shown efficacy in treating vasomotor symptoms [66, 67]. One of the negative soy trials [62] was done on survivors of breast cancer most of whom were being treated with tamoxifen. While this is a population who could truly benefit from an effective alternative treatment for vasomotor symptoms of menopause, it is hard to know what effect the tamoxifen had on the ability of the isoflavones to bind to the estrogen receptors. The other negative trial [61] was done on peri-menopausal women within 12 months of their last menstrual cycle and experiencing at least 10 hot flushes a week. Most of the other studies have used post-menopausal women who are at least 12 months past their last menstrual bleed and having several hot flashes a day. Isoflavones may not have as potent an estrogenic effect in women who still may have some significant levels of circulating endogenous estrogens.

Efficacy data of Soy and Isoflavones on lipids and cardiovascular disease

It has been well established that soy supplementation has beneficial effects on lipids and may have other effects that reduce the risk of cardiovascular disease. After a review of the available evidence in October 1999, the FDA authorized a health claim that including 25 grams of soy protein in a diet low in saturated fat may also reduce the risk of heart disease. The approval of this claim allows this information to be used on labels for foods that contain at least 6.25 grams of soy per serving and also meet the requirements for low fat and low cholesterol content. The claim includes foods that use whole soy products and excludes other phytoestrogens and isoflavone extracts [68]. Phytoestrogens have not yet been approved as a food additive.

Soy protein has consistently been shown to lower total cholesterol and LDL-c. A meta-analysis of 38 randomized controlled trials of soy protein consumption found that soy lowered total cholesterol by an average of 9.3%, LDL by 12.9% and triglycerides by 10.5%. Soy protein raised HDL by an average of 2.4% which was not statistically significant [69]. The lipid lowering effect was smaller in subjects with normal cholesterol than in those with hypercholesterolemia who achieved a 10% reduction in cholesterol levels. More recently, Crouse found a stepwise decrease in total and LDL cholesterol levels with increasing isoflavone dose in both men and women [70]. Potter found that 40 grams of soy protein a day for 6 months produced a cholesterol lowering effect similar to that seem with ERT [71]. The ability of soy to raise HDL has been less consistent.

Table 25.5. Studies evaluating soy, isoflavones for treatment of menopausal symptoms

Study	N(#)	Intervention	Isoflavone dose	Length of study	Study design	Outcomes measured	Effect flushes	Effect vag cyt	Misc.
Washburn	51	soy protein supplement	34 mg QD 17 mg BID	3–6 wk periods	DBRCT crossover	hot flash frequency, severity, lipids	+ BID group	N/A	LDLß 7% in treatment group
Albertazzi	104	soy protein supplement	76 mg QD	3 months	DBRCT Multi-center	#hot flashes/day Kupperman Index	+	N/A	
Murkies	58	Soy flour supplement	(45 gm flour)	6 wks	DBRCT	menopausal sxScore	+	–	control-wheat flour
St. Germain	69	soy protein isolate	80 mg QD	24 wks	DBRCT	menopausal index	–	N/A	control-Whey protein
Quella	177	soy supplement Tablets	50 mg TID	9 wks	DBRCT	hot flash freq, side effects	–	N/A	Pts s/p Breast CA 156 on tamoxifen
Brzezinski	145	phytoestrogen-Rich foods	(80 gm tofu, miso 10 gm linseed)	12 wks	unblinded randomized	hot flashes, menopause scale, vaginal dryness	+	+	total menopause score not signif.D
Scambia	?	standardized Soy extract (Soyselect)	50 QD	6 wks	DBRCT	Greene climacteric scale transvaginal ultrasound	+	–	no effect on endometrium
Upmalis	177	isoflavone Extract	50 mg QD	12 wks	DBRCT	Freq, severity of flashes Ebx, FSH, SHBG, lipids	+	–	no effect on labs, endometrium
Baber	51	isoflavone Extract from Red clover	40 mg QD	2–12 wk phases	DBRCT cross-over	Greene Menopause score FSH, SHBG, transvag. US	–	–	no effect on labs, endometrium
Knight	37	isoflavone Extract from Red clover	40 mg QD160 mg QD	12 wks	DBRCT	Greene Menopause score FSH, SHBG, transvag. US	–	–	no effect on labs endometrium

The effect of soy on lipid levels seems to apply only to soy protein. [72]. Studies done using isoflavones alone and isoflavone extracts have been largely ineffective [51]. One exception to this has been studies done using isoflavone extracts made from red clover. In one study [73], HDL levels rose significantly by 15–28% in three groups given different doses of the red clover extract for 6 months. However, the effect did not follow a dose-response relationship. In the study by Knight [67], a post-hoc analysis showed a statistically significant increase in HDL in the 40 mg red clover extract group.

Soy's potential cardiovascular benefits may lie with other mechanisms besides their lipid lowering effects. Many but not all studies show that soy affects the oxidative susceptibility of LDL [72]. There have also been a few studies showing that soy and red clover derived isoflavones improve arterial compliance [51, 74].

Effects of Isoflavones on osteoporosis

A diet high in soy and isoflavones is sometimes credited with the low rate of hip fractures in Asian women despite their relatively low bone mineral density. While isoflavones may play some role, epidemiological data suggest that the low hip fracture rate may be largely due to the short hip axis length of Asians. [51, 72]. Several research groups have shown that isoflavones can preserve or increase BMD in ovariectomized rat models [51]. The primary proposed mechanism for this effect is the ability of isoflavones to bind to estrogen receptors in the bone. Some data suggests that at least one of the isoflavones, genistein directly inhibits osteoclast activity [51]. There have been no long-term studies looking for an effect on rate of fracture and very few studies done in humans measuring bone density. One study randomized 66 postmenopausal women to one of three 40 gram protein diets. The control group received a milk protein supplement and the two intervention groups received either moderate or high dose isoflavone supplements for 6 months. The group receiving the high isoflavone dose experienced a 2.5% increase in spine BMD but no effect of femoral neck BMD [71]. This study supports the theory that isoflavones mimic estrogen's more pronounced effect on trabecular bone. Another study using three different doses of isoflavone extract from red clover (Rimostil TM) for 6 months reported a 4.1% and 3.0% rise in BMD of the proximal radius and ulna in the groups receiving the middle and higher doses respectively [73]. A third study using soy protein over 24 weeks was able to show attenuation of the BMD loss seen in the placebo group [75]. There is some preliminary evidence to suggest that isoflavone supplementation may have a beneficial effect on bone. Larger studies using consistent interventions are needed.

Safety of Isoflavones: Effect on Endometrium and Breast

The data from animal studies on isoflavone's effect on the endometrium have been mixed. While isoflavones have been shown to induce uterine growth in mice, rats and cows, a soy-based diet has not had this effect in ovariectomized rats or rhesus macaques [51].

One epidemiological case-control study in Hawaii found that a plant-based diet high in legumes (especially soybeans) in a multi-ethnic population reduced the risk of endometrial cancer [76]. Many of the studies evaluating the use of isoflavones on vasomotor symptoms in postmenopausal women have also assessed the effect on the endometrium using either transvaginal ultrasound or endometrial biopsy (see Table 25.5). None of those [64–66] have found an effect but have only treated with isoflavones for a maximum of 12 weeks. While more long-term human data is needed to feel confident that postmenopausal women are not at risk of an estrogenic effect on the endometrium, the evidence to date appears fairly promising.

Data from animal models looking at isoflavones effect on the breast has produced very mixed results. Most of the work has been done with genistein. In some animal models genistein has been shown to be protective against the development of breast cancer in animals exposed to large quantities of carcinogens and in other models genistein has been shown to have a stimulatory effect on breast cancer [51]. Epidemiological data and several case-control studies have shown high levels of soy intake to be protective against the development of breast cancer in humans [77–79] although the effect seems to be stronger for pre-menopausal women than postmenopausal women. In summary, no firm conclusions can be made about the effect of isoflavones and soy on the risk of breast cancer.

Ipriflavone: A synthetic isoflavone

Studies using a synthetic isoflavone, ipriflavone, have produced the strongest evidence of the isoflavones ability to prevent bone loss. Ipriflavone was developed as part of a research project to synthesize isoflavones with androgenic and not estrogenic activity. 7-isopropoxyisoflavone (ipriflavone) was selected and has been found to have several mechanisms of action that enhance bone density. Animal studies evaluating ipriflavone's effect on bone began in 1974 with human studies being done as of 1981. From the 1980s until 1997 there had been 60 trials (many of them randomized and placebo-controlled) done with a total of 2769 subjects [80].

Ipriflavone has been found in trace amounts in bee propolis but is for all practical purposes synthesized in the laboratory. It is metabolized in the liver and completely excreted in the kidney within 120 hours without any accumulation in the body [80]. Ipriflavone has several mechanisms of action on bone. Its inhibition of bone resorption is dose-dependent and involves inhibition of oseteoclasts. Receptors for ipriflavone have been found on osteoclasts and osteoclast precursor cells [80]. Ipriflavone also stimulates bone formation by stimulating osteoblast differentiation and maturation. Ipriflavone has little intrinsic estrogen effect and is not displaced from its receptors by estradiol [80].

Ipriflavone has several metabolites one of which is daidzein. The other metabolites have been found to have a variety of effects like increasing alkaline phosphatase levels, inhibiting parathyroid hormone stimulated bone resorption and enhancing collagen formation [81].

Animal studies on ipriflavone have shown an increase in bone density in the rat with glucocorticoid induced osteoporosis model [82]. There have been several small trials in postmenopausal women with rather consistent findings. In these randomized-controlled trials, ipriflavone has been shown to significantly protect against the bone loss seen in the placebo groups. This prevention of bone loss has been accompanied by a decrease in urinary biochemical markers of bone resorption [83, 84]. A larger, 2 year, multi-center randomized controlled trial using an intent-to-treat analysis done in Italy found similar results. 453 postmenopausal women who received ipriflavone 200 mg TID plus 1 gram of calcium a day experienced no significant loss of either vertebral or radial bone while the women receiving calcium alone lost 1.2% bone mineral density [85].

Several studies have looked at whether isoflavones can augment estrogen's effect on bone. Two randomized controlled trials found that when ipriflavone was added to 0.3 mg CEE, there was a significantly greater increase in bone mass than that seen with 0.3 mg of CEE alone [86– 88]. There is also some suggestion that ipriflavone may also augment vitamin D's protective effect against bone loss [89].

While the data on ipriflavone's effect on bone mineral density has been consistent, there still remains a lack of data on its effect on the incidence of fractures. One small and poorly reported study suggests that ipriflavone may decrease the rate of fractures in women who have a history of osteoporotic fractures [90].

The Ipriflavone Multi-center European Fracture Study recently reported its results [91] and did not find a significant difference in bone mineral density with ipriflavone. Unfortunately, there were a large number of dropouts (474 patients randomized and only 292 completed the trial) with more of them coming from the treatment group and the study did not have the power to detect a difference in fracture rate. The reason for many of the dropouts in this study was lymphocytopenia. Lymphocytopenia had been sporadically reported previously with ipriflavone but in this trial it was seen in 12.4% (n=29) of the patients. 81% of the lymphocytopenia resolved after 2 years and the rest eventually resolved spontaneously without any clinical related events (i.e. infections) being reported. Except for the lymphoctopenia, ipriflavone is otherwise very well tolerated. Occasional GI side effects and self-limited increases in LFTs have been reported and there has been a report of increased INR in patients on acenocoumarol but not coumadin [80].

Despite the fact that ipriflavone is chemically synthesized in the laboratory, it is currently marketed as a dietary supplement. This may inhibit the kind of large multi-center trials that could more firmly establish ipriflavone's role in the treatment of osteoporosis. While the problem of lymphocytopenia clearly needs to be better characterized, ipriflavone shows great promise as a treatment for osteoporosis.

Combination Products

As complementary and alternative medicine has increased in popularity so have the plethora of dietary supplement products aimed at older women. Many of these products are combinations of herbs, soy protein or isoflavones, vitamins and minerals. While some of these individual components are mentioned in this chapter, none of these combinations have been tested for efficacy. There is no way to know how the individual effects of any of these components can affect the activity of the others. Some of the more commonly sold products as well as their ingredients are listed in Table 25.6.

Table 25.6. Combination dietary supplement products for women

Product	Herbs	Soy/Isoflavone	Vitamins	Minerals	Misc
Estroven	Black Cohosh Kava root extract	Isoflavones from soy and pueraria root (kudzu)	E, B12, B6, thiamin-niacin, folate, riboflavin	Calcium, selenium boron	Mammary gland power Ovary gland powder Adrenal gland powder Pituitary gland powder
Rejuvex	Dong Quai	–	E, B6, thiamin, niacin, Riboflavin	Magnesium, selenium manganese	
One-a-day Menopause Remifemin plus	Black Cohosh Black Cohosh St.John's Wort	Soy extract	E	Calcium	Lecithin
FEM Support	Black Cohosh Chasteberry Dong Quai Licorice Root	Soy Red Clover	E, D, B6, B12, thiamin, niacin	Calcium, Magnesium	
Estrologic	Black Cohosh Chasteberry Sage Vervain extract Astragalus extract				Wild yam extract
GNC Menopause VitaPak	Evening Primrose Oil Black Cohosh	Red Clover Blossom Isoflavones	A, C, D, E, B12, B6	Calcium Selenium, Boron, Copper Chromium, Selenium, Zinc Manganese	

Table 25.6. *continued*

Product	Herbs	Soy/Isoflavone	Vitamins	Minerals	Misc
Natrol Menopause Formula	Black Cohosh Red Rasberry Licorice root Gotu Kola Dong Quai Horse Chestnut Ginkgo Biloba Chasteberry Kava and kava extract	Soy isoflavones Red Clover extract		Calcium, Magnesium	Wild yam extract
Women's Natural Replacement	Cranberry	Soy protein			

Natural Progesterone

Introduction

There are two very prevalent myths surrounding natural progesterone products. The first myth is that they are natural. The second is that they are present "naturally" in wild yams. Many women, therefore, are using wild yam creams and taking wild yam pills that have no progesterone in them at all. The two most commonly used natural progesterone products are oral micronized progesterone and progesterone creams.

Transdermal Progesterone Cream

Many progesterone creams are made from diosgenin, a substance found both in soybeans and in inedible wild Mexican yams. Diosgenin has no hormonal activity and cannot be converted to progesterone in the body. In the laboratory it can be used as the substrate in a chemical synthetic process that results in a progesterone which is identical to endogenous human progesterone. Transdermal progesterone can also made from a micronized form of endogenous progesterone. In most preparations, 1/4 tspn has 20 mg of progesterone. The recommended dose is 1/4–1/2 tspn per day. There is some controversy as to whether the dosing of progesterone cream can be adjusted based on serum or salivary progesterone levels.

Claims that salivary progesterone levels are a more accurate reflection of bioavailable progesterone are made with little supportive data [92]. There is some evidence, however, that both serum and urinary progesterone levels vary widely in women after the use of transdermal progesterone [93].

There are 3 relevant clinical questions about the use of transdermal progesterone that have been addressed in the literature. The first is whether it is a viable alternative to medroxyprogesterone as a protector of the endometrium for postmenopausal women on hormone replacement therapy. The data here is scarce and conflicting. One study used both vaginal and transdermal preparations of micronized progesterone in postmenopausal women on daily 0.625 mg CEE. The groups receiving the progesterone creams demonstrated a significant anti-proliferative effect on endometrial biopsy at 4 weeks [94]. The opposite findings were seen in a study with women on the estrogen patch and using three different strengths of the progesterone cream for 3 months [95].

The second question is whether transdermal progesterone is effective for vasomotor symptoms in postmenopausal women. One randomized-controlled study done by Leonetti [96] found that 83% of the group using transdermal progesterone cream for a year had improvement or resolution of their vasomotor symptoms while only 19% of the placebo group improved. This finding is impressive but needs to be replicated by other studies.

The third question that has been addressed is whether transdermal progesterone has a beneficial effect on bone. There are progesterone receptors on bone and progesterone is able to stimulate osteoblasts in vitro [97]. However, very little work has been done looking at the ability of progesterone cream to increase bone density. The study mentioned above by Leonetti [96] also did DEXA scans on their subjects and found no benefit of progesterone cream after treatment for a year.

Progesterone creams are being used widely with little to no evidence that they are efficacious or safe. Women using these products should use caution. There will hopefully be more evidence soon to help us answer the above clinical questions.

Oral Micronized Progesterone

Oral micronized progesterone is a product that was developed to overcome the poor GI absorption of endogenous progesterone and the unwanted side effects of the synthetic progestogens currently in use. These synthetic progestogens (i.e. medroxyprogesterone, levogestrel, norethindrone) are used for oral contraception and hormone replacement are not ideal for use as a progesterone but are very well absorbed when taken orally. As we all know they have varying degrees of androgenic activity. Oral micronized progesterone can be absorbed effectively because of an emulsification process termed micronization using peanut oil. Its half life is not as short as unprocessed endogenous progesterone (T 1/2 =5 min) but not as long as the progestogens (T 1/2=10–12 h). Being prepared in an oil base, oral micronized progesterone does not mix well with crystalline agents. It can therefore not be combined into tablets with estrogen [99].

Oral micronized progesterone was developed and became available in Europe in the 1980s. In 1995 it was released in Canada and was approved by the FDA in 1998. Even before that time it was available in compounding pharmacies in the U.S. and marketed by and available by mail from the women's health pharmacy (Madison Pharmacy Associates) in Madison Wisconsin. When converting the dose, 100 mg of oral micronized progesterone is roughly equivalent to 5 mg of medroxyprogesterone. It is recommended that it be given at night as it has a mildly sedating effect [98].

There are also vaginal and rectal preparations of micronized progesterone, which are dosed at about 1/3 of the oral dose.

The evidence supporting oral micronized progesterone's use in lieu of medroxyprogesterone by postmenopausal women on HRT is quite good. The best data comes from the PEPI trial [3]. PEPI was a multi-center, randomized, double-blind controlled trial that tested the effects of 4 HRT regimens over 3 years in 875 postmenopausal women. The women were randomized to receive 0.625 mg CEE alone, 0.625 mg CEE with continuous medroxyprogesterone 2.5 mg/day, 0.625 CEE with cyclical medroxyprogesterone and 0.625 mg CEE with cyclical oral micronized progesterone 200 mg for 12 days of the month.

Micronized progesterone was found to:

▶ Preserve the beneficial effects of estrogens on lipids (increase in HDL) while medroxyprogesterone did not.
▶ Share the same protective effect on the endometrium as medroxyprogesterone.
▶ Share the same positive effect on bone density as all the treatment arms.
▶ Result in fewer reported side effects.

This progesterone shows great promise as an alternative to the synthetic progestogens in widespread use. It is almost identical to endogenous human progesterone and seems to convey all the benefits of progestogens without the unwanted negative effects. With more interest in this area, there will hopefully be more studies which can guide its integration into use in women's health care.

Natural Estrogens

There are many «natural « products currently being marketed to women. There are dietary supplements being sold as alternatives to estrogen and then there are actually products being called «natural estrogen». Estriol or tri-estrogen (TriEst) are two of those products. Estriol is a weak, short-acting estrogen. TriEst is a mixture of estrone, estradiol and estriol (1:1:8). The recommended dose is 2.5–5.0 mg/day. There is no evidence to back any claims of anti-cancer effects. There is data, however, to refute claims of endometrial safety. A national population-based, case-control study of 789 women in Sweden found that estriol use of 1–2 mg a day increased the risk of endometrial cancer and endometrial hyperplasia with odds ratios of 3.0 and 8.3 respectively [99]. «Natural estrogens» should not be recommended for routine use until there is more data to establish its efficacy and safety.

Lifestyle and Diet

Lifestyle factors such as diet, vitamin and mineral supplements, caffeine and alcohol use, cigarette smoking, and exercise, can have an impact on symptoms of menopause as well as a number of health problems occurring primarily in the postmenopausal years. A high fat diet, for example, has been associated with the development of coronary artery disease and explored as a risk factor for breast and other cancers. While many interventional studies have now been done looking at the effect of soy intake and supplementation, there is only a small amount of epidemiological data evaluating the association between dietary intake of sodium, protein, caffeine and alcohol on the incidence of osteoporosis. The data establishing a role for calcium, vitamin D, exercise and smoking is much more convincing.

Dietary Sodium

Excessive sodium intake has been theorized to have a negative effect on bone mineral density by increasing the urinary excretion of calcium. In a study of 29 healthy young women, 8 were found to have increased urinary calcium excretion when given an increasing dietary load of sodium [100]. These same women were compared with sodium-non-sensitive subjects for the effects of a high and low sodium diet on markers of bone metabolism. Although the sodium-sensitive subjects had increased urinary calcium excretion (by an average of 73%) with the 180 mmol/day sodium diet, biochemical markers of bone resorption and bone formation were unchanged. Another study assessed the effects of dietary sodium intake on calcium excretion and bone turnover in pre-and postmenopausal women [101]. Eleven women in each group followed a high sodium (300 mmol/day) and a low sodium (50 mmol/day) diet for one week each. In this study, all subjects on the high sodium diet exhibited a significant increase in 24 hours urinary sodium and calcium levels relative to creatinine. While there was no change in the biochemical markers of bone metabolism in the premenopausal women, the postmenopausal women showed evidence of an increase in bone resorption. Although these studies are small and only of short duration, the effect of sodium on blood pressure alone is compelling enough to recommend that older women limit their sodium intake.

Dietary Protein

Excessive dietary protein is theorized to cause deleterious effects on bone metabolism because of its high potential renal acid load. Bone acts as a buffer to acid by releasing carbonate, citrate and calcium [102]. A study of 16 healthy premenopausal women showed that the consumption of a high protein diet (2.1 g/kg/d) resulted in a significant increase in urinary calcium excretion, as well as a rise in urinary N-telopeptide (a marker of bone resorption). There was no change in either serum osteocalcin or bone-specific alkaline phosphatase (markers of bone formation) [103].

Observational epidemiologic studies have demonstrated a negative effect of a high protein diet on bone density. The Nurses' Health Study, a prospective study of 85, 900 women assessed fracture risk and dietary protein [104]. In women who consumed more than 95 g of protein per day, there was an increased risk of forearm fracture compared to women who consumed less than 68 g/d (RR 1.22, 95% CI 1.04–1.43, p=0.01). The consumption of red meat was also associated with an increased risk of forearm fracture (RR for 5 or more servings of red meat vs. less than 1 per week was 1.23, 95% CI 1.01–1.50). Interestingly, when the women were asked to recall their consumption of protein or red meat during their teen years, there was no increased risk of fracture with increased consumption during that period. No association was found between protein intake and hip fracture, though the power of the study to assess this was low. In a similar observational study of a cohort of men and women in Norway, 19, 752 women and 20, 035 men were followed for 11 years [105]. Women with the highest intake of animal protein and the lowest calcium intake were found to have a higher risk of hip fracture (RR for highest quarter of protein intake and lowest quarter of calcium intake vs. the three lower quarters of protein intake and three higher quarters of calcium intake = 1.96, 95% CI 1.09–3.56). Protein malnutrition should also be avoided, as severely reduced protein intake has been associated with lower femoral neck density in hospitalized elderly patients [106]. Over time, this could increase the risk of hip fracture.

One protein, which may positively affect bone metabolism, is milk basic protein (MBP). It is the basic fraction of milk whey protein. In vitro studies of MBP on bone showed a dose-dependent suppression of the number of pits formed by osteoclasts [107]. A randomized, controlled trial of 33 health women receiving either 40 mg/d of MBP or placebo showed a significantly higher rate of gain of bone mineral density of the calcaneus in the women receiving MBP [108]. There was a significant decrease in the excretion of N-telopeptides in the women receiving MBP but no change in osteocalcin or bone-specific alkaline phosphatase. This compound deserves further study.

There is currently a growing popularity for high protein, high fat, low carbohydrate diets such as the Atkins diet. More work needs to be done to assess the safety of these diets given the possible adverse effects on bone from high protein intake in women.

Caffeine

Caffeine intake has been theorized to increase the risk of osteoporotic fractures based upon its effect on urinary excretion of calcium. A two-year prospective study of caffeine use and bone mineral density in 92 nonsmoking postmenopausal women found no association between caffeine consumption and total body or femoral neck bone density at baseline [109]. There was no correlation between caffeine intake and longitudinal changes in total body or femoral neck bone density. The Iowa Women's Health Study was a survey of 34,703 postmenopausal women, which assessed the effect of alcohol and caffeine on fracture risk [110]. After a follow-up of 6 years, 4378 women reported at least one fracture. There was no association between caffeine intake and total fracture risk (RR for highest vs. lowest quintile of caffeine use 1.0, 95% CI 0.99–1.21). Wrist fractures, however, were associated positively with caffeine consumption (RR 1.37, 95% CI 1.11–1.69). It appears, therefore, that although the effect of caffeine on the bones may be small, it would be prudent to limit intake in women at high risk of fracture.

Smoking

Cigarette smoking has been linked to an earlier age at menopause as well as an increased risk of osteoporotic fractures [111, 112]. The National Osteoporosis Risk Assessment was a study of 200,160 postmenopausal women ages 50 and older without any previous history of osteoporosis [113]. Subjects were interviewed to determine presence or absence of risk factors for low bone mineral density (BMD). Peripheral bone densitometry measurements were done of the heel, finger, or forearm. Seven percent of the sample met the World Health Organization criteria for osteoporosis (T score of <or = -2.5). Cigarette smoking was associated with an increased risk of osteoporosis. The odds ratio (OR) for current smokers was 1.58 (95% CI 1.48–1.68), and the OR for former smokers was 1.14 (95% CI 1.10–1.19). In a recent case-control study, 1328 women with hip fractures were compared to 3312 controls [114]. Current smokers were found to have a significantly increased risk of hip fracture with an age-

adjusted odds ratio of 1.66 (95% CI 1.41–1.95). Duration of smoking was a more power-ful variable than amount smoked. There was a 6% increase in age-adjusted risk per 5 years smoked. Postmenopausal smoking appeared more detrimental to the bones. The OR per 5 years of postmenopausal smoking was 1.10 (95% CI 1.04–1.17) compared to an OR of 1.06 (95% CI 1.00–1.12) per 5 years of premenopausal smoking.

In addition, the risk of hip fracture decreased with duration of cessation. Fourteen years after quitting smoking, the risk of fracture drops to the level of nonsmokers. It is imperative that women be encouraged to quit smoking to decrease their risk of osteopenia, osteoporosis, and subsequent fracture in addition to respiratory disorders and cancer.

Alcohol

The risks of low bone mineral density and osteoporotic fractures with alcohol intake were evaluated in the following studies with conflicting results. The National Os-teoporosis Risk Assessment study found that alcohol consumption was associated with a decreased likelihood of osteoporosis [113]. The age-adjusted OR for osteoporosis in women who consumed 1–6 alcoholic drinks per week was 0.85 (95% CI 0.80–0.90). The risk of fracture for the same intake level was 0.85 (95% CI 0.75–0.96). Increasing levels of consumption appeared to negate the protective effect of alcohol. Consuming 7 to 13 alcoholic beverages weekly was associated with a risk of 0.90 (95% CI 0.74–1.09); more than 14 drinks per week was associated with a risk of 1.00 (95% CI 0.78–1.30). The case-control study showed an age-adjusted OR of 0.80 (95% CI 0.69–0.93) for subjects who drank alcohol, but there was no difference in level or risk with differing amounts of alcohol consumed [114]. On the other hand, the Iowa Women's Health Study found a relative risk (RR) of 1.55 for all fracture sites for the highest quintile of alcohol use as compared to the lowest (95% CI 1.25–1.92) [110].

There are many other health reasons for women to limit their use of alcohol. The current recommendation is that women limit their alcohol intake to 3–4 drinks a week. This number may need to decrease as women age and their ability to metabolize alcohol decreases.

Vitamins and Minerals

Vitamin E

Vitamin E has been a popular remedy for hot flashes. A placebo-controlled, random-ized, crossover trial of vitamin E supplementation was performed in 105 breast cancer survivors with hot flashes [115]. There was a small but statistically significant ($p<0.05$) decrease in the frequency of hot flashes with vitamin E. Treatment with 800 IU of vitamin E resulted in one less hot flash per day. No other vitamins have been examined in clinical trials for their effects on hot flashes.

B Vitamins

There has been much work done on the role of the B vitamins, especially folic acid, in cardiovascular disease. Folic acid is now being used to lower high homocysteine levels which has been identified as a potent risk factor for cardiovascular disease [116]. Homocysteine levels increase sharply in women after menopause. Estrogen may play a role in controlling the levels of homocysteine. Adequate levels of vitamins B_6, B_{12} and especially folic acid are necessary for the conversion of homocysteine into harmless metabolites. It has been suggested that deficiencies of these vitamins accounts for the majority of high homocysteine levels in older people [117]. Older women with a high risk for cardiovascular disease or those not getting an adequate amount of these B vitamins in their diets should consider taking a daily supplement with 4–8 mg of folic acid, 3–6 mg of vitamin 6 and 6,000–12,000 IU of vitamin B_{12}. Women who smoke and drink large amounts of coffee may need higher doses [118].

Minerals

Supplements containing minerals such as magnesium, calcium, and copper may be beneficial in limiting bone loss. A review of dietary magnesium intake and its relation to bone mineral density found a positive correlation between BMD and magnesium intake [119]. It also discussed a few small studies of magnesium supplementation, which showed an increase in BMD. Copper supplements may prove to be useful in preventing bone loss after menopause. A small study of rats showed those who received a diet supplemented with copper after ovariectomy did not lose any bone at L5 or in the femur [120]. No studies in humans have been done to establish the safety or efficacy of copper supplementation.

Calcium and Vitamin D

Calcium supplementation has been extensively studied and has been consistently shown to prevent bone loss in postmenopausal women [121] and reduce the incidence of fractures [122]. Sixteen observational studies were pooled to give an odds ratio of fracture of 0.96 (95% CI 0.93–0.99) with supplementation of 300 mg/day of calcium. While calcium is not as effective at reducing bone loss as antiresorptive agents such as bisphosphanates, calcitonin, estrogen, and raloxifene, it potentiates the action of these agents when used in combination.

Vitamin D 400–600 IU daily is essential for the absorption of calcium from the gut. It has been shown that in women from northern latitudes, bone loss has been greatest during the winter months when serum 25-OH vitamin D levels are the lowest [123]. Calcium supplementation with 1000 mg of calcium carbonate or increased dietary calcium intake (4 glasses of milk daily) prevents bone loss of the hip and spine in elderly women during the winter [123]. Calcium supplementation must be maintained to ensure continued benefit. A randomized, controlled trial of calcium and vitamin D in elderly men and women showed significant improvement in bone mineral density of the femoral neck, spine and total body [124]. There was a decreased risk of fracture in the group receiving the supplements. The subjects then discontinued the supplements and were followed along with the control subjects for an additional 2 years [125]. There was no lasting benefit of cal-cium and vitamin D in women on either bone mineral density or on the biochemical markers of bone metabolism when the supplementation was stopped. Similarly, a randomized controlled trial of calcium supplements given to postmenopausal women for 4 years showed a sustained reduction in the rate of bone loss over the 4-year period [126].

After reviewing the data regarding calcium's role in preventing and treating osteoporosis, and its effects on hypertension, colorectal cancer, obesity and nephrolithiasis, the North American Menopause Society issued a consensus opinion recommending that all women have an adequate intake of calcium of at least 1200 mg daily either through diet or supplements [127]. Women older than 65 years should take in 1500 mg of calcium daily. There appears to be equal absorption and bioavailability of calcium carbonate, encapsulated calcium carbonate, and calcium citrate [128]. A cost benefit analysis therefore suggests the least expensive product is the best choice.

Physical Activity and Exercise

Exercise is another aspect of a healthy lifestyle that can have a positive impact on health problems seen in older women. Sedentary lifestyle is a well-established risk factor for cardiovascular disease and has been associated with an increased risk of breast cancer [129]. In addition, participation in an exercise program has been shown to significantly improve feelings of psychological well being as well as self-perceived health [130].

Exercise has also been shown to have a positive impact on vasomotor symptoms of menopause. A survey of 793 women in Sweden found that those women who were highly physically active were significantly less likely to have experienced severe hot flashes at the time of menopause than were women who were sedentary, 5% vs. 15% respectively [131]. Similarly, another group of 142 women participating in organized physical exercise was compared to 1246 controls and were found to be less likely to have moderate to severe hot flashes with sweats (21.5% vs. 43.8% for controls) [132].

Exercise has been postulated to prevent or alleviate hot flashes by raising beta-endorphin levels in the hypothalamus. Beta-endorphins are involved in temperature regulation. Hot flashes are clearly related to a relative deficiency of estrogen and steroid hormones affect the metabolism of beta-endorphins. In an estrogen-deficient state, vigorous exercise may increase the level of beta-endorphins in the hypothalamus, thus stabilizing the thermoregulatory center [133].

Regular physical exercise is essential for developing and maintaining peak bone mass. Because the hormone changes of menopause shift the normal homeostasis of bone to involution, it is important to maximize peak bone mass. Regular physical exercise begun after menopause can improve bone density and prevent bone loss. A meta-analysis of randomized, controlled trials published from 1966 to 1996 assessed the effect of exercise on BMD of the lumbar spine and femoral neck [134]. There was a consistent positive effect of exercise in preventing or reversing almost 1% of bone loss per year.

Quadriceps strength has been found to be significantly related to BMD in elderly men and women [135]. Women in the top tertile of quadriceps strength and dietary calcium intake had 15% higher bone mineral density than those in the lowest tertile. Quadriceps strength is enhanced by weight bearing exercise. However, there is also evidence that regular physical activity such as walking can have a positive effect on the bones. A survey of 580 postmenopausal women found that stair climbing and regular walking were significantly associated with higher bone density at the trochanter hip site and total body bone density [136]. In women who reported regular brisk walking of at least a mile, there was a significant positive association with bone density at the proximal femur. Regular walking has also been shown to decrease the risk of fracture. In a study of 3110 men and women over the age of 70, habitual physical activity was associated with a decreased risk of fracture [137]. For women who walked for at least 1 mile three times weekly, the RR of fracture was 0.76 (95% CI 0.50–1.15).

Strength training may be more beneficial at preventing bone loss than fitness training. A study comparing strength training with increasing weights was compared with fitness training (minimal increase in load, identical set of exercises) and a non-exercise control [138]. Subjects were followed for two years. The strength-training group had a significant positive change in the BMD of the total and inter-trochanter hip sites while the fitness and control groups did not. Strength training has other benefits as well. A study of 40 sedentary postmenopausal women found that high intensity strength training had a positive effect on several risk factors for osteoporotic fractures: bone density, muscle mass, muscle strength, and dynamic balance [139]. Exercise has also been shown to decrease falls in elderly women by 25% [140]. Regular exercise may therefore reduce the risk of fractures by increasing bone density, increasing muscle mass and strength and decreasing falls. It should be recommended for women of all ages but especially to those in the peri and post-menopausal years.

Mind-Body Therapies

Relaxation Therapy

Mind-body therapies such as paced respiration and applied relaxation can be helpful at reducing stress. The frequency and intensity of hot flashes are worsened by stress [141]. There are few studies of relaxation therapies for hot flashes, and the small number of subjects limits their usefulness. Two studies, however, are worth mentioning [142, 143]. The first [142] examined instruction in paced respiration vs. instruction in muscle relaxation vs. alpha-wave electroencephalographic feedback. This last treatment was a placebo because it causes subjective feelings of relaxation without any physiologic effects. Subjects all underwent 24-hour ambulatory monitoring of sternal skin conductance to assess number of hot flashes per day. Only the group who learned paced respiration experienced a significant decrease in hot flash frequency. The second study [143] examined relaxation response instruction in women with at least 5 hot flashes per day. The relaxation response group had significant reductions in hot flash intensity compared to their symptoms prior to the training. Although the studies are small, and the effect is minimal, the techniques described are easily taught, easily performed, have no side effects, and can be used in any stressful situation with some benefit.

Yoga

Yoga is becoming extremely popular with its combination of philosophy, stretching, and meditation. Although no formal studies have been done with yoga and its effect on hot flashes, it may be beneficial because of stress reduction [144].

Acupuncture

Acupuncture has been used extensively in menopausal women with hot flashes [145]. There are however, few randomized, placebo-controlled trials assessing acupuncture's effects on vasomotor symptoms. One small study of 10 patients measured complaints of menopausal symptoms and randomized patients to acupuncture or placebo-acupuncture [146]. The acupuncture done with a standardized combination of acupuncture points resulted in a significant reduction in complaints and an improvement in well being. In a study of the efficacy of acupuncture in treating hot flashes, men who had undergone orchiectomy for prostate cancer, and were experiencing vasomotor symptoms, underwent acupuncture treatment weekly for 10 weeks [147]. There was a substantial decrease in the frequency of their symptoms, with an average decrease of 70%. This was not a blinded, controlled study, and there is a well-established placebo effect on vasomotor symptoms. On the other hand, a decrease of 70% is substantial, and makes further study of acupuncture essential as an alternative for men and women who cannot use hormones to treat their hot flashes.

Conclusion

Many older women are using alternative therapies. Herbs, vitamins, minerals and soy products marketed for postmenopausal women are available in pharmacies, supermarkets and health food stores. The current regulatory environment for dietary supplements does not encourage the productions of well-standardized or reliable products. This situation will hopefully improve. There is no evidence to support the use of Don Quai, Evening Primrose Oil or Ginseng. Black Cohosh, however, shows some promise as a treatment for postmenopausal vasomotor symptoms. Kava and Valerian may be useful as sleep aides or mild anxiolytics but should both be used with caution. Cranberry is safe and efficacious for the prevention of urinary tract infections.

The literature on the clinical effects of a soy-enriched diet and isoflavone supplements is large and growing. The lipid (LDLc) lowering effects of soy protein has been consistently seen in studies with that claim recently supported by the FDA. The data supporting the ability of soy and isoflavones to alleviate hot flashes is largely positive but less robust. There is some preliminary evidence to suggest that isoflavone supplementation may have a beneficial effect on bone. Larger studies using consistent interventions are needed. A synthetic isoflavone currently marketed as a dietary supplement, ipriflavone, shows great promise as a treatment for osteoporosis. It can cause lymphocytopenia so needs to be used with caution. More long-term safety data is needed to make any firm conclusions about the effect of soy and isoflavones on the endometrium and breast.

Two commonly used "natural" hormone products are oral micronized progesterone and progesterone cream. While they contain a progesterone identical to endogenous human progesterone, they are both produced synthetically. There is little evidence that progesterone creams are efficacious or safe. Conversely, oral micronized progesterone shows great promise as an alternative to the progestogens used in postmenopausal hormone replacement regimens. It may convey all the benefits of progestogens without the unwanted effects. There is no evidence to support the use of "natural" estrogens such as estriol.

There is a small amount of data suggesting an association between the association between the excessive intake of dietary sodium and protein, caffeine and alcohol on the incidence of osteoporosis. There is one study that found a positive correlation between magnesium intake and bone mineral density. Smoking is well-established risk factor for osteoporosis. Regular exercise and adequate intakes of calcium and vitamin D are clearly essential in preventing it.

Vitamin E, applied relaxation techniques, acupuncture and exercise may be useful in alleviating postmenopausal hot flashes.

References

1. Weiss NS (1980) Decreased risk of fractures of the hip and lower forearm with postmenopausal use of estrogen. NEJM; 303: 1195–1198
2. Genant HK (1997) Low-dose esterified estrogen therapy: Effects on bone, plasma estradiol, endometrium and lipid levels. Arch Intern Med; 157: 2609–2615.)
3. The PEPI investigators (1995) Effects of estrogen or estrogen/progestin regimens on heart disease risk factors in postmenopausal women. JAMA 273: 199–208.
4. Mendelsohn ME (1999) The protective effects of estrogen on the cardiovascular system. NEJM; 340: 1801–1811.
5. Utian WH (1999) Efficacy and safety of low, standard and high dosages of an estradiol transdermal system compared with placebo on vasomotor symptoms in highly symptomatic menopausal patients. Am J Obstet Gynecol; 181: 71–79
6. Grodstein F (1999) Postmenopausal hormone use and risk for colorectal cancer and adenoma. Ann Intern Med;128: 705–712), cognitive decline and dementia
7. LeBlanc ES (2001) Hormone replacement therapy and cognition: systematic review and meta-analysis. JAMA; 285: 1489–1499.
8. Wluka AE (2000) Menopause, oestrogens and arthritis. Maturitas; 35: 183–199.
9. Fantl JA (1994) Estrogen therapy in the management of urinary incontinence in postmenopausal women: A Meta-analysis: First report of the hormones and urogenial therapy committee. Obstet Gynecol; 83: 12–18
10. Cauley JA (1990) Prevalence and determinants of estrogen replacement therapy in elderly women. Am J Obstet Gynecol; 163: 1438–1444.
11. Menopause 2001; 8 (6): 433–440
12. Alternative Medicine; Expanding Medical Horizons. A report to the NIH on Alternative Medical Systems and Practices in the United States. US Gov't Printing Office 017–040–00537–7
13. Eisenberg D, Kessler RC, Foster C, Norlock FE, Calkins DR, DelBanco TL. (1993) Unconventional medicine in the United States-prevalence cost and patterns of use. NEJM; 328: 246–252.
14. Eisenberg DM et al (1990) Trends in Alternative Medicine use in the U.S. 1990–1997. JAMA; 280: 1569–75.
15. Landmark Healthcare, Sacramento, CA; The Integrator for the Business of Alternative Medicine. 1999; vol3.
16. Palinkas LA et al. (2000) The use of CAM by primary care patients. J Fam Pract; 49: 1121–1130.
17. Mathuna DP (2000) Where to with herbals. Alternative Therapies. 6: 34–35.

18. Foster S, (1999) Black Cohosh: A literature review. Herbalgram; 45: 35–49.
19. Duker EM (1991) Effects of extracts from Cimicifuga racemosa on gonadotropin release in menopausal women and ovariectomized rats. Planta Med.; 57: 420–424
20. Liske E (1998) Therapy of Climacteric Complains with Cimicifuga racemosa. Menopause; 5: 250.
21. Liske P (1998) Therapeutic efficacy and safety of Cimicifuga racemosa for gynecological disorders. Advances in Therapy; 15: 45–53.
22. Stoll W (1987) Phytopharmacon influences atrophic vaginal epithelium: double-blind study – cimicifuga vs. estrogenic substances. Therapeuticum; 1: 23–31.
23. Ozaki Y, (1990) Inhibitory effects of tetramethylpyrazine and ferulic acid on spontaneous movement of rat uterus in situ. Chem Pha; 38: 1620–1623.
24. Rotblatt MD (1999) Dong Quai: A review.; 1: 65–72.
25. Hirata JD et al. (1997) Does Don quai have estrogenic effects in postmenopausal women? A double-blind, placebo-controlled trial. Fertil Steril; 68: 981–6
26. Blatt MHG, Wiesbader H, Kupperman HS (1953) Vitamin E and climacteric syndrome: failure of effective control as measured by menopausal index. Arch Intern Med; 91: 792–9.
27. Natural Medicines Comprehensive Database compiled by the editors of Prescriber's Letter and Pharmacists Letter. Published by Therapeutic Research Faculty, Stockton, California. 2000 p.422
28. Chenoy R Effect of oral gamolenic acid from evening primrose oil on menopausal flushing. BMJ 1994; 308: 501–503.)
29. Natural Medicines Comprehensive Database compiled by the editors of Prescriber's Letter and Pharmacists Letter. Published by Therapeutic Research Faculty, Stockton, California. 2000 p. 1053.
30. Hardy ML. (1999) Valerian Root for Insomnia. Alt Med Alert.; 2: 85–96.
31. Donath F et al. (2000) Critical evaluation of the effect of valerian extract on sleep structure and sleep quality. Pharmacopsychiatry 33: 47–53.
32. Garges HP et al. (1998) Cardiac complications and delirium associated with Valerian Root withdrawal. JAMA; 280: 1566–1567.
33. Pittler MH and Ernst E. (2000) Efficacy of kava extract for treating anxiety: systematic review and meta-analysis. J Clin Psychopharmacol; 20: 84–9.
34. Natural Medicines Comprehensive Database compiled by the editors of Prescriber's Letter and Pharmacists Letter. Published by Therapeutic Research Faculty, Stockton, California. 2000 p.626.
35. Almeida JC et al. (1996) Coma from the health food store: interaction between kava and alprazolam. Ann Intern Med; 125: 940–941.
36. Herbal Rx Promises and Pitfalls. Consumer Reports. March 1999, pp 44–48.
37. Herbal Roulette. Consumer Reports. November 1995: 698–705.
38. Natural Medicines Comprehensive Database compiled by the editors of Prescriber's Letter and Pharmacists Letter. Published by Therapeutic Research Faculty, Stockton, California. 2000. p.733.
39. Vogler BK (1999) The efficacy of ginseng. A systematic review of randomized clinical trials. Eur J Clin Pharmacol. 55: 567–575
40. Vuksan V et al. (2000) American ginseng reduces postprandial glycemia in nondiabetic subjects and subjects with type 2 diabetes. Arch Intern Med; 160: 1009–1013.
41. Hopkins MP, et al. (1983) „Ginseng ace cream and unexplained vaginal bleeding. Am J Obstest Gynecol 1988; 159: 1121–2, Greenspan EM „Ginseng and vaginal bleeding" JAMA; 249: 2018.
42. Miller LG (1998) Herbal Medicinals. Arch Intern Med; 158: 2200–2211.
43. Tyler VE, Herbs of Choice. Pharmaceutical Products Press, NY 1994, p.80.
44. Howell AB (1998) Inhibition of the adherence of P-fimbriated E. coli to uroepithelial cell surfaces by proanthocamidin extracts from cranberries NEJM; 339: 1085–1086
45. Avorn J (1994) Reduction of bacteriuria and pyuria after ingestion of cranberry juice. JAMA; 271: 751–4
46. Kontiokari T (2001) Randomised trial of cranberry-lingonberry juice and Lactobacillus GG drink for the prevention of urinary tract infections in women. BMJ; 322: 1571–3.
47. Terris MK (2001) Dietary supplementation with cranberry concentrate tablets may increase the risk of nephrolithiasis. Urology: 57: 26–29.
48. Vincent A, Fitzpatrick LA. (2000) Soy Isoflavones: Are they Useful in Menopause? Mayo Clin Proc; 75: 1174–1184.
49. Murkies AL (1998) Phytoestrogens J Clin Endocrinol Metab; 83: 297–303.
50. Tham DM. (1998) Potential Health Benefits of Dietary Phytoestrogens: A Review of the Clinical, Epidemiological and Mechanistic Evidence. J Clin Endocrinol Metab; 83: 2223–2235.
51. NAMS Consensus Opinion (2000) The Role of Isoflavones in Menopausal Health: Consensus Opinion of The North American Menopause Society. Menopause; 7: 215–229.
52. Nisly N (1999) Phytoestrogens for the prevention and treatment of osteoporosis. Alt Med Alert; 2(12): 138–142.
53. Schreiber MD (2001) Dietary inclusion of whole soy foods results in significant reductions in clinical risk factors for osteoporosis and cardiovascular disease in normal postmenopausal women. Menopause; 8: 384–392.
54. Kim H (1998) Mechanisms of action of the soy isoflavone genistein. Am J Clin Nutr; 68: 1418S-1425S.
55. Hutchins (1995) Vegetables, fruits and legumes: effect on urinary isofavonoid phytoestrogen and lignan excertion. J Am Diet Assoc; 95: 769–774.
56. Aldercreutz H (1997) Phytoestrogens and Western diseases. Ann Med; 29: 95–120.

57. Gold EB (2000) Relation of demographic and lifestyle factors to symptoms in a multi-racial/ethnic population of women. Am J Epidemiol; 152: 463–83.
58. Washburn S (1999) Effect of soy protein supplementation on serum lipoproteins, blood pressure and menopausal symptoms in perimenopausal women. Menopause; 6(1): 7–13.
59. Albertazzi P (1998) The effect of dietary soy supplementation on hot flashes. Obstet Gynecol; 91: 9–11.
60. Murkies AL (1995) Dietary flour supplementation decreases post menopausal hot flushes: effect of soy and wheat. Maturitas; 21: 189–195.
61. St. Germain A (2001) Isoflavone-rich or isoflavone-poor soy protein does not reduce menopausal symptoms during 24 weeks of treatment. Menopause 8: 17–26.
62. Quella SK (2000) Evaluation of soy phytoestrogens for the treatment of hot flashes in breast cancer survivors. J Clin Onc; 18(5): 1068–74.
63. Brzezinski A (1997) Short-term effects of phytoestrogen rich diet on postmenopausal women. Menopause; 4(2): 89–94.
64. Scambia G (2000) Clinical effects of a standardized soy extract in postmenopausal women: a pilot study. Menopause; 7(2): 105–111.
65. Upmalis DH (2000) Vasomotor symptom relief by soy isoflavone extract tablets in postmenopausal women: a multi-center, double-blind, randomized, placebo-controlled study. Menopause; 7(4): 236–242.
66. Baber RJ (1999) Randomized placebo-controlled trial of an isoflavone supplement and menopausal symptoms in women. Climacteric. 2: 85–92.
67. Knight DC (1999) The effect of Promensil, an isoflavone extract, on menopausal symptoms. Climacteric; 2: 79–84.
68. FDA talk paper: FDA approves new health claim for soy protein and coronary heart disease.
69. Anderson JW (1995) Meta-analysis of the effects of soy protein intake on serum lipids. N Engl J Med; 333: 276–82.
70. Crouse JR (1999) A randomized trial comparing the effect of casein with soy protein on plasma concentrations of lipids and lipoproteins. Arch Intern Med; 159: 2070–76.
71. Potter SM (1998) Soy protein and isoflavones: their effects on lipids and bone density in postmenopausal women. Am J Clin Nutr; 68: 1375S-1379S.
72. Lu LJW (2001) Phytoestrogens and healthy aging: gaps in knowledge. Menopause; 8: 157–170.
73. Clifton-Bligh PB (2001) The effect of isoflavones extracted from red clover (Rimostil) on lipid and bone metabolism. Menopause; 8: 259–265.
74. Nestle PJ (1999) Isoflavones from red clover improve systemic arterial compliance but not plasma lipids in menopausal women. J Clin Endocrinol Metab; 84: 895–8.
75. Alekel DL (2000) Isoflavone-rich soy protein isolate attenuates bone loss in the lumbar spine of perimenopausal women. Am J Clin Nutr; 72: 844–52.
76. Goodman MT (1997) Association of soy and fiber consumption with the risk of endometrial cancer. Am J Epidemiol 146: 294–306.
77. Murkies A (2000) Phytoestrogens and breast cancer in postmenopausal women: a case control study. Menopause 7(5): 289–96.
78. Ingram D (1997) Case-control study of phyto-estrogens and breast cancer. Lancet. 350: 990–994.
79. Wu AH (1998) Soy intake and risk of breast cancer in Asians and Asian Americans. Am J Clin Nutr. 68 (6suppl): 1437S-43S.
80. Balk JL (2000) Ipriflavone for prevention of osteoporosis. Alternative Medicine Alert 3(12): 133–144.
81. Nisly N (2000) Ipriflavone: Mechanism and safety. Alternative Therapies in Women's Health. 2(9): 65–72.
82. Yamazaki I (1986) Effects of ipriflavone on glucocorticoid-induced osteoporosis in rats. Life Sci 38: 951–8.
83. Gennari C (1998) Effect of ipriflavone on bone mass loss in the early years after menopause. Menopause 5: 9–15.
84. Valente M (1994) Effects of one year treatment with ipriflavone in postmenopausal women with low bone mass. Calcif Tissue Int 54: 377–380.
85. Melis GB (1992) Ipriflavone and low doses of estrogens in the prevention of bone mineral loss in climacterium. Bone Miner 19 (suppl 1): S49–56.
86. Agnuside D (1995) Prevention of early postmenopausal bone loss using low dose conjugated estrogen and ipriflavone. Osteoporosis Int 5: 462–6.
87. Gennari C (1997) Effect of chronic treatment with ipriflavone in postmenopausal women with low bone mass. Calcif Tissue Int 61(S1): 19–22
88. Gambacciani M (1997) Effects of combined low dose ipriflavone and ERT on bone mineral density and metabolism in postmenopausal women. Maturitas; 28: 75–81.
89. Ushiroyama T (1995) Efficacy of ipriflavone and vertebral vitamin D for the cessation of bone loss Int J Gynecol Obstet; 48: 283–288.
90. Maugeri D (1994) Ipriflavone treatment of senile osteoporosis: Results of a multi-center double-blind randomized trial of 2 years. Arch Gerentol Geriatr; 19: 253–63.
91. Alexandersen P (2001) Ipriflavone in the treatment of postmenopausal osteoporosis. JAMA 285: 1482–1488.
92. Lee JR (1998) Use of Pro-Gest cream in postmenopausal women. Lancet. 352: 905–6
93. Carey BJ (2000) A study to evaluate serum and urinary hormone levels following short and long term administration of two regimens of progesterone cream in postmenopausal women. BJOG 107: 722–6.
94. Anasti JN (2001) Topical progesterone cream has antiproliferative effect on estrogen-stimulated endometrium. Obstet Gynecol 97 (4 Suppl 1): S10

95. Wren BG (1999) Micronised transdermal progesterone and endometrial response. Lancet 354: 1447–8.
96. Leonetti HB (1999) Transdermal progesterone cream for vasomotor symptoms and postmenopausal bone loss. Obstet Gynecol 94(2): 225–8.
97. Fugh-Berman A (1999) Progesterone cream for osteoporosis. Alt therapies in women's health 1: 33–36.
98. Langer RD (1999) Micronized progesterone: A New Therapeutic Option. Int J Fertil 44: 67–73.
99. Weiderpass E (1999) Low-potency oestrogen and risk of endometrial cancer: A case-control study. Lancet, 353: 1824–1828.
100. Ginty F, Flynn A et al. (1998) The effect of dietary sodium intake on biochemical markers of bone metabolism in young women. Br J Nutr; 79 (4): 343–50.
101. Evans CE, Chughtai AY et al. (1997) The effect of dietary sodium on calcium metabolism in premenopausal and postmenopausal women. Eur J Clin Nutr; 51 (6): 394–9.
102. Barzel US, Massey LK. (1998) Excess dietary protein can adversely affect bone. J of Nutr; 128 (6): 1051–3.
103. Kerstetter JE, Mitnick MA et al. (1999) Changes in bone turnover in young women consuming different levels of dietary protein. J Clin Epidem and Met; 84 (3): 1052–5.
104. Feskanich D, Willet WC et al. (1996) Protein consumption and bone fractures in women. Am J Epidemiol; 143(5): 472–9.
105. Meyer HE, Pedersen JI et al. (1997) Dietary factors and the incidence of hip fractures in middle-aged Norwegians. A prospective study. Am J Epidemiol; 145(2): 117–23.
106. Bonjour JP, Schurch MA et al. (1997) Proteins and bone health. Pathol Biol (Paris); 45(1): 57–9.
107. Toba Y, Takada Y et al. (2000) Milk basic protein: a novel protective function of milk against osteoporosis. Bone; 27 (3): 403–8.
108. Aoe S, Toba Y et al. (2001) Controlled trial of the effects of milk basic protein (MBP) supplementation on bone metabolism in healthy adult women. Biosci Biotechnol Biochem; 65 (4): 913–8.
109. Lloyd T, Johnson-Rollings N et al. (2000) Bone status among postmenopausal women with different habitual caffeine intakes: a longitudinal investigation. J Am Coll Nutr; 19(2): 256–61.
110. Hansen SA, Folsom AR et al. (2000) Association of fractures with caffeine and alcohol in postmenopausal women: the Iowa Women's Health Study. Public Health Nutr; 3(3): 253–61.
111. Baron JA, La Vecchia C et al. (1990) The antiestrogenic effect of cigarette smoking in women. Am J Obstet Gynecol; 162(2): 502–14.
112. Black DM, Cooper C. (2000) Epidemiology of fractures and assessment of fracture risk. Clin Lab Med; 20(3): 439–53.
113. Siris ES, Miller PD et al. (2001) Identification and fracture outcomes of undiagnosed low bone density in postmenopausal women: results from the National Osteoporosis Risk Assessment. JAMA; 286(22): 2815–2822.
114. Baron JA, Farahmand BY et al. (2001) Cigarette smoking, alcohol consumption, and risk of hip fracture in women. Arch Int Med; 161(7): 983–988.
115. Barton DL, Loprinzi CL et al. (1998) Prospective evaluation of vitamin E for hot flashes in breast cancer survivors. J Clin Oncol; 16 (2): 495–500.
116. Welch GN. (1998) Homocysteine and atherothrombosis. NEJM; 338: 1009–15.
117. Selhub J. (1993) Vitamin status and intake as primary determinants of homocysteinemia in an elderly population. JAMA; 270: 2693–8.
118. Seibel MM (1999) The role of nutrition and nutritional supplements in women's health. Fertil Steril; 72: 579–91.
119. Rude RK. (2000) Dietary magnesium intake and osteoporosis. Alt Therapies in Women's Health; 2(10): 73–77.
120. Rico H, Roca-Botran C, et al. (2000) The effect of supplemental copper on osteopenia induced by ovariectomy in rats. Menopause; 7(6): 413–6.
121. Cumming RG. (1990) Calcium intake and bone mass: a quantitative review of the evidence. Calcif Tissue Int; 47(4): 194–201.
122. Cumming RG, Nevitt MC. (1997) Calcium for prevention of osteoporotic fractures in postmenopausal women. J Bone Miner Res; 12 (9): 1321–9.
123. Storm D, Eslin R et al. (1998) Calcium supplementation prevents seasonal bone loss and changes in biochemical markers of bone turnover in elderly New England women: a randomized placebo-controlled trial. J Clin Endocrinol Metab; 83 (11): 3817–25.
124. Dawson-Hughes B, Harris SS et al. (1997) Effect of calcium and vitamin D supplementation on bone density in men and women 65 years of age or older. NEJM; 337: 670–6.
125. Dawson-Hughes B, Harris SS et al. (2000) Effect of withdrawal of calcium and vitamin D supplements on bone mass in elderly men and women. Am J Clin Nutr; 72 (3): 745–50.
126. Reid IR, Ames RW. (1995) Long term effects of calcium supplementation on bone loss and fracture in postmenopausal women: a randomized controlled trial. Am J Med; 98 (4): 331–5.
127. The role of calcium in peri- and postmenopausal women: consensus opinion of The North American Menopause Society. (2001) Menopause; 8 (2): 84–95.
128. Heaney RP, Dowell SD et al. (2001) Absorbability and cost effectiveness in calcium supplementation. J Am Coll Nutr; 20 (3): 239–46.
129. Friedenreich CM. (2001) Influence of physical activity in different age and life periods on the risk of breast cancer. Epidemiol; 12 (6): 604–12.
130. Bravo G, Gauthier P et al. (1996) Impact of a 12-month exercise program on the physical and psychological health of osteopenic women. JAGS; 44: 756–62.

131. Ivarsson T, Spetz AC et al. (1998) Physical exercise and vasomotor symptoms in postmenopausal women. Maturitas; 29(2): 139–46.
132. Hammar M, Berg G et al. (1990) Does physical exercise influence the frequency of postmenopausal hot flashes? Acta Obstet Gynecol Scand; 69(5): 409–12.
133. Hammar ML, Hammar-Henriksson MB et al. (2000) Few oligo-amenorrheic athletes have vasomotor symptoms. Maturitas; 34: 219–25.
134. Wolff I, van Croonenborg JJ et al. (1999) The effect of exercise training programs on bone mass: a meta-analysis of published controlled trial in pre- and postmenopausal women. Osteoporosis Int; 9(1): 1–12.
135. Nguyen TV. (2000) Osteoporosis in elderly men and women: effects of dietary calcium, physical activity, and body mass index. J Bone Miner Res; 15 (2): 322–31.
136. Coupland CA, Cliffe SJ et al. (1999) Habitual physical activity and bone mineral density in postmenopausal women in England. Int J Epidemiol; 28(2): 241–6.
137. Sorock GS, Bush TL et al. (1988) Physical activity and fracture risk in a free-living elderly cohort. J Gerontol; 43(5): M 134–9.
138. Kerr D, Ackland T et al. (2001) Resistance training over 2 years increases bone mass in calcium-replete postmenopausal women. J Bone Miner Res; 16(1): 175–81.
139. Nelson ME, Fiatarone MA et al. (1994) Effects of high-intensity strength training on multiple risk factors for osteoporotic fractures. A randomized, controlled trial. JAMA; 272: 1909–14.
140. NIH Consensus Statement. March 27–29, 2000. Osteoporosis prevention, diagnosis and therapy; 17 (1): 1–45.
141. Gannon L, Hansel S et al. (1987) Correlates of menopausal hot flashes. J Behav Med; 10(3): 277–85.
142. Freedman RR, Woodward S. (1992) Behavioral treatment of menopausal hot flushes: evaluation by ambulatory monitoring. Am J Obstet Gynecol; 167: 436–9.
143. Irvin JH, Domar AD et al. (1996) The effects of relaxation response training on menopausal symptoms. J Psychosom Obstet Gynecol; 17(4): 202–7.
144. Wood C. (1993) Mood change and perceptions of vitality: a comparison of the effects of relaxation, visualization, and yoga. J R Soc Med; 86 (5): 254–8.
145. Wu L, Zhou X. (1998) 300 cases of menopausal syndrome treated by acupuncture. J Tradit Chin Med; 18(4): 259–62.
146. Kraft K, Coulon S. (1999) Effect of a standardized acupuncture treatment on complaints, blood pressure and serum lipids of hypertensive, postmenopausal women. A randomized, controlled clinical study. Forsch Komplement-armed; 6(2): 74–9.
147. Hammar M, Frisk J et al. (1999) Acupuncture treatment of vasomotor symptoms in men with prostatic carcinoma: a pilot study. J Urol; 161(3): 853–6.

26 The Use of Phytotherapy in the Treatment of Men with Benign Prostatic Hyperplasia

N.F. Alsikafi, G.S. Gerber

Plants and plant extracts have been used to treat a variety of medical problems since ancient times. Presently, the use of herbal agents in men with benign prostatic hyperplasia (BPH) varies widely in different parts of the world. In countries, such as France and Germany, phytotherapeutic products are available by prescription and are among the most commonly used initial therapies for men with lower urianry tract symptoms (LUTS) secondary to BPH. In contrast, herbal agents are available without prescription in the U.S. and few physicians recommend such therapy for men with BPH. In addition, all costs associated with the use of phytotherapeutic therapies are paid by the patient rather than by insurance companies or other third party payers. Despite these limitations, it is estimated that $500 million to $1 billion is spent each year in the United States for non-prescription herbal treatments [1]. Unfortunately, despite the widely held perception among lay persons that „natural" remedies are helpful in treating many chronic medical conditions, such as BPH, there is limited or no scientific evidence to support the use of these agents in many cases.

In most cases, herbal therapies used in the treatment of BPH have not been subjected to rigorous scientific testing. However, in recent years, there have been an increasing number of well-conducted studies concerning these products. Many of these trials have been carried out in Europe by companies who have proprietary rights to these products and stand to benefit financially if efficacy can be demonstrated. Since medicinal botanicals are generally categorized as food additives in the U.S. and are not subject to patent protection, there is little financial incentive for American companies to support large trials of these agents. Due to restrictions placed by the Food and Drug Administration, most European companies have elected not to pursue approval of their phytotherapeutic products in the United States.

Other limitations to the use of herbal therapies in the U.S. include the lack of standardization of these products. In many cases, this leads to marked variation in the chemical composition of phytotherapeutic products that are sold by different companies. The reliability of such products and the assurance that they actually contain the ingredients listed on the label is largely at the discretion of each manufacturer since there is little or no oversight of production. In the treatment of BPH, saw palmetto is the most commonly used herbal agent in the U.S. More than 30 companies produce and distribute saw palmetto, which is often sold as a combination product containing other herbs, vitamins and minerals. A number of consumer watchdog groups and Internet sites have investigated the reliability of saw palmetto and other herbal products. In many cases, these groups have found wide discrepancies between the actual and stated composition of these products. In Europe, the most commonly marketed form of saw palmetto is Permixon, which is a patented product produced by a French company. Most of the larger studies that have been conducted concerning saw palmetto and BPH have used Permixon. However, the results of these studies may have little bearing on the treatment outcome to be expected by American consumers using other saw palmetto products. Most patients are not aware of the significant differences that may exist between the chemical composition and efficacy of products that may have similar or identical names.

Herbal Therapy and BPH- Proposed Mechanisms of Action

A number of different herbal agents and plant extracts have been used in the treatment of men with BPH and are listed below.

Commonly Used Herbal Therapies in Men with Benign Prostatic Hyperplasia

▶ Saw palmetto (Serenoa repens)
▶ Pygeum Africanum (African plum)
▶ Beta-sitosterol
▶ Pollen extracts
▶ Stinging nettles (Urtica dioica)
▶ Pumpkin seeds
▶ Radix Urticae

In most cases, these products contain a variety of fatty acids, plants oils and phytosterols [2]. It is generally believed that it is the phytosterols that are largely responsible for the efficacy of these herbal agents [2]. Beta-sitosterol is felt to be the most important phytosterol, which are a class of compounds related to cholesterol [2]. A number of proposed mechanisms have been suggested to be associated with phytosterols, including anti-androgenic effects, direct inhibition of prostatic growth and 5-alpha reductase activity [1, 2].

Possible Mechanisms of Action of Herbal Therapies Used in the Treatment of Men with Benign Prostatic Hyperplasia

▶ Anti-inflammatory effects
▶ Inhibition of 5-alpha reductase (conversion of testosterone to dihydrotestosterone)
▶ Anti-androgenic effects
▶ Anti-estrogenic effects
▶ Effects on bladder function in response to outlet obstruction
▶ Growth factor inhibition
▶ Reduction in sex hormone binding globulin

A number of in vitro studies have been conducted demonstrating these effects. However, supra-physiologic doses of these agents have been used in many of these trials, which limits the ability to draw conclusions regarding the true mechanism by which improvement in clinical parameters may occur. For example, it is widely believed that saw palmetto is a natural 5-alpha reductase inhibitor acting in similar fashion as the prescription drug, finasteride (Proscar) [1]. A number of in vitro studies have demonstrated 5-alpha reductase activity with saw palmetto, in the form of Permixon [3, 4]. However, clinically relevant 5-alpha reductase effects, such as prostate shrinkage or decreases in serum prostate specific antigen (PSA) levels, generally have not been demonstrated in clinical studies of saw palmetto [5, 6]. These discrepancies, as well as a lack of clear understanding of the mechanism of action of many phytotherapeutic products, have led to skepticism among many clinicians concerning the true effectiveness of herbal products used to treat BPH.

Saw Palmetto

Saw palmetto is the most popular herbal therapy used in the treatment of men with BPH and is derived from the berry of the American dwarf palm tree which is found in the southeastern United States [1, 2]. Permixon is the most extensively investigated form of saw palmetto and is widely used in Europe but it is not available in the U.S. permixon is a liposterolic extract of the berry containing free fatty acids, phytosterols and other compounds [5]. Human and animal studies have demonstrated that some of the compounds in Permixon are absorbed through the gastrointestinal tract and may accumulate in normal and hyperplastic prostatic cells [5, 7, 8]. A variety of mechanisms by which saw palmetto may improve voiding symptoms have been suggested, including anti-estrogenic effects, anti-androgenic effects mediated through androgen-receptor blockade, growth factor inhibition and others [1–4, 9, 10]. It is most commonly believed, however, that saw palmetto works by inhibition of 5-alpha reductase, which is responsible for the conversion of testosterone (T) to its active form in the prostate, dihydrotestosterone (DHT) [1–4]. Using human skin fibroblasts, primary cultures of human BPH cells and other models, a number of in vitro studies have been performed with Permixon which have generally demonstrated inhibition of type 1 and type 2, 5-alpha reductase activity leading to a decrease in DHT levels [3, 4, 9, 10].

A number of attempts have been made to demonstrate 5-alpha reductase activity in human subjects. In a trial of 33 men awaiting open prostatectomy for BPH, three months treatment with finasteride, flutamide (an anti-androgen), placebo or Permixon was randomly administered [11]. After surgical removal of the prostate, growth factor levels along with T and DHT measurements were carried out. All 3 measured factors were found to be highest in the periurethral prostatic tissue and lowest in the subcapsular zone of the prostate. DHT and growth factor levels were markedly decreased overall with no difference in intraprostatic distribution among men receiving finasteride or Permixon. In those men treated with flutamide, there was no change in T or DHT levels, although growth factor levels decreased throughout the prostate. Although this was a small study, it appeared that both finasteride and Permixon led to important changes in androgen levels primarily within the prostatic tissue adjacent to the urethra. In contrast to these findings, other investigators have not been able to demonstrate significant 5-alpha reductase activity with saw palmetto [12, 13]. In one study, rats were stimulated with T or DHT and it was noted that finasteride, but not Permixon, inhibited prostatic growth [12]. Among 32 healthy male volunteers without BPH, treatment with finasteride for 7 days led to a decrease in serum DHT levels which was not seen with treatment with Permixon [12]. Other investigators have also been unable to demonstrate changes in serum DHT levels among men treated with Permixon [13]. Even if one were to accept that saw palmetto has in vivo 5-alpha reductase activity, several human trials call into question the clinical relevance of this activity [5, 6, 14]. Although finasteride will lead to an approximate 50% decrease in serum PSA levels, this effect does not occur with saw palmetto [5, 6, 14]. In addition, while finasteride will lead to a 20–30% reduction in prostate size when administered for 6–12 months, minimal or no reduction in prostate size has been shown in large clinical trials using saw palmetto [5, 6, 14].

A number of other potential mechanisms of action of saw palmetto have also been proposed. In addition to androgen receptor blockade, which has been demonstrated using human foreskin fibroblasts [9] there is evidence to suggest that saw palmetto may have anti-estrogenic effects [15]. Di Silverio, et al, performed a placebo controlled trial in which men with BPH were treated for 3 months with Permixon prior to surgery [15]. Those receiving the saw palmetto formulation had a marked drop in estrogen receptor activity in comparison with men receiving placebo. It was suggested that by competitive inhibition of the cytosoloic estrogen receptors that there was a decrease in estrogen mediated prostatic growth. Anti-inflammatory effects of saw palmetto within the prostate have also been demonstrated in a limited study of patients who later underwent open prostatectomy [16]. A significant decrease in congestive prostatitis, stromal edema and intraglandular congestion were noted in patients receiving saw palmetto as compared to those men who were treated with placebo.

Clinical Studies of Saw Palmetto

A number of clinical trials using saw palmetto in men with BPH were published in the 1980's. However, the findings of many of these studies are limited by the inclusion of small numbers of patients often treated for brief intervals of one to three months [17–31]. In a study of 110 men, Champault, et al, found that saw palmetto led to marked improvement in nocturia and dysuria [17]. A significant increase in the peak urinary flow rate was also noted in the men receiving saw palmetto. However, the duration of this study was only one month and validated questionnaires, such as the International Prostate Symptom Score (I-PSS), were not yet available. Using a similar study design, Smith et al. reported no significant difference in the improvement of any subjective or objective measures among patients with BPH receiving saw palmetto or placebo [22]. Due to these conflicting findings, as well as the limitations of small patient numbers and brief treatment intervals, there remained skepticism regarding the efficacy of saw palmetto.

Following a period of very limited study of saw palmetto, several larger scale clinical trials of this agent were performed during the last 5–7 years [5, 6, 14, 23]. Using Permixon in a non-randomized study of 505 men with mild to moderate voiding symptoms, it was noted that the mean peak urinary flow rate increased from 9.8 ml/sec to 12.2 ml/sec [14]. In addition, symptom scores improved from a baseline of 19.0 to 12.4 after treatment with saw palmetto for 3 months. At the end of the study, approximately 88% of patients and physicians deemed the treatment to be successful. A small, but statistically significant decrease in prostate volume of 9.2% was also found among men treated with saw palmetto in this study. Although this was a large-scale study, the lack of placebo controls makes it difficult to draw conclusions regarding the effectiveness of saw palmetto.

At the University of Chicago, we have also conducted an open label study of saw palmetto in men with BPH [6]. Patients received saw palmetto for six months and underwent urodynamic evaluation at the onset and completion of the study. Although the mean symptom score improved from 19.5–12.3, no improvement in any urodynamic parameter, including peak flow rate, detrusor pressure or post-void residual was noted. The saw palmetto was well tolerated and no changes in serum PSA level were noted. Subsequent to this study, we conducted a randomized, placebo-controlled study of saw palmetto in men with BPH [24]. A significant improvement in symptom score was noted in men treated with the active agent as compared with those receiving placebo, but no difference in urinary flow rate was noted between the two groups. Finally, Wilt et al. have published the results of a meta-analysis of 2939 men treated with saw palmetto [23]. This study involved the results of 18 trials and the authors concluded that men treated with saw palmetto had an overall improvement of 1.9 ml/sec in peak urinary flow rate and a drop of 1.4 points in symptom score as compared with controls. However, the findings of this analysis are limited because the mean duration of the 18 studies used was only 9 weeks, and several of the trials did not include a placebo group or involved the use of saw palmetto in combination with other herbal agents.

The largest single study of saw palmetto was a randomized comparison between 1,098 men receiving Permixon or finasteride for six months [5]. This multicenter trial was conducted in Europe and did not include a control group. There was a statistically significant improvement in symptom score and peak urinary flow rate in both groups, although the flow rate increase was slightly greater among men treated with finasteride. While there were few side effects in either group, patients receiving finasteride had a greater incidence of sexual dysfunction. Prostate size was measured by transrectal ultrasound at the outset and completion of the study and decreased by 18% and 6% in those treated with finasteride and Permixon, respectively. In addition, there was no change in serum PSA levels seen with Permixon and a mean decrease of 41% in this serum marker associated with finasteride. These findings suggest that saw palmetto has little or no clinically relevant 5-alpha reductase activity in men with BPH. The investigators in this large trial subsequently stratified their results according to prostate size and noted no significant difference in outcome based on this parameter [25]. The results of the VA Cooperative Trial [26], conducted in the U.S., must be taken into account when assessing the findings of this European trial comparing Permixon and finasteride. In the VA trial, in which men were randomized to receive terazosin, finasteride, both drugs or placebo, the results suggested that finasteride was no more effective than placebo. Therefore, it is possible that the findings of the European study may largely indicate a placebo effect in men receiving Permixon as well as those treated with finasteride.

Marks et al. studied the use of a saw palmetto herbal blend in 44 men who underwent histologic evaluation of the prostate before and after treatment for six months [27]. In this randomized trial, there was no significant difference in the change in symptom score, flow rate or post-void residual urine volume between those treated with the herbal blend or placebo. However, there was a significant increase in prostatic epithelial contraction and in the percentage of atrophic glands among those receiving saw palmetto as compared to those treated with placebo. This is one of the first studies to convincingly demonstrate saw palmetto induced histologic changes in the prostate and may begin to help explain symptomatic improvement in men with BPH treated with this agent.

Saw Palmetto – Summary

Saw palmetto is used by a large number of men in the United States and Europe to help control symptoms related to BPH. Few, if any, adverse effects have been noted with saw palmetto and it has been well demonstrated that this agent has no effect on serum PSA levels. Increasing evidence suggests that saw palmetto leads to histologic changes within the prostate and may have efficacy beyond a placebo effect. However, the precise mechanism of action of saw palmetto in men with BPH remains unclear. At present, men considering the use of saw palmetto can be told that it is safe, will not mask the detection of prostate cancer and may lead to mild to moderate improvement in voiding symptoms.

Pygeum Africanum

Another popular herbal product used by men with BPH is Pygeum Africanum, which is derived from the bark of the African plum tree. The major components of Pygeum that are felt to be active are phytosterols, triterpenoids and linear alcohols [1, 2]. Anti-inflammatory effects may also be seen with Pygeum and these may be mediated by inhibition of prostatic fibroblast proliferation [27, 28]. The phytosterols present in Pygeum may also have an inhibitory effect on prostaglandin E2 and F2 alpha production which may improve voiding symptoms via a decrease in vascular congestion and local hyperemia within the prostate.

Studies have also suggested that Pygeum may improve urinary symptoms through actions on the detrusor muscle of the bladder rather than through direct action on the prostate [29, 30]. Investigators have studied the effect of Tadenan, a Pygeum extract available in Europe, on the detrusor response to bladder outlet obstruction in animal models [29, 30]. In men with bladder outlet obstruction, the bladder muscle hypertrophies which may lead to reduced bladder capacity and hypercontractility. These effects may have a major impact on voiding symptoms due to BPH. Studies in animals have demonstrated that the experimental creation of partial bladder outlet obstruction leads to collagen deposition within the bladder wall as well as smooth muscle hypertrophy [30]. There is biochemical evidence of bladder dysfunction in such animals as demonstrated by a decrease in citrate synthase and calcium ATP'ase activities [29]. In addition, Tadenan has been shown to inhibit growth factor mediated fibroblast hyperproliferation, which may help counteract bladder outlet obstruction induced fibroblast hyperplasia in the prostate [29]. Levin et al. have used Tadenan in rabbits and then created partial bladder outlet obstruction [30]. When compared with control animals, those receiving Tadenan had significantly less detrusor dysfunction suggesting a protective effect on the bladder musculature using this agent. In a subsequent study it was shown that rabbits pre-treated with Tadenan had less metabolic dysfunction within the bladder muscle as compared to control animals after a period of bladder outlet obstruction [29].

Another animal study was performed in which Tadenan was given to rats prior to subcutaneous injection of DHT [31]. It appeared that Tadenan helped to partially block the development of bladder outlet obstruction mediated by DHT. In addition, histologic evidence from the prostates of rats given Tadenan suggested that there was a suppression of growth of the ventral lobes of the prostate. Therefore, it appears that Tadenan may help to counteract DHT mediated prostate growth. Although these findings are provocative and may indicate alternative mechanisms by which Pygeum may help men with BPH, it is difficult to draw conclusions regarding these animal studies. In general, the dosages used in these studies were well above physiologic levels that would be used in humans. In addition, it is not feasible to treat men with Tadenan prior to the development of bladder outlet obstruction. It is not clear whether this agent might reverse long-standing changes in the detrusor muscle if given after urinary symptoms develop.

Clinical Studies

A small number of clinical trials have been published concerning the use of Pygeum in men with BPH [32–34]. Most of these studies have involved a limited number of patients treated for brief intervals. Dufour et al. treated 120 men with Pygeum for 6 weeks and reported a significant improvement in urinary symptoms, such as nocturia, hesitancy and sense of incomplete bladder emptying, as compared with patients receiving placebo [32]. In another trial of 263 men treated for 2 months, "significant symptomatic improvement" was noted in 66% of those receiving Pygeum as compared with 31% of men who were randomized to the placebo arm [33]. Finally, in a study of 235 men with symptomatic BPH, Chatelain et al. randomized men to receive one of two different dosages of Pygeum [34]. Both groups had significant improvement in the mean symptom score and urinary flow rate, although no difference in outcome was noted based on the dosage of Pygeum. Overall, there is a suggestion that Pygeum leads to improvement in urinary symptoms. However, further study is needed to provide convincing evidence concerning the efficacy of this agent.

Phytosterols

Phytosterols are believed to be the most important compound in a variety of herbal products used by men with BPH. A number of different mechanisms of action have been associated with phytosterols, including 5-alpha reductase inhibition, anti-androgenic effects, growth factor inhibition, anti-estrogenic effects and others [1, 35]. Among the phytosterols, beta-sitosterol has been suggested to be the most important for men with lower urinary tract symptoms and BPH [35, 36]. In one of the best conducted studies of herbal therapies in men with enlarged prostates, a form of beta-sitosterol sold in Germany (Harzol) was tested in 200 men at multiple medical centers [36]. Among men receiving Harzol, the symptom score improved from a mean 14.9 to 7.5 after treatment for six months. In comparison, those men given placebo had a mean symptom score decrease from 15.1 to 12.8. The difference between the two treatment groups was statistically significant ($p<0.01$). There was also a significantly greater increase in the peak urinary flow rate and decrease in the post-void residual urine volume seen in the Harzol group. No change in prostate size occurred with Harzol and no severe adverse effects were noted.

Further study with Harzol included an open-label extension among the same patient population reported above [37]. After 18 months, those patients who continued to take Harzol had stable measurements for all outcome variables. However, those patients not receiving further therapy had continued worsening of their urinary symptoms and post-void residual urine volume. In addition, those patients initially randomized to receive placebo were crossed over to the Harzol group after the completion of the trial. Among these patients, similar subjective and objective improvements were seen as in those men initially randomized to receive the active agent. Other studies using alternative beta-sitosterol preparations have also been presented and have generally demonstrated similar results as those seen with Harzol [38–40].

Pollen Extract

Cernilton is a product composed of the pollen extract of several plants that is available in Sweden and some other European countries. A small number of clinical trials have suggested that Cernilton may be of benefit in men with BPH [1, 41]. As is true for most herbal products used to treat urinary symptoms, phytosterols are felt to be the most important component of Cernilton [41]. In animal studies, Cernilton has been demonstrated to lead to epithelial atrophy in the prostate, as well as a decrease in prostatic acid phosphatase and zinc levels [42]. In addition, inhibition of human cell line growth of prostatic cells and down regulation of hormone stimulated growth of transplanted BPH tissue have also been seen with Cernilton in animal models [41, 43].

Buck et al. have studied the use of Cernilton in men awaiting surgery for BPH [41]. In this placebo controlled trial, 60 men received either Cernilton or placebo for six months. A statistically significant improvement was seen in urinary symptoms among patients receiving the active agent as compared with those treated with placebo (69%

vs. 29%, p<0.009). While no change was seen in urinary flow rate in either group in this study, post-void residual urine volume decreased significantly in those men treated with Cernilton as compared with controls. In addition, a decrease in prostate size was noted among patients receiving Cernilton.

The role of Cernilton has also been investigated among men with chronic prostatitis and prostatodynia [44]. In a non-randomized, uncontrolled study, a subjectively favorable response was noted in 78% (56/72) of men with chronic perineal pain, dysuria and frequency, who had no objective evidence of infection [44]. Finally, in a study comparing the effectiveness of Cernilton in comparison with the Pygeum extract, Tadenan, superior subjective and objective results were seen with the pollen product [45].

Other Phytotherapeutic Products

A number of other plant products have been used to treat men with BPH. In most cases, very limited information is available regarding the effectiveness of these agents. Bazoton is a product that has been tested in Hungary and consists of an extract from the plant Radix urticae [46]. It appears that Barzoton may be an inhibitor of intracellular sex hormone binding globulin receptors and in limited, uncontrolled study leads to subjective and objective improvement in men with BPH [46].

Stinging nettles (Urtica dioica) have been used extensively in Germany and have been suggested to suppress prostate cell growth and metabolism, among other actions, in men with BPH [47, 48]. Similar to other infrequently used agents, improvement in urinary symptoms and flow rates have been shown in small, brief clinical trials of stinging nettles [49]. Other trials have investigated the efficacy of herbal agents in combination [50, 51].

However, the value of these studies has generally been limited by small numbers of participants and short treatment intervals. Other agents that have been suggested to be of benefit in men with BPH but have not been tested include unicorn root, rye pollen and pumpkin seeds.

Summary

The use of alternative medications to treat a variety of conditions continues to grow in the United States. Unfortunately, most physicians have limited knowledge of the use of these products and are thus unable to provide advice to their patients. Many factors have increased the interest in alternative agents among American consumers, including the proliferation of health food stores, aggressive marketing in a variety of media outlets and the growing popularity of the Internet. Men with BPH may be considered ideal candidates to use herbal therapies since the condition is chronic and the primary goal of treatment in most cases is improvement in subjective symptoms and quality of life. Standard medical and surgical therapies for BPH may be associated with side effects and many patients also feel that "natural remedies" are inherently more desirable for a variety of reasons.

Although there is increasing scientific evidence to suggest that saw palmetto, pygeum and beta-sitosterol may be effective in men with BPH beyond a placebo effect, much work needs to be done to further our understanding of these agents. A number of proposed mechanisms of action have been suggested for these products, but clinical evidence to support these actions is largely lacking. Additional difficulties in advising patients regarding the use of herbal therapies include the lack of standardization of these agents. Since there is little if any oversight of the production and distribution of non-prescription products in the U.S., there are likely to be significant discrepancies in the content of similar products sold by different companies. This issue may be further confused by the widespread availability of combination products that often contain vitamins and minerals in addition to a variety of plant extracts. A number of consumer watchdog groups and Internet sites have tested herbal products and many of these products have been demonstrated to contain insufficient quantities of the active ingredients. Despite these limitations, the growing popularity of herbal therapies for BPH is likely to continue and it is important for physicians to educate themselves regarding these agents so that they can speak knowledgeably with their patients.

References

1. Lowe FC and Ku JC. Phytotherapy in treatment of benign prostatic hyperplasia: a critical review. Urology 1996; 12–20.
2. Mowrey DB. Herbal tonic therapies. New Canaan: Keats Publishing, Inc., 1993.
3. Delos S, Iehle C and Martin PM. Inhibition of the activity of basic 5-alpha reductase (type 1) detected in DU 145 cells and expressed in insect cells. J Steroid Biochem Mol Biol 1994; 48: 347–352.
4. Bayne CW, Grant ES, Chapman K and Habib FK. Characterisation of a new co-culture model for BPH which expresses 5-alpha reductase types 1 and 2: the effects of Permixon on DHT formation. J Urol 1997;157 (supp. 4): abstract 755.
5. Carraro JC, Raynaud JP, Koch G et al. Comparison of phytotherapy (Permixon) with finasteride in the treatment of benign prostate hyperplasia: a randomized international study of 1098 patients. Prostate 1996; 29: 231–240.
6. Gerber GS, Zagaja GP, Bales GT, Chodak GW and Contreras BA. Saw palmetto (Serenoa repens) in men with lower urinary tract symptoms: effects on urodynamic parameters and voiding symptoms. Urology (in press).
7. Chevalier G, Benard P, Cousse H and Bengone T. Distribution study of radioactivity in rats after oral administration of the lipido/sterolic extract of Serenoa repens (Permixon) supplemented with $(1-1^4 C)$-lauric acid or $(4-1^4C)$-sitosterol. Eur J Drug Metab Pharmacokin 1997; 22: 73–83.
8. De Bernardi di Valserra M, Tripodi AS, Contos S, Germogli M. Serenoa repens capsules: a bioequivalent study. Acta Toxicol Ther 1994; 15 (1): 21–39.
9. Sultan C, Terraza A, Devillier C, Carilla E, Briley M, Loire C, Descomps B. Inhibition of androgen metabolism and binding by a liposterolic extract of "Serenoa repens B" in human foreskin fibroblasts. J Steroid Biochem 1984; 20: 515–519
10. Carilla E, Briley M, Fauran F, Sultan C, Duvilliers C. Binding of Permixon, a new treatment for prostatic benign hyperplasia, to the cytosolic androgen receptor in the rat prostate. J Steroid Biochem 1984; 20: 521–523.
11. Silverio F, Sciarra A, D'Eramo G, Casale P, Di Nicola S, Buscarini N, Sciarra F. Response to tissue androgen and epidermal growth factor concentrations to the administration of finasteride, flutamide, and Serenoa repens in patients with BPH. Eur Urol 1996; 30 (supp. 2): abstract 317.
12. Rhodes L, Primka RL, Berman C, Vergult G, Gabriel M, Pierre Malice M, Gibelin B. Comparison of finasteride (Proscar), a 5-alpha reductase inhibitor, and various commercial plant extracts in In vitro and In viv 5-alpha reductase inhibition. Prostate 1993; 22: 43–51.
13. Strauch G, Perles P, Vergult G, Gabriel M, Gibelin B, Cummings S, Malbecq W, Pierre-Malice M. Comparison of finasteride Proscar) and Serenoa repens (Permixon) in the inhibition of 5-alpha reductase in healthy male volunteers. Eur Urol 1994; 26: 247–252.
14. Braeckman J. The extract of Serenoa repens in the treatment of benign prostatic hyperplasia: a multicenter open study. Curr Ther Res 1994; 55: 776–785.

15. Di Silverio F, D'Eramo G, Lubrano C, Flammia GP, Sciarra A, Palma E, Caponera M, Sciarra F. Evidence that Serenoa repens extract displays an antiestrogenic activity in prostatic tissue of benign prostatic hypertrophy patients. Eur Urol 1992; 21: 309–314.

16. Helpap B, Oehler U, Weisser H, Bach D, Ebeling L. Morphology of benign prostatic hyperplasia after treatment with sabal extract IDS 89 or placebo. J Urol Path 1995; 3: 175–182.

17. Champault G, Patel JC, Bonnard AM. A double-blind trial of an extract of the plant Serenoa repens in benign prostatic hyperplasia. Br J Clin Pharmacol 1984; 18: 461–462.

18. Cukier J, Ducassou J, Le Guillou M, Leriche A et al. Serenoa repens extract vs. placebo. Pharmacol Clin 1985; 4: 15–21.

19. Descotes JL, Rambeaud JJ, Deschaseaux P, Faure G. Placebo controlled evaluation of the efficacy and tolerability of Permixon in benign prostatic hyperplasia after exclusion of placebo responders. Clin Drug Invest 1995; 9: 291–297.

20. Emile E, Lo Cigno M, Petrone U. Clinical results on a new drug in the treatment of benign prostatic hyperplasia (Permixon). Urologia 1983; 50: 1042–1049.

21. Plasker GL, Brogden RN. Serenoa repens (Permixon). A review of its pharmacology and therapeutic efficacy in benign prostatic hyperplasia. Drugs and Aging 1996; 5: 379–395.

22. Smith HR, Memon A, Smart CJ, Dewbury K. The value of Permixon in benign prostatic hypertrophy Br J Urol 1986; 58: 36–40.

23. Wilt TJ, Ishani A, Stark G, MacDonald R, Lau J and Mulrow C. Saw palmetto extracts for treatment of benign prostatic hyperplasia. A systematic review. JAMA 280:1604–1609, 1998.

24. Gerber GS, Kuznetsov D, Johnson BC and Burstein JD. Randomized, double-blind, placebo-controlled trial of saw palmetto in men with lower urinary tract symptoms. Urology (in press).

25. Chopin DK, Perrin P, Authie D, Deschaseaux P, Perier A and Raynaud JP. Prostatic volume does not correlate with efficacy of treatment for mild to moderate benign prostatic hyperplasia using either finasteride or phytotherapy (Permixon). Presented at the 4th International Consultation on BPH, Paris, 1997.

26. Lepor H, Williford WO, Barry MJ, Brawer MK et al., The efficacy of terazosin, finasteride, or both in benign prostatic hyperplasia. New Engl J Med 1996; 335: 533–539.

27. Yablonsky F, Nicolas V, Riffaud JP, Bellamy F. Antiproliferative effect of Pygeum africanum extract on rat prostatic fibroblasts. J Urol 1997; 157: 2381–2387.

28. Paubert-Braquet M, Monboisse JC, Servent-Saez N, Serikoff A, Cave A, Hocquemiller R, Cupont C, Fourneau C, Borel JP. Inhibition of bFGF and EGF-induced proliferation of 3T3 fibroblasts by extract of Pygeum africanum (Tadenan). Biomed Pharmacother 1994; 48 (supp. 1): 43–47.

29. Levin RM, Riffaud JP, Bellamy F, Rohrmann D, Habib M, Krasnopolsky L, Haugaard N, Zhao Y, Wein AJ. Effects of Tadenan pretreatment on bladder physiology and biochemistry following partial outlet obstruction. J Urol 1996; 156: 2084–2088.

30. Krasnopolsky L, Zhao Y, and Wein AJ. Protective effect of Tadenan on bladder function secondary to partial outlet obstruction. J Urol 155: 1446–1470, 1996.

31. Choo MS, Bellamy F and Constantinou CE. Functional evaluation of Tadenan on micturition and experimental prostate growth induced with exogenous dihydrotestosterone. Urology 55: 292–298, 2000.

32. Dufour B, Choquenet C, Revol M, Faure G and Jorest R. Controlled study of the effects of Pygeum africanum extract on the functional symptoms of prostatic adenoma. Ann Urol 18: 193–195, 1984.

33. Barlet A, Albrecht J, Aubert A, Fischer M, Grof F, Grothuesmann HG, Masson JC, Mazeman E, Mermon R, Reichelt H. Wirksamkeit eines Extraktes aus Pygeum africanum in der medikamentosen Therapie von Miktionsstörungen infolge einer benignen Prostathyperplasie: Bewertung objektiver und subjektiver Parameter. Wie Klin Wochenschr 1990; 102: 667–673.

34. Chatelain C, Autet W, Brackman F. Comparison of Once and Twice Daily Dosage Forms of Pygeum africanum Extract in Patients with Benign Prostatic Hyperplasia: A Randomized, Double Blind Study, with Long Term Open Label Extension. Urology 1997; 54(3): 473–8.

34a. Berges RR, Windeier J, Trampisch HJ, Senge T. Randomised, placebo-controlled, double-blind clinical trial of beta-sitosterol in patients with benign prostatic hyperplasia. Lancet 1995; 345: 1529–1532.

35. Carbin BE, Larsson B, Lindahl O. Treatment of benign prostatic hyperplasia with phytosterols. Br J Urol 1987; 66: 639–641.

36. Berges RR, Windeier J, Trampisch HJ and Senge T. Randomised, placebo-controlled, double-blind clinical trial of beta-sitosterol in patients with benign prostatic hyperplasia. Lancet 345: 1529–1532, 1995.

37. Berges RR, Kassen A, Senge T. Treatment of Symptomatic Benign Prostatic Hyperplasia with B-Sitosterol: An 18 Month Follow-up. Br J Urol 2000; 85: 842–6.

38. Dreikorn K, Richter R and Schonhofer PS. Konservative, nicht-hormonelle Behandlung der benignen Prostatahyperplasia. Urologe 29: 8–16, 1990.

39. Klippel KF, Schipp B. A placebo-controlled, double-blind clinical trial of B-sitosterol (phytosterol) for the treatment of benign prostatic hyperplasia. 4th International Consultation on BPH, Paris, Abstract 5, 1997.

40. Klippel KF, Hiltl DM, Schipp B. Randomized, double blinded placebo controlled trial to evaluate the efficacy of B-sitosterol (phytosterol) in patients with obstructive and irritative symptoms due to BPH. 4th International Consultation on BPH, Paris, Abstract 42, 1997.

41. Buck AC, Cox R, Rees WM, Ebeling L, John A. Treatment of outflow tract obstruction due to benign prostatic hyperplasia with the pollen extract, Cernilton. A double-blind, placebo-controlled study. Br J Urol 1990; 66: 398–404.

42. Ito R, Ishii M, Yamashita S. Cernitin pollen-extract (Cernilton): antiprostatic hypertrophic action of Cernitin pollen-extract (Cernilton). Pharmacometrics 1986; 31: 1–11.

43. Habib FK, Buck AC, Ross M. In vitro valuation of the pollen extract, Cernitin T-60, in the regulation of prostate cell growth. Br J Urol 1990; 66: 393–397.

44. Rugendorff EW, Weidner W, Ebeling L, Buck AC. Results of treatment with pollen extract (Cernilton N) in chronic prostatitis and prostatodynia. Br J Urol 1993; 71: 433–438.

45. Dutkiewicz S. Usefulness of Cernilton in the treatment of benign prostatic hyperplasia. Int Urol Nephrol 1996; 28: 49–53.

46. Romics I. Observations with Bazoton in the management of prostatic hyperplasia. Int Urol Nephrol 1987; 19: 293–297.

47. Hryb DJ, Khan MS, Romas NA, Rosner W. The effects of extracts of the roots of the stinging nettle (Urtica dioica) on the interaction of SHBG with its receptor on human prostatic membranes. Planta Med 1995; 61: 31–32.

48. Wagner W, Willer F, Samtleben R, Boos G. Search for the antiprostatic principle of stinging nettle (Urtica dioica) roots. Phytomedicine 1994; 1: 213–224.

49. Konrad L, Muller HH, Lenz C et al. Anitproliferative Effect on Human Prostate Cancer Cells by a Stinging Nettle Root (Uritica dioica) Extract. Planta Med 2000; 66(1): 44–7.

49a. Vontobel HP, Herzog R, Rutishauser GH. Ergebnisse einer Doppelblind studie uber die Wirksamkeit von ERU-Kapseln in der konservativen Behandlung der benignen Prostatahyperplasie. Urologe (A) 1985; 24: 49–51.

50. Carbin BE, Larsson B, Lindahl O. Treatment of benign prostatic hyperplasia with phytosterols. Br J Urol 1990; 66: 639–641.

51. Metzker H, Martin C. Efficacy and safety of the Sabal Urtica combination PRO 160/120 in the treatment of patients with benign prostatic hyperplasia (a placebo-controlled double-blind long term clinical trial). 1997; 4th International Consensus on BPH, Paris, abstract 15.

27 Alternative and Complementary Methods in Cancer Treatment, Palliation, and Prevention

N.S. Cherniack

Introduction

Cancer is the leading cause of death in the United States with lung, colon, breast and prostate cancer being the most common cancers in both whites and blacks. Conventional treatments of surgery, radiation, and chemotherapy often produce serious adverse effects. It's not surprising then that studies show that about 50% or more of patients with cancer use some form of alternative therapy [1–4]. About 60% of those using unconventional treatments used some form of psychological or spiritual therapy. Fifty percents use various vitamins and nutrients. Half of the patients use herbals. There are probably many more who use alternative and complementary methods to reduce the risk of cancer. There have been no specific studies of the use of alternative methods by the elderly.

Frequently patients do not inform their primary physician or their oncologist of this use. For example a study of 453 cancer patients showed that 83 percent used at least one form of complementary/alternative medicine [2]. Even when psychotherapy and spiritual practices were excluded 69 percent had used a form of alternative medicine in their cancer treatment. Some alternative therapies may interfere with chemotherapy while others may mask the occurrence of symptoms. The forms of alternative medicine used include nutritional methods including specific diets as well as nutritional supplements, herbal, medicinal including enzymes, and certain polypeptides and amino acids, naturopathic which uses only natural treatments, homeopathic, body movement and manipulation usually based on the belief that life forces or "chi" blockage leads to illness that can be unblocked by treatments such as acupressure, acupuncture, yoga, and therapeutic touch, and finally psychological and spiritual techniques which use counseling,visualization of positive situations, meditation, art and music therapy, and religious rituals [4].

In general alternative and complementary treatments are used to prevent, to treat, and to palliate cancers. In most cases alternative and complementary methods have been assessed for their action in cancer in general. More recent and in ongoing NIH supported evaluations have focused on specific cancer types. Also there have been increasing numbers of studies using herbals or other alternative medicine products in vitro against specific cell types. Even though some herbal extracts and other agents have an anti proliferative effect in cell cultures of tumor cells, clinical trials have not been encouraging in most instances where they have been attempted. There are so far no established alternative methods of cancer treatment [4].

Cancer Prevention

There is suggestive evidence that some diets reduce cancer risks [5–16]. No vitamins or nutritional supplements have been shown to definitely prevent cancers, but data about such supplements has generally arisen from studies concerned with the evaluation of some other treatment as their main objective and may have been too brief to fully assess preventive effects.

Alternative and Complementary Approaches that have been Claimed to Prevent Cancer

▶ Dietary high fiber diets, low red meat consumption, low fat diets, broccoli consumption, macrobiotic diets
▶ High doses of vitamins c, e, d, beta-carotene, co enzyme q10, selenium and zinc
▶ Use of herbals and other plant products such as green tea, grape seed extracts, citrus flavenoids, soybeans
▶ Smoking cessation
▶ Abstinence from alcohol

Prevention takes two forms; avoiding cancer risks, and detoxifying or nullifying in some way the effects of carcinogens

Avoiding Cancer risks

A diet rich in fresh fruits and vegetables, high in fiber, containing minimal amounts of red meat seems to reduce the risks of cancer of the epithelia [5, 6, 8–10]. Fruits and vegetables contain nutrients such as vitamin A and C, which may have antioxidant effects [13–23]. Vitamin C has been advocated as an adjuvant in cancer treatment as well as a preventative, but controlled studies have failed to find a treatment benefit [13, 19, 23]. Vitamin A and related carotenoids have also been claimed to be of benefit in cancer prevention and treatment [14–16]. A number of different studies have found Vitamins A, C, and E to have anti tumor growth effects in cell lines and an association between intake and the occurrence of cancers. Excessive intake of vitamin A has toxic effects [14, 15].

1-alpha 25-dihydroxy vitamin D, the active metabolite of vitamin D, has been demonstrated to have an anti-proliferative- effect in prostate cancer cell lines. Because the vitamin causes hypercalcemia it is not widely employed in chemotherapy [22].

Preserved and smoked foods and beer have been reported to increase the risk of some cancers presumably by conversion of nitrites and nitrates to carcinogenic nitrosamines. Diets rich in fat have been related to the occurrence of many cancer particularly colon and prostate. The chances of getting breast cancer may be increased High fiber seem to lower the occurrence of colon as compared to low fiber diets but they also generally are low in fats. Obesity itself may be a risk factor for some cancers. Red meat consumption has been implicated in some cancers like those of the renal cell [10–14].

Diets rich in certain phytocemicals, on the other hand, may reduce cancer risks [24–26]. One polypenolic flavenoid, isolated from the fruits of milk thistle, silymarin, has been used as a skin cancer preventative in laboratory animals.

Broccoli ingestion also may reduce cancer risks. It is rich in both vitamins A and C, but in addition has isothiocyanates, which have anti-cancer properties blocking the growth of melanoma cells in culture [18, 19]. Broccoli is a member of the cruciferous family of vegetables, which include cauliflower, cabbage, and kale) which may all have some protective action against cancer. Indole-3-carbinol found in broccoli and cabbage is an anti-oxidant.

Smoking cigarettes not only is the main cause of respiratory tract cancers but also substantially elevates the risks of bladder, and kidney cancer. There are associations between cigarette smoking and increased stomach, liver, prostate, colon, rectal, and cervical cancer. Users of smokeless tobacco and pipe and cigar smokers have increased chances of developing cancers of the oral cavity, larynx, and esophagus [27–29].

Caffeine in large amounts may increase the risk of pancreatic cancer. But coffee and tea consumption are risk factors for urinary tract cancers. Cigarette smoking and excessive use of alcohol are associated [28, 29]. But alcohol by itself in quantities greater than four drinks per day increases the risks or oral and pharyngeal cancers. Folio acid has said to decrease any cancer risk presented by alcohol. In the Calvados region of France, the increased incidence of esophageal cancer has been linked to apple brandy consumption. Moonshine whisky may also increase risks for esophageal cancer. The incidence of liver cancer may be associated with excess alcohol consumption.

Psychological stress has been said to predispose to the occurrence of cancer with little or no evidence. It's been claimed that the loss of a parent, a sibling or even a pet can give rise to cancer

Agents Used to Counteract Cancer Risks

Oxygen radical formation has been implicated both in aging and as cause of DNA damage. Anti-oxidants might mitigate the effects of some mutagens. Many of the agents that have been advocated in cancer prevention are anti-oxidants Diets rich in flavenoids have been associated with a reduced risk of cancer. Vitamin C, Vitamin E, beta-carotene, selenium, coenzyme Q10, zinc and bioflavenoids are anti-oxidants found in foods, and in massive doses have been used as cancer preventives [30–35].

Macrobiotic diets are used as part a system for maintaining general health and relieving cancer. They are said to consist of an optimal mixture of yin and yang foods, and is mainly composed of whole grains, vegetables, nuts and seeds [36].

A number of products derived from plants may have anti-oxidant actions of varying potency and have been touted as cancer preventatives [14, 15, 26, 37–40]. These include green tea, grape seed extract, and ginkgo bilbo, but the evidence is not strong has not been uniformly positive Epidemiological studies show an association between green tea consumption and a reduced risk of various cancers in humans. The polyphenols in green tea mainly epigallocatechin-3-gallate (EGCg) are good anti-oxidants, but have other biological properties [26]. They inhibit the production of pro-inflammatory prostaglandins and leukotrienes. They seem to have thermogenic properties and may aid in weight control programs. Recent studies in human glioblastoma cells suggest that EGCg inhibits matrix metalloproteins both in vitro and in vivo and could thus prevent tumor spread [26]. In vitro EGCg may inhibit the gene activator AP-1 and interfere with cell signal transduction. However the mechanisms that produce any anti-cancer properties of green tea remain largely uncertain. Although green tea has low toxicity it does contain caffeine, anywhere from 15 to 50 mgm per cup.

The citrus flavenoid, naringenin found in grapefruits inhibited growth in a human breast cancer line as did hesperetin found in orange juice [14, 15]. While rats fed high fat diets developed more mammary tumors than rats fed diets low in fat those given orange juice or diets supplemented with naringenin had smaller tumor burdens even though the rats themselves were larger.

Products derived from grape seeds contain proanthocyanins, a group of polyphenolic bioflavenoids that have anti-oxidant properties [37, 38]. PCO a bioflavenoid complex that can be extracted from grapes, blueberries, and pine bark has several compounds that have anti-oxidant effects and has been advocated for the prevention of ulcers, cataracts, cardiovascular, and other disease as well as cancer mainly on the basis of anecdotal reports.

Soybeans contain isoflavone phytoestrogens like genistein that inhibit mammary cell growth and suppress the development of anthracene induced breast cancer. Genisten may have anti-oxidant actions. It can inhibit tyrosine kinase and tropisomerasse II. Isoflavones may also inhibit angiogenesis [14, 15].

There is a long list of other substances, which have been reported at one time, or another to have anti-cancer effects. For example some amino acids like cysteine may inhibit tumors and protect against the damaging effects of radiation and certain forms of chemotherapy. Restriction in the diet of tyrosine and phenylalanine may also slow tumor growth, but on the other hand tryptophane and glutamine may stimulate tumor growth.

Likewise acidophilus, bacteria found in the normal gastrointestinal tract and in yogurt, has been claimed to have anticancer as other health promoting actions.

Treatment of Cancer

There are no alternative or complementary treatments of cancer that have been accepted as efficacious [3]. Some of the techniques and agents used have according to their proponents anti-oxidant, immune stimulating or anti-angiogenic actions. With others the effects claimed have been more general such as body strengthening or detoxifying. Treatments that have been proposed consist primarily of whole body and dietary regimens, the use of certain herbal mixtures, animal products such as shark and bovine cartilage, and compounds such as laetrile Some studies in cell cultures using extracts of herbs or cartilage have had positive effects. However, controlled studies in humans when they have been performed have been negative or inconclusive. Studies using shark cartilage as an adjuvant in treating lung cancer are on going.

Alternative and Complementary Approaches that have been Advocated for the Treatment of Cancer

▶ Whole body regimens such as those proposed by Revici, Gerson, Issel, Kelley etc.
▶ Herbal and other plant products such as essiac tea, iscador (mistletoe extract), pc-spes, milk thistle extracts, laetrile, resveratrol, lentinam, psk
▶ High doses of vitamins
▶ Animal products, like fish oils and other polyunsaturated fats, bovine and shark cartilage, krebiozen
▶ Drug mixtures like cancell
▶ Physical techniques like acupuncture, aromatherapy, massage, shiatsu, therapeutic touch
▶ Psychological techniques like meditation, hypnotherapy, and relaxation therapy

The "whole body" regimes aim at strengthen the body's natural defenses and at detoxification. The following are some examples of treatment regimens.

In Issel's whole body therapy, teeth, which contain mercury amalgam, are removed, and the diet reordered to contain only natural materials. Tobacco, tea, and coffee are forbidden. Oxidation therapy is given and vaccines and hyperthermia may be also used while psychotherapy is encouraged. In Revici therapy the aim is to improve the balance between anabolic and catabolic activities. Selenium, copper, and oxygen are given. Gerson therapy administers a special diet which involves hourly consumption of crushed fruit and vegetables mainly apples and carrots. Caffeine is given rectally 3–4 times a day. The idea is to reduce body sodium content and remove dead cells. Pepsin, potassium, pancreatin, and thyroid extracts are also given. Kelley's nutritional-metabolic therapy uses a diet consisting of whole grains, fruits, and vegetables with pancreatic enzyme administration. Detoxification procedures are also employed [3].

Herbal mixtures and plant products have been used in treating cancer. When tested no effectiveness in cancer treatment has been demonstrated. Examples of such agents are Essiac tea, PC-SPES and mistletoe extracts [3, 41–47].

Essiac tea is an herbal mixture developed by Renee Casisse, a Canadian nurse who claimed it was based on traditional Native American medicine. Essiac tea is not freely marketed either in the United States or Canada. A number of companies now sell competing Essiac teas since Caisse never made her formula public. Recipes for making Essiac tea are available on the Internet. They generally consist of four major ingredients, burdock Indian rhubarb, sorrel, and slippery elm. These substances have been studied separately in vitro. Some chemicals extractable from Indian rhubarb and from burdock have some anti-tumor effect. Some cases of toxicity from drinking burdock root tea have been reported [3].

Mistletoe treatment for cancer seems to have been advocated first by Rudolf Steiner who advocated a system of thought known as antroposopy, a kind of holistic medicine. He believed mistletoe would work because it expresses itself in a rhythm, which is opposed to the growing rhythm of the other plants and could exert a regulating effect on tumors. Currently it is thought that mistletoe may act by binding of mistletoe lectin by its B chain to the cell membrane, followed by endocytosis and enzymatic inhibition of ribosomes. Mistletoe lecitin extract has been claimed to have immune-modulating actions, inducing tumor necrosis factor, increasing natural killer cell activity, activating macrophages, and increasing production of interleukin-1 thereby inhibiting the spread of cancer cells in studies of mice with skin melanomas. It is sold commercially as Iscar or Iscador with additional ingredients sometimes added [42, 43, 45].

It is usually given by injection for several months several times a week. It is widely used in Central Europe but its efficacy has not been verified in clinical studies where it had no beneficial effect.

In a study by Stuer-Vogt in which 407 patients were studied, the deaths due to tumor were about the same in treated and untreated groups but slightly higher in the mistletoe treated group. Relapse rate and the development of distant metastases was not influenced by mistletoe lecithin treatment

PC-SPES is a commercially available mixture of eight herbs that has an estrogenic effect and has a beneficial effect in patients with prostate cancer [46, 47]. But it has potent side effects that include breast tenderness, venous thrombosis, and loss of libido. It contains isatis, Panax-pseudo ginseng, Chrysathemum, licorice, saw palmetto, skullcap, ganoderma lubiium, and rabdosia rubescens. In a prostate epithelial cell line LNCaP it reduced cell growth, increased apoptosis, and decreased secreted and intracellular levels of PSA. Clinical trials showed reductions of PSA, but levels rose again when PC-SPES was discontinued and there was no effect on prostate growth. Because the use of PC-SPES is unregulated there is concern that it use could confound interpretation of the results of more standard treatments.

Silymarin, a phytochemical, that can be extracted from milk thistle is used in Europe to treat liver and gall bladder diseases but also causes regression of skin tumors in mice [3, 44].

Laetrile, "vitamin B_{17}," a purported anti-cancer remedy is related chemically to amygadalin, which is found in apricot pits [39, 40]. Amygdalins can be enzymatically broken down to glucose, benzaldehyde, and cyanide. Amygdalin is the main constituent of products sold as laetrile. It is a member of a class of compounds, beta-cyanogetic glucosides, which are found in common vegetables such as maize, sorghum, lima, kidney beans, and almonds among others.

One theory proposed that cancer cells are rich in an enzyme, which causes amygdalin to release cyanide killing the cancer cells. This enzyme is also found in trophoblasts, but not in non-cancerous cells. A 1982 trial of laetrile sponsored by NCI examined the effect of the agent in 175 patients with cancer. Amygdalin was injected for 21 days. Vitamins and pancreatic enzymes were also given. All of the patients showed disease progression 7 months after completing treatment. NCI concluded that the laetrile was not effective. It is not approved by the FDA for use in the United States but is manufactured and can be obtained in Mexico.

Resveratrol is a phytoalexin found in many plants including grapes and peanuts, and has an anti-cancer action. It is a powerful antioxidant, which can inhibit several enzymes such as DNA polymerase and cyclooxygenase 1 and 2 [38, 47]. It's not clear whether resveratrol exerts its effect in an androgen –independent manner. In a human prostate cell line resveratrol depressed cell proliferation. It also inhibited the growth of both hormone sensitive and hormone refractory breast cell cultures.

CanCell is a liquid which is claimed to eradicate cancer by lowering the voltage of cancer cells causing them to be digested. CanCell contains inositol, nitric acid, sodium sulfite, potassium hydroxide, sulfuric acid and catechol. The NCI in1991 reported it could not find evidence that CanCell was useful in treating cancer [3].

Hydrazine sulfate based on early studies was believed to produce regression of tumors and improvement in symptoms in cancer patients but this has not been confirmed by later investigations [48,49].

Bio-oxidative therapies are based on the belief that cancer is caused by oxygen deficiency and that cancer can be cured if the neoplastic tissue is exposed to high concentrations of oxygen by producing ozone or hydrogen peroxide. There is no experimental evidence that supports the usefulness of this concept in cancer therapy [49].

Polyunsaturated fatty acids (PUFA) in biological systems can undergo lipid peroxidation with the formation of free radicals [21, 24, 32 ,33]. The lipid peroxides rapidly break down giving rise to aldehydes, which can reduce the rate of cellular growth and proliferation. Low levels of PUFA are cytostatic but higher levels can kill cells. Studies in laboratory animals fed a diet containing peroxidized fish oil show reduced tumor growth that is partially but not entirely reversed by anti-oxidants. This suggests that all of the actions of PUFA are not due to oxidation. Investigation in cell cultures showed that the toxic effects of doxorubicin and cisplatin were enhanced by PUFA. These observations support the idea that PUFA may enhance the effect of some neoplastic agents.

Lentinan and PSK are products derived from mushrooms, that have been claimed to have an anti-tumor action by stimulating the immune system. PSK is used extensively in Japan where it is sometimes given in conjunction with standard chemotherapy. It can be taken orally, while lentinan is injected [45].

Krebiozen is prepared from the serum of horses injected with an extract of actinomyces bovis. The serum is extracted with an organic solvent to obtain a substance, which has antigrowth properties. After extensive study of documents submitted to the NCI twenty years ago by the Krebiozen Foundation, the drug was judged to be ineffective [50].

Other methods, which attempt to stimulate the immune system, have also been tried. For example, fevers produced by the injections of chemicals and organic materials have been used to retard the growth of cancers. This approach includes the injection of mixed bacterial vaccines (Coley's Toxins) [3].

Bovine and shark cartilage have been used to treat cancer because in studies in cell culture they have an angiogenesis inhibiting action [51–54]. In published human studies however the results have been inconsistent, and an NIH supported study to evaluate shark cartilage as a component of cancer treatment is in progress.

Bovine and shark cartilage have been evaluated as treatments for psoriasis and arthritis, in addition to cancer. It has been proposed that cartilage stimulates the immune system and kills cancer cells.

There is some evidence that glycosasminoglycan in cartilage has some effect in inhibiting the growth of new blood vessels possibly by inhibiting matrix metalloproteins Two relatively small proteins have been purified which inhibit matrix metallproteinase in vitro. More than 40 different brands of shark cartilage are sold in the United States as powders or liquid extracts and are marketed as dietary supplements. Reported side effects of shark cartilage treatment include hypercalcemia, hypotension, and hypoglycemia.

Palliative Treatment of Cancer

Palliative treatment can be considered to be the care of patients whose disease is not responsive to treatment [55–58]. Control of symptoms to maintain the best quality of life for the patient is the main objective. In one survey, 84 percent of cancer patients near death experience severe pain while 33 percent had nausea and 49 percent had shortness of breath Complementary and alternative techniques are frequently used to alleviate symptoms because they have or are believed to have fewer side effects than traditional therapy.

Cancer patients in order to palliate their illness have used acupuncture, physical techniques such as massage, and a variety of mental approaches such as mediation [55, 59–65].

Acupuncture has been widely used in the United States since the 1972 visits of President Nixon to China [59–66]. Acupuncture has been used in China at least since the time of the Yellow Emperor around 200 BC. The needles used in acupuncture are regulated by the FDA and certification courses for acupuncturists are available in many states. The World Health Organization has listed a number of conditions that may benefit from acupuncture treatment including relief of pain, addiction to alcohol and tobacco and other drugs, treatment of pulmonary diseases such as asthma and bronchitis and in rehabilitation patients who have suffered strokes. Promising results have been obtained in treating cancer pain and the nausea and vomiting caused by cancer chemotherapy. The occurrence of adverse effects with acupuncture is rare [59]. More than one million Americans use acupuncture annually. A majority of the States provide licensure or registration for acupuncturists. It is estimated that there are more than 10,000 acupuncturists in the United States While there are no Medicare payments for acupuncture, acupuncture is reimbursed by some HMO's. Acupuncture is just one form of therapy within Chinese medicine that includes special exercises such as Tai Chi and QiGong, as well as the use of herbal mixtures, and dietary regulation.

Greatly simplified acupuncture is based on the concept that health depends on the unimpeded flow of vital energy "Qi" which must occur to maintain energetic balance within pathways known as meridians or channels [61]. The acupuncturist influences health by stimulating key points, "acupoints" along these meridians with fine steel needles placed just under the skin. Originally 365 points were identified corresponding to the days of the year, but currently there are more than 2000. In treatment the selection of points takes into account not just the symptoms to be relieved but what I can be thought of as the entire energy balance of the patient. The aim is always to adjust or readjust the flow of vital energy so that the proper amount reaches the right place in the right time. Many other forms of stimulation can be used in addition to just needle insertion in acupuncture including electricity, magnetism, lasers, and herbs.

But sometimes just pressure, acupressure, is applied to crucial points [60, 62]. In moxabustion burning dried leaves or sticks are applied either to the skin directly or to the needle. In cupping a partially evacuated glass or bamboo cup is applied to the acupoint and a partial vacuum created inside the cup by a flame.

Each person it is believed is influenced by opposing forces of yin (female, dark, cold, passive forces) and yang (light, male, hot active forces) [61]. Disease occurs when the two are not in balance. Acupuncture helps restore that balance which varies among people. Chinese medicine recognizes five elements, water, wood, fire, earth, and metal that are dissimilar combinations of yin and yang. Each individual consists of a different balance of these five elements. Too much or too little of one of the elements cause specific symptoms. Illness in this philosophy can result from diseases that block channels or affect the organs, which are classified as Zang and Fu. Zang organs are yin organs and Fu organs are yang. In diseases that affect channels, the acupuncturist selects local tender (Ah Shi) points and a distal point on a channel that traverses the affected local area. In diseases of Zang and Fu organs the acupuncturist decides what organ is involved using traditional diagnostic methods. If the acupuncturist diagnosis is that the organ is too cold for example, the acupuncturist will apply heat using moxabustion or cupping. There are shu or points on the back and mu or front points that are the surface representation of specific organs. The back points are believed to be more effective in yin organ disease, and the front in yang. Yaun points near the wrists and ankles are source points of channels are used often in the treatment of organ disease. There are also Luo connecting points where channels are connected internally or externally to other channels. Each channel also has a point that represents one of the five elements. These points can be used to tone up or calm down organs.

The acupuncture needle is always placed beneath the skin and may be as much as about an inch deep. It is inserted until a so-called "deqi" or needling sensation is felt which depending on the acupoint may vary in character from burning, pricking, bursting, or numbing.

Although acupuncture is base on a rather complex philosophy of health and disease, this philosophy has very little or no scientific support. Acupuncture however does produce observable biologic effects, which may be useful in treating illness. There is a substantial amount of support for the idea that the analgesic effects of acupuncture involve the endogenous opiod system [57]. Acupuncture also seems to stimulate hypothalamic neuronal groups and give rise to a broad range of systemic effects. Alterations in the secretion of neurohormones and neurotransmitters both centrally and peripherally have been observed. There are also reported changes in immune function.

In China, acupuncture is used widely for many diseases [63]. In the United States it has been used as a complementary treatment in cancer patient. There is no evidence that acupuncture has any effect on the tumor itself. An unstable spine and severe clotting disorders may be contraindications to the use of acupuncture. As discussed in the chapter on lung disease appropriate sham controls for acupuncture has been difficult to develop complicating studies of the clinical efficacy of acupuncture [57, 58, 65]. Many studies of acupuncture relief of pain in cancer patients have been uncontrolled. For example, 183 patients in a cancer pain clinic were treated with acupuncture in 5–15 minute sessions 1 to 4 times a week. About half the patient reported more than 3 days of pain relief and/or an increase in mobility. In a more recent study 92 cancer patients with abdominal pain due to local invasive or metastatic cancer were treated every day for one to two weeks. In all the patients with mild to moderate pain by the WHO scale, pain control was achieved, as it was in three-quarters of the patients with severe disease.

In another study 20 patients with peripheral or central neuropathic pain were treated by auricular acupuncture using electrical stimulation. Eleven of the patients had post-mastectomy brachial plexus pain. Average pain intensity decreased, with no patient experiencing pain worsening. Some felt well enough to stop all other analgesic treatment [57, 58]

Using an acupressure wristband versus a placebo or no wristband at all failed to make a significant difference in the intensity of nausea felt by cancer patients. But only 6 patients were involved and 2 of them never had nausea [66].

Feelings of stress, anxiety and depression are common in cancer patients. It's not surprising that psychotherapeutic approaches have been used in cancer patients and have included for example various relaxation therapies often with imagery training in which pleasant situations are visualized mentally. Uncontrolled studies have been encouraging.

There are several kinds of alternative treatments based on mind body interactions that have been thought to act in part at least through the immune system so called psycho-immunology and there have been reports of longer survival in cancer patients using these techniques [67–73]. These vary from simple breathing and relaxation exercises to meditation and self-hypnosis. Self-hypnosis in an unblinded control study in women with advanced breast cancer was reported to produce a significant improvement in pain. Finally spiritual counseling, music therapy, and the establishment of self-help groups seem to be useful for cancer patients.

Although there are no controlled studies in cancer patients massage therapies like shiatsu, a Japanese form of massage related in philosophy to acupuncture, in some cancer patients seems to relieve anxiety and reduce symptoms. Aromatherapy involves the use of different sorts of oils during massage with supposedly different effects, for example cedar wood oil for relaxation an rosemary for invigoration. Therapeutic touch and healing touch are two methods, which use supposed energetic healing approaches that are sometimes used in nursing. Actual physical contact need not occur. They have been mainly used as a nursing technique to reduce anxiety.

Conclusions

There are seemingly an endless number of treatment modalities that have been or are being used to prevent, treat, and/or palliate cancer. There have been very few randomized controlled studies of the efficacy of any of them and when such studies have been carried out even fewer have had a positive result. There is epidemiological evidence that the risk of developing cancer is reduced by diets rich in fruits and vegetables and by high fiber diets There is also some studies that suggest that ingestion of large quantities of smoked fish can be harmful increasing the risk somewhat of some cancers. Chicken and fish may be better than red meat.

There is no convincing evidence that any alternative or complementary treatment is useful in the treatment of cancer but perhaps enough studies of sufficient size have not as yet been done.

There is evidence that acupuncture helps in relieving cancer pain and in suppressing nausea. There is also at least anecdotal evidence that various forms of massage and meditation can improve the quality of life of some cancer patients

References

1. Tough SC, JohnstonDW, Verhoef MJ, Arthur K, Bryant H. (2002) Complementary and alternative medicine use among colorectal cancer patients in Alberta, Canada. Alt Ther. Health Med. 8: 58–64
2. Richardson MA, Sanders T, Palmer JL, Geisinger A, Singletary SE. (2000) Complementary/alternative medicine use in a comprehensive cancer center and the implications for oncology. J. Clin Oncol.27: 623–630
3. Giovannucci E, Sampfer MJ, Colditz GA et al.(1998)Multivitamin use, folate, and colon cancer in women in the Nurse's Health Study. Ann. Intern. Med.129: 517–524
4. American Cancer Society (1993). Questionable methods of cancer treatment. Atlanta: American Cancer Society
5. The ABTC cancer prevention study group; (1994) The effects of Vitamin E and beta-carotene on the incidence of lung cancer and other cancers in male smokers. N. Eng. J. Med. 330: 1029–35
6. Block G, Patterson B, and Subar A (1992) Fruits, vegetables, and cancer prevention. A review of the epidemiological evidence. Nutr. Cancer 18: 1–29
7. Marquat-Moulin G et al. (1991). Cancer and polyps of the colorectum and lifetime consumption of beer and other alcoholic beverages. Am. J. Epidemiol. 134: 157–166
8. Hill MJ. (1997) Cereals, cereal fibre and colorectal cancer risk: a review of the epidemiological literature. Eur. J Cancer Prev.6: 219–225
9. Earnest DL, Einspahr JG, Alberts DS. (1999) Protective role of wheat bran fiber: data from marker trials. Am J. Med 106: 32S-37S
10. Fuchs CS, Giovannucci EL, Colditz GA et al (1999) Dietary fiber and risk of colorectal cancer and adenomas in women. Eng J. Med. 340: 169–176
11. Sinha R, Kulldorf M, Curtin J et al. (1998) Fried, well-done red meat and the risk of lung cancer in women (United States) Cancer Causes Control 9: 621–630
12. Gann PH, Hennekens CH, Sacks FM et al. (1994) Prospective study of plasma fatty acids and risk of prostate cancer. J. Natl. Cancer Inst: 86:281–286
13. Bostick RM, Potter JD, Kushi LH et al. (1994) Sugar, meat, fat intake, and non-dietary risk factors for colon cancer incidence in Iowa women (United States). Cancer Causes Control 5: 38–52
14. Lamson DW, Brignall MS. (1999) Antioxidants in cancer therapy; their actions and interactions with oncologic therapies. Altern. Med Rev.4: 304–329
15. Lamson DW, Brignall MS (2000) Antioxidants and cancer therapy I: quick reference guide. Altern. Med. Rev. 5: 152–163
16. Knept P et al.(1991)Dietary anti-oxidants and the risk of lung cancer. Amer. J. Edidem. 145: 4–9
17. Schwartz J, Shklar G (1992). The selective cytotoxic effects of carotenoids and alpha-tocopherol on human cancer cell lines in vitro. J. Oral Maxillofac. Surg.50: 367–373
18. Zhang Y, Talay P, Cheon-Gyu, C, Posner G. (1992). A major inducer of anti-carcinogenic protective enzymes from broccoli: Isolation and elucidation of structure. Proc. Nat. Acad. Sci. 89: 2394–2398
19. Fahey JW, Zhang Y, Talay P. (1997) Broccoli sprouts: An exceptionally rich source of inducers of enzymes that protect against chemical carcinogenesis. Proc. Nat. Acad. Sci. 94: 10367–10372
20. Cameron E, Pauling L. (1978) Supplemental ascorbate in the supportive treatment of cancer: reevaluation of prolongation of survival times in terminal human cancer. Proceed. Nat. Acad Science. 75: 4538–4542.
21. Block G. (1991) Vitamin C and cancer prevention. The epidemiological evidence. Am J. Clin .Nutr.53: 270S–282S.
22. Hedlund D, Moffat KA, Uskokovic MR, Miller GJ (1997) Three synthetic vitamin D analogues induce prostate-specific acid phosphatase and prostate specific antigen while inhibiting the growth of human prostate cancer cells in a Vitamin D receptor-dependent fashion. Clin. Cancer Res: 3: 1331–1338
23. Creagan ET et al. (1979) Failure of high dose vitamin C (ascorbic acid) therapy to benefit patients with advanced cancer. A controlled trial. New. Eng. J. Med. 301: 687–690
24. Yam D, Peled A, Shinitzky M. (2001) Suppression of tumor growth and metastasis by dietary fish oil combined with vitamin E and C and cisplatin. Cancer Chemother. Pharmacol. 47:34–40
25. Yang, CS, Landau JM, Huang MT, Newmark HL (2001). Inhibition of carcinogenesis by dietary polyphenolic compounds. Annu. Rev. Nutr. 21: 381–406
26. Annabi B, Lachambre M-P, Bousqet-Gagnon N, Page M, Gingras D, Beliveau R.(2002) Green tea polyphenols(-)-epigallocatechin 3-gallate inhibits MMP-2 secretion and MT1-MMP-driven migration in glioblastoma cells. Biochem. Biophys. Acta1 542: 209–220

27. Anonymous (1996) Tobacco control: reducing cancer incidence and saving lives. J. Clin. Onc.14: 1961–1963

28. Franceschi S, Talamini R, Barra S, Baron AE, Negri E, Bidoli E, Serraino D, La Vecchia C (1992) Smoking and drinking in relation to cancers of the oral cavity, pharynx, larynx, and esophagus in Northern Italy. Cancer Res. 50: 6502–6507

29. Garro AJ, Espina, N, Lieber CS (1992) Alcohol and cancer. Alcohol Health and Research World 16: 81–86

30. Dianzani MU (1995). Lipid peroxidation and cancer. Crit Rev. Oncol. Hemat. 15:125–147

31. Chandra J, Samali A, Orrenius S (2000) Triggering and modulation of apoptosis by oxidative stress. Free Rad. Biol. Med. 29: 323–333

32. Gonzalez MJ, Schemmel RA, Dugan L Jr. et al (1993). Dietary fish oil inhibits human breast carcinoma growth: a function of increased lipid peroxidation. Lipids 28: 827–832.

33. Rose DP. (1997) Dietary fatty acids and cancer. Am. J. Clin. Nutr, 66:998S-1003S

34. Rose DP, Connolly JM. (1999) Omega-3 fatty acids as cancer chemopreventive agents. Pharmacol. Ther. 83: 217–244

35. Sinha BK (1989) Free radicals in anticancer drug pharmacology. Chem Biol Interactions 69: 293–317

36. Dwyer J. (1990) The macrobiotic diet: No cancer cure. Nutrition Forum &: 9–11

37. Foldeak S, Dombradi G (1964). Tumor-growth inhibiting substances of plant origin. I. Isolation of the active principle of Arctium lappa. Acta Phys Chem. 10: 91–93

38. Mgbonyebi OP, Russo J, Russo IH (1998) Antiproliferative effect of synthetic resveratrol on human breast epithelial cells. Int. J. Oncol.12: 865–869

39. Wilson B. (1998) The rise and fall of laetrile. Nutrition Forum 7: 33–40

40. Moertel C et al. (1982) A clinical trial of amygdalin (laetrile) in the treatment of human cancer. New Eng. J. Med.: 306:201–206

41. Bussing A. (1997): Mistletoe (a story with an open end. Anti-cancer Drugs (Suppl) 8: S1–2

42. Hajto T, Hostanska K, Frei K, Rordorf C Gabius H-J. (1990) Increased secretion of tumor necrosis factor alpha, Intrerleukin I and Interleukin mononuclear cells exposed to b-galactoside-specific Lectin from clinically applied mistletoe extract. Cancer Res. 50: 3322–3326

43. Salzer G (1994). 70 years of mistletoe therapy and no proof of efficacy? JAMA 11: 23–26

44. Singh RP, Tyagi AK, Zhao J, Agarwal R.(2002) Silymarin inhibits growth and causes regression of established skin tumors in SENCAR mice via modulation of mitogen – activated protein kinases and induction of apoptosis. Carcinogenesis 23: 499–510.

45. Landanyi A, Timar J, Lapis K. (1993) Effect of lentinan on macrophage cytoxicity against metastatic tumor cells. Cancer. Immunol. Immunother. 36: 123–126.

46. Dixon SC, Knopf KB, Figg WB. (2001) The control of prostate specific antigen expression and gene regulation by pharmacological agents. Pharmacol. Rev. : 573–99

47. DiPaola RS, Zhuang H, Lambert GH, Meeker R.Lietra E et al. 1998. Clinical and biologic activity of an estrogenic herbal combination (PC-SPES) in prostate cancer. New Eng J Med: 339: 785–789

48. American Cancer Society (1993) Questionable methods of cancer management. Hydrogen peroxide and other hyperoxygenation therapies. CA – a cancer journal for clinicians43: 47–55

49. Loprinzi C et al. Randomized placebo-controlled study of hydrazine sulfate in patients with newly diagnosed non-small cell cancer Clin. Oncologyu12: 1126–1129

50. Holland JF (1977) The Krebiozen therapy: Is cancer quackery dead? JAMA200: 213–218

50a. Austin S, Dale EB, DeKadt S. (1994) Long-term follow-up of cancer patients using Conteras, Hoxsey and Gerson therapies. J. Naturopathic Med. 5: 74–76

51. Davis PF,He Y,Furneaux RH et al.(1997) Inhibition of angiogenesis by oral ingestion of powdered shark cartilage in a rat model. Microvascular Res. 54: 178–182

52. Suzuki F (1999). Cartilage-derived growth factor and anti-tumor factor:Past,present, and future studies. Biochem Biophys Res. Communic. 259: 1–7

53. Moses Ma Sudhalter J, Langer R. (1992) Isolation and characterization of an inhibitor of neovascularizatin from scapular cartilage. J. Cell Biol. 119: 475–482

54. Miller DR et al. (1998) Phase I/II trial of shark cartilage in the treatment of advanced cancer. J. Clin. Oncol. 16: 3649–3655

55. Calman SK, Hanks G, Doyle D, Hanks GWC eds. (1998) Oxford Textbook of Palliative Care, 2nd edition: Oxford University Press Oxford

56. Pan CX, Morrison RS, Ness J, Fugh-Berman A, Leipzig RM (2000) Complementary and Alternative Medicine in the management of pain, dyspnea, nausea, and vomiting near the end of life. A systematic review. J. Comp. Altern. Med. 20: 374–387

57. World Health Organization. Cancer Pain and Relief (1990) (Technical Report Series 804) World Health Organization Geneva

58. Portnoy RK, LePage P. Management of cancer pain (1999). Lancet 333: 1695–1700

58a. Seale C, Cartwright A. (1994) The year before death. Brookfield, VT

59. Acupuncture. NIH consensus statement, NIH vol.15: Nov 3–5, 1997

60. Alimi D, Rubino C, Leandri EP, Brule SF (2000) Analgesic effects of auricular acupuncture for cancer pain. J Pain Symptom Management 19: 81–82

61. Pockert M, Ullmann C (1988) Chinese Medicine (Howson M, translator) (1st US edition) NewYork: Morrow

62. Gadsby JG, Franks P, Jarvis P et al. (1997) Acupuncture-like transcutaneous electrical nerve stimulation within palliative care: a pilot study. Complement Threrap. Med. 5: 13–18

63. Xu S, Liu Z, Li Y.(1995) Treatment of cancerous abdominal pain by acupuncture in Zuslani: a report of 92 cases. J Tradit. Chin. Med. 15: 189–191

64. Fishlie J, Redman D. (1986) Acupuncture and malignant pain problems. Eur. J. Surg. Oncol.11: 389–394

65. Fishlie J, Penn S, Ashley et al. (1996) Acupuncture for the relief of cancer related breathlessness. Palliat. Med.10: 145–150

66. Brown S, North D, Marvel MK, Fons R (1992). Acupressure wrist bands to relieve nausea and vomiting in hospice patients: do they work? Am. J. Hosp. Palliat. Care 9: 26–2

67. Gellert G, Maxwell RM, Siegel BS (1993). Survival of breast cancer patients receiving adjunctive psychosocial support therapy: A 10-year follow-up study. J. Clin. Oncol. 11: 66–69

68. Havas H et al. (1990) The effect of bacterial vaccine on tumors and immune response of ICR/Ha mice. J. Biol. Res. Mod. 9: 194–204

69. Keen AR,Frelick RW (1990). Response of tumors to thermodynamic stimulation of the immune system. Del. Med. J. 62: 1115–6

70. Weinrich SP, Weinrich MC. (1990) The effect of massage on pain in cancer patients. Appl. Nurs. Res. 3: 140–145

71. Wilkinson S. (1995) Aromatherapy and massage in palliative care. Int. J. Palliat. Nurs.1: 21–30

72. Fleming U. (1985) Relaxation therapy for far-advanced cancer. Practitionmer 229: 471–475

73. Curtis S. (1986) The effect of music on pain relief and relaxation of the terminally ill. J. Music Ther. 23:10–14

28 Dementing Illness and Complementary and Alternative Medicine

R. McCarney, J. Warner

Introduction

Dementia is a common illness in older people and has major implications for individuals with the disease, their carers and society. The recent development of conventional therapies for dementia has spurred interest in all forms of treatment and led to a new era of therapeutic optimism. This chapter outlines the clinical and epidemiological features of the principal types of dementia and reviews the evidence base for CAM treatments.

There is a paucity of quality research into CAM treatments of the dementias. However there are a number of CAM therapies that are providing some interesting preliminary results. *Ginkgo biloba* is an exception, with a sizeable evidence base that is quite promising, although more research of this herbal treatment needs to be done, for example addressing issues such as its prophylactic potential, its comparability to conventional treatments and its effectiveness in primary care. Goals of treatment range from symptomatic improvement with herbal preparations such as *Ginkgo*, to providing palliation with therapies such as massage and aromatherapy. Although there are many herbs and dietary supplements to which memory and attention enhancing properties are attributed [1], we will only focus on those for which there is some degree of evidence. The scope of the chapter is intentionally wide as the boundaries between CAM and conventional treatment are sometimes blurred, for example vitamin supplementation may or may not be considered CAM depending on dose. The boundaries are slightly extended to include treatments where there is this uncertainty.

The potential for CAM therapies is large as current conventional treatments for mild to moderate dementia (cholinesterase inhibiting drugs such as donepezil, rivastigmine and galantamine) are expensive and have limited efficacy for individuals with dementia and their carers [2–4]. Cholinesterase inhibitors also have a significant incidence of adverse effects, which may be observed in as many as a third of patients on rivastigmine.

Definition

Dementia is characterised by a decline in verbal and non-verbal memory, a decline of other cognitive abilities such as judgement, planning and processing of information and a change in emotion, motivation or social behaviour without clouding of consciousness [5, 6]. Age-associated memory impairment may portend dementia in some people, but the stigma and nihilism often associated with the label dementia impels clinicians to be accurate about the diagnosis. Other disorders that may mimic dementia include depression and delirium (acute confusional states).

There are many causes of dementia, but the three most common types are Alzheimer's disease, vascular dementia and dementia with Lewy bodies (DLB), together accounting for at least 95% of all cases. Less common causes include fronto-temporal dementia, Creutzfeldt-Jakob disease, Huntington's disease, and dementia arising as a consequence of other disorders (for example, hypothyroidism, alcohol misuse, syphilis, B-group vitamin deficiency and multiple sclerosis). Rarity and nosological difficulties have limited the evidence-base for treatment of these dementias.

Aetiology

The cause of Alzheimer's disease is unknown, although an early pathological process appears to be deposition of an abnormally insoluble form of amyloid in the central nervous system [7]. A rare subtype is early onset Alzheimer's disease which manifests before age 60. This is a familial disorder with an autosomal dominant inheritance due to mutations on presenelin or amyloid precursor protein genes. Later onset dementia is sometimes clustered in families, but specific gene mutations have not been identified. Head injury, Down's syndrome and lower premorbid intellect may be risk factors for Alzheimer's disease. Vascular dementia is often related to cardiovascular risk factors, such as smoking, hypertension, and diabetes.

Epidemiology

A meta-analysis of population based studies in Europe found the prevalence of dementia in individuals over 65 was 6.4%. Nearly 70% of cases were Alzheimer's disease and 25% were vascular dementia. The prevalence of dementia rises sharply with increasing age; 0.8% for those aged 65–69, rising to 28.5% of those aged 90 or over [8]. Alzheimer's disease affects women more than men, although the greater mortality of men from other causes may account for some of this difference. The age-standardised prevalence of dementia may be less in developing countries, although the explanations for these differences, if they are real, remain unclear [9]. Over the last decade or so, dementia with Lewy bodies has become increasingly recognised and probably accounts for around 15% of cases [10].

Clinical Features

Although the symptoms and signs of dementia are numerous and protean, most types of dementia have symptoms in common. There is a large diversity of symptoms between individuals, and in one individual over time. The impact of these symptoms can vary between individuals and their carers. These are divisible into features of decline in cognitive abilities and the non-cognitive features, known collectively as Behavioural and Psychological Symptoms of Dementia (BPSD). It is useful to consider which symptoms are prominent in an individual when assessing which CAM intervention may be most suitable.

The principal cognitive features in the early stages are deterioration in: memory, especially for more recent events; orientation; abstract thought (planning and problem solving ability) and judgement. Later symptoms include dysphasia, agnosia and apraxia.

Over the course of dementia individuals are highly likely to experience at least some behavioural or psychological symptoms. The psychological symptoms of BPSD include depression, occurring in around up to 28% of individuals, anxiety, hallucinations (in up to 28%) and paranoid ideas (in up to 73%). Behavioural symptoms and signs include agitation (40%), aggression (18–20%), wandering (18%) incontinence and apathy (63%) [11].

Carers will often attribute problematic symptoms such as apathy or incontinence to the individual being lazy or "difficult" rather than as part of the disease process. Similarly, psychological symptoms such as depression may, when recognised, be regarded as part of the dementing process. Recognition of depression is difficult and should be treated if suspected. Paranoid ideas are commonly focussed on theft, but can include delusions of infidelity or persecution. They are often understandable in the context of a poor memory. A common example is the patient who accuses carers of stealing her pension because she cannot remember spending it. BPSD symptoms do not have the predictability or stability of the cognitive ones and account for significant distress for the individual with dementia and their carers. The consequence of this pathoplasticity is that patients should be carefully monitored and new treatments sought as symptoms emerge. Furthermore, the necessity of established treatments should be revised as the disease progresses.

Alzheimer's Disease

The principal features of Alzheimer's disease are progressive loss of memory, reasoning and planning with alteration of personality including emotional and motivational changes. The onset is usually insidious, and the disease may be difficult to diagnose in the early stages. As the disorder progresses, learned skills such as language and fine motor tasks are lost. Depression, quasi-psychotic phenomena and behavioural problems such as wandering and aggression are common. In the later stages, individuals become incontinent, immobile and totally dependent. Death usually occurs in 7–10 years after diagnosis.

Vascular Dementia

Vascular dementia often has an abrupt onset and more unpredictable, stepwise progression. The clinical picture may vary according to the site and pattern of vascular disease, but focal neurological signs, abnormal gait, changes in personality or mood and retention of insight are may be more frequent than in early Alzheimer's disease. Vascular risk factors, such as diabetes, hypertension and smoking are usually present. In practice, vascular and Alzheimer pathology often co-exist, and vascular disease may be an independent risk factor for Alzheimer's disease.

Dementia with Lewy Bodies

Dementia with Lewy bodies is usually associated with features of Parkinson's disease (tremor, rigidity, bradykinesia, abnormal gait), which may predate the onset of dementia. Other features include fluctuating cognitive abilities, which may be dramatic and rapid, visual hallucinations and a propensity to falls [12]. Comprehensive cognitive testing may reveal disproportionate loss of visuo-spatial abilities. The prognosis of DLB appears slightly worse than Alzheimer's disease, with an interval between diagnosis and death of around 6 years. The aetiology of DLB is uncertain, but key neuropathological features include the presence of Lewy bodies in the cortex identical to those found in the substantia nigra of individuals with Parkinson's disease.

Therapies

Herbal Preparations

Ginkgo biloba

Background. *Ginkgo biloba* extract is derived from the dried leaves of the ginkgo tree (*Ginkgo biloba* L.; more commonly known as the 'maidenhair' tree), the last remaining member of the ginkgoaceae family. This tree, native to China, has survived unchanged for more than 200 million years and is widely cultivated ornamentally around the world. In the west it is generally the leaf which is used medicinally, whereas in China it is the seed, of which there is a history of its medicinal use for almost 5000 years [13]. It is currently a popular drug in Europe for circulatory conditions [14] and the evidence is now growing for its use in the symptomatic treatment of dementia.

The pharmacological activity (including vaso- and tissue-protective action) of standardized leaf extract are attributed to the flavonoids and highly oxidized terpene trilactones (ginkgolides and bilobalide) [15].

Therapeutic target. Symptomatic improvement of cognitive functioning.

Evidence. Two good reviews of *Ginkgo* trials have been published [16, 17]. Oken's systematic review [16] included English and non-English articles which use a patient population with a clear diagnosis of Alzheimer's disease, clearly stated exclusion criteria, use of standardized *Ginkgo* extract, randomised, placebo-controlled and double-blinded design, objective assessment of cognitive function as an outcome measure and sufficient detail to allow a meta-analysis. Of fifty articles identified, four studies were included and showed a small but significant effect that translated into a 3% difference between *Ginkgo* and placebo in the ADAS-Cog (objective assessment of cognitive function). Ernst's review [17] again did not restrict by language and included randomised, placebo-controlled and double-blinded trials of *Ginkgo* extract for dementia. Nine studies were reviewed of varying methodological quality but a meta-analysis was not performed. The conclusion made was that the majority of trials support the notion that *Ginkgo* can delay the decline in symptoms but whether this translates into a clinically meaningful difference is questionableunclear. Finally both reviews call for more research in the area, Oken's [16] in trials to determine whether there is functional improvement and optimum dosage and Ernst's [17] to establish the clinical value of *Ginkgo*.

A comparison was made by Wettstein [18] between (separate) studies of cholinesterase inhibitors and *Ginkgo* extracts. This was a difficult comparison, with the author conceding that an equivalence trial would be required to reach definite conclusions as to the relative performance of the two medications. As such a study was unavailable then the next best thing, the results of separate randomised, placebo-controlled, double-blind trials were evaluated. In all, six studies were included (four of cholinesterase inhibitors versus placebo, two of *Ginkgo* versus placebo). Only the intent-to-treat analyses data were compared and no evaluation of the effects of age or gender in the study populations were made. The results were that symptoms were delayed for similar time periods and a similar response rate (difference between verum and placebo) were obtained with both cholinesterase inhibitors and EGb 761 (the *Ginkgo* extract used in the two *Ginkgo* trials). Although Wettstein could not comment on statistical equivalence or non-equivalence, he does concluded that the use of both groups of substances in treating dementia is justified.

To date, most studies on the treatment of dementia have been undertaken in hospital-based populations, sponsored by pharmaceutical companies. Consequently the generalisability of these studies to routine clinical care is limited.

Number-Needed-to-Treat (NNT) and Intent-to-Treat (ITT) Analyses. Based on the data from Le Bars study [19], Ernst [17] reports that seven patients will need to take *Ginkgo* rather than placebo for one year for see an improvement of to observe a difference of four points on the 70-point ADAS-Cog scale in one patient (the equivalent of six-months delay in progression of the disease), or for a family member of one of the patients to notice improvement in daily living and social behaviour.

Le Bars conducted an intent-to-treat analysis [19] again on the data from his earlier study [20], and concluded that 26% of the *Ginkgo* group had a clinically significant improvement in cognitive functioning (four points on the ADAS-Cog), with the same improvement occurring in 17% of the placebo group; on the relatives rating instrument 30% of the *Ginkgo* group improved and 17% worsened, compared to 25% improving and 37% worsening in the placebo group. No differences were reported between the two groups in terms of safety.

Applicability. Existing studies have focused on Alzheimer's and vascular dementia.

Safety. Adverse events associated with *Ginkgo* may be no greater than those linked to placebo [20]; there are however a number of potential interactions and contraindications [21].
 Interactions reported in the literature include:
- Anticoagulants,
- thiazide diuretics,
- trazodone,
- warfarin,
- drugs metabolized by CYP type enzymes (e.g. CYP1A2, CYP2D6 and CYP3A4).

Moreover theoretically possible interactions include:
- Insulin,
- monoamine oxidase inhibitors.

Contraindications include:
- bleeding disorders,
- diabetes (theoretical),
- epilepsy (theoretical),
- infertility (theoretical).

Dosage. To date studies have generally used standardized extracts doses of 120 mg or 240 mg, containing 24% flavenoids (Ginkgo-flavoneglycosides) and 6% terpenoids (3.1% ginkgolides A, B and C, 2.9% bilobalide) although it is unclear which is the optimum dose. Indeed the need for more research on efficacy of relevant dosages has been expressed [16]. Kayne [21] reports that the literature does not show evidence for other dosage forms or low concentration extracts made from the leaf.

How to obtain. Available over the counter. A number of products are available, so care must be taken as there can be variation in quality in the numerous brands available. The extraction process originally patented (now expired) by Schwabe Pharmaceuticals (Germany) is commonly used with a standardized content of 24% flavonoids and 6% terpenoids. Research to date has mainly used the Schwabe product, Tebonin (EGb 761) although Ginkyo (LI 1370) developed by Lichtwer Pharma (Germany) has been used in some studies. Other brand names such as Kaveri, rökan and Tanakan are commercial best sellers in Europe.

Conclusion. The existing evidence for *Ginkgo* is encouraging. Its effect on cognitive functioning and relative-rated behavioural functioning is greater than that observed on placebo; the improvement is similar to that on cholinesterase inhibitors but with fewer side effects.

Silymarin

Background. Silymarin is an extract of milk thistle (*Silybum marianum* L.), a tall herb with prickly leaves and a milky sap [13]. Native to the Mediterranean region of Europe it is now naturalized in California and the eastern United States. The components of Silymarin include a large number of flavonoglicans purported to have antihepatotoxic effects.

Therapeutic target. Reduction of side effects experienced with Tacrine, a cholinesterase inhibitor with a significant risk of hepatotoxic adverse effects.

Evidence. A randomised, double-blind, placebo-controlled trial [22] compared tacrine and silymarin to tacrine and placebo (silymarin and placebo assigment was double-blinded), in patients with mild to moderate dementia. Tacrine-induced hepatic dysfunction was evaluated by measuring amino-transferase levels (ALAT, ASAT); the study found Silymarin was unable to prevent elevation of these levels. However cholinergic side effects and notable gastrointestinal problems were reduced in this group, leading to the conclusion that co-administered Silymarin could help improve tolerability of tacrine therapy in the early stages.

Safety. Toxic effects have not been reported (although transient gastrointestinal side effects have been reported in observational studies); it is considered to be well-tolerated [13].

Dosage. The study team administered 420 mg of Silymarin per day.

How to obtain. Marketed as a dietary supplement in the form of capsules containing 200 mg of a concentrated extract representing 140 mg of Silymarin [13].

Conclusion. Seems useful in reducing side-effects in de novo tacrine-treated patients (and, the authors speculate, in future cholinesterase inhibitors) although this is based on one trial involving 217 patients.

Other Herbal Preparations

Two Kampo mixtures (a Japanese variant of Chinese traditional medicine), Choto-san (which contains 11 medicinal plants) and Kami-Umtan-To (KUT) (which contains 13 different plants) have been the subject of investigation [23, 24]. The Choto-san paper reports on two studies, one of which was a randomised, placebo controlled, double-blind trial with 139 participants (the other study, involving 60 patients, was not blinded). This trial reported a statistically significant improvement global improvement over 12 weeks in patients with vascular dementia. The positive KUT review reports (in the English abstract) that an open clinical trial found cognitive decline was slower in group given the KUT preparation but the methodological quality is unclear.

The Chinese traditional medicine herbal Yizhi capsule (YZC) has also been the subject of investigation [25, 26]; unfortunately the full paper was unavailable in English for one of these [25, 26]. Both studies used patients with vascular dementia, and although both report positive results, the methodological quality of the studies is poor.

Further studies on all these preparations seems warranted.

Aromatherapy and Massage

There is some evidence that aromatherapy, either alone or in combination with massage, is effective in treating behavioural disturbances in dementia. One well conducted but small randomised controlled trial [27] compared aromatherapy and massage, aromatherapy and conversation, and massage only. Using a novel outcome measure [28] it found excessive motor behaviour was reduced significantly by aromatherapy and massage in combination at one of the measurement time points [29]. Another well-conducted study investigated lavender oil versus placebo (in an aromatherapy stream) with a cross-over design on a ward of 15 patients with dementia [30]. Agitation as rated by a blinded assessor showed a small but significant improvement when compared to placebo sessions. The benefit of aromatherapy and massage [31] and expressive physical touch (affective touch behaviour generally including gentle massage) [32] have also been reported by uncontrolled studies, although one review reported inconclusive findings [33].

Music Therapy

A Cochrane review of music therapy for dementia (that is currently being reworked) [34], reported no randomised controlled trials in this area. They do conclude however that based on the available evidence, music therapy may be beneficial in treating dementia symptoms and improving quality of life in patients and caregivers. A systematic review of music therapy reported results on 21 studies, (most with weak methods). Music therapy versus control interventions significantly improved reported outcomes and significant effects were noted with different types of music therapy (active vs. passive, taped vs. live) [35].

Acupuncture

A number of studies have addressed the use of acupuncture for treating dementia of the Alzheimer's type [36, 37], vascular dementia [38–40] and traumatic dementia [41]. These Chinese studies all report positive effects but all are uncontrolled and/or of low methodological quality. One further small, uncontrolled study investigated the treatment of associated mental problems (anxiety and depression) in dementia [42]. It found a significant improvement in anxiety and depression scores and insignificant cognitive decline amongst the patients. Randomised, controlled trials are needed to confirm these positive preliminary findings.

Dietary Supplements

Antioxidants

Evidence is growing (supported by theoretical work) for the idea that oxidative stress to the central nervous system is a contributory factor in the development of Alzheimer's disease; and as such this area has been the subject of a number of reviews [43–46]. A number of antioxidants have shown positive effects, in particular *Ginkgo* (see above), alpha-tocopherol (vitamin E), selegiline and idebenone.

One study examined vitamin E (2000 units daily), selegiline (10 mg daily) or a combination versus placebo in 341 patients with moderately severe Alzheimer's disease for a two year period [47]. The results were only significant in an analysis adjusted for baseline cognition, an analysis that has not escaped criticism [46], as the baseline cognitive functioning score was higher in the placebo group. Furthermore the accompanying editorial [48] points to the lack of effect on progression of the disease. Falls and syncope were more common in the active treatment group (although this did not lead to an increase in number of withdrawals). As Praticò reports [46] the authors do suggest replication of the study to confirm their positive results.

A multi-centre, random-ised, double-blind, placebo controlled trial investigating the possible prevention of dementia in patients with mild cognitive impairment effects by taking vitamin E daily is underway [45].

A study of idebenone (a coenzyme Q_{10} analogue), that found it to have a dose-dependent positive effect in mild to moderate Alzheimer's disease [49] reporting safety and tolerability to be similar to placebo. Positive effect and safety were still good at 2 years.

Omega-3 fatty acids

Freeman's review of dietary fatty acids [50] found no controlled trials. From the evidence found from basic research, postmortem assessment, naturalistic studies and a case study, however, he concluded that omega-3 fatty acids could play a role in prevention and treatment. Controlled trials would be needed to confirm this.

General Nutrition

Although there is no evidence that dietary factors are implicated in the aetiology of Alzheimer's disease, weight loss in patients with Alzheimer's disease is a recognised problem complication and seems to be through lack of attention to proper nourishment rather than part of the disease process [51]. Dietary supplementation can produce a significant increase in mean body weight amongst patients with dementia, as found by a randomised, controlled trial with an active vitamin placebo in a psychiatric hospital ward [52].

Nutritional awareness is important for the elderly in general: one randomised, double-blind, placebo-controlled trial on 96 healthy individuals aged 65 or over found that dietary supplementation of vitamins and trace elements improved cognitive function [53].

Melatonin and Bright Light Therapy

The hormone melatonin, released by the pineal gland and considered important in regulating sleeping behaviour, has been cited as a beneficial supplement for patients with sleep disturbances. Sleep disorders and disruptive nocturnal behaviour associated with dementia present a significant clinical problem [54]. A characteristic pattern of sleep disturbance referred to as "Sundowning" has been described in people with dementia [55]. Sundowning presents with increased arousal, usually in the late afternoon, evening or night and is a cause of increased stress by caregivers.

There is considerable theoretical evidence to support the use of melatonin as a novel treatment for sleep disturbance associated with dementia [54]. Melatonin is a hormone implicated in the control of the sleep wake cycle. It is stimulated during darkness and suppressed by light. While the effects of melatonin have been extensively studied in photoperiodic animals such as birds, reptiles and some mammals, there is growing evidence that melatonin is also involved in the regulation and control of circadian rhythms in humans [56]. Dementia appears to be associated with flattening of the circadian rhythm of melatonin secretion [57].

One well conducted but small cross-over study [58] evaluated the effect of bright light therapy in combination with melatonin or placebo on motor restless behaviour. Bright light therapy was found to have a positive effect on motor restless behaviour, but the addition of melatonin negated the effect. Further research in the use of bright light therapy amongst this patient group is necessary. The review of psychosocial interventions for dementia [58] found evidence to support the use of light therapy from four small studies (combined $n=45$), although this again calls for replication of the findings.

Preventing Dementia

This is currently the subject of trials of *Ginkgo biloba* [59] and vitamin E [45]. Nourhashémi et al. [60] concludes from a number of studies that good nutrition, in the form of vitamins, minerals and other micronutrients, may prevent cognitive decline.

Conclusion

Based on current evidence it appears CAM can be of benefit and assist in the treatment of dementia. In the main this is in the form of standardised extract of *Ginkgo biloba* for symptomatic treatment. However, many other CAM approaches in dementia show promise and more high-quality research is needed. Research sponsors and funders should consider giving a higher priority tto this area of research.

References

1. Ott, Brian R, Owens NJ (1998) Complementary and alternative medicines for Alzheimer's disease. Journal of Geriatric Psychiatry & Neurology 11(4): 163–173.
2. Birks JS, Melzer D, Beppu H. Donepezil for mild and moderate Alzheimer's disease (Cochrane Review). In: The Cochrane Library, Issue 2 2002. Oxford: Update Software.
3. Birks J, Grimley Evans J, Iakovidou V, Tsolaki M (2002) Rivastigmine for Alzheimer's disease (Cochrane Review). In: The Cochrane Library, Issue 2 2002. Oxford: Update Software.
4. Wilcock G, Lilienfield S, Gaens E (2000) Efficacy and safety of galantamine in patients with mild to moderate Alzheimer's disease: multicentre randomised controlled trial. British Medical Journal 321: 1–7.
5. World Health Organisation (1993) ICD-10: International Statistical Classification of Diseases and Related Health Problems (10th Revision). WHO, Geneva.
6. Crook T, Bartus RT, Ferris SH, et al. (1986) Age associated memory impairment: proposed diagnostic criteria and measures of clinical change. Developmental Neuropsychology 2: 261–76
7. Hardy J (1991) Molecular classification of Alzheimer's disease. Lancet 337: 1342–1343.
8. Lobo A, Launer LJ, Fratiglioni L et al. (2000) Prevalence of dementia and major subtypes in Europe: A collaborative study of population-based cohorts. Neurology 54: S4–9.
9. Prince M (2000) The epidemiology of Alzheimer's disease. In: O'Brien, Ames and Burns (eds) Dementia (2nd edition). Arnold, London.
10. Perry RH, Irving D, Blessed G, et al. (1989) Senile dementia of Lewy body type and spectrum of Lewy body disease. Lancet 1: 1088.
11. Finkel SL (1998) Signs of behavioural and psychological symptoms of dementia. Clinician 16: 33–42.
12. McKeith IG, Galasko D, Kosaka K et al. (1996) Consensus guidelines for the clinical and pathological diagnosis of dementia with Lewy bodies (DLB): report of the consortium on DLB International workshop. Neurology 47: 1113–1124.
13. Foster S, Tyler VE (1999) Tyler's honest herbal: a sensible guide to the use of herbs and related remedies (4th edition). The Haworth Herbal Press, New York.
14. Schilcher H (1988) Zeitschrift für Phytotherapie 9:119–127. Comment in: Foster S, Tyler VE (1999) p184.
15. van Beek T, Bombardelli E, Morazzoni P, Peterlongo F (1998) Ginkgo biloba L. Fitoterapia LXIX (3): 195–244.
16. Oken B, Storzbach D, Kaye J (1998) The efficacy of Ginkgo biloba on cognitive function in Alzheimer disease. Archives of Neurology 55: 1409–1415.
17. Ernst E, Pittler M (1999) Ginkgo biloba for dementia: A systematic review of double-blind, placebo-controlled trials. Clinical Drug Investigations 17(4): 301–308.
18. Wettstein A (2000) Cholinesterase inhibitors and Ginkgo extracts- are they comparable in the treatment of dementia? Comparison of published placebo-controlled efficacy studies of at least six months' duration. Phytomedicine 6(6): 393–401.
19. Le Bars P, Kieser M, Itil K (2000) A 26-week analysis of a double-blind, placebo-controlled trial of the ginkgo biloba extract EGb 761® in dementia. Dementia and Geriatric Cognitive Disorders 11(4): 230–7.
20. Le Bars P, Katz M, Berman N, et al (1997) A placebo-controlled, double-blind, randomized trial of an extract of Ginkgo biloba for dementia. JAMA 278: 1327–1332.
21. Kayne S (2001) Ginkgo biloba: potential concern. Good Clinical Practice Journal 8(11): 8–10.
22. Allain H, Schuck S, Lebreton S, et al. (1999) Aminotransferase levels and silymarin in de novo tacrine-treated patients with Alzheimer's disease. Dementia and Geriatric Cognitive Disorders 10(3): 181–5.
23. Itoh T, Shimada Y, Terasawa K (1999) Efficacy of Choto-san on vascular dementia and the protective effect of the hooks and stems of Uncaria sinensis on glutamate-induced neuronal death. Mechanisms of Ageing and Development 111(2–3): 155–73.
24. Arai H, Suzuki T, Sasaki H, et al (2000). A new interventional strategy for Alzheimer's disease by Japanese herbal medicine (Japanese) Japanese Journal of Geriatrics 37(3): 212–5.
25. Chen K, Chen KJ, Zhou WQ (1997) Clinical study of effect of yizhi capsule on senile vascular dementia (Chinese). Chung-Kuo Chung Hsi i Chieh Ho Tsa Chih 17(7): 393–7.
26. Xu H, Shao N, Cui D, et al. (2000) A clinical study of yi zhi capsules in prevention of vascular dementia. Journal of Traditional Chinese Medicine. 20(1): 10–3.
27. Smallwood J, Brown R, Coulter F, et al. (2001) Aromatherapy and behaviour disturbances in dementia: a randomized controlled trial. International Journal of Geriatric Psychiatry 16: 1010–1013.
28. Smallwood J, Irvine E, Coulter F, Connery H. (2001) Psychometric evaluation of a short observational tool for small-scale research projects in dementia. International Journal of Geriatric Psychiatry 16: 288–292.
30. Holmes C, Hopkins V, Hensford C, et al. (2000) Lavender oil as a treatment for agitated behaviour in severe dementia: a placebo controlled study. International Journal of Psychogeriatrics 13 (suppl 2): pp277.
31. Brooker DJ, Snape M, Johnson E, et al. (1997) Single case evaluation of the effects of aromatherapy and massage on disturbed behaviour in severe dementia. British Journal of Clinical Psychology 36(Pt 2): 287–96.
32. Kim EJ, Buschmann MT (1999) The effect of expressive physical touch on patients with dementia. International Journal of Nursing Studies 36(3): 235–43.

33. Opie J, Rosewarne R, O'Connor D W (1999) The efficacy of psychosocial approaches to behaviour disorders in dementia: a systematic literature review. Australian and New Zealand Journal of Psychiatry 33(6): 789–799.

34. Vink AC, Bruinsma MS, Scholten R. (2002) Music therapy in the care of people with dementia (Protocol for a Cochrane Review). In: *The Cochrane Library*, Issue 2, 2002. Oxford: Update Software.Koger SM, Brotons M (2000) Music therapy for dementia symptoms. Cochrane Database of Systematic Reviews.

35. Koger S M, Chapin K, Brotons M (1999) Is music therapy an effective intervention for dementia: a meta-analytic review of literature. Journal of Music Therapy 36(1): 2–15.

36. Geng J (1999) Treatment of 50 cases of senile dementia by acupuncture combined with inhalation of herbal drugs and oxygen. Journal of Traditional Chinese Medicine 19(4): 287–9.

37. Xudong G (1999) The influence of acupuncture modalities on the treatment of senile dementia: a brief review. American Journal of Acupuncture 24: 105–109.

38. Liu HA, Hou DF, Diao ZY, Wang Y (1997) Observation on the clinical curative effects of turbit clearing and intelligence-improving acupuncture therapy on vascular dementia and the study onits mechanisms. Chinese Acupuncture and Moxibustion 17(9): 521–525.

39. Lai XS (1997) Observation on curative effects of senile vascular dementia treated by acupuncture. Chinese Acupuncture and Moxibustion 17(4): 201–202.

40. Jiang ZY, Li CD, Li YK (1999) Treatment of vascular dementia with scalp acupuncture. International Journal of Clinical Acupuncture 10(1): 15–21.

41. Zhang AR, Pan ZW, Lou F (1995) Effect of acupuncturing houxi and shenmen in treating cerebral traumatic dementia (Chinese). Chung-Kuo Chung Hsi i Chieh Ho Tsa Chih 15(9): 519–21.

42. Emerson Lombardo NB, Vehvilainen L, Ooi WL et al. (2000) Acupuncture to treat anxiety and depression in Alzheimer's disease and vascular dementia: a pilot feasibility and effectiveness trial. Conference proceedings World Alzheimer Congress; 9–13 July, Washington DC.

43. Vatassery GT, Bauer T, Dysken M (1999) High doses of vitamin E in the treatment of disorders of the central nervous system in the aged. American Journal of Clinical Nutrition 70(5): 793–801.

44. Launer LJ, Kalmijn S (1998) Anti-oxidants and cognitive function: a review of clinical and epidemiologic studies. Journal of Neural Transmission Supplementum 53: 1–8.

45. Grundman M (2000) Vitamin E and Alzheimer disease: the basis for additional clinical trials. American Journal of Clinical Nutrition 71(2): 630S-636S.

46. Praticò D, Delanty N (2000) Oxidative injury in diseases of the central nervous system: focus on Alzheimer's disease. American Journal of Medicine 109(7): 577–85.

47. Sano M, Ernesto C, Thomas RG, et al. (1997) A controlled trial of selegiline, alpha-tocopherol, or both as a treatment for Alzheimer's disease. New England Journal of Medicine 336: 1216–1222.

48. Drachman DA, Leber P (1997) Treatment of Alzheimer's disease: searching for a breakthrough, settling for less. New England Journal of Medicine 336: 1245–1247.

49. Gutzmann H, Hadler D (1998) Sustained efficacy and safety of idebenone in the treatment of Alzheimer's disease: update on a 2-year double-blind multicentre study. Journal Neural Transmission 54(suppl):301–310.

50. Freeman MP (2000) Omega-3 fatty acids in psychiatry: a review. Annals of Clinical Psychiatry 12(3): 159–65.

51. Gillette-Guyonnet S, Nourhashémi F, Andrieu S, et al. (2000) Weight loss in Alzheimer disease. American Journal of Clinical Nutrition 71(suppl): 637S-42S.

52. Carver AD, Dobson AM (1995) Effects of dietary supplementation of elderly demented hospital residents. Journal of Human Nutrition and Dietetics 8(6): 389–394.

53. Chandra RK (2001) Effect of vitamin and trace-element supplementation on cognitive function in elderly subjects. Nutrition 17(9): 709–12.

54. McGaffigan, S., Bliwise, DL. (1997) The treatment of sundowning: A selective review of pharmacological and nonpharmacological studies. Drugs and Aging, 10(1), 10–17.

55. Rindlinsbacher P and Hopkins RW (1992) An investigation of the sundowning syndrome. International Journal of Geriatric Psychiatry, 7, 15–23.

56. Lewy AJ. Sack RL. Blood ML. Bauer VK. Cutler NL. Thomas KH. (1995) Melatonin marks circadian period position and resets the endogenous circadian pacemaker in humans. Ciba Foundation Symposium. 183: 303–17; discussion 317–21.

57. Uchida K. Okamoto N. Ohara K. Morita Y. (1996) Daily rhythm of serum melatonin in patients with dementia of the degenerate type. Brain Research. 717(1–2): 154–9.

58. Haffmans PM, Sival RC, Lucius SA, et al. (2001) Bright light therapy and melatonin in motor restless behaviour in dementia: a placebo-controlled study. International Journal of Geriatric Psychiatry 16(1): 106–10.

59. DeKosky ST, et al. (2000) Ginkgo Biloba Prevention Trial in Older Individuals. http://clinicaltrials.gov

60. Nourhashémi F, Gillette-Guyonnet S, Andrieu S, et al. (2000) Alzheimer disease: protective factors. American Journal of Clinical Nutrition 71(2): 643S-649S.

29 Depression in the Elderly

N.S. Cherniack, E.P. Cherniack

Overview of Psychiatric Disorders in the Elderly

Depressive disorders affect about 19 million people in the United States and are a common reason for disability in the aged [1]. Women tend to be affected more than males (about two times more frequently). Men seem to be less likely to admit to depression than women but about 3 to 4 million men are affected of all ages. While some studies have defined a relatively low incidence, others describe depression as occurring in fifteen to twenty percent of community-dwelling older persons [2]. The incidence of depression varies by the population studied; approximately three percent of community dwelling outpatients suffer from depression [3, 4], about fifteen percent of all nursing home patients [3,4] and as many as roughly forty percent of all in medical inpatients [5].

About one to two percent of those over 65 living in the community suffer from major depression; and another two percent have less severe depression [1]. Thirteen to 27 percent of older adults have subclinical depression and are at increased risk of mental and physical disability.

Suicide is more common in the elderly. The rate of suicide is much higher in men than women. After age 70 the rate of suicide increases steadily in men rising after age 85. In 1996 the rate of suicide in white males over 85 was six times the nation average.

Symptoms of depression are listed below.

Symptoms of Depression

▶ Persistent sad mood
▶ Loss of appetite and/or body weight
▶ Difficulty sleeping or oversleeping
▶ Physical slowing or agitation
▶ Loss of energy
▶ Feelings of worthlessness or inappropriate guilt
▶ Difficulty thinking or concentrating
▶ Recurrent thought of death or suicide

If five or more of these symptoms exist in the same 2-week period, the patient is considered to have a major depressive disorder (unipolar major depression). Geriatric depression often manifests itself differently than depression at other ages. Typically, the geriatric patient may complain of loss of interest in daily activities, be fatigued, or have sleep disturbance. The elderly may relate symptoms of memory disturbance and impaired concentration. There can be difficulty discriminating between depression and dementias, and some patients early in the onset of their dementing illness might become depressed. Some older individuals develop psychotic features together with depression. Usually periods of depression reoccur over a lifetime.

In bipolar or manic-depressive disorder, periods of depression alternate with periods persistently elevated mood, touchiness, talkativeness, distractibility and sleeplessness (mania). Dysthymia is a more chronic form of depression that is less severe.

Depression often co-exists with other anxiety disorders such as panic disorders, obsessive-compulsive behavior, social phobia, and post-traumatic stress syndrome. These disorders also need to be appropriately treated. Depression often occurs together with serious physical ailments and can complicate treatment and worsen prognosis.

Depression can be treated with certain types of psychotherapy (cognitive-behavioral and interpersonal therapy); medications such as serotonin reuptake inhibitors, tricyclic antidepressants or monamine oxidase inhibitors; and in its severe forms with electroconvulsive therapy. The pharmaceutical agents seem to act on monamine neurotransmitters in the forebrain such as serotonin, norepinephrine, and dopamine. They often take several weeks to show an effect, which may not be much greater than with placebo treatment. Cognitive-behavioral therapy attempts to change negative ways of thinking and behavior; while interpersonal therapy concentrates on repairing poor interpersonal relationships. Electroconvulsive therapy is the most effective treatment and research has greatly reduced the incidence of side effects

Because of the possibility of side effects and the high costs of conventional treatments, interest in alternative medicine approaches to the treatment of depression is high. Alternative treatments include herbals particularly St.John's wort, massage, aromatherapy (with cloves, calamus and/or camphor), meditation, homeopathic preparations (such as essence of mustard), nutritional supplements such as 5-hydroxytryptamine, fish oils (because of their omega 3 fatty acids) and vitamins (mainly B vitamins). There are on-going federally funded studies of St. John's Wort in obsessive compulsive disorder, omega-3 fatty acids in bipolar disorder, and massage in the treatment of depression in HIV patients(NCCAM web page).

St. John's Wort

By far the most extensively studied of the alternative medicine treatments of depression is St. John's Wort [6–15]. (Other herbal preparations used are listed below.)

Herbal Remedies Used in the Treatment of Depression

- ▶ St. John's Wort (Hypericum perforatum)
- ▶ Kava kava (piper methysticum)
- ▶ Valerian Root
- ▶ Ayurvedic mixtures, which contain for example herbs like shavateri (asparagus racemosus) jatamansi (nordostachys jatamansi) brahmi (gotu kola) and gudachi (tinospora cordifolia)

▶ Mimosa tree bark (albizzia julbrissin) a traditional Chinese herbal
▶ Ginko Bilboa
▶ Ginseng

St. John's Wort is a flowering perennial and grows to one to three feet in height in un-cultivated areas both in woods and meadows in many parts of the world. It is a wild growing plant in California, southern Oregon, and Colorado. It has pale green oblong leaves with oil glands, which can be detected by holding the leaf to the light. Its flow-ers are yellow. It blooms from June to August, followed by numerous small round black seeds that have a bitter taste and a resinous smell. Its scientific name hypericum comes from the Greek and means "over an apparition" coming from the idea that the odor of the plant would cause evil spirits to disappear. Its been used since ancient times for a variety of complaints including gastrointestinal disorders, wound healing, kidney and lung ailments It has been claimed recently to have anti-viral properties. However, now it is used mainly as an anti-depressant.

St. John's Wort is widely prescribed in Germany and in other parts of Europe. It can be purchased over the counter in the United States as tablets, which contain about 300 mg of the herb. While many different doses are used, usually a tablet is taken three times a day. It is made from an extract of the dried flowering tops of the plants; and contains a mixture of many different chemical but principally flavenoids and nap-thodianthrones [6]. The main active ingredient is hypericin a polycyclic quinone. St. John's Wort is also available in water and oil infusions mainly as topical applications for skin rashes. A *Good Housekeeping* Institute Study in 1998 found a several-fold difference in the amount of hypericin and pseudohypericine actually contained in over the counter products and the amount listed on the label. Studies of extracts of St. John's Wort particularly hypericin in vitro and in animal preparations indicate that it inhi-bits synapatosomal uptake of norepinephrine, serotonin, and dopamine and induces beta receptor down regulation [6]. It does have side effects, which include increased photosensitivity. It should not be used in patients with HIV and it interferes with the effectiveness of indinavir, reducing inidinavir levels by fifty percent [7]. It also inter-feres with the activity of the immunosuppressive (cyclosporin) and the anticoagulant warfarin [8–10]. Many patients with epilepsy also use it and its safety in those patients is not clear. However a recent study in eight healthy volunteers who received the anti-epileptic carbamazepine together with St. John's wort showed no effect of the herb on the meta-bolism of carbamazepine [11]. The FDA has issues an advisory on St. John's Wort warning that the herb appears to an inducer of the cytochrome P450 pathway and should not be used with drugs that are metabolized by that pathway [6]. It should not be used with other anti-depressant drugs.

A meta-analysis of 23 randomized placebo controlled studies of the efficacy ex-tracts of St. John's Wort in mildly to moderately depressed patients was reported by Linde et al. in 1996 [12]. They found that the extracts were significantly better than placebo and as effective as standard antidepressant pharmaceuticals. Despite these promising results, differences in dosages used in the different studies and their re-latively short duration led the authors to believe that further clinical trial should be conducted to determine whether St. John's wort was better at treating some depressive disorders than others, produced less side effects, and to determine optimum dosage.

Wheatley in 1997 compared the efficacy of an extract of St. John's Wort with amitryptiline in depressed patients [13]. The Hamilton Depression Scale response rate was not statistically different in the two treatment groups. Side effects were twice as frequent in the amitryptiline treated group suggesting that the superior tolerability of the herb extract was a real advantage. Since then, larger randomized double-blind studies have been completed comparing St. John's Wort extracts with placebo or sertraline again using changes in depression scales as the main criteria for change [14, 15]. In one study no difference was observed between St. John's Wort and placebo in the treatment of outpatients with depression [14].

No difference between St. John's extract and placebo was found in 340 adults with moderately severe major depression followed for at least eight weeks in a second study. But on the other hand sertraline was also no better than placebo although the dose used may have been too small [15].

Thus it still remains difficult to decide whether standard pharmaceuticals are superior to St. John's Wort in the treatment of milder forms of depression.

References

1. Lebowitz BD, Pearson JL, Schneider LS. (1997) Diagnosis and treatment of depression in late life: consensus statement update, Journal of the American Medical Association 278: 1186–90
2. Gurland BJ, Cross PS, Katz S. (1996) Epidemiological perspectives on opportunities for treatment of depression. American Journal of Geriatric Psychiatry 4(4): S7–S13.
3. Hay DP, Franson KL,. Linda Hay George T. Grossberg. (1998) "Depression " in Duthie, EH. Practice of Geriatrics, 3rd ed., (W. B. Saunders Company: Philadelphia): 286–293.
4. U.S. Department of Health and Human Services: Consensus Statement: National Institute of Mental Health Consensus Development Conference: The diagnosis and treatments of depression in late life. (1991) Bethesda, MD, U.S. Department of Health and Human Services, pp. 1–6.
5. Koenig HG, Blazer DG. (1996) Minor depression in late life. American Journal of Geriatric Psychiatry 4(4): S14–S21.
6. Singer A, Wonneman M, Muller WE. (1999) Hyperforin: a major antidepressant constituent of St. John's Wort Inhibits serotonin uptake by elevating free intracellular sodium ion. Pharmacology 3: 1363–68
7. Piscitelli SC et al. Indinavir concentrations and St. John's Wort. (2000) Lancet 355: 547–8
8. Ruschitzka F et al. (2000) Acute heart transplant rejection due to Saint John's Wort. Lancet 355: 548
9. Jobst KA et al. (2000) Safety of St. John's Wort. Lancet; 355: 576.
10. Lumpkin MM. Risk of drug interactions with St. John's wort and indinavir and other drugs. FDA Health Advisory Feb.10, 2000.
11. Burstein AH, Horton RL, Dunn T. (2000) Lack of effect of St. John's Wort on carbamazepine pharmacokinetics in healthy volunteers. Clinical and Pharmacological Therapeutics 68: 605–12
12. Linde K et al. (1996) St John's Wort for depression – an overview and meta-analysis of randomized clinical trials. British Medical Journal 313: 253–8
13. Wheatley D. (1997) LI160, an extract of St. John's Wort, versus amitriptyline in mildly to moderately depressed outpatients-a controlled 6-week trial. Pharmacopsychiatry Suppl.2: 77–80
14. Shelton RC, Keller MB, Gelenberg AJ et al. (2001) Effectiveness of St. John's Wort in major depression. JAMA 285: 1978–86
15. Hypericum Depression Trial Study Group. Effect of Hypericum perforatum (St. John's Wort) in major depressive disorder: a randomized, controlled trial JAMA; 2002; 287:1807–14

30 Complementary and Alternative Medicine in Neurology

S. Kaufman, M. Rubin

Introduction

Neurology certainly has its fair share of incurable illness, inviting complementary and alternative (CAM) therapeutic modalities as a source of succor if not cure. Interestingly, even when help *is* available, patients continue to seek CAM therapies. This is not the result of dissatisfaction with conventional medicine. Rather, they seek options more "congruent with their values, beliefs, and philosophies", to provide a more "holistic" approach to life and health [1].

In this article we review the recent literature on complementary and alternative medicine in neurology using a disease oriented approach. The field is large and we have not tried to be inclusive. Rather we have chosen to highlight those areas either most in need of an alternative therapy due to the lack of something better, or those currently receiving attention due to ongoing research. Dementia and mental illness are treated elsewhere in this text.

Headache

Along with back pain and the common cold, headaches are among the most common ailments for which patients seek useful, and sometimes unconventional, remedies. A panoply of alternative therapies exist, all purporting to relieve headache, some with legitimate scientific merit, others with nothing more than anecdotal, "medicine-man" rumor (heard through relatives or the internet). CAM therapies include vitamins, minerals, botanicals, homeopathy, acupuncture, biofeedback, physical manipulation, and stress reduction methods, and they may be divided by the headache type they are professed to help, including migraine, cluster, and tension.

CAM treatments for migraine are available for both acute pain relief and long term prophylaxis. Magnesium and riboflavin supplementation has been shown to prevent migraine in a few controlled trials. Fifty-five patients with migraine headache were randomized to either 400 mg/day of riboflavin or to placebo taken for three months. Significantly, the number of patients who improved by at least 50 percent was 15 percent in the placebo group and 59 percent in the riboflavin group [2]. Side effects in the riboflavin group included diarrhea and polyuria.

Migraine patients have been found to have reduced erythrocyte magnesium levels compared to normal controls [3]. Among a group of 81 patients with migraine headache randomized to either 600 mg/day magnesium or placebo for three months, attack frequency was reduced by 15.8% in the placebo group and 41.6%in the magnesium group [4]. Side effects in the magnesium group included diarrhea and gastric irritation.

Botanicals such as feverfew, gingko (a herbal therapy used by the Chinese for millennia, mostly for asthma), and ginger have also been reported to be effective in the treatment of migraine. The medicinal use of feverfew (tanacetum parthemium) dates back to Greek and Roman times, its name derived by its use as a febrifuge (fever reducer). Its active ingredient is thought to be parthenolide (sesquiterpene lactones) which is felt, among its other anti-inflammatory actions, to block serotonin. Treatment with feverfew is still controversial due to the variability of outcomes found in the controlled trials performed so far.

In a cross-over trial, 72 patients with migraine were randomized to receive either one capsule of dried feverfew leaf per day or placebo for four months. They were then switched to the other treatment arm. Treatment with feverfew reduced the mean number and severity of attacks and the degree of vomiting [5]. In a 1998 systematic review of four randomized, double blind, placebo controlled trials of feverfew preparations, high levels of statistical significance were found to favor feverfew over placebo for migraine prophylaxis [6]. None of these trials tested feverfew against conventional prophylactic therapy and larger controlled trials are needed to establish which dose and formulation is safe and effective.

There are several case reports describing the use of ginkgo as a preventive therapy and ginger as an abortive therapy, taken at the onset of visual aura. No satisfactory controlled trials have been performed to date. Of note, feverfew, ginkgo, and ginger all have the potential to alter bleeding time and should not be used with warfarin [7].

A variety of physical techniques have been applied to migraine with some success, including acupuncture, cupping, biofeedback and spinal manipulation. Among 27 clinical trials evaluated in one review, 23 found acupuncture to be beneficial in the treatment of migraine and tension headaches [8]. Another literature review examined 14 clinical trials comparing sham acupuncture with true acupuncture for the treatment of recurrent migraine or tension type headaches. A trend in favor of acupuncture was found but did not reach statistical significance [9].

Other researchers compared acupuncture to conventional prophylactic therapy. Hesse and colleagues randomized 85 patients with migraine to either

▶ acupuncture and placebo tablets or
▶ placebo stimulation and metoprolol 100 mg/day for 17 weeks [10].

Both groups exhibited a significant reduction in attack frequency. No difference was found between groups regarding frequency or duration of attacks. However, metoprolol was found to be statistically superior in reducing severity of attacks.

Due to the large variations in study size, design, control groups, and statistical significance of results, a need remains for larger, more standardized, randomized controlled trials to firmly establish whether acupuncture is truly effective in the treatment of migraine and other headaches.

There are reports that spinal manipulation and homeopathy are effective in the treatment of headache. One study of 218 patients found spinal manipulation to be comparable in effectiveness to amitriptyline for the treatment of migraine and tension-type headache [11]. A recent review of 9 trials supported this observation. However the 9 trials varied widely in sample size, use of control groups, methodology, and outcome measures, raising questions as to whether a valid conclusion could be drawn from the data [12].

A review of homeopathic prophylaxis for migraine identified three double-blind, randomized, controlled trials with a total of 220 patients. No significant difference between homeopathy and placebo was found for all outcomes studied, including headache frequency, severity, and duration of attacks [13]. No study has yet compared homeopathic therapy to conventional prophylactic medication.

Melatonin has been used as a treatment for cluster headache based on previously observed relationships between cluster headache and circadian rhythms. Plasma melatonin levels are decreased in cluster headache patients [14]. In one double-blind pilot study, 20 patients with cluster headache were treated for two weeks with either melatonin 10 mg/day or placebo [15]. Headache frequency was significantly reduced and a strong trend was seen towards reduced analgesic consumption in the melatonin treatment group. However, the response rate overall was lower than that for established prophylactic medications, such as verapamil and lithium. Larger controlled trials are needed to determine if melatonin has a beneficial adjunct or alternative role in the management of cluster headache.

Stroke

Botanicals, acupuncture and hyperbaric oxygen are CAM therapies that have been applied to stroke management and rehabilitation. Botanical extracts of ginkgo biloba and kava have been analyzed for their potential effect in reducing cerebral ischemia. Ginkgo biloba has been shown in numerous studies to inhibit platelet activation and adhesion [16], to reduce production of free radicals [17], and to increase cerebral blood flow. In hypertensive rats, ginkgo biloba leave extract increased blood perfusion, altered vasomotor function, and decreased peripheral resistance, thereby reducing systolic blood pressure [18]. A significant reduction in the volume of brain tissue infarcted was seen in mice subjected to reversible middle cerebral artery occlusion after treatment with ginkgo biloba extract for seven days [19]. In another study, gingko biloba extract reduced vasospasm and cerebral ischemic damage in the rat by decreasing nitric oxide in brain tissue [20].

Kava has also been found to reduce ischemia in animal models. A significant reduction in infarct area was found in kava-treated mice 48 hours after induced left middle cerebral ischemia [21]. These studies position gingko biloba and kava as potential neuroprotective agents in humans. However, the few clinical trials of these botanicals to date are varied in design, with varied methods and outcomes. They remain unconvincing. One double-blind, placebo-controlled trial of 55 acute stroke patients, confirmed with computerized tomography (CT), examined gingko versus placebo taken every 6 hours for two and four weeks. No significant difference in clinical improvement was seen among these patients [22].

Other antioxidants including garlic and vitamin E have been shown to reduce cholesterol and may be useful in stroke prevention [23, 24].

A 1997 National Institutes of Health (NIH) Consensus Statement concluded that acupuncture might be useful as an adjunct or alternative treatment in stroke rehabilitation [25]. A clinical trial of electrical acupuncture in hemiplegic patients demonstrated improved neurological and functional outcomes and reduced hospital stay [26]. Among 20 patients who received acupuncture following stroke, 8 showed significant improvements in knee flexion, knee extension, and shoulder abduction [27]. Other reports also note that acupuncture might be helpful in restoring function in subacute stroke patients [28]. However, most trials showing benefit have involved control groups receiving no intervention. A follow up study reported no significant difference in functional outcomes between groups of stroke patients who received acupuncture or transcutaneous electrical nerve stimulation compared to those who received subliminal electrostimulation [29]. Similarly, a controlled trial randomized 106 stroke patients with moderate to severe motor impairment to either standard post-stroke rehabilitation or to traditional Chinese manual acupuncture [30]. No significant differences were observed between the two groups after 10 weeks of therapy. Two meta-analyses of acupuncture currently in progress may clarify its potential role in post-stroke care.

The use of hyperbaric oxygen in acute stroke is controversial. It has been observed to reduce ischemic brain damage in rats subjected to middle cerebral artery occlusion [31]. In one double blind pilot study of human stroke patients, a positive outcome trend, not statistically significant, was found in favor of hyperbaric oxygen therapy [32].

There are anecdotal reports and case studies of music therapy, massage, hypnosis, biofeedback, electromagnetic therapy, homeopathy, energy healing and meditation as beneficial to the recovery of stroke patients. However, no satisfactory controlled trials have been performed of these techniques.

Parkinson's Disease

In a study of 201 patients with Parkinson's disease at Boston University School of Medicine and Johns Hopkins University, 40 percent reported using a least one type of CAM therapy such as herbs, vitamins, massage, or acupuncture [33]. Vitamin E, which was shown in a 1993 New England Journal of Medicine study to have no beneficial effect on Parkinson's disease, was the most popular choice among patients using vitamins and herbs at a mean dose of 93 mg/day. Vitamin E has antioxidant properties that may potentially protect the brain from free-radical induced oxidative stress. Support for this therapeutic role can be found in several animal studies, including one that found a significant protective effect of vitamin E in the substantia nigra of a rat model of Parkinson's disease [34]. Nevertheless, in human studies this benefit has not been borne out.

Fahn reported a pilot trial of 21 patients with early Parkinson's disease. He noted that high dose vitamin E (3200 IU/d) with vitamin C (3000 mg/d) over a 6–19 year period was effective in delaying the need for levodopa by a mean of 2.5 years [35]. However, the multicenter, controlled, DATATOP trial (Deprenyl and Tocopherol Antioxidative Therapy of Parkinsonism) revealed no evidence for any beneficial effect of vitamin E (2000 IU/day) in slowing progress of the disease or improving clinical symptoms. Nicoletti and colleagues, investigating the possible role of vitamin E in the pathogenesis of Parkinson's disease, found no significant difference in the plasma levels of vitamin E between Parkinson's disease patients and age and sex matched controls [36].

Another antioxidant being investigated for its potential neuroprotective effect in Parkinson's disease is coenzyme Q10. Shults et al found that the level of coenzyme Q10 was significantly lower in mitochondria from patients with Parkinson's disease than in age and sex matched controls [37]. In a follow-up pilot study of 15 patients with Parkinson's disease, he reported no change in the mean score on the motor portion of the Unified Parkinson's Disease Rating Scale after treatment with oral coenzyme Q10 for one month at three different dosages [38].

The broad bean (vicia faba) contains intrinsic dopamine in therapeutic levels. Several case reports describe its clinical effect. Rabey found that, in six patients with Parkinson's disease, ingestion of 250 g of cooked faba beans produced a significant increase in L-dopa plasma levels and was associated with substantial clinical improvement [39]. Faba beans have also been observed to prolong "on" periods in Parkinson's disease patients who have "on-off" fluctuations [40].

Several therapies have been reported as beneficial but predominantly in case reports and rarely in controlled trials. Electromagnetic therapy has been applied to Parkinson's disease with mixed results. Several case reports have demonstrated improvement in a range of Parkinson's symptoms including motor disability, mood, sleep, cognitive functions, appetite, and gait [41]. Melatonin and biofeedback have been observed to reduce levodopa-induced dyskinesiae. The Alexander Technique, a discipline which focuses on posture and movement, was shown in an uncontrolled pilot study to improve motor function and depression in Parkinson's patients [42]. Music therapy was shown in one randomized, controlled, single-blind study to improve bradykinesia, activities of daily living, and emotional functions [43]. There are also anecdotal reports of benefit from acupuncture, massage, nicotine, and sleep deprivation but no satisfactory controlled trials to date.

Multiple Sclerosis

In a survey of 569 patients with multiple sclerosis (MS), one-third reported having visited a practitioner of unconventional therapy within the last six months [44]. Massage, diet, acupuncture, biofeedback, botanicals, therapeutic touch, melatonin, yoga, chelation, chiropractic, cannabis, and bee-venom have all been reported to help patients with MS symptoms. No adequate controlled trials have been performed testing any of these therapies.

Treatment of MS patients with a diet of very low saturated fat and high polyunsaturated fatty acids was initiated in the late 1940's. In 1990 this diet was reported to have resulted in a significant reduction in the severity and frequency of exacerbations in a group of 144 MS patients followed for over 34 years [45]. However, no satisfactory controlled trials have been performed to establish if a diet, low in saturated fats, is beneficial for patients with MS.

Mercury in dental amalgam has been implicated in numerous diseases including MS, lupus, arthritis, headache, epilepsy, Parkinson's disease and brain tumors. There are no controlled trials that support the claim that removing dental fillings improves MS symptoms or reduces exacerbations. A case-control comparison of 132 MS patients and 423 controls who were age, sex, and residence matched, found no association between MS and the number of dental amalgam fillings or the duration of exposure to amalgam [46].

Extrapolating from "Uthoff's phenomenon", the observation that warming produces worsening of MS symptoms, cooling should improve MS symptoms. In one controlled trial of ten patients with MS, patients were dressed in a cooling garment for one hour (with coolant at 7 degrees centigrade). Three hours after cooling they were found to have less fatigue, improved lower limb muscle strength, and improved postural stability [47]. In another study of 10 patients with MS, cooling suits improved walking, transferring, and bladder function [48]. The benefits found in these studies are hindered by the very small sample size. Results from a ongoing, large, multicenter trial begun in 1999 involving approximately 100 patients will hopefully clarify the role of cooling suits in the care of MS patients [49].

Procarin, a transdermal preparation of caffeine and histamine, has been reported to improve numerous MS symptoms. There is one uncontrolled report that found that 67% of MS patients who used Procarin for six weeks had improvement in weakness, numbness, gait, pain, fatigue, and depression [50]. No randomized controlled trials of procarin have been performed to date.

There are several case reports which describe the effectiveness of pulsed electromagnetic fields (EMFs) in the management of various MS symptoms including fatigue, diplopia, gait ataxia, bladder dysfunction, and pain [51]. No controlled trials have been performed to date.

Therapeutic horseback riding (known as hippotherapy), the Feldenkrais Method (a discipline which encourages self-awareness of body parts and movement patterns), T'ai Chi (a traditional Chinese martial art) and yoga have all been observed to reduce stress and improve mood in MS patients. Evidence is limited to anecdotal reports and case studies. No adequate controlled trials have been performed to date.

Epilepsy

The ketogenic diet, a high-fat, low carbohydrate, low protein diet, is perhaps the most widely known CAM therapy for epilepsy. The ketogenic diet's effectiveness has been regarded in one 2000 evaluation "as good or better than any of the newer medications" [52].

Developed in the 1920's, its efficacy is well supported in the literature for the alternative or adjunct management of both generalized and focal seizure disorders, especially for refractory cases. Hemingway and colleagues at John Hopkins followed a group of 150 children who enrolled, prospectively, into a cohort study evaluating the efficacy and tolerability of the ketogenic diet. Three to six years after initiation, 13% of enrollees were seizure-free and an additional 14% had a 90–99% decrease in their seizure frequency [53]. A similar prospective study of 51 children found at least a 50% decrease in seizure frequency in 28 (51%) patients after six months on the diet [54]. However, metabolic and biochemical alterations induced by the ketogenic diet have been associated with a few, albeit rare, complications, including prolonged QTc interval [55], pancreatitis [56], gastrointestinal complaints [57], and excessive bruising [58].

Melatonin has been proposed as a treatment for seizures based on its antioxidant properties and its anticonvulsant activity in animals. In one uncontrolled trial of six young patients with intractable seizures, five patients reported significant clinical improvement in seizure activity after taking 3 mg/d for 3 days as a supplement to their conventional antiepileptic regimen [59]. Others have observed its pro-convulsant effects in children [60]. With such contradictory results and no placebo-controlled trials, it is still unclear what role, if any, melatonin has in the management of epilepsy.

Music therapy is an evolving technique that is also reported to improve seizure frequency. One investigation of the "Mozart effect", as music therapy is popularly referred to, found a significant decrease in EEG epileptiform activity in 23 of 29 patients with focal discharges, or bursts of generalized spike and wave complexes, who listened to the Mozart piano K448 [61].

Acupuncture, yoga, meditation, art therapy, pet therapy, aromatherapy, homeopathy, and chiropractic are reported to be beneficial in the management of seizure disorders. However, most of the information concerning these therapies remains anecdotal.

Back Pain

Based on a literature review of randomized controlled trials, acupuncture appears to be of no significant benefit for the treatment of nonspecific low back pain [62]. No difference was appreciated between transcutaneous electrical nerve stimulation (TENS) or trigger point injection and acupuncture. Placebo and sham acupuncture were no worse than true acupuncture.

Meta analysis of randomized controlled trials in the literature up to June 2000 similarly provided no evidence to support TENS alone for the treatment of chronic low back pain [63].

Low intensity (1.06 microm) neodynium:yttrium-aluminum-garnet (Nd:YAG) laser, administered three times per week for four weeks demonstrated only moderate benefit for 63 low back pain patients in a randomized, double-blind, placebo controlled study [64]. Such improvement as was reported, however, diminished by one month of follow-up.

Percutaneous electrical nerve stimulation (PENS) uses an acupuncture-like needle positioned in soft tissues or muscle to electrically stimulate dermatomal areas which correspond to levels of radicular pathology. In a single-blind, sham controlled, cross over study of 60 low back pain patients, PENS was found superior to both TENS and flexion extension exercises. PENS was more effective in reducing both visual analog scale (VAS) scores for pain and daily nonopioid analgesic drug use [65]. It also significantly improved the level of physical activity, sleep quality, and sense of well being.

Osteopathic spinal manipulation was comparable to medical care (muscle relaxants, analgesics, anti-inflammatory medication, physical therapy, ultrasound, diathermy, corset use, and TENS) in producing similar beneficial results among 173 low back pain patients, tested in a randomized controlled fashion [66]. Less medication and less physical therapy were needed in the osteopathy group to achieve improvement and the cost difference was significant.

Among 321 patients with nonspecific low back pain for more than one week, chiropractic manipulation and the McKenzie method of physical therapy provided similar benefits at similar cost [67]. However, almost as much relief was obtained when the patient simply received an educational booklet on the causes and prevention of low back pain and at a fraction of the cost, raising doubts as to the cost effectiveness of the formal treatments.

Low back pain patients treated with willow bark extract required less tramadol for pain control than placebo treated patients [68]. Benefit was evident by one week and only one patient suffered a severe allergic reaction, suggesting it is a safe and useful treatment for low back pain. Further studies are warranted.

Craniocerebral and Spinal Cord Trauma

Ginkgo biloba has been experimentally used to treat numerous disorders including impotence, deafness, vertigo, depression, and myocardial reperfusion injury [69]. In the rat model of bifrontal traumatic brain injury it enhanced recovery. In the rat model of cortical hemiplegia it improved motor function. It is not used in practice for brain trauma.

Fatigue, depression and anxiety were significantly reduced in 10 traumatic brain injury patients treated with H. niger homeopathy. Vertigo and headache were diminished by hypnosis among 155 such patients. Total resolution of symptoms was reported in 50% and significant improvement was reported in another 20%.

Hyperbaric oxygen (HBO) has not been shown to significantly improve function following brain trauma. In HBO animal studies of memory, balance, and motor skills pre- and post-focal brain contusion, behavioral testing showed mixed results with hippocampal CA3 region pathological analysis showing no significant difference in pyramidal cell counts 10 days post-contusion on the injured side of either group [70].

References

1. Astin JA. Why patients use alternative medicine JAMA 1998; 279; 1548–1553
2. Schoenen J, Jacquay J, Lenaerts M. Effectiveness of high dose riboflavin in migraine prophylaxis. A randomized controlled trial. Neurology 1998; 50: 466–470
3. Gallai V, Sarchielli P, Abbritti G. Red blood cell magnesium levels in migraine patient. Cephalgia 1993; 13: 81–94
4. Piekert A, Wilimzig C, Kohne-Volland R. Prophylaxis of migraine with oral magnesium: results from a prospective, multi-center, placebo-controlled and double blind randomized study. Cephalalgia 1996; 16: 257–263

5. Murphy JJ, Heptinstall S, Mitchell JR. Randomized double-blind controlled trial of feverfew in migraine prevention. Lancet 1988; 2: 189–192

6. Vogler BK, Pittler MH, Ernst E. Feverfew as a preventive treatment for migraine: a systemic review. Cephalalgia. 1998; 18: 704–708

7. Miller LG. Herbal medicinals: selected clinical considerations focusing on known or potential drug-herb interactions. Archives of Internal Medicine. 1998; 158: 2200–11

8. Manias P, et al. Acupuncture in headache: a critical review. Clinical Journal of Pain 2000; 16: 334–9

9. Melchart D et al. Acupuncture for recurrent headaches: a systematic review of randomized controlled trials. Cephalgia 1999; 19: 779–86

10. Hesse J et al. Acupuncture versus metoprolol in migraine prophylaxis: a randomized trial of trigger point inactivation. Journal of Internal Medicine 1994; 235: 451–6

11. Nelson CF et al. The efficacy of spinal manipulation, amitriptyline and the combination of both therapies for the prophylaxis of migraine headache. Journal of Manipulative and Physiological Therapeutics 1998; 21: 511–19

12. Bronfort G et al. Efficacy of spinal manipulation for chronic headache: a systematic review. Journal of Manipulative and Physiological Therapeutics 2001; 24: 457–66

13. Ernst E. Homeopathic prophylaxis of headache and migraine: a systematic review. Journal of Pain and Symptom Management 1999; 18: 353–357

14. Leone M, et al. Twenty-four-hour melatonin and cortisol plasma levels in relation to timing of cluster headache. Cephalalgia 1995 Jun; 15: 224–9

15. Leone M, et al. Melatonin versus placebo in the prophylaxis of cluster headache: a double-blind pilot study with parallel groups. Cephalalgia. 1996 Nov; 16: 494–6

16. Braquet P, et al. Is there a case for PAF antagonists in the treatment of ischemic disease? Trends in Pharmacol Sci 1989; 10: 23–30

17. Oyama Y, et al. Myricetin and quercetin, the flavonoid constituents of Ginkgo biloba extract, greatly reduce oxidative metabolism in both resting and Ca^{2+}-loaded brain neurons. Brain Res 1994; 635(1–2): 125–9

18. Zhang WR, et al. Protective effect of ginkgo extract on rat brain with transient middle cerebral artery occlusion. Neurology Research 2000; 22(5): 517–21

19. Clark WM, et al. Efficacy of antioxidant therapies in transient focal ischemia in mice. Stroke 2001; 32(4): 1000

20. Sun BL, et al. Effects of Ginkgo biloba extract on somatosensory evoked potential, nitric oxide levels in serum and brain tissue in rats with cerebral vasospasm after subarachnoid hemorrhage. Clin Hemorheol Microcirc 2000; 23 (2–4): 139–44

21. Backhauss C, Krieglstein J. Extract of kava (Piper methysticum) and its methysticin constituents protect brain tissue against ischemic damage in rodents. Eur J Pharmacol 1992; 215: 265–9

22. Garg RK, et al. A double blind placebo controlled trial of gingko biloba extract in acute cerebral ischemia. J Assoc Physicians India 1995; 43(11): 760–3

23. Stevinson C, Pittler MH, Ernst E. Garlic for treating hypercholesterolemia. A meta-analysis of randomized clinical trials. Annals of Internal Medicine 2000; 133: 420–9

24. Pruthi S, et al. Vitamin E supplementation in the prevention of coronary heart disease. Mayo Clin Proc 2001; 76(11): 1131–6

25. NIH Consensus Statement 1997; 15: 1–34

26. Wong AM, et al. Clinical trial of electrical acupuncture on hemiplegic stroke patients. American Journal of Physical Medicine and Rehabilitation 1999; 78: 117–22

27. Naeser MA, et al. Acupuncture in the treatment of paralysis in chronic and acute stroke patients – improvement correlated with specific CT scan lesion sites. Acupuncture Electrotherapy Research 1994; 19: 227–49

28. Johansson K, Lindgren I, Widner H, Wiklund I, Johansson B. Can sensory stimulation improve functional outcome in stroke patients. Neurology 1993; 43: 2189–2192

29. Johansson BB, et al. Acupuncture and transcutaneous nerve stimulation in stroke rehabilitation: a randomized, controlled trial. Stroke 2001; 32: 707–13

30. Sze FK, et al. Does acupuncture have additional value to standard post-stroke motor rehabilitation? Stroke 2002; 33(1): 186–94

31. Chang CF. Hyperbaric oxygen therapy for treatment of post-ischemic stroke in adult rats. Exp Neurol 2000; 166 (2): 298–306

32. Nighoghossian N, et al. Hyperbaric oxygen in the treatment of acute ischemic stroke. Stroke 1995; 26(8): 1369

33. Rajendran et al. The use of alternative therapies by patients with Parkinson's disease. Neurology 2001; 57: 790–794

34. Roghani M, et al. Neuroprotective effect of vitamin E on the early model of Parkinson's disease in rat: behavioral and histochemical evidence. Brain Res 2001; 892(1): 211–7

35. Fahn S. An open trial of high-dosage antioxidants in early Parkinson's disease. Am J Clin Nutr 1991; 53(1 Suppl): 380S–382S

36. Nicolletti G, et al. Plasma levels of vitamin E in Parkinson's disease. Arch Gerontol Geriatr 2001; 33: 7–12

37. Shults CW, et al. Coenzyme Q10 levels correlate with the activities of complexes I and II/III in mitochondria from parkinson and nonparkinson subjects. Annals of Neurology 1997; 42(2): 261–4

38. Shults CW, et al. Absorption, tolerability, and effects on mitochondrial activity of oral coenzyme Q10 in parkinsonian patients. Neurology 1998; 50: 793–5

39. Rabey JM, et al. Broad bean (Vicia faba) consumption and Parkinson's disease. Adv Neurol. 1993; 60: 681–4

40. Apaydin H. Broad bean (Vicia faba)–a natural source of L-dopa–prolongs "on" periods in patients with Parkinson's disease who have "on-off" fluctuations. Mov Disord. 2000; 15: 164–6

41. Sandyk R. Treatment of Parkinson's disease with magnetic fields reduces the requirement for antiparkinsonian medications. Int J Neurosci. 1994; 74: 191–201
42. Stallibrass C. An evaluation of the Alexander Technique for the management of disability in Parkinson's disease – a preliminary study. Clin Rehabil. 1997; 11: 8–12
43. Pacchetti C, et al Active music therapy in Parkinson's disease: an integrative method for motor and emotional rehabilitation. Psychosomatic Medicine 2000; 62: 386–93
44. Schwartz CE, Laitin E, Brotman S, LaRocca N. Utilization of unconventional treatments by persons with MS: is it alternative or complementary? Neurology 1999; 52(3): 626–9
45. Swank RL, Dugan BB. Effect of low saturated fat diet in early and late case of multiple sclerosis. Lancet 1990; 336: 37–39
46. Casetta I, Invernizzi M, Granieri E. Multiple sclerosis and dental amalgam: case-control study in Ferrara, Italy. Neuroepidemiology 2001; 20(2): 134–7
47. Beenakker EAC, et al. Cooling garment treatment in MS: clinical improvement and decrease in leukocyte NO production. Neurology 2001; 57(5): 892
48. Flesner G, Lindencrona C. The cooling-suit: case studies of its influence on fatigue among eight individuals with multiple sclerosis. Journal of Advanced Nursing 1999; 29: 1444–1453
49. Bowling A. Alternative Medicine and Multiple Sclerosis. 2001. Demos Medical Publishing. NY. 66–67
50. Gillson G, Wright JV, Ballasiotes G. Transdermal histamine in multiple sclerosis: part one – clinical experience. Altern Med Rev 1999; 4: 424–428
51. Sandyk R. Long-term beneficial effects of weak electromagnetic fields in multiple sclerosis. Int J Neurosci. 1995; 3(1–2): 45–57
52. LeFevre F, Aronson N. Ketogenic diet for the treatment of refractory epilepsy in children: a systematic review of efficacy. Pediatrics 2000; 105(4): E46
53. Hemingway C, Freeman JM, Pillas DJ, Pyzik PL. The ketogenic diet: a 3- to 6-year follow-up of 150 children enrolled prospectively. Pediatrics 2001; 108: 898–905
54. Vining EPG, Freeman JM et al. A multicenter study of the efficacy of the ketogenic diet. Archives of Neurology 1998; 55: 1433–1437
55. Best TH, et al. Cardiac complications in pediatric patients on the ketogenic diet. Neurology 2000; 54: 2328–30
56. Stewart WA, et al. Acute pancreatitis causing death in a child on the ketogenic diet. Journal Child Neurology. 2001; 16: 633–5
57. Katyal NG et al. The ketogenic diet in refractory epilepsy: the experience of Children's Hospital of Pittsburgh. Clinical Pediatrics. 2000; 39: 153–9
58. Berry-Kravis E, et al. Bruising and the ketogenic diet: evidence for the diet induced changes in platelet function. Annals of Neurology. 2001; 49: 98–103
59. Peld N, et al. Melatonin effect on seizures in children with severe neurological deficit disorders. Epilepsia. 2001; 42: 1208–9
60. Sheldon SH. Pro-convulsant effects of oral melatonin in neurological disabled children. Lancet. 1998; 351: 1254
61. Jenkins JS. The Mozart effect. Journal of the Royal Society of Medicine. 2001; 94: 170–172
62. van Tulder MW; Cherkin DC; Berman B; Lao L; Koes BW. The effectiveness of acupuncture in the management of acute and chronic low back pain. A systematic review within the framework of the Cochrane Collaboration Back Review Group. Spine 1999; 24: 1113–23
63. Brosseau L, Milne S, Robinson V, Marchand S, Shea B, Wells G, Tugwell P. Efficacy of TENS for the treatment of chronic low back pain. Spine 2002; 27: 596–603
64. Basford JR; Sheffield CG; Harmsen WS. Laser therapy: a randomized, controlled trial of the effects of low-intensity Nd:YAG laser irradiation on musculoskeletal back pain. Arch Phys Med Rehabil 1999; 80: 647–52
65. Ghoname EA, Craig WF, White PF, Ahmed HE, Hamza MA, Henderson BN, Gajraj NM, Huber PJ, Gatchel RJ. Percutaneous electrical nerve stimulation for low back pain: a randomized crossover trial. JAMA 1999; 281: 818–823
66. Andersson GBJ, Lucente T, Davis AM, Kappler RE, Lipton JA, Leurgans S. A comparison of osteopathic spinal manipulation with standard care for patients with low back pain. N Engl J Med 1999; 341: 1426–1431
67. Cherkin DC, Deyo RA, Battie M, Street J, Barlow W. A comparison of physical therapy, chiropractic manipulation, and provision of an educational booklet for the treatment of patients with low back pain. N Engl J Med 1998; 339: 1021–1029
68. Chrubasik S, Eisenberg E, Balan E, Weinberger T, Luzzati R, Conradt C. Treatment of low back pain exacerbations with willow bark extract: a randomized double-blind study. Am J Med 2000; 109: 9–14
69. Ernst E. The risk benefit profile of commonly used herbal therapies: ginkgo, St. John's wort, ginseng, echinacea, saw palmetto, and kava. Ann Intern Med 2002; 136: 42–53
70. Tinianow CL; Tinianow TK; Wilcox M. Effects of hyperbaric oxygen on focal brain contusions. Biomed Sci Instrum 2000; 36: 275–81

31 Acupuncture Effect on Pain

Wen-Hsieh Wu, Jiang Ye

Acupuncture has been used in China for thousands of years to maintain the health status and treat diseases by adjusting and balancing the negative, Yin, and positive, Yang, energy. It has also been used to treat different types of pain disorders. In this chapter, the effort will be devoted to summarize the scientific basis for its use in pain control. The discussion will be divided into the following sections:

▶ the current knowledge of acute and chronic pain mechanisms,
▶ possible explanation for acupuncture/electro-acupuncture (EA) effect on these mechanisms, and
▶ the critical and scientific review on highly discriminated clinical investigations for its effectiveness.

Current Understanding of Acute and Chronic Pain Mechanisms

Acute Pain

Nociception is transduced to neural signals and transmitted through different sizes and types of nerve fibers ending in various Laminae of the spinal cord, then, follows the paleospinothalamic track to the midbrain, hypothalamus, and the sensory cortex.

Chronic Pain

Once the acute pain becomes chronic pain, the involved mechanism becomes complex. It can be discussed below under the headings of peripheral sensitization, central sensitization, descending inhibitory circuit, processing in limbic system, and cerebral responses.

Sensitization

When nociception or neural injury is transduced into neural signal, it activates the sodium channel and depolarizes the axon. The signal propagates along the axon toward the central nervous system. Simultaneously, the neural injury triggers an inflammatory reaction. Products of this process include algogenic substances such as H^+ and bradykinin and sensitizing substances such as serotonin and norepinephrine. When partial neural injury occurs, sprouting from the injured terminal is limited and most of the regenerated fibers will reach the distal neural tubules to grow into them in an orderly fashion. However, in case of severely damaged or severed nerve terminals, the sprouting becomes rather disorganized. It can grow distally, proximally toward the axon, or even toward the neighboring nerve fibers, thereby forming ephatic excitation. When the nociceptive input becomes frequent and persistent beyond physiological limits, peripheral sensitization (a reduced pain threshold) occurs, coupled with loss of inhibitory interneurons at the cord levels and spontaneous firing from the neurons in the dorsal root ganglion and dorsal horn. These processes are called central sensitization.

High threshold ummyelinated pain transmitting C-fiber afferents terminate in Lamina 1 (marginal layer) of the dorsal horn of the spinal cord, while low threshold thinly myelinated Aδ-fibers terminate in Lamina 5. When an excessive barrage of peripheral nociceptive signals arrives in Lamina 5, it triggers 2nd and 3rd messengers to promote neuronal growth expanding to Laminae 1. Inhibitory interneurons with a wide dynamic range, which can be excited with a variety of stimuli, are present in Lamina 5 and posses NMDA receptors, which regulate intracellular calcium. Excess intracellular Ca^{2+} can eventually cause apoptosis of these inhibitory inter-neurons. It is known that stimulation of Aδ or Aβ fibers can inhibit the C-afferent input (Gate Control Theory 1965). This mechanism potentially involves the NMDA receptor system.

It also has been shown experimentally, that stimulation of the Aδ fiber or sympathetic neurons in the intermediate lateral funiculus of the spinal cord can generate neuronal connections between the two regions in a reciprocal manner. This explains how persistent sympathetic excitation can initiate hyperalgesia and nociception can evoke sympathetic response. Central sensitization of the spinal cord results in expansion of the receptive field. This expansion develops not only in the segmental level of the signal input (sagital expansion) but also expands cephaled and caudad (axial expansion). It is essential to recognize that the expansion of the receptive field develops in two dimensions. This information renders the concept of neuroablation to control pain invalid. The nociceptive signals of the dorsal horn following the neo-spinothalamic track travel to the peri-aqueductal and midbrain regions. At this level, the sensory input is processed in the limbic system to integrate the past experiences and also activate the descending inhibitory seratoninergic and GABAnergic neurons, which descend to the spinal level for modulating the sensory input from the periphery. The processed signals from the limbic system are then transmitted to the cerebrum to be interpreted in three domains, namely, sensory discriminative, affect emotional and cognitive behavioral.

Possible Mechanisms of Acupuncture Involving Pain Control

Effective acupuncture generates a sensation, named "De-qi" during needling. If one eliminates this sensation by injecting local anesthetic into the acupoint or using sham, abrogates no acupuncture effect would occur. This "De-qi"s transmitted through C- and Aδ fibers into the dorsal horn. This input could activate the Gate Control mechanism, namely, activation of A-δ fibers inhibits the input from C-fiber.

Acupuncture and Endogenous Opioid System

The association of acupuncture with modulation of endogenous opioid system has been well documented. The narcotic antagonist naloxone has been found to reduce the analgesia induce by electro-acupuncture (EA) in humans, monkeys, and mice (Mayer et al. 1977; Sjolund and Eriksson 1979), monkeys (Ha et al. 1981), mice (Ho et al. 1978; Pomerantz and Chiu 1976), rats (Fan et al. 1982) and rabbits (Han et al. 1984). In addition, extensive animal studies revealed that high and low frequency electro acupuncture (EA) is mediated by different opioid peptides (Han et al. 1984). While 2 Hz EA induced release of endogenous morphine, enkephalins and beta-endorphin, which act on mu and delta receptors in the brain and spinal cord, 100 Hz EA induced only the release of dynorphins, which act on kappa receptors in the spinal cord (Han et al. 1999). Furthermore, the 2 Hz EA produced endorphin release into the CSF. This mode of stimulation leaves residual analgesia after discontinuation of the EA. Higher frequency (150 Hz) produced immediate onset of analgesia without residual effect after its discontinuation, suggesting that this involves a neural competitive entry mechanism (Gate Control Theory 1965). Simultaneous application of 2 Hz and 100 Hz releases all three neurotransmitters, thus, strengthens the EA effects (Han 1999).

Needling sympathetic structures such as the stellate ganglion can produce ilipsolateral hemifascial warming and upper extremity vasodilatation. Electrical stimulation of the celiac plexus can reduce pain generated from the upper abdominal organs, such as pancreas and liver. These types of stimulation may cause super-depolarization of the sympathetic structure, therefore interrupt the sensory input via sympathetic fibers, and thus reducing pain.

Tolerance to Electroacupuncture Stimulation

The optimal duration of EA stimulation has been found to be 30 minutes, which is the induction period necessary for the full development of acupuncture analgesia in humans (Research Group of Acupuncture Anesthesia 1973). On the other hand, stimulation lasting for more than 1 to 2 hours would inevitably result in a gradual decease of the analgesic effect. This can be comparable to the development of morphine tolerance when multiple injections were given at short time intervals, hence the term acupuncture tolerance (Han et al. 1981).

An interesting finding was that rats made tolerant to 2 Hz EA were still reactive to 100 Hz, and vice versa. This is understandable because 2 Hz and 100 Hz EA analgesia are mediated by different types of opioid receptors, i.e., activation of μ/δ opioid receptors by enkephalin and endorphin in low-frequency EA, and activation of κ-opioid receptors by dynorphin in high-frequency EA (Chen and Han 1992). In the HANS device, a 30-minute auto-off mechanism has been installed to prevent unintentional excessive prolongation of the stimulation. For severe chronic pain or cancer pain patients who need multiple treatments, it is advisable that the HANS be used no more than 3 to 4 times (30 minutes for each session) a day.

The mechanisms for the development of EA tolerance are many-fold, two of them have been clarified:

▶ repeated EA elicits a down regulation of the gene expression of opioid receptors in identified brain area (Wang et al., unpublished data);

▶ the release of large amount of opioid peptide in the CNS triggers the release of another kind of neuropeptide, cholecystokinin octapeptide (CCK-8), to counteract the opioid effect (Zhou et al. 1993a, b).

Indeed, the central administration of the CCK receptor antagonist L-365260, or the antibody against CCK can postpone the development of tolerance to EA.

Low Versus High Responders for Electroacupuncture Analgesia

When a large group (>100) of rats is given a standard session of EA, one can easily find a bimodal distribution of the analgesic effect. Cluster analysis revealed two distinct groups i.e. high responders (HR) and low responders (LR). This phenomenon is reproducible at least within 2 days. Interestingly, the rats had a LR to EA also had a LR to low dose (3 mg/kg) of morphine, and vice versa (Tang et al. 1997).

The causes of LR are at least two: a low rate of release of opioid peptides in the CNS and a high rate of release of CCK-8 that is a very potent anti-opioid. An LR rat can be changed into an HR by injection of a CCK antisense RNA into the brain to block the expression of the gene coding for CCK (Tang et al. 1997), or by the administration of a compound L-365260 characterized as an antagonist to the CCK-B receptor (Tang et al. 1996). On the other hand, a breed of rat called P77PMC rat, bred to be highly susceptible to audiogenic seizure, was found to be an HR to EA analgesia. These rats were found to contain high level of β-endorphin and low level of CCK in the brain. They can be changed into LRs by the central administration of a vector containing CCK cDNA that induces an overexpression of CCK in the CNS (Zhang et al. 1992). Thus, a dynamic balance between opioid peptides and anti-opioid peptides in the CNS seems to be a cardinal factor determining the effectiveness of EA analgesia.

It should be stressed, however, that CCK-8 is just one of the members of the family called anti-opioid peptides. A new member was discovered recently called orphanin FQ (OFQ), a peptide with 17 amino acid residues. That OFQ may be functioning as another negative feedback control mechanism for EA analgesia is evidenced by our recent finding that blockade of OFQ gene expression by central administration of OFQ antisense RNA produced a dramatic augmentation of EA-induced analgesia (Tian, Xu, Grandy, Han, abstract for the 1996 International Narcotic Research Conference, Jul. 2–25, 1996, Long Beach, USA).

Mechanisms responsible for the low- and high-responders appear to be based on CCK-8. The peptide CCK-8 has been shown to form a negative feedback control for opioid analgesia. Elevated level of opioids triggers the gene transcription, protein synthesis, and ultimate release of CCK, thus, checking excessive opioid analgesia (Hang 1995a). Several studies have been conducted to explore the molecular mechanisms involved (Han 1995b).

▶ Cross-talk between opioid and CCK receptors: CCK-8 was shown to decrease the number and to lower the affinity of opioid receptors, as evidenced by the decrease of B_{max} and an increase of Kd in receptor-binding assays.

▶ Patch-clamp study provided direct evidence to show that opioid suppression of voltage-gated calcium current can be reversed by CCK-8, indicating that opioid/CCK interaction takes place at the membrane of one and the same neuron (Liu et al. 1995; Xu et al. 1996).

▶ CCK-8 seems to induce an uncoupling of opioid receptors from their relevant G protein, thus interfering with the transmembrane signal transduction induced by opioid peptides (Zhang et al. 1993).

▶ Activation by CCK-8 of the phosphoinositide (Fl) signaling system in the CNS (Zhang et al. 1992), which increases the intracellular free calcium concentration by mobilization of intracellular calcium stores, whereas the opioid effect lowers intracellular free calcium levels (Wang et al. 1992).

Optimization of Acupuncture Treatments

Some acupuncturists claim that the therapeutic effects produced by multiple acupuncture treatments once a week (QW) is better than that of once a day (QD). In normal rats we have compared the analgesic effect induced by EA administered QD, Q4D, and Q7D, and found that in the Q4D regime, the EA analgesia showed a trend of gradual strengthening accompanied with a gradual increase of the concentration of monoamines in the spinal perfusate, whereas in the QD regime, there was a gradual decrease of the analgesia effect, i.e., development of tolerance (Ye and Xu, unpublished data). This treatment schedule may be different in various disease states, which warrants future stay.

Acupuncture and Opioid Detoxification

The opioid peptides release in the CNS by EA could be used to treat opioid addiction by replacing exogenous opiates. Morphine-dependent rats exhibited less withdrawal symptoms with acupuncture (Han and Zhan 1993). This led to exploring acupuncture for the treatment of heroin addiction.

In heroin addicts, acupuncture treatment (30 min/session, 1–3 sessions/day for seven days) produced a significant reduction of the withdrawal syndrome. The DD (2/100 Hz) wave was significantly more efficient than the constant low (2 Hz) or constant high (100 Hz) wave in ameliorating tachycardia, insomnia, and reducing craving. All three treatment groups using 2-, 100-, and 2/100 Hz stimulation, respectively, were equally effective in increasing the body weight as compared with the placebo group in which a gradual decrease of body weight was observed in the first week of drug abstinence (Han et al. 1994, 1995). After the detoxification period of 7 to 10 days, Acupuncture can be used for the treatment of postdetoxification syndromes including insomnia and various kinds of pain. An acceleration of the release of endogenous opioid peptides in the CNS may account for the mechanisms underlying acupuncture detoxification. It should be remembered that 2/100 Hz DD waves releases not only enkephalins and β-endorphin, which work in much the same way as morphine, but also dynorphin that may interact with κ-opioid receptors resulting in a suppression of the abstinence syndrome (Wu et al. 1995).

Selection of Electroacupuncture Parameters Should be Tailored According to Disease Category and Individual Cases

DD waves have been shown to be the best choice for pain control for most cases, but it may not be the standard solution in all cases. This can be seen in the acupuncture treatment of pain resulting from muscle spasticity caused by spinal injuries (Han et al. 1994). Intrathecal injection of dynorphin has been shown to produce analgesic effects in the dorsal horn and may produce paralytic effects in the ventral horn (Xue et al. 1995a, b). In spinal spasticity, the anterior horn neurons are in a state of hyperexcitability. It was hypothesized that an increased release of dynorphin in the spinal cord by high-frequency (100 Hz) EA might be helpful to suppress the excitability of spinal motor neurons. This was tested in clinical cases of spinal spasticity. The best therapeutic effect was obtained by using HANS of 100 Hz; that of DD mode (2/100 Hz) was only half effective; 2 Hz EA was totally without therapeutic effect, and may even produce a negative effect. The therapeutic effect of 100 Hz EA became increasingly prominent over 5 days and remained stable after 12 days (Han et al. 1994).

Another issue worth mentioning is that a LR rat at 2 Hz EA may not be a low responder at 100 Hz EA, and vice versa. Therefore, unless the best parameter for the treatment of an identified case is known, the DD wave should be tried first.

Effects of Acupuncture on CNS Neurons

The effect of acupuncture on the CNS have been well documented. Using functional MRI (fMRI), Cho and colleague (PNAS 1998) found activation of occipital cortex of human when the vision-related acupoint (VA1), located in the lateral aspect of the foot, was stimulated. However, stimulation of nonacupoints 2 to 5 cm away from the vision-related acupoints on the foot did not activate the occipital lobes. Much evidence comes from animal studies. Using single unit recording in the amygdaloid nucleus of rabbit brains, Lar et al. (1989) showed that the signals of acupuncture at Neiguan (PC6) reached the amygdaloid nucleus and altered the neuronal electrical activity. Most relevant to the current review is the finding that many animal studies have demon-strated that acupuncture reversed or attenuated changes of neuronal activity induced by diseases or conditions. For example, in a study of rabbits, acupuncture of PC6 reversed the alterations of electrical activity of dorsal horn neurons induced by acute myocardial ischemia (Liu et al. 1994). In a rat study with the extracellular recording technique, Huang et al. (1995) found that after acupuncture on "Zusanli (St 36)" and "Sanyinjiao (Sp 6)", the discharges of pain-excitatory neurons (firing increases when pain signal arrives) of the hypothalamic dorsomedial nucleus were profoundly de-creased, and the spontaneous firing rate of pain-inhibitory units neurons (firing decreases when pain signal arrives) was increased. A similar result was observed in rostral ventromedial medulla neurons. Ao et al. (1996) found that 2 Hz EA on bilateral "Zusanli (St 36)" inhibited the pain response of sensitive neurons.

In addition to the alteration of neuronal electrical activity induced by acupuncture, Ying and Cheng (1994) found that acupuncture at "Feng-fu (Du 16)" and "Jin-suo (Du 8)" for 30 minutes substantially potentiated the induction of C-FOS protein like immu-noreactivity (CFPLI) in hippocampal neurons following transient global ischemia, especially in CA1 of gerbils. At the same time, acupuncture can prevent most of the CA1 cells from delayed degeneration after ischemia. These results indicate that acupuncture has a protective effect on neurons of hippocampus after cerebral ischemia. Despite that it is still unclear how these changes occur, this may be one of the mechanisms under-lying the efficacy of acupuncture therapy for stroke rehabilitation.

Acupuncture/EA is known to cause relaxation and anxiolytic effects. It is probable that this is a result of the interaction of acupuncture and limbic system processing. The acupoints yielding these effects are usually peripheral to the head and neck. Therefore, its effect must be through the neuroendocrine or the neurotransmitter system. The sympatholytic and relaxation effects of acupuncture may imply the reduction of endo-genous catecholamine release, therefore reduce its sensitizing effect in the peripheral nerve endings.

Other effects produced by EA include dopaminergic, and oxytocin-modulating effects. Dystonia from insufficient dopaminergic neuronal activities could be improv-ed by EA. Therefore, it might be feasible to use EA to treat myofascial pain caused by muscle spasms.

References

1. Ao M, Wei J, Tan Z, Hu Q, Tang J. [The influence of EA with different frequencies on the discharges of neurons in rostral ventromedial medulla on rats]. Zhen Ci Yan Jiu. 1996; 21(4): 41–5.
2. Chen XH, Han JS. Analgesia induced by electroacupuncture of different frequencies is mediated by different types of opioid receptors: another cross-tolerance study. Behav Brain Res. 1992; 47(2): 143–9.
3. Cho ZH, Chung SC, Jones JP, Park JB, Park HJ, Lee HJ, Wong EK, Min BI. New findings of the correlation between acupoints and corresponding brain cortices using functional MRI. Proc Natl Acad Sci U S A. 1998; 95(5): 2670–3.
4. Fan SG, Qu ZC, Zhe QZ, Han JS. GABA: antagonistic effect on electroacupuncture analgesia and morphine anal-gesia in the rat. Life Sci. 1982; 31(12–13): 1225–8.
5. Gao M, Wang M, Li K, He L. Changes of mu opioid receptor binding sites in rat brain following electroacupuncture. Acupunct Electrother Res. 1997; 22(3–4): 161–6.
1. Ha H, Tan EC, Fukunaga H, Aochi O. Naloxone reversal of acupuncture analgesia in the monkey. Exp Neurol. 1981; 73(1): 298–303.
6. Han JS, Xie GX, Zhou ZF, Folkesson R, Terenius L. Acupuncture mechanisms in rabbits studied with microinjec-tion of antibodies against beta-endorphin, enkephalin and substance P. Neuropharmacology. 1984; 23(1): 1–5.
7. Han JS, Zhang RL. Suppression of morphine abstinence syndrome by body electroacupuncture of different fre-quencies in rats. Drug Alcohol Depend. 1993; 31(2): 169–75.

8. Han JS. The neurochemical basis of pain relief by acupuncture. 1998 Hubei Science and Technology press. China.

9. Han JS. Mechanisms of acupuncture analgesia. 1999 Brain Science series Shanghai, China.

10. Han Z, Jiang YH, Wan Y, Wang Y, Chang JK, Han JS. Endomorphin-1 mediates 2 Hz but not 100 Hz electroacupuncture analgesia in the rat. Neurosci Lett. 1999; 274(2): 75–8.

11. Henry P, Baille H, Dartigues JF, Jogeix M. Headache and acupuncture. In Pfaffenrath V, Lundberg PO, Sjaastad O. ed. Updating in Headache. Berlin: Springer Verlag, 1985.

12. Herz A. Endogenous opioid systems and alcohol addiction. Psychopharmacology, 1997; 129: 99–111.

13. Ho WK, Wen HL, Lam S, Ma L. The influence of electro-acupuncture on naloxone-induced morphine withdrawal in mice: elevation of brain opiate-like activity. Eur J Pharmacol 1978; 49(2): 197–9.

14. Huang Z, Tong Z, Sun W [Effect of electroacupuncture on the discharges of pain-sensitive neurons in the hypothalamic dorsomedial nucleus of rats].Zhen Ci Yan Jiu. 1995; 20(1): 20–3. Chinese.

15. Hui KK, Liu J, Makris N, Gollub RL, Chen AJ, Moore CI, Kennedy DN, Rosen BR, Kwong KK. Acupuncture modulates the limbic system and subcortical gray structures of the human brain: evidence from fMRI studies in normal subjects. Hum Brain Mapp. 2000; 9(1): 13–25.

16. Kim MR,Yoon SS, Kwon YK, Kim KJ, Shim I, Lee HJ, Kang GH, Yang CH. Acupuncture-mediated reduction in ethanol-induced dopamine release in the rat nucleus accumbens. Abstract (980.5), Society for Neurosci. 2001.

17. Lar ZF, Cao QS, Chen SP, Han ZJ. Effect of electro-acupuncture of "Neiguan" on spontaneous discharges of single unit in amygdaloid nucleus in rabbits. J Tradit Chin Med. 1989; 9(2): 144–50.

18. Lewith GT, Machin D. On the evaluation of the clinical effects of acupuncture. Pain. 1983; 16(2): 111–27. Review.

19. Liu J, Han Z, Chen S, Cao Q. [Influence of electroacupuncture of neiguan (PC 6) on ami-induced changes in electrical activity of dorsal horn neurons]. Zhen Ci Yan Jiu. 1994; 19(1): 37–41. Chinese.

20. Ma QP, Zhou Y, Han JS. Electroacupuncture accelerated the expression of c-Fos protooncogene in dopaminergic neurons in the ventral tegmental area of the rat. Int J Neurosci. 1993; 70(3–4): 217–22.

21. Margolin A, Kleber HD, Avants SK, Konefal J, Gawin F, Stark E, Sorensen J, Midkiff E, Wells E, Jackson TR, Mayer DJ, Price DD, Rafii A. Antagonism of acupuncture analgesia in man by the narcotic antagonist naloxone. Brain Res. 1977; 121(2): 368–72.

22. Melzack R. Acupuncture and related forms of folk medicine. In: Melzack R, Wall PD, ed. Textbook of Pain. London: Churchill Libvingstone, 1984.

23. Mihic SJ. Acute effects of ethanol on $GABA_A$ and glycine receptor function. Neurochem Int. 1999; 35(2): 115–23. Review.

24. Miriam Melis, Rosana Camarini, Mark A. Ungless, and Antonello Bonci Long-Lasting Potentiation of GABAergic Synapses in Dopamine Neurons after a Single In Vivo Ethanol Exposure. J. Neurosci. 2002; 22: 2074–2082

25. Ng L. Auricular acupuncture in animals: effects of opiate withdrawal and involvement of endorphins. J Altern Complement Med. 1996, 2(1): 61–3.

26. Ng LK, Douthitt TC, Thoa NB, Albert CA. Modification of morphine-withdrawal syndrome in rats following transauricular electrostimulation: an experimental paradigm for auricular electroacupuncture. Biological Psychiatry, 1975, 10, 575–580.

27. Pomeranz B, Chiu D. Naloxone blockade of acupuncture analgesia: endorphin implicated. Life Sci. 1976; 19(11): 1757–62.

28. Pomeranz B, Warma N. Electroacupuncture suppression of a nociceptive reflex is potentiated by two repeated electroacupuncture treatments: the first opioid effect potentiates a second non-opioid effect. Brain Res. 1988; 452 (1–2): 232–6.

29. Pomeranz B. 1987. Scientific basis of acupuncture:text book and atlas. Berlin, Germany: Springer-Verlag.

30. Pontieri FE, Tanda G, Orzi F, Di Chiara G. Effects of nicotine on the nucleus accumbens and similarity to those of addictive drugs. Nature. 1996; 382(6588): 255–7.

31. Price DD, Mayer DJ. Evidence for endogenous opiate analgesic mechanisms triggered by somatosensory stimulation (including acupuncture) in man. Pain Forum 1994; 4: 40–43.

32. Qian XZ, Progress in scientific research on acupuncture, moxibustion and acupuncture anesthesia by integrating traditional Chinese and Western medicine. Ed. Zhang XT, Research on acupuncture, moxibustion, and acupuncture anesthesia, Science press, Beijing, 1986; 1–18.

33. Richardson PH, Vincent CA. Acupuncture for the treatment of pain: a review of evaluative research. Pain. 1986; 24(1): 15–40. Review

34. Robbins TW, Everitt BJ. Neurobehavioural mechanisms of reward and motivation. Curr Opin Neurobiol. 1996; 6(2): 228–36. Review.

35. Sjolund BH, Eriksson MB. The influence of naloxone on analgesia produced by peripheral conditioning stimulation. Brain Res. 1979; 173(2): 295–301.

36. Stux G, Hammerschlag R (Eds) 2000. Clinical acupuncture: Scientific basis. Berlin, Germany: Springer-Verlag.

37. Tang D, Advances of research on the mechanism of acupuncture and moxibustion. Acu Res. 1987, 4: 278–284.

38. Thorer H, Volf N. Acupuncture after alcohol consumption: a sham controlled assessment. Acupunct Med 1996; 14(2): 63–7.

39. Vazquez J, Munoz M, Caceres JL.Modifications in the distribution of met-enkephalin in the limbic system of the cat brain after electroacupuncture. An immunocytochemical study. Histol Histopathol. 1995; 10(3): 577–82.

40. Vincent CA. A controlled trial of the treatment of migraine by acupuncture.Clin J Pain. 1989; 5(4): 305–12.

41. Vincent, C and Lewith, G: Placebo controls for acupuncture studies J Roy Soc Med 1995, 88: 199–202.

42. Wang B, Luo F, Xia YQ, Han JS Peripheral electric stimulation inhibits morphine-induced place preference in rats. Neuroreport. 2000; 11(5): 1017–20.
43. Weight FF, Li C, Peoples RW. Alcohol action on membrane ion channels gated by extracellular ATP (P2X receptors). Neurochem Int. 1999; 35(2): 143–52. Review.
44. Wen HL, Cheung SYC. Treatment of drug addiction by acupuncture and electrical stimulation. Asian J. of Med. 1973; 9: 138–141.
45. Wu LZ, Cui CL, Han JS. Effects of electrical acupuncture on the heart rates in human with morphine withdrawal syndrome. Journal of Chinese pain medicine. 1996; 2: 98–102.
46. Wu LZ, Cui CL, Han JS. Suppression of morphine abstinence syndrome by body acupuncture of different frequencies in human. Journal of Chinese pain medicine, 1995; 1: 30–38.
47. Wu LZ, Cui CL, Tian JB, Ji D, Han JS. Suppression of morphine withdrawal by electroacupuncture in rats: dynorphin and kappa-opioid receptor implicated. Brain Res. 1999; 851(1–2): 290–6.
48. Yang CL, Shin I, Lee HI, Jin C, Kim MR, Roh HJ, Song JH, Yoon SS, Kwon YK, Lim S, Golden GT . Acupuncture attenuates cocaine-induced dopamine release in the nucleus accumbens and locomotor activity of the rats. Soc. Neurosci 2000; 26 (part 1): 795, abs 293.17.
49. Ying SX, Cheng JS. Effects of electro-acupuncture on C-FOS expression in gerbil hippocampus during transient global ischemia.Acupunct Electrother Res. 1994;19(4): 207–13.
50. Zhu W, Xi G, Ju J. Effect of acupuncture and Chinese medicine treatment on brain dopamine level of MPTP-lesioned C57BL mice]. Zhen Ci Yan Jiu. 1996; 21(4): 46–9.

D Appendix

Index

E

Printing (Computer to Plate): Saladruck Berlin
Binding: Stürtz AG, Würzburg

3